Blood Relations

'The philosophers have only interpreted *the world in different ways; the point is to* change it.'

Karl Marx, Theses on Feuerbach: XI *(1845)*

Blood Relations

Menstruation and the Origins of Culture

Chris Knight

Yale University Press
New Haven and London 1991

To my children,
Rosie, Olivia and Jude

Set in Garamond by Excel Typesetters Co., Hong Kong

ISBN 0–300–04911–0 (hbk.)
ISBN 978-0-300-06308-0 (pbk.)
Library of Congress Catalog Number 90–71194

Printed in the United States of America

Contents

Preface to the Paperback Edition

By 40,000 years ago, the effects of a symbolic explosion – an efflorescence of human art, song, dance and ritual – were rippling across the globe. The bearers of symbolic culture were recent immigrants from Africa, dispersing so rapidly to encompass the globe that the process has become known as 'the human revolution'. Enough data and sophisticated neo-Darwinian theory now exists to begin to explain this most momentous revolution in history.

Simplistic, sexist stereotypes on the model of 'Man the Hunter' or 'Man the Toolmaker' contravene Darwinian theory. Females are not appendages; they pursue their own independent reproductive strategies, which typically diverge from those of males.

Primate societies are systems of alliances through which individuals pursue their fitness interests. Group-living places a premium on social intelligence, setting up selection pressures for large brains. But among primates, this process is constrained by the very high thermoregulatory, metabolic and obstetric costs of such brains. The exponential increase in brain size characterising the evolution of *Homo sapiens* indicates that, in some radical way, these constraints were overcome.

The costs of brain growth fall over-whelmingly on the female. In the human case, not only did mothers have to secure more and better quality food, they had to accomplish it whilst weighed down by heavily dependent infants. The problem is: how did they cope?

We now know the basic answer. Evolving women succeeded in gaining unprecedented levels of energetic investment from their mates. Success went to mothers who could reward more attentive, heavily investing partners at the expense of would-be philanderers.

A philandering male maximises his reproductive fitness by fertilising as many females as possible. He achieves this by reducing the time spent searching for each fertilisable female, and the time spent with her to ensure impregnation. The human female appears well-designed by evolution to waste the time of any philanderer by witholding information about her true fertility state. Concealment of ovulation and loss of oestrus with continuous receptivity deprives the male of information on whether his mate is likely to have been impregnated. The longer a male takes to impregnate any one female, the smaller his chances of being able to fertilise another.

A further means of thwarting philanderers is reproductive cycle synchrony. If females synchronise their fertile moments, no single male can cope with guarding and impregnating a whole group. He must concentrate on one at a time. The effect is to maximise the number of males in the breeding system, and hence the amount of male investment available. Ovulatory synchrony in local populations drives the ratio of sexually active males to females in groups towards one-to-one. Sustained male/female bonds on this basis mean greater paternity confidence, hence greater inclination on the part of males to invest in offspring. The evolutionary effect is to discriminate against philanderers in favour of more committed males.

Once ovulation was concealed and oestrus lost in the human lineage, menstruation acquired new significance as a cue. This, however, threatened the stability of the female strategy of withholding information from philanderers. Menstruation in the human case is particularly profuse. It is not something a female can easily hide. In fact it is a complete give-away. It signals a female's imminent fertility – and hence by contrast the *infertility* of neighbouring females who, whilst pregnant and nursing, are not displaying such blood. Males would have been drawn towards any such fertile female within the local area, competing to bond with her at the expense of pregnant or nursing females. Mothers with heavy childcare burdens, lacking the menstrual signal, would then have lost out just when they most needed help.

Cosmetics, according to recent research, were the answer. If there is a menstruating female in the neighbourhood, why not join her? Why not *appear* to be as fertile, painting up with blood-red colours? Ethnographic and historical records show how hunter-gatherer women across southern Africa prevented any young menstruant in their midst from being perceived as an isolable individual. Conjoining with her in a ritual dance, they used red ochre body-paint not only to signal menstruation and fertility, but *simultaneously* to indicate inviolability or taboo, their basic message being: 'No meat, no sex!'. We know that in Africa, anatomically modern humans were intensively mining, preparing and liberally applying red ochre body-paint 110,000 years ago.

Human symbolic culture emerged out of struggle. Its rituals and myths were expressions of 'counterdominance' – signals for thwarting exploitation by males. The signallers were females, allied with their male kin; their targets were their mates. Culture, in short, was a female invention for the provisioning of babies. Through it, womankind resisted and brought to an end the male's time-honoured biological status as the leisured sex.

January 1995

Acknowledgements

This book could not have been completed without help from many sources.

A Thomas Witherden Batt Scholarship and grants from the Folklore Society and the Royal Anthropological Institute (Radcliffe-Brown Award) are gratefully acknowledged.

I thank Mary Douglas for much personal encouragement and for launching me on my research project in 1976–7 while I was a diploma student at University College London. Thanks also to Alan Barnard for his exceptionally conscientious tutoring during the same period and subsequent twelve years of informal help and encouragement with all aspects of my book. Without such support, my effort to turn myself into an anthropologist would have had to be abandoned at an early stage.

Acknowledgements are due to the British Medical Anthropology Society, the Scottish Branch of the Royal Anthropological Institute, the Institute for Contemporary Arts, the Traditional Cosmology Society and the organisers of the 1986 World Archaeological Congress and the Fourth International Conference on Hunting and Gathering Societies for inviting me to present papers which subsequently became incorporated into this book. In each case, the resulting discussion and criticism allowed me to improve the arguments immensely.

I acknowledge supportive specialist criticism from Tim Buckley (on the Californian Yurok), Vieda Skultans (on medical and menstrual anthropology), Alain Testart (on the 'ideology of blood'), Maurice Godelier (on Baruya menstrual symbolism), Kenneth Maddock (on Dua/Yiritja duality and other aspects of symbolism in Arnhem Land), Roy Willis (on cross-cultural snake symbolism), Joanna Overing (on menstrual myths and many aspects of cross-cultural gender construction) and Stephen Hugh-Jones (on Barasana menstrual rites). At an early stage of the research I benefited particularly from discussions with David McKnight (on the own-kill rule in Cape York Peninsula), and with James Woodburn (on normative menstrual synchrony among the Hadza). Marilyn Strathern, while editor of *Man*, made extensive comments on an article for that journal which became incorporated into Chapter 12 of this book; it was she who first drew my attention to Tim Buckley's work. Howard Morphy provided information on Yolngu symbolism and suggested the term 'transformational template' to describe my model. Bernard Campbell made valuable and firmly supportive comments on a paper on cultural origins which was later expanded to form Chapter 9 on human origins. Monique Borgerhoff Mülder also constructively (if more stringently) criticised the same paper. Robin Dunbar, Clive Gamble, Graham Richards, Chris Stringer, Robert Kruszynski and Elaine Morgan all read selected chapters within their various fields of competence, offering much extra information and making the final text (whatever its inadequacies) considerably more error-free than it might otherwise have been. None of this implies, of course, these specialists' agreement with what I eventually came to write.

Among many of my students who helped, Max Pearson gave me versions and details of traditional myths from which the argument substantially benefited, while Ian Watts helped me in keeping up to date with the recent palaeontological and archaeological literature on human origins. Lionel Sims read every chapter as it was written and offered many helpful suggestions. Other research assistance came from Chris Catton, Sue Walsh, Isabel Cardigos, Nick Kollerstrom and many others. The text benefited much from Beth Humphries' eagle-eyed and sometimes painfully stringent copy-editing. My Ph.D. supervisors at University College London, first Andrew Strathern and then Philip Burnham, were astonishingly patient with my slow progress in completing the thesis on which this book was eventually to be based. Finally, my warm thanks for the good advice, encouragement and almost equally astonishing patience of Robert Baldock at Yale University Press.

I am often told that the basic idea of my book is 'entirely original'. This is generous but not quite true. I was fortunately able to discuss and correspond with Elaine Morgan over the past ten years, an experience which led me to realise with ever-increasing astonishment the precariousness of the prevailing savannah hypothesis of hominid origins. Close familiarity with the aquatic hypothesis as it developed helped to give evolutionary depth to my initial suspicion that tidal synchrony may have been involved in both the biological *and* sociopolitical dimensions of cultural origins. My appreciation of menstruation as a potentially empowering experience, on the other hand, derived in part from my reading in 1966–7 of Robert Briffault's *The Mothers*. Ten years later, Denise Arnold introduced me to a series of papers on the same theme by members of the Matriarchy Study Group. A year or so after that, the poets Peter Redgrove and Penelope Shuttle published *The Wise Wound*, a literary work of great originality and insight, one of its main themes being the centrality of menstrual symbolism to any cross-cultural understanding of ritual and myth. I had already tentatively reached related conclusions on the basis of rather different lines of evidence, but the germs of many of my ideas may be traced in part to that book. The authors have since given me invaluable friendship, inspiration and advice.

On a different level, Graham Bash, Keith Veness, Ken Livingstone, Jane Stockton and Ann Bliss — none of them anthropologists — were among the political as well as personal friends and comrades who helped provide the support system necessary to sustain so daunting and unorthodox a research project. My children — Rosie, Olivia and Jude — have been a constant source of strength. Many others over the years — my parents, kin, friends and comrades too numerous to mention — gave me insights, courage and support.

More material in her support than anyone, however, was Hilary Alton, who made it a seven-year personal commitment to see to it that I actually finished. Hilary read every line of this book as it was written, sometimes many times; her insights into my reasoning and her judgements on presentation came to seem to me unerringly perceptive and authoritative. Without her firmness and loving encouragement, these pages would still be one more stack in an apparently unending sequence of never-to-be-finished notes, versions and drafts.

Chris Knight, Lewisham, November 1990

Introduction

Modern bourgeois society with its relations of production, of exchange and of property, a society that has conjured up such gigantic means of production and of exchange, is like the sorcerer, who is no longer able to control the powers of the nether world whom he has called up by his spells.

Karl Marx and Friedrich Engels, *The Communist Manifesto* (1848)

Humanity now has the power to destroy not only itself but most of the more complex forms of life on earth. No one can measure the scale of threat posed by our unplanned global economy as it hurtles along on its present course. What seems certain is that the future of our planet now depends on conscious planning decisions which we do not yet know ourselves to be capable of taking.

No scientific story about our distant past can avoid this troubling fact about our present, nor escape being shaped by it. Western scientific/ industrial culture now holds the rest of creation in its shadow. During the four billion years since life itself first evolved, no living subject has ever held such power or been vested with such responsibility. It is a realisation expressed eloquently by the anthropologist Robin Fox fifteen years ago, when the Cold War was still at its height. 'In the past', he wrote then,

> it has not mattered greatly what people believed about themselves and their societies, since nothing that followed from these beliefs could have endangered the species. Man is now rapidly approaching the point – and it will come in the lifetimes of his children – when, unless he takes his survival consciously into his own hands, he may not survive as a species. This requires a revolution in thinking as serious as the Copernican revolution. Man has to move to a *species-centred* view of the human world he inhabits. And he has to do it quickly – within the next fifty years or even less.

'Anthropology, if it chooses to fulfil its mandate', Fox concluded then, 'can make a more significant contribution to this change in man's view of himself than any other science' (Fox 1975a: 271).

Fifteen years later, with the Cold War replaced by new, less stable structures of conflict, the science historian Donna Haraway has taken this argument a bold step further. She asks: What does it *mean* to be species-centred, rather than merely western-centred or middle-class or masculinist in one's scientific outlook? Her book, *Primate Visions* (Haraway 1989), was published in that 'year of revolutions' when the Stalinist project of 'socialism in one country' finally collapsed, opening up a new and fearsome era of global instability but hopefully allowing the workers' struggle internationally to resume at last its own more autonomous, planet-oriented, course. As if the earth-moving events of 1989 were not enough, Haraway in that year shook the western primatological and palaeoanthropological establishment to its roots by unmasking the contemporary political roots of even the most 'scientific' of modern theories of human origins and human nature.

I was at the inaugural meeting of the Human Origins Interdisciplinary Research Unit in Sheffield early in 1990 when I realised that behind the scenes, Haraway's book – never mentioned in the formal sessions – was being talked about in hushed, almost reverential, tones. 'It's hard to avoid agreeing', I heard a senior colleague confide, 'that we are all just telling politically motivated fairy-tales'. Haraway has stripped away the fig-leaves, showing that when palaeoanthropologists wrestle with one another over what it means to be human and over how it was that human life first emerged, they are articulating the most deep-seated contemporary cultural longings whilst simultaneously promoting massively powerful (and of course over-whelmingly western) vested interests. As they argue over the meaning of a grooming bout between baboons, over an enigmatic scratch on a fossilised molar or over some vestigial Middle Palaeolithic lunch, what they and their constituencies are really contesting is the right to close off debate about human potentiality – and thereby determine the future of our planet. The primary ideological battleground on which this contest is being waged is that staked out in contemporary sociobiological and other debates over 'human nature', over what it means to be human and over how human life first emerged. 'The Territorial Imperative', 'The Selfish Gene', 'Man the Hunter', 'Woman the Gatherer' – the weaving of such origin myths is a struggle for power.

This book is an intervention in that discourse. Haraway's work has freed me to be explicitly rather than implicitly political. Although employing many of the narrative techniques of my sociobiological and anthropological professional colleagues, mine is a story rather different from the familiar ones. It is told, ultimately, for another audience, to whom I wish to be accountable. Science is, as it has always been, information which gives us power. But *whose* power? Haraway has demonstrated that if it is just men, or just middle-class people, or just Westerners – then there can be nothing very objective about the 'science'. As a rule, the breadth of the constituency of scientists determines the precise mix of ideology and objectivity in their paradigms. A narrow base yields narrow, biased science; a wider accountability helps correct such distortions of perspective. Science as I understand the term therefore must be, among other things, both anti-racist and feminist (Haraway 1989). More generally, it cannot exist outside the empowerment of oppressed humanity. Human culture has not always been capitalist; neither has it always been dominated by persons with light-coloured skins. In these pages it will be argued further that culture was not invented by – and has not always been dominated by – men.

We humans – according to the narrative I favour – are a very recently evolved species (Stringer 1988; Mellars and Stringer 1989b; Binford 1989). Anatomically modern humans are known to have existed in Africa and the Near East at most 130,000 years ago; humanity's surviving linguistic and other cultural traditions can be traced back, probably, no more than some 45,000 to 90,000 years. The closeness in time of our biological origins and the apparently explosive pace at which cultural evolution subsequently took over have led many modern writers to describe our origins in terms of a 'revolution' – the 'human revolution', as it is often called (Mellars and Stringer 1989a).

This book is a revolutionary Marxist's reconstruction of that event. I am making my political motivation clear on the understanding that the reader has the right to information of this kind. In the wake of Haraway's extraordinarily liberating work, no palaeoanthropologist can any longer write about the 'Origins of Man' (or indeed of 'Woman') as if it were a matter of dispassionate disclosure of 'the facts'. There are no facts in this field – other than those released by courtesy of fiercely contested theories which are in turn packed with political dynamite.

Admitting this at the outset, let me say that from my own chosen political vantage point, virtually everything primatologists and palaeoanthropologists have been saying about human origins since twentieth-century science began addressing this topic has been wrong – and not just wrong in detail, but utterly wrong! On all the major issues, I think that we would get nearer the truth by systematically positing the exact opposite of what the functionalist and (more recently) sociobiological establishments have been telling us.

For example, whilst most authorities still portray the earliest hominids as they were being pictured many decades ago – as tool-using, meat-seeking bipeds striding out with their new technology from dense forest on to the hot, dry savanna – I prefer what is as yet a minority view. I see them as part-time tree climbers, walkers and, in general, as super-adaptable creatures who amongst other things enjoyed swimming and diving in rivers, lakes, estuaries and along marine shores (Hardy 1960; Morgan 1982). Whilst with dreary unanimity the establishment still posits the 'nuclear family', Victorian-style, as the basic, primordial cultural institution (see Chapter 14), I would posit the reverse – gender solidarity on a scale sufficient to keep husband and wife in separate camps for much of the time. Whilst they stress female 'loss of oestrus' and 'continuous sexual receptivity' (see Chapter 6), I spotlight menstruation and its associated marital and other cultural taboos. Whilst they stress 'Man the Hunter' or his *alter ego*, 'Woman the Gatherer' (Chapter 5), I see evolving palaeowomen using their increasing solidarity to shape the structure of both hunting and gathering, in addition to much else in life.

A final, very important, difference concerns dating. Whilst most socio-biologists and palaeoanthropologists still perpetuate a tradition according to which culture emerged some two or three million years ago, very gradu-ally and contemporaneously with the manufacture of the first stone tools (Holloway 1969; Leakey and Lewin 1977), I would follow Binford (1989) in shifting the dates forward several million years. 'Culture' as contemporary hunter-gatherers might understand such a term is much, much more than the ability to make a stone tool and pass on the tradition. Symbolic culture involves very widespread levels of synchronised co-operative action. It is not merely an 'adaptation'; it does not appear 'naturally' when large-brained, two-legged hominids are set down in a congenial environment. It requires community members' participation in a universe of shared meanings which are not merely technological but also (and here lie the greater challenges) social, sexual, political, mythological and ritual. I think that this multi-levelled intensity of sociality and mental sharing – and this is what I mean by 'culture' in the following pages – was universally and stably achieved at most 90,000 and more probably some 40,000 to 45,000 years ago (Binford 1989; Trinkaus 1989). I also think that it emerged not gradualistically but in a massive social, sexual and political explosion – 'the creative explosion', as it has been called (Pfeiffer 1982).

When palaeontologists and archaeologists nowadays speak of 'The Human Revolution', it is to this relatively *recent* series of momentous events that they are by common consent referring (Mellars and Stringer 1989a). Of course, there are other stories: many specialists would prefer a much more gradualist version of events. But the chief value of a study of human origins, from my political perspective, is that it demonstrates, firstly, that early life was communist (Engels 1972 [1884]; Lee 1988). Secondly, it teaches us that revolution lies at the very heart of what we are. Far from it being the case that 'no revolution can change human nature', everything distinctively *human* about our nature – above all, our capacities for language, self-consciousness, symbolically regulated co-operation and creative work – are precisely the products of that immense social, sexual and political revolution out of whose travails we were born. Whilst this process was finally consummated perhaps 40–45,000 years ago, in the earliest phases of the period known as the Upper Palaeolithic, it seems to me self-evident that so massive a human achievement has relevance for those of us hoping for revolutionary change leading to a more peaceful, sustainable and co-operative world order as the condition of our survival today.

In that sense – because I am motivated politically – I am of course constructing a myth. I am doing what all palaeoanthropological storytellers have been doing since the birth of their science (Landau 1991). The test of a good myth, however, is that it is both widely and enduringly believed. Very few of the stories that palaeoanthropologists have so far constructed have passed this particular test. The stories are always changing, and in detail, as I show in this book, they do not add up. This matters: even a fictional plot must work internally if the audience is to suspend disbelief at all.

But while internal coherence may be an important aspect of a narrative's plausibility, it is not the only one. In the game of scientific discourse, despite all the contestants' many disagreements and conflicts, the players have no choice but to adhere, for the duration of particular debates and contests, to at least some agreed ground rules. The rules that matter are those for disputing what kinds of observation are to count as data. 'The facts' themselves will never be stably agreed upon or there would be no game. But the procedures for constructing and verifying them must be shared as common currency at least up to a point. Were it not for some such agreement, in any event, it would be impossible to speak of a scientific community at all (Kuhn 1970). I am one of those who would accept that palaeoanthropology and sociobiology are disciplines which in the main have overcome this particular hurdle; whatever their limitations, they are not just pseudo-sciences. Most importantly, their relationship with a rather widely pooled, commonly accessible database ensures that there are countless antibodies inoculating participants from excess gullibility, constraining rather rigidly the kinds of stories which can nowadays be told.

I write under such constraints. I fully expect my narrative to be vigorously contested. Like any scientific storyteller, however, I live in at least the faint hope that my own particular myth may turn out to become accepted so widely that – whilst it can never be the final word – it forms part of the kernel of all subsequent stories. In our own culture, such a myth would be termed 'science'. In saying this, there is no intention to belittle science, nor to deny its superiority to myth-making. One story is certainly *not* as good as another (Haraway 1989). I am simply registering my view that the ultimate test can only be a social one. Whilst both science and myth are means through which humans become aware of their power, the first differs from the second in that its data confer power upon more than just one minority section of humanity in opposition to the rest. In general, people nowadays will *not* feel sustainably empowered by a story that evades the rigorous testing in the light of evidence which modern science – at least in principle –

demands. The corollary is that if a story survives such testing and in consequence feels so empowering to so many people that conflict over it is largely brought to an end, then it must be a good myth – and under the rules of modern discourse *deserves* to be termed 'science' (see Chapter 14).

Sociobiology: Political Economy of the 1990s

Founded on the premises of methodological individualism, modern sociobiology is – as Donna Haraway (1989) among others has shown us – the supreme mental expression in the life sciences of the inner logic of late capitalism. In this hyper-liberal perspective, social groups, communities, corporations, institutions, cartels, families, mother–child dyads, hordes, troops and even species all disappear. In their place – within a given 'population' – stands the rational, calculating, profit-maximising individual subject.

This entity has nothing to do with the rounded-out organism of commonsense perception, located in space and time, embedded in relationships and subject to death. For sociobiology, the flesh-and-blood individual – the phenotype – is pure agency. What animates it is a set of shadier, more mysterious entities – complex and usually unique sets of molecular, protein-building instructions known as 'genes', whose spatial locations transcend the physical boundaries of individual organisms, and whose only law is to survive death in one form or another and 'stay in the game' at the expense of all contradictory sets of instructions (Dawkins 1976).

Sociobiology triumphed in the life sciences at the start of the 1980s, a decade symbolised, in Britain and the United States, by the coming to power of governments expressing a new, coherent and explicit conservative ideology often known as the New Right (Rose *et al.* 1984: 3). Sociobiological writers characterised the activities of their 'Selfish Genes' (Dawkins 1976) in terms remarkably similar to those used to describe the enterprising moneymakers central to the new current's political manifestos. Even the most austerely academic of books and articles constantly resorted to metaphors derived in the most obvious manner from liberal economics and from modern military theory – giving us, for example, genetic 'arms races', 'investment strategies', 'cost-benefit calculations', 'payoffs' and so on. To many on the left during the 1970s and 1980s, these concepts seemed so ruthlessly bourgeois and right-wing as to preclude the possibility that feminists, socialists, green activists or others could possible learn anything from them (Sahlins 1977; Rose *et al.* 1984).

In the 1990s, however, this situation has begun to change. It has begun to be realised that capitalism is not all negative, and that its vigorous, explicit manifestation in thought can do us all much good. Once again, Donna Haraway is central here, for her book has probably done more than any other single work to clarify for the left what sociobiology has actually achieved. Particularly in her chapters on the work of sociobiologically trained feminist primatologists (Haraway 1989: 176–9; 349–82), she has taken us beyond the left's knee-jerk complaints about 'biological reductionism' to a new understanding of the paradoxically liberating role which this uncompromisingly 'late capitalist' school of thought has played.

Central to *Blood Relations* is the firm belief that sociobiology's achievements are to a modern Marxist analysis of sociality what the constructs of classical pre-Marxist political economy were to Marx himself. They are the corrosive acid which eats away at all illusions, all cosy assumptions about 'the welfare of the community' or 'the brotherhood of man', all unexamined prejudices about how 'natural' it is for humans to co-operate with one another for the good of all. There is much that is useful in this.

Sociobiology came on to the scene in triumphant opposition to the well-meaning functionalist theory according to which biological organisms are genetically selected for their ability to act for the good of their social groups. This functionalist theory was essentially social-democratic and corporatist: it saw the 'species' or 'group' very much as the prevailing political currents of the period (including Stalinism) saw 'the state'. Just as the various constituent bodies of the 'welfare state' or 'nation' were supposed to pull together for the good of the whole, so the individual organisms making up biological social units were supposed to be 'by nature' inclined to work for the common good.

Like a powerful solvent, the sociobiological paradigms of the 1980s tore into all this, eating away at the supposed co-operative bonds holding together 'species', 'communities', 'hordes', 'mother–child units' and other sentimentally conceived 'holistic entities'. In doing so, sociobiology produced results which to my ears recall Marx's and Engels' words written in 1848 in the *Communist Manifesto* (Marx and Engels 1967 [1848]: 82):

> The bourgeoisie, wherever it has got the upper hand, has put an end to all feudal, patriarchal, idyllic relations. It has pitilessly torn asunder the motley feudal ties that bound man to his 'natural superiors', and has left remaining no other nexus between man and man than naked self-interest, than callous 'cash payment'. It has drowned the most heavenly ecstasies of religious fervour, of chivalrous enthusiasm, of philistine sentimentalism, in the icy water of egotistical calculation. It has resolved personal worth into exchange value, and in place of the numberless indefeasible chartered freedoms, has set up that single, unconscionable freedom – 'Free Trade'.

Now, the point is that Marx found *within* this logic of capitalism – not from something external – the revolutionary antithesis he was seeking. He analysed the works of Adam Smith, Ricardo and the other classical political economists carefully on the understanding that such authors were the leading social scientists of their time, their work representing the cutting edge of *scientific* thought on the issues which concerned him. Refashioned in the hands of Marx, the findings of these champions of free-market economics were transubstantiated – into a body of theory which validated as never before the notion of men and women as intrinsically, necessarily social, and the future as intrinsically, necessarily communist.

Sociobiology may have a comparable significance for our age. Ideologically right-wing through and through, it incorporates nonetheless much of what is most advanced in current scientific thought on the nature of life. Not only does it seem obvious to me that its political metaphors actually work – that is, they are enlightening, clearly engaging with something actually going on in the natural world. It is equally apparent that the old, functionalist and group-selectionist biological paradigms – counterparts in science of social democracy in politics – in their time were like bad book-keeping. They made it impossible to see what needed to be seen.

When primate social groups were seen as 'functional wholes', the forms of data on which this book depends were simply concealed from view. No one could pick up conflicts of interest between males and females, between parents and offspring, or indeed between social group-members of any kind, since the members of each biological 'community' were seen by definition as harmoniously integrated on the model of the heart, lungs and other parts of a single organism. It took sociobiology with its calculus of genetic interest to reveal female primates, for example, not as passive valuables herded about and organised by dominant males – but as agents in their own right, active strategists fighting for their own genetic goals (Haraway 1989: 176–9). It took sociobiology to dispense with confusing and sentimental terms such as 'the mother–infant dyad', showing that in fact an infant can have rather different genetic interests from its mother – as (for example) when a female needs to wean an existing child in order to make room for another.

Sociobiology does not insist that all individuals are selfish. It would be a crass misreading to confuse the molecular 'selfishness' of sets of genetic instructions with selfishness at the behavioural level on the part of flesh-and-blood individuals. Nonetheless, sociobiology (like revolutionary Marxism) is about struggle and conflict. Whilst not denying altruism in nature, it insists that this constitutes a challenge to our understanding – a *seeming* anomaly which cries out to be *explained*. How much more helpful this is, scientifically, than the view that co-operation is the default condition, so 'natural' that explanation is not really necessary! Had it not been for Barbara Smuts, Shirley Strum, Sarah Hrdy and other sociobiologically informed primato-logical fieldworkers (see Haraway 1989), many of them what I would term 'bourgeois feminists', the basic concepts of Marxism – of struggle, conflict, contradiction and revolution – would have been inapplicable to the study of monkeys and apes. The relevant data on conflict would simply have been lacking. By the same token, without sociobiology, Marxism would have remained (as it has remained for many decades) inapplicable to palaeo-anthropology and to the study of human origins. The concept of 'class struggle' in particular would have remained boxed in by bourgeois ideology, denied all claims to universality, confined strictly and mechanically to recent cultural history – instead of being seen (as it is in this book, cf. Engels 1964 [1873–86]) as a construct with resonances echoing far back into our evolutionary past.

Gradualism, Genes and 'Memes'

A modern tale of human origins must conform to various narrative conventions if it is to be heard. Usually, this involves an element of gradualism. The gradualism which seems inescapable stems from the need for consistency with contemporary Darwinian theory. My story will convince no one if it seems to be contradicted by the basic laws of genetic inheritance, random mutation and non-random differential selection which – as I am quite capable of accepting – have governed evolution on this planet since life itself began some 3–4,000 million years ago.

Admittedly, many palaeontologists and evolutionary biologists nowadays describe themselves as 'punctuationists'. But even those who see in the evolutionary record long periods of stability which are on rare occasions 'punctuated' by sudden bursts of change (Eldredge and Gould 1972) hold that their 'sudden' changes are in fact strung out over immense periods, each quantum leap or 'speciation-event' consisting of barely perceptible modifications stretched across hundreds of thousands if not many millions of years. No one can tell a story about a new species of primate, for example, which leaps into existence from one generation to the next. All evolutionary theory is inherently gradualist in this basic sense, and must remain so if it is to have any credibility at all.

On the other hand, virtually all evolutionary biologists are believers in radical and – on a geological timescale – 'sudden' change, although some may feel that such events are extremely rare. Richard Dawkins in his bestseller, *The Selfish Gene* (1976), stresses two such very rare or 'abnormal' events – two events in the course of which something utterly new seems to have appeared in the known universe. One of these is the origin of life. The other is the origin of culture. Since (as Dawkins himself suggests) the first may have something to teach us concerning the second, it is perhaps worth touching on the problem of life before pursuing any further the main topic of this book.

Almost all biologists agree that life as we know it had only *one* origin, giving rise to a *single* history, characterised by shared derived characteristics such as the genetic code and the universal molecular symmetry of metabolised sugars (see, e.g., Margulis 1982). A much-contested contemporary scientific question is whether *modern humanity* and *culture* as we now understand this term had a single origin and a single history in something like the same way (Mellars and Stringer 1989a).

What might there be in common between life's origins and the emergence of culture? Many thinkers have linked these two processes. If we accept Dawkins' version, as presented in *The Selfish Gene* (1976: 208), the 'genetic takeover' accomplished at life's birth was not to be the only one ever to occur:

> As soon as the primeval soup provided conditions in which molecules could make copies of themselves, the replicators themselves took over. For more than three thousand million years, DNA has been the only replicator worth talking about in the world. But it does not necessarily hold these monopoly rights for all time. Whenever conditions arise in which a new kind of replicator *can* make copies of itself, the new replicators *will* tend to take over, and start a new kind of evolution of their own. Once this new evolution begins, it will in no necessary sense be subservient to the old.

With the origin of culture, according to Dawkins, there was launched just such a novel form of evolution, based on the immortality not of the gene but of the 'meme'.

A successful 'meme', according to Dawkins, is a portion of cultural tradition — say, a tune, an idea or a catch-phrase — which survives in the memories of successive generations of humans and is capable of evolution at a very rapid pace. Just as genes propagate themselves in the gene pool by leaping from cell to cell, so according to this view, memes propagate themselves in the meme pool by being transmitted from brain to brain through a process which, in the broad sense, can be called 'learning' or 'imitation'.

History or cultural change, in this view, is basically the evolution of memes. Because the differential selection and preservation of memes has little to do with the genetic constitutions of the individuals who memorise them, it follows that cultural evolution is in Darwinian terms a quite peculiar thing, and that in gaining an understanding of it 'we must begin by throwing out the gene as the sole basis of our ideas on evolution' (Dawkins 1976: 205). Some rudimentary examples of 'cultural' or 'memic' evolution can be found in birds and in monkeys, but as Dawkins (1976: 204) points out, ' . . . . these are just interesting oddities. It is our own species that really shows what cultural evolution can do.' The appearance of humanity, in this view, opened the door to a 'new takeover' by memes — in effect a seizure of power by the new replicators, ending or at least transcending the tyranny of the old, blind genetic replicators (Dawkins 1976: 208, 215). It was rather like the origin of life all over again — but on a new, higher level. In any event, something utterly new had once again begun to happen. There was a leap to a new level of determinism, requiring for its analysis a distinct — more-than-biological — kind of science.

I intend to draw on this parallel between 'genes' and 'memes' not because I find the analogies to be entirely convincing (for variations on the theme see

Cavalli-Sforza and Feldman 1981; Lumsden and Wilson 1981; Boyd and Richerson 1985; Rindos 1985, 1986), but because this way of looking at matters helps to validate my own narrative of a 'human revolution' which transported evolution *beyond the parameters of ordinary Darwinism*. The 'memes' concept implies that just as a theory of life's origin must explain where Darwinian principles came from when they had never operated within our part of the universe before, so my book must explain where the still more complex phenomenon of memic immortality came from. Dawkins stresses that no theory of life's origin can 'contradict the laws of physics'. But he also stresses that such a theory will have to 'deploy these laws in a special way that is not ordinarily discussed in physics textbooks' (Dawkins 1988: 15). The corresponding logic applies to the task I have set myself here. Naturally, *Blood Relations* must not contradict the laws of Darwinian natural selection. But it must deploy these laws '*in a special way that is not ordinarily discussed in biology textbooks*'. Biology – even sociobiology – will not be enough.

Nature and Culture

It will be clear that the notion of a human revolution both validates and to an extent depends upon the peculiarly western cultural construct of a domain called 'nature' which stands in polar opposition to a different domain known as 'culture'. Since I am convinced that it stands for something real, I like this distinction and intend to respect it. With his notion of 'memic immortality', Dawkins has both replicated this cultural construct and refined it, helping those of us who value it to perform the difficult task of determining precisely where the boundary between 'nature' and 'culture' should be drawn.

An implication of Dawkins' argument is that in deciding whether palaeoanthropological events belong on one side or the other of the divide, what matters is not whether memes are occasionally replicated. What matters is (a) their centrality in maintaining the continuity of social structure and (b) whether true immortality is open to them. As noted earlier, many creatures can pass down memorised patterns from one generation to the next. Vervet monkeys in the Amboseli National Park, Kenya, for example, have been observed to dip dry *tortilis* pods during a drought into the sap-filled well of a *tortilis* tree, a technique which makes the parched pods much more nutritious and edible (Hauser 1988). This technique is not an element in the ordinary species-specific behavioural repertoire of the vervets; it has to be invented by an individual during a particular drought and then passed on to others via imitation. Why, then, can we not speak of vervet monkeys as having 'culture'?

Part of the reason is that such learning-dependent skills are peripheral to the political determinance of structure. However great their survival value, they are marginal to the maintenance of social-structural continuity from one generation to the next. This means that although behavioural patterns may fluctuate, seasonally or in other ways, there can be no real, cumulative *social evolution* beyond that which is chained to the slow evolution of genes.

Linked to this limitation, such learned skills tend to circulate only in limited pockets of time and space before being forgotten. In the case of Hauser's vervets, social groups are so small that the pod-dipping technique 'has a high probability of disappearing by chance alone' (Hauser 1988: 341). A period of drought has only to end for this element of collective wisdom to get forgotten, although it will very probably be reinvented by some other individual or individuals in a subsequent drought and shared within one or more small groups all over again. The important point here is that memes under such conditions can experience no real evolution. There is no widespread, universalistic information pooling and therefore no progressive accumulation of memes – only the endless rediscovery within small groups of what previous generations may already have known.

It is this kind of limitation which – according to my origins narrative – anatomically modern humans transcended in the course of those momentous events which led up to and were consummated in the Upper Palaeolithic revolution whose reverberations began rippling across the world between 40,000 and 45,000 years ago. Whilst chimpanzees have been shown to have preserved and developed a surprisingly rich traditional knowledge of the use of medicinal plants (Sears 1990), and whilst there can be little doubt that archaic humans such as the Neanderthals had palaeotraditions, palaeolanguages and perhaps also palaeorituals (Marshack 1989), my point is that communication between local groups prior to the Upper Palaeolithic was poor (Gamble 1986a). Memes could replicate themselves and accumulate, but only patchily, within small, circumscribed, scattered and often isolated social units. The real breakthrough – the 'creative explosion', as it has been called (Pfeiffer 1982) – was made when new and extended patterns of social interaction allowed such local boundaries to be transcended. At that point, in a process which we might liken to 'freedom of the press' or 'ideational free trade', memes could circulate freely over such distances that it no longer mattered (from a memic point of view) whether a particular local population survived: so many intercommunicating populations preserved at least something of the basic pool of memes that memic immortality as such was now assured. In my story, the human revolution was finally consummated when – paralleling life's establishment of the infinite immortality of genes – events opened up channels for the transmission of memes across what were in principle indefinite expanses of space and of time.

Agreements, Contracts and the Cultural Domain

Symbolic culture as I understand the term, then, has its basis in the immortality of whole sets of extremely complex memes – culture-constituting instructions shaped not just by behavioural interaction between organisms and their environments, and derived not only from the genetically based phylogenetic conservatism of the species, but shaped also through the relationship between these and a highly specific, rich and accumulating fund of collective wisdom or tradition materialised in technology, design, language, art, ritual, kinship and so on.

What were the conditions which had to be established to enable such complex memic patterns to be preserved? Central to my argument is politics. There could be no memic immortality in the absence of the essentially *political* capacity to establish agreements, rules and contracts. No human kinship system, no economic system, no religious community and indeed no cultural institution of any kind could function without these. Although my focus will be essentially upon the notion of 'blood' contract, let me for the moment leave aside this dimension and consider 'contract' in general as a novel evolutionary possibility.

Not even the simplest of collectively agreed or sanctioned contracts can occur in nature. Despite constructs such as kin selection (Hamilton 1964) and (in the case of large-brained creatures) reciprocal altruism (Trivers 1971), sociobiological theory insists that plants and animals do not and cannot adhere to 'agreements'. Instead, each organism is programmed to pursue its genetic interests and – except when mistakes are made – to allow nothing to get in its way. This (according to sociobiological doctrine) remains the case no matter how great may be the ultimate costs of such activities to the group or community to which each individual belongs.

Dawkins (1988: 184) drives home this point vigorously in a fascinating anti-socialist discussion concerning plants. 'Why for instance, are trees in forests so tall?', he asks, and replies:

> The short answer is that all the other trees are tall, so no one tree can afford not to be. It would be overshadowed if it did.

Dawkins points out how difficult we morally minded humans find all this. As we examine the situation at any point in the course of the struggle for sunlight, it becomes obvious that the tree community as a whole has gained no more light than would have been available had each tree stayed short. We might well ask: Why don't the trees co-operate? As Dawkins puts it:

> if only they were *all* shorter; if only there could be some sort of trade union agreement to lower the recognized height of the canopy in forests, *all* the trees would benefit. They would be competing with each other in the canopy for exactly the same amount of sunlight, but they would all have 'paid' much smaller growing costs to get into the canopy. The total economy of the forest would benefit, and so would every individual tree.

Yet this seemingly logical solution has never been hit upon. Neither trees nor any other plants or animals have ever come to realise the immense potential benefits which, theoretically, could stem from mutual self-restraint and solidarity in the interests of all. Disappointingly for those who would root a co-operative world political system in a benevolent 'nature', there is never in the animal world a collectivity capable of imposing global harmony or 'rational planning'. Such planning might seem 'objectively necessary', but as Dawkins continues in his tree discussion: 'Unfortunately, natural selection doesn't care about total economies, and it has no room for cartels and agreements.' There has simply been an 'arms race' in which forest trees became larger as the generations went by. At each stage, there was no intrinsic benefit in being tall. The only point was to be always just that little bit ahead of one's neighbours.

I have characterised Dawkins' discussion here as 'anti-socialist'. In a way, at least by implication, it is. But Dawkins makes his case without for a moment suggesting that it therefore makes no sense for humans to take collective action, form trade unions or collaborate to protect the global environment. He is not against – say – trying to save the large whales (whose genes are quite different from ours) from becoming extinct. His point is simply that no other species would artificially and through collective action try to impose self-denying regulations to curb the long-term effects of short-term competitive profit-seeking.

To me, it seems fruitless to deny this. But the implications are not necessarily 'reactionary'. They must seem so only to those who require their constructs of what is 'moral' or 'socialist' to match a model supposedly afforded by 'nature'. What logic is there in this? Surely, the point is that we speaking primates are not plants or animals but culturally organised *humans*. This means, on the one hand, that we have evolved to a potentially catastrophic degree the power to upset the balance of nature on our planet, destroying the Amazonian and other tropical rain forests, puncturing the ozone layer, polluting our atmosphere, altering the climate and threatening our own and many other biological species with complete extinction in the event of nuclear war. But it also means that the competitive pursuit of short-term 'selfish' interests is emphatically *not* the only political logic of which we are or have been capable.

Solidarity and Memic Immortality

Blood Relations is designed to show how it was that in evolving our bio-logically improbable languages, kinship systems, rituals and taboos, we humans have shown that we *are* capable of establishing 'artificial' rules which are in the interests of whole clans, interconnected bands, villages or entire communities, and enforcing respect for these. Although there is always some tension between personal interests and wider collective ones, we are and always have been capable of precisely that concern for 'total economies', and precisely that power to form trade unions or other contractual alliances which, as Dawkins points out, are not to be found in the natural world.

It would be a truism to say that solidarity in a general sense – including clan solidarity, tribal solidarity, ethnic rebellion, nationhood, class solidarity and other forms – has been a vastly important component of all human history up until now. No human sociobiology which failed to take account of such phenomena could claim to have much of interest to say to social historians or sociologists. Yet of course there are good reasons why sociobiologists have chosen not to focus on such things. Their science is an attempt to explain all social life in terms of constraints imposed by the 'selfish' self-replicatory interests of genes. This works well in the study of insects, and even in the study of primates. Up to a point, it also works in the study of ourselves. But only up to a point.

'We, alone on earth', Dawkins writes in concluding *The Selfish Gene* (1976: 215), 'can rebel against the tyranny of the selfish replicators'. The difference between ourselves and other creatures is that we *can* transcend the level of determinism which is represented by competition between genes. Unlike trees competing for sunlight, we humans *can* form trade unions or comparable bodies. We *can* act with conscious foresight in our collective long-term interests, instead of remaining wrapped up in our short-term individualistic pursuits. Where the 'total economy' of our planet is concerned, the idea of taking collective responsibility for it may seem a novel and daunting political challenge, which we have barely begun to rise to. Yet it may be precisely such a new cultural 'leap' that is required if our own and many other species' genes are to have any future at all.

In any event, it is part of the argument of this book that our power to make and to enforce life-enhancing collective agreements has been with us since the very inception of culture. My task in the chapters which follow is to investigate how such abilities could have arisen.

Language

Politics must be centre stage in any discussion of 'memes'. This is because a condition of memic immortality is at least a *relative* absence of political conflict. If two primates are fighting, then for the duration of hostilities there will be little 'meeting of minds' and therefore little if any memic sharing or interchange. By contrast, two close allies – perhaps in a coalition directed against a third – are likely to be sharing and exchanging memes as a matter of course. Where a coalition is large, the likelihood of memic survival within it becomes magnified correspondingly.

It is an obvious point, but one which has been all too often missed. It has a bearing on the question of the origins of language – 'the most remarkable and characteristic of all human creations' (Renfrew 1987: 1). With many others, I take the view that our species did not become fully human until the abilities of advanced reasoning that language helps to foster were fully developed (Binford 1989: 36; Mellars and Stringer 1989b; Renfrew 1987: 1; Cavalli-Sforza *et al.* 1988).

However uncertain the results, it is intriguing to examine fossil hominids such as the Neanderthals for signs of the physical ability to articulate the range of sounds which modern humans can pronounce (Arensburg *et al*. 1989; Lieberman and Crelin 1971; Lieberman 1988, 1989). It is also useful to seek to identify the basic 'design features' common to all human languages – features distinguishing them from the communications systems of animals (Hockett 1960; Hockett and Ascher 1964), or to debate whether the primary channel for earliest human language was gestural or vocal (Hewes 1974; Hill 1974). But such questions concerning the mechanics of language are obviously secondary as far as the real theoretical problems are concerned.

A human linguistic system is made up of 'memes'. In the case of language, these are phonetic rules, syntactical rules, semantic rules and 'pragmatics' – sets of conventionally agreed relationships between what participants hear or say and what they are supposed, consequently, to do. If these latter rules – insufficiently discussed in theories of language origins – are not respected, language itself cannot evolve. In short, the creativity behind language 'arises not from linguistic skills narrowly conceived but from sociality and the social matrix in which one lives' (Carrithers 1990: 202). Or as the linguistic philosophers Bennett (1976) and Grice (1969) among others have shown, human speech is possible only against a *logically prior background of social interaction and sociality*.

Language is 'a product of the collective mind of linguistic groups' (De Saussure 1974 [1915]: 5). It 'exists only by virtue of a sort of contract signed by the members of a community' (De Saussure 1974 [1915]: 14), and has no existence apart from that contract. It has frequently been observed (for example by Wescott 1969: 131) that the word 'communication' comes to us from the Latin adjective *communis*, 'common'. This word, in turn, is derived from a reconstructed Indo-European verbal root *mey-*, 'to share' or 'to exchange'. For a speech community to emerge, it is necessary that intelligent hominid individuals should *share understandings*, and that these mental sharings should extend even to those sensitive areas – such as food and sex – which are most liable to provoke the kinds of conflict which would otherwise lead to blows. The sharing of understandings, the sharing of wealth such as food and a downgrading of the role of violence are all in this context interconnected. 'Language', as the French anthropologist Pierre Clastres (1977: 36) has cogently put it, 'is the very opposite of violence'; speech 'must be interpreted . . . as the means the group provides itself with to maintain power outside coercive violence; as the guarantee repeated daily that this threat is averted'.

Such a capacity for transcending physicality has obviously less to do with the genetic constitution of individuals than with the political/social/sexual situation in which they find themselves. To the extent that, in any community, issues between individuals or groups are decided purely or primarily physically, language not only cannot evolve – it loses all its relevance.

This was perhaps the most important lesson to emerge from the many attempts made some years ago to teach chimpanzees to speak (for a survey see Desmond 1979). For example, when Roger Fouts (1975: 380) and his colleagues taught American Sign Language to the chimpanzees 'Booee' and 'Bruno', explaining to them how to ask politely for food, everything worked well − for as long as it was *humans* who were called upon to make the culturally required responses. Once the animals were left to give and take food or other valuables between themselves, their newly learned skills were left hanging in a cultural vacuum, deprived of any meaning or use:

> The food eating situation has turned out to be somewhat of a one-way ASL communication because neither of the two males seems to want to share food with the other. For example, when one of the two chimpanzees has a desired fruit or drink the other chimpanzee will sign such combinations as GIMME FRUIT or GIMME DRINK. Generally, when the chimpanzee with the desired food sees this request he runs off with his prized possession. (Fouts 1975: 380)

So much for asking. Any chimp seriously wanting food or drink, then, must forget linguistic subtleties and fight for its objectives using hands, feet or whatever other instruments are available.

It is undeniable that compared with chimpanzees, humans have more highly evolved speech areas in the brain, and that the capacity to learn any language has a major genetic component. But this must not obscure the essential fact that the conditions for language's relevance have always been political. The problem for Booee and Bruno was not their inadequate linguistic competence or training. It was their lack of involvement in a wider system of cultural meanings. The two animals were not citizens within a chimpanzee republic; neither were they 'classificatory brothers' within a chimpanzee counterpart of an exogamous clan. Their rights and duties were not codified in the name of a higher authority; neither had they entered into any moral contract regarding the sharing of valuables such as food or sex. It was for these reasons that they lacked a social universe capable of making human language even remotely worth learning − except, of course, for those periods during which they were entirely cocooned as individuals within an artificial, fully cultural, human foster-family. Just as one does not speak to one's enemies, so there would be little to be gained from conversing with a calculating rival who opposed one's own interests at every point. A growing child who got hit in the face by its parents on requesting love or support would develop only the most stunted of linguistic skills. No one can sustain the use of speech for very long unless there are others ready not only to listen, but to act with at least reasonable predictability in accordance with agreed rules on the basis of what is said.

Human language is in this context utterly dependent on the rest of culture, and has no function in its absence. 'Without language, culture could not exist; but without the rest of culture, language would have no function' (Trager 1972: 6). For language to work, in short, there has to be a deeper, sub-linguistic level of mutual understanding already built up in relation to the most important things and underpinning any agreement on the more superficial level of purely linguistic usage.

It is for this reason (and not just out of considerations of space) that I have chosen in this book not to concentrate heavily on the topic of language, despite its evident centrality. Instead, I have focused on what I consider to be the political conditions essential for language's emergence. I have stressed that languages are spoken effectively only within coalitions which can evolve into stable 'speech communities', and that therefore the important thing is to explain how coalitions of the necessary stability and scope could have been formed.

Primeval Soups and Coalitions

Primates' calculations of genetic self-interest frequently induce them to form coalitions. These are not exactly 'trade unions' or contractual 'agreements', but they seem to be the closest we can get to these in the natural world. When one primate forms a coalitionary alliance with another, each member of the alliance supports his or her partner when in conflict with a third party, *on the understanding that this will be reciprocated should the need or opportunity arise.* It is possible for individuals to 'renege' on such understandings, but there can be no doubting their reality for those who enter into them. An animal who reneges on a coalition partner is taking a risk, since the victim will remember the event and perhaps refuse needed support in the future (see, for example, Harcourt 1988).

Within stable coalitions, evolving protohumans could have shared certain understandings and passed on proto-cultural traditions such as methods of foraging or tool use (Wynn 1988; Hauser 1988). By contrast, where individuals were left to fend for themselves in a behaviourally stark battle of each against all, 'memes' – to return to Dawkins' term – would not have had a favourable medium within which to replicate themselves.

Some kinds of memes may have been transmissible even between hostile individuals. A particular weapon-using technique, for example, might have been copied by one contestant following defeat at the hands of a better-armed rival. However, memic immortality even on this level would be favoured by defensive coalitions and alliances – male chimpanzees probably accomplish their highest cognitive levels in the course of 'warfare' between rival co-operative groups (see references in Alexander 1989). More neutrally, technical foraging tricks may have been relatively easily transmitted, the only requirement being sufficient mutual tolerance to allow imitation to take place. Again, however, the likelihood would be that even these would soon be forgotten unless the techniques were dispersed widely within coalitions which met frequently and in mutually supportive contexts.

Much more resistant to transmission, however, would have been memes *which specified something about how society should be organised*. These could never have percolated through a population riven by boundary disputes, inequalities or power conflicts, for the simple reason that the dominant and subordinate, those in one coalition and those in the next, would have had such very different interests and perspectives. Wherever a *political* or *sexual-political* meme travelled from brain to brain, replicating itself in identical copies, it could only have been because the individuals so connected already possessed much in common. They must already have shared the same social and political interests, providing them with a common vantage-point from which to view their world. In this context, the fact that so many widely dispersed contemporary populations of hunter-gatherers (among other peoples) share mythologically and ritually codified memes of this kind says much about the scope of coalition-forming which the human revolution must have entailed.

A coalition is a situation-dependent, temporary and informal agreement to share power, rather than fight over it. To the extent that individuals share power, political memes can be freely transmitted between them. In this context, we can posit a simple relationship: the stronger, the more stable and the broader each coalition the greater the likelihood of the spread of rudimentary political and other memes within it. Extensive and strong coalitions would have been the complex components of the new 'primeval soup' – as Dawkins (1976: 206) terms it – within which culture's 'new replicators' could have begun to evolve towards take-off point.

Emergence of the Human Coalition-forming Capacity

The specific *sexual-political* concept of coalition-forming central to this book represents the development and extension of an idea first suggested by the biological anthropologist Paul Turke (1984). Turke's field of interests explains my subtitle, *Menstruation and the origins of culture*. His aim was to explain the emergence of the human female reproductive system; his basic finding was that somewhere along the road towards fully human status, evolving hominid females must have systematically formed coalitions of a particular kind. What was special about these coalitions was that the females within them *synchronised their ovulatory cycles with one another*.

Published in the journal *Ethology and Sociobiology*, Turke's article was a contribution to a long-standing debate on the evolution of human female reproductivity. I had long felt that there was something explicitly competitive about the manner in which female chimpanzees and many other primates display their brightly coloured, swollen genitals at or around the time of ovulation. By the same token, my guess had been that the human condition of ovulation concealment and absence of sexual swellings had evolved in the context of a less behaviourally competitive sexual-political dynamic. To be more precise: I had long felt that inter-female *gender-solidarity* had had something to do with the unusual and characteristic features which the human female showed.

Turke's article seemed to me to translate such intuitive guesses into the language of science. A system in which a few 'alpha-males' monopolise the bulk of the female population may not be as common as was once thought (for a discussion, see Haraway 1989: 304–15; 349–67), but neither is it usual for all males in a population to have equality of access to the available mates. To the extent that the receptive females in a given primate community tend to be monopolised by only the more dominant males – Turke pointed out – they must tend to keep *out* of phase with one another. This is because each dominant male can adequately satisfy the females he consorts with only on condition that they come into receptivity not simultaneously but in turn. Should all of his females come into oestrus simultaneously, their demands over the next few days would be unmanageable and he would risk losing them to neighbouring rival males.

Turke is prominent among those sociobiologists who have looked at human evolution from a female-centred theoretical standpoint, viewing evolving protohuman females not as passive reproductive resources but as active agents in their own right. He argues that evolving protohuman females would have had compelling reasons to reject anything resembling an 'alpha-male' system. Such a system would in effect have 'wasted' the potential usefulness of all the unmated, less-dominant males. Faced with heavy child-care burdens and requiring as much male provisioning and parenting assistance as possible, evolving protowomen would have needed to approximate towards a situation in which inter-male differentials (in terms of reproductive success) were minimised. Selection pressures on biological features such as duration of sexual receptivity would have acted to favour those females who resisted their separation from potentially useful males, including males behaviourally less inclined towards fighting and/or direct struggles for dominance.

Imagine, writes Turke, a group of evolving hominid females who are under pressure to maximise their harnessing of the energies of even the least dominant adult males, each insisting on the support of at least one male for herself. It would then be logical for them to synchronise their ovulatory cycles with one another in groups – a course which at the same time would lessen direct sexual competition among themselves. In these circumstances, pronounced sexual swellings would not be predicted. Indeed, Turke goes on to show that it would be in such females' interests – if they wished to keep their partners with them – to dampen their signals markedly, eventually concealing the moment of ovulation completely and extending receptivity uniformly throughout the cycle. This, of course, is what human females do.

Without entering into the details of this argument here (see Chapters

6–9), let it be said simply that on reading Turke I felt that this model had more than the virtues claimed for it by its author. Firstly, it seemed to me to represent a sociobiologist's discovery of the virtues of a kind of 'egalitarianism', in that it envisaged a levelling process in which inter-male as well as inter-female status differentials were progressively minimised. Females and males according to Turke's model still had counterbalanced gender-specific interests, but within each gender group, enhanced levels of mutual tolerance and reciprocity must by implication have prevailed. Involvement in the synchrony envisaged by Turke would have demanded of each individual – male and female – a very high degree of co-operative *awareness of others*. Although he himself did not treat the emergence of large, gender-specific coalitions as a factor underpinning the transmission of memes, it seemed to me that Turke had successfully defined some of the basic sexual-political preconditions under which memic evolution could have evolved towards take-off point.

Secondly and equally importantly, I soon realised that with its emphasis on *ovulatory synchrony*, this particular model solved a number of theoretical problems I had been grappling with for years. These were not restricted to evolutionary biology; they extended to palaeontology, archaeology and to my own more familiar terrain of social and symbolic anthropology.

The Myth of Matriarchy

To explain the full significance to me of Turke, I must retrace my steps a little and return to the subject of political belief.

The myth on the basis of which I first became drawn to anthropology was that of Friedrich Engels in *The Origin of the Family, Private Property and the State* (Engels 1972 [1884]). Any reader of this book will without difficulty recognise my narrative as a version of that tale. Human society was originally communist; men and women were free and equal; sexual and other forms of oppression were at first unknown.

Engels (1972 [1884]: 49) argued that whilst primate societies were sexually competitive and incapable of sustaining solidarity, the transition to earliest human life placed solidarity first. This solidarity was not just a matter of technical co-ordination or co-operation in the hunt. So powerful were the first forms of solidarity that even sexual jealousy was transcended: whole groups of kin-related women were 'married', collectively, to whole groups of men (Engels 1972 [1884]: 49–50).

Because of such 'group marriage', according to the Engels myth, no one could know who the father of a particular child was: only the mother was known. Consequently, kinship tended to be traced only through the female line. The result – skipping a few stages in Engels' argument – was 'the matrilineal clan', whose features Engels derived from Lewis Morgan's account of matriliny among the Iroquois Indians. The 'matrilineal clan' or 'mother-right gens' (as Lewis Morgan usually termed it) was a group of women and men united by blood, descended from a common ancestral mother, sharing joint ownership in land, longhouses, children and other valuables, and based on a strict rule stipulating marriage outside the clan. Following Morgan, Engels characterised the internal life of an Iroquois longhouse as a form of 'communism'.

Clan solidarity – according to this view – always split or cut across the biological family, since a husband would always belong to and owe his primary loyalties to one clan while his wife and children belonged to another. Following Morgan, Engels insisted that it was vital to an understanding of human history and prehistory to accept this priority of the unilineal clan over 'the family'. In the beginning, marriage as modern Europeans understand this term was unknown. A husband acquired neither unconditional property rights in nor authority over his wife and her children. Instead, a man's kinship rights were in his sister and her children, just as his shared rights in clan property were rights in the resources of his own matrilineal clan, not his wife's. The virtue of this system, for Engels, was that it precluded the exploitation and oppression associated, at a later historical stage, with the emergence of 'the family, private property and the state'.

In my early twenties, when my political allegiances were just forming, I needed this myth because without it I could see no way of making communism seem either reasonable or possible. All the other accounts, as far as I could see, were so many different anthropological ways of rooting the contemporary social order in 'nature' or in the very foundations of earliest cultural life. Belief in these other myths, it seemed to me, must rule out any hope for real change in our contemporary world. If it was true that the nuclear family – basic cellular unit of modern capitalist society – was also central to nature and to all historical forms of kinship organisation to date, what hope was there of replacing it nowadays by something else? If male dominance in the family had always existed, what hope was there for fundamental sexual change? If domestic life could never be social and collective, with real love and solidarity extended beyond its contemporary nuclear family bounds, what hope was there for self-organised community life, sustainable workers' power or a future without the state?

But although I needed Engels' wonderful myth, I could not make it work. In my mid-twenties it rapidly became evident to me that bourgeois anthropology had gained complete hegemony in this area in the period since Engels' death, and that by the late 1960s no Marxist had made even a faintly credible attempt to keep abreast of developments in order to keep the story alive. As I began tussling with the literature, I realised that my political world was divided between comrades who knew nothing about anthropology but supported Engels all the same, and others who were familiar with the recent literature and had therefore abandoned the myth.

My main need was to find some real evidence for that sex-related 'solidarity' at the heart of earliest culture which had seemed to me to be the fundamental, indispensable kernel of the Engels myth. If necessary I could dispense with virtually any other aspect of the story; for political reasons I could not let go of that.

Engels Regained

In 1966, perhaps three or four years after assimilating Engels, I discovered an article by Marshall Sahlins in the *Scientific American* entitled 'The Origin of Society' (Sahlins 1960). The tone seemed weighty and authoritative, the article's privileged positioning within the journal signalling (as I thought) Sahlins' status as a leading expert on this issue. I at once realised the piece was exactly what I needed.

Just as Engels had written, primate societies were hierarchical, competitive, ridden with conflicts over sex and food. There were echoes here of the situation under capitalism, but – according to Sahlins – traditional hunter-gatherer societies were quite different. They were strongly egalitarian, based on a sharing way of life, and at their heart were rules or taboos which ensured that values such as sexual access and food were not nakedly fought over, with the strongest monopolising the most, but distributed fairly. Sahlins implied that a revolution – 'the greatest reform in history' – had been responsible for the momentous transition from a primate to a human way of life. Under the logic of what Sahlins termed 'primate dominance', sex had organised pre-human society. With the establishment of earliest culture, society at last succeeded in organising sex.

With the Sahlins model firmly in my head, it now seemed easy to save my basic myth, evolving it directly from the Marxist political vision to which I was by now attached. I concluded that in primatology there were two sexes – just as under capitalism there were two contending classes. Only one of these two groups was responsible for the *material* production which sustained life's continuance over the generations. It seemed clear to me that the responsibilities involved in female pregnancy and lactation were as heavy as the male's sperm contribution was light, and that in this context one could think of males on a biological level as the 'leisured sex', escaping most of the costlier tasks associated with the replication of their genes by getting females to do the work for them. Female primates, in other words, functioned in my mind as 'Labour'. The fact that, nonetheless, male dominance among primates could be pronounced was also not unfamiliar: did not the leisured classes in history usually dominate those whose labour sustained social reproduction as a whole?

As I structured the field through these and similar political preconceptions, I found that the most fruitful course was to be completely uninhibited in applying my Marxist grid. In this context, while female reproductivity was 'Labour', primate male dominance functioned in my mind as 'Capital'. Dominance was the primate mothers' own reproductive produce – their own male offspring – alienated so as to act as a force opposed to themselves. In Marxist terms, I saw nothing unorthodox about these ideas. In his Preface to the first edition of *The Origin of the Family*, Engels (1972 [1884]: 26) had written that 'production' in the first instance includes pregnancy and childbirth – 'the production of human beings themselves, the propagation of the species'; moreover, he himself (albeit in a rather different context) had emphasised (p. 75) that the first class oppression known to history coincided with that of the female sex by the male.

Other aspects of my grid seemed to fit. Some years before sociobiology had stressed the inevitability of conflict between female and male gene-replicating strategies, I was ready to assume on doctrinal grounds the divergence of 'Labour's' interests from those of 'Capital'. As I read up on primate politics – discovering dominance hierarchies, 'alpha' males controlling 'harems' of females, infanticidal males tussling with lactating mothers to decide the fate of rival males' offspring, breeding season battles between male sexual 'haves' and their rival 'have-nots' – I saw irreconcilable contradictions and class struggle everywhere. One of the very earliest books I had read had been Solly Zuckerman's harrowing description of what he termed 'the social life of monkeys and apes' (in reality the story of a pathologically distorted Hamadryas baboon community artificially created in the London Zoo). As I read this in 1967, it reminded me of some of Lenin's descriptions (which I happened to be reading simultaneously) of inter-imperialist rivalries exploding at the expense of workers everywhere during the First World War. On the bloody battlefields of Monkey Hill in Regent's Park Zoo, the males fought one another so viciously for the right to control females that within a few weeks most mothers and their offspring had been killed (Zuckerman 1932).

Becoming human, it seemed obvious to me, meant escaping all this via some kind of revolution. I took this idea literally. It meant the overthrow of Capital by the Proletariat – which I translated as the overthrow of Primate Male Dominance by Female Reproductive Labour. In what follows, I will refer to this as my 'mythical' version of the story central to this book. It was *Blood Relations* before I began worrying about what specialists in the field might have to say on such topics – my story in the period before I had started testing it and transforming it under collective pressure from comrades, friends and, eventually, professional colleagues.

Within this myth-like 'initial version' of the theory, the culture-inaugurating overthrow of Dominance could only be accomplished by Solidarity. The oppressed category of females had to resist their former sexual/reproductive exploitation and found a new, egalitarian order. They had to end the situation in which they had to do all the work. *They had to force the leisured sex to help in child care for the first time.* The obvious thing for them to do in this context was what any oppressed, revolutionary class in such a situation must do – win over to its side those members of the ruling class who in fact have an interest in change. I pictured the females as reaching out to the 'outcast' males – those excluded sexual failures who had lost out in the battle for females. These were the ones who had nothing to lose.

I soon realised that I could introduce at this point an economic element: meat. The outcast males, cut off from sexual attachments, would be mobile and free. The 'overlords' would be immobilised – chained down by the need to guard jealously their 'private property' in the form of females and slow-moving young. Because hunting (as I reasoned) requires unfettered mobility, the outcasts would occupy the most privileged position from which to exploit this new source of food. My conclusion was that any circumstances which might make meat-eating worthwhile would turn the tables on the dominant males in any group, destabilising the political hierarchy by enhancing the bargaining power of the formerly subordinate hunter-males. It all seemed to me so simple: in such a situation, the females would have needed meat; the meat-possessing subordinate males would have needed sex. What would have prevented the two sides from coming together? Only the sexual jealousy of the Tyrant Male. He had to go. He was duly overthrown. The transition to culture was consummated in that revolutionary act.

From this point on, the narrative evolved on the basis of its own mythic logic. Having thrown off one Tyrant Male on account of his uselessness as a hunter, the females – I reasoned – would have needed to continue to rely on the same revolutionary gender solidarity to prevent yet another male from occupying the old Tyrant's place. The solution seemed obvious, and again stemmed directly from my political grid. Organise strike action! This was the way for the females to demonstrate that *their bodies now belonged to themselves.* Just as the females in effect must have sexually boycotted the defeated Tyrant, so they would again have had to go on sex strike given any future signs of dominance-like behaviour in any of the males who were now allied to them sexually. More precisely: any male who approached seeking sex *without* first joining his comrades in the hunt would have had to be met with refusal. No meat: no sex. I already knew that in hunter cultures in the ethnographic record, a preliminary period of sexual abstinence was usually thought central to success in the chase, whilst bride-service was almost always the condition of men's on-going marital rights.

No matter how great the females' potentiality to *enjoy* sex, I reasoned, this would not have been the point. Babies – and therefore feeding them – would ultimately have had to come first. Sex would have had to be subordinated to economics. And the logic of strike action would have necessitated collective vigilance in this respect: within any female group, the sexuality of each would have become – by the inherent logic of strike action – the concern of all. Women *as a collectivity* now would have possessed and been responsible

for the value their sexuality represented. This seemed to me to conform
nicely with Sahlins' (1960) formulations in connection with the need for
'society' for the very first time to organise 'sex'. In my narrative, however, it
was not 'society' in a general sense which had organised the sexual availability of its female members: it was women themselves.

Organising a sex strike meant joint action. No individual could freely
offer herself to a male as and when it suited her. The living 'instruments of
production' were now socialised – self-socialised. I was intrigued by the
thought that this idea had the potential to explain not only the morality-
laden intersection of sex and economics in all cultural institutions of marital
alliance, but also those complexes of sexual self-control, self-awareness,
potential 'shame' and 'embarrassment' so central to all human cultures –
features obviously unknown (as I had noted as a young boy when visiting
zoos) among monkeys or apes.

For the first culturally organised humans, sexuality could no longer be
under purely personal control. The availability of one's body was of potential
concern to *the whole group*. There were elements of repression in this. Freud
(1965 [1913]) on this score had not been entirely wrong. But there was
nothing necessarily patriarchal about the repressive forces which now came
into play. The culturally necessary inhibitions came from within. Contrary
to the Victorian myths, so-called 'modesty' or 'morality' had not been
imposed on earliest women by men: women had imposed it on themselves
(producing mirror-image responses among culturally organised men) as a
condition of their own solidarity and power.

The model gave me the cultural incest/exogamy taboo. Women imposing
their sex strike did so – according to my model – to inhibit the sexual
advances of all non-hunter males. Their own adolescent male offspring would
have come into this category, and the forms of sex-excluding solidarity so
generated would have endured to produce unilineal clans. Finally, the same
story gave me matrilineal descent. I was pleased to discover from my myth
that, contrary to Engels, the internal solidarity of the matrilineal clan was
based on much more than 'ignorance of paternity'. It was an inescapable
political consequence of the gender solidarity central to the revolution and to
the cultural logic which this had set up. Men were not included in the same
political camp as their wives and children for the simple reason that camps
were defined by gender solidarity. Naturally, whenever women went on sex
strike. they *included* their male offspring within the boundaries of their
coalition but *excluded* their male sexual partners. Inevitably, this meant at
least two matrilineal 'coalitions' or 'clans'.

Matriliny: a Fathers' 'Own Offspring' Taboo

Impressed with the internal logic of the model, I nonetheless knew that I
would have to learn something about recent developments in anthropology,

archaeology and palaeoanthropology to see whether it all worked. In other words, satisfied though I was by my myth as pure myth, almost entirely independent of any modern data, I did retain a sufficient sense of perspective to realise my story's private status and total incommunicability to others in the absence of sufficient actual knowledge.

I began with the matrilineal clan. If my theory were right, then matriclans in the ethnographic record would be predicted to operate in a certain way, exogamy rules and food-sharing rules interlocking according to an underlying structural pattern specified in my myth. By the time I had combed through Robert Briffault's *The Mothers* (1927) and then Schneider and Gough's *Matrilineal Kinship* (1961), I felt broadly satisfied that my story was safe. The logic apparently worked. In a matrilineal clan system husbands can usually be divorced easily, and tend not to have rights in either children or *food-stocks* in their wives' households. On the other hand, these husbands *have to provide food for these households*, often under the authority of wives' brothers who have a stake in the home. A frequent reason for divorce or sexual refusal is alleged laziness on the part of an in-marrying husband.

This logic was exactly what my model had already given me: a situation in which women and their male kin organise a sexual rebuff to 'outsider' males unless they provide food (in the model's case, meat). The food which is taken in from these 'outsiders' then becomes the shared property of matrilineal 'insiders' – offspring and uterine kin of the woman. Drawing out the implications of my model, I reasoned that if the in-marrying males were to be allowed to eat meals in their wives' household, it ought to be as a favour and on sufferance, not as a matter of their rights in the food-stocks as such. This should not be a problem for men, however, provided they could always go to their sisters' or mothers' households and be sure of rights there.

I drew a diagram (figure 1) to illustrate two matrilineal moieties interconnected in this way. The conceptual grid seemed to accommodate the data, with a little squeezing here and there. Virtually every account of a matrilineally organised community that I consulted confirmed that men *did* retain rights throughout life in the household property and offspring of their mothers/sisters, and that there *were* various taboos or inhibitions against helping themselves to provisions within the households of their wives. The logic of matriliny, I decided, implied on an economic level that what husbands produced for their wives or wives' kin was food which they themselves had no right to appropriate, while that over which they exercised shared rights (in their mothers' or sisters' households) was always produced by other men than themselves. The same applied to children: those whom men fathered were never 'theirs', while 'their own' children were those born to their sisters – having been fathered, of course, by other men.

My diagram brought out the fact that these rules dovetailed into one another to define the logic of what I termed – following Mauss (1954) – 'total exchange'. In this, the rule *denying men rights in the produce of their own labour*

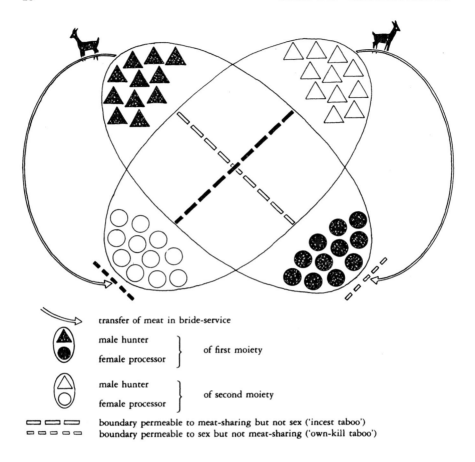

transfer of meat in bride-service

male hunter
female processor } of first moiety

male hunter
female processor } of second moiety

▭ ▭ ▭   boundary permeable to meat-sharing but not sex ('incest taboo')
▭ ▭ ▭ ▭   boundary permeable to sex but not meat-sharing ('own-kill taboo')

Figure 1   Mutual dependence of marital exchanges and the exchange of meat. 'Total exchange' results as each moiety is prohibited from appropriating its own 'flesh', whether human or animal. Just as humans born in one moiety can be maritally enjoyed only by the other, so the privilege of distributing meat produced (hunted) by men in one moiety is reserved for members of the other.

was an economic counterpart to the exogamy rule which *prevented people from having sex with their own kin*. In each case, what was at issue was a principle of exchange – this always resting, of course, on some factor acting to inhibit people from consuming their own productive or reproductive output. None of these exchange rules, it seemed important to note, would have had to be constructed through arriving at specific, separate, 'agreements' or 'contracts'. They were no more than emergent properties or dynamic consequences of that basic commitment which was rooted in the logic of the strike.

But of course, I quickly became aware that matrilineal clan systems are somewhat unusual in the ethnographic record, and that very few social anthropologists any longer give credence to the view that matriliny was once universal. Although my myth *yielded* matriliny, duality and exogamy, I was aware that with few exceptions twentieth-century social anthropology was no longer in conformity with Morgan or Engels in treating such things as central to culture's initial situation, and that informed critics would seize on this to marginalise my story should I prematurely attempt to publish it.

Reviewing the great early twentieth-century controversy over 'matrilineal priority', I felt far from satisfied with the mid-century and contemporary consensus on this issue. Boas' material on supposedly recent patriliny-to-matriliny changes among the Kwakiutl Indians I soon found to be by general consent irrelevant, since neither unilineal recruitment nor exogamy characterised descent groups in the region (see, for example, Harris 1969: 305). And the other main allegedly seminal contribution — Radcliffe-Brown's (1924) paper, 'The Mother's Brother in South Africa' — had long ago been demolished by G. P. Murdock (1959), who had succeeded in showing, firstly, that Radcliffe-Brown's new 'solution' to the problem of the avunculate was little more than a play on words whilst, secondly, the tribes Radcliffe-Brown was discussing almost certainly *were* matrilineal in the relatively recent past. It seemed to me strange that late twentieth-century anthropologists should continue to accept the anti-evolutionist paradigms of theorists such as Radcliffe-Brown and Boas on the matriliny issue even though the grounds on which these conclusions had been arrived at were now known to be at least questionable and at worst spurious.

Still, I felt that the nineteenth-century myths about a 'primitive matriarchy', along with their *ways* of arguing for the more scientific concept of matrilineal priority, were now past history. Despite my lingering sympathy with these myths in some of their aspects, I did not relish the idea of taking on the modern social anthropological establishment by attempting directly to revive them. I chose instead another tack.

The Hunter's 'Own-kill' Rule

I concentrated on the economic implications of my model. If matriliny was, in effect, an 'own-offspring rule' — a rule denying men rights in their own sexual 'produce' — then the economic counterpart of this (in my model's terms) was an 'own-produce rule', denying men rights in whatever they themselves had produced by way of food. In the context of a hunter-gatherer lifestyle, this translated into a rule prohibiting hunters from appropriating their own kills.

When I had first formulated my model, it was without any evidence for any such rule in the ethnographic record. I had been made aware of 'sharing', but that was not the same. My model specified that central to human culture's initial situation — indeed, just as central as the incest taboo itself — was the expectation that men should not have kinship rights in the

household property of their wives, and that this should imply their inability
to appropriate for their own use the meat which they themselves had killed.
Men killed game animals, not to eat the meat, but to surrender it to the
opposite sex as a condition of their sexual rights. If my origins story was to
survive I had to find evidence, at some level within the cultural domain, for
the centrality of this complex in which sex and economics intertwined.

Anyone who turns to the ethnographic record determined to prove the
existence of what she or he wishes to find will rarely be disappointed, and I
was no exception. Over several years during spare moments in a life taken up
mostly with political activism, combing through all the ethnographies I
could find, I piled up example after example of what I termed 'the hunter's
own-kill taboo', writing patiently and in neat handwriting in a series of very
thick, hard-backed, notebooks. By the time I arrived as a diploma student in
the Anthropology Department at University College London, I had collected
scores of these; they appear in this book as the basis of Chapter 3. My first
tutor, Alan Barnard, appreciated the 'own-kill' concept in structuralist terms
and helped me to integrate it effectively with Lévi-Strauss' (1969a) con-
ceptualisation of incest prohibitions as rules of exchange in *The Elementary
Structures of Kinship*.

It was in this period that I made what for me seemed an advance. I
succeeded in recodifying 'totemism' (cf. Lévi-Strauss 1969b) as an expression
of the same principle of exchange. Over the years, it had become clear to me
that most hunters in hunter-gatherer cultures in fact *do* quite often eat their
own kills, or eat their kills of certain species, or eat certain parts of the
animals which they kill. If my rule existed at all, then it was as if people in
most cultures had long since concluded that *rules are there to be broken*. But to
break a rule is not to deny its existence on any level. I was aware of reports
from all over the world of hunters' apparent feelings of guilt over the taking
of life or the killing of bears, deer or other game 'for base motives'. Hunters
in classical accounts would apologise to the animals before killing them, or
offer prayers or gifts to them after their death (Hallowell 1926). And of
course, I also knew of rituals of 'sacrifice' in accordance with which people
took the life of an animal in order, not just to eat it, but to make an explicit
gift of its life 'to the gods' (Hubert and Mauss 1964).

Increasingly, I felt able to discern my 'hunter's own-kill rule' in all of
these manifestations. What they expressed in common was a reluctance on
the part of hunters simply to *kill and eat*. Although my taboo as such was not
universal, in other words, its logic – its underlying 'structure', to use Lévi-
Strauss' term – apparently was. The rule as such was still visible, *even in the
stratagems through which it was evaded or negated*. I reasoned that if economic
conditions had changed from those of culture's 'initial situation', then there
may have occurred a collapse or weakening of the earlier chains of reciprocity
necessary if the old exchange rules were to work. In these circumstances,
people may have have felt compelled to begin breaking the rule against

eating one's own kill, just as features such as strict exogamy, duality or matriliny also broke down. Under such conditions, the ethnographic record as actually found could well have been arrived at.

Faced with difficulties, hunters would violate neither their extensive incest taboos nor the own-kill rule suddenly or wholesale, in an all-or-nothing way. Instead, they would eat away at these rules' more inconvenient consequences whilst retaining others, evading the stricter interpretations whilst on a formal level respecting them, making 'exceptions' – in the case of the own-kill taboo – of this species or that one, this part of a killed animal or that one, apologising always to 'the spirits' for infringements which seemed particularly difficult to justify.

Anthropologists had not properly understood the welter of different 'respect' or 'avoidance' relationships towards animals or their flesh in traditional cultures, I felt, because they had apprehended each institution separately, as if it were a particular local anomaly. The reality was that all of these avoidances were central to culture's default condition. In that context, they were not anomalous. They were as 'natural' (given culture) as the incest taboo. In other words, given culture in its default state, all meat was 'avoided', 'taboo', 'totemic', 'sacrificial' and so on. All raw or unprepared meat was exchange value, not use value. If people in *contemporary* hunter-gatherer and other cultures felt free about killing-in-order-to-eat with respect to *any animals at all*, then it was this weakening of the 'own-kill' taboo – not the logic of gift-giving behind 'sacrifice', 'totemism' and so on – which was the 'anomaly' to be explained.

In this book I have chosen to begin with this account of 'totemic' phenomena because it helps illustrate, perhaps better than anything else could, the distinctiveness of my palaeoanthropological aim. I am seeking to get beneath the ethnographic record to an underlying structure which helps explain its more seemingly anomalous features. I want my model to illuminate the hunter-gatherer ethnographic record as a whole, shedding light not only on kinship and economics but also on dance and trance, myth and magic, ritual and art. But above all, I want *Blood Relations* to seem to the reader to constitute a satisfying explanation for the genesis of *this structure itself*. That would make it a narrative adequate to the *richness, variability and specificity of culture*, rather than a model which seemed helpful in accounting for just a few selected, highly generalised, statically conceived 'universal features' such as (to take some examples from conventional palaeoanthropological accounts) 'the sharing way of life', 'pair-bonding' or 'consciousness'.

Sociobiology and Feminism

It was only from the late 1970s onwards – a decade or so after I had first glimpsed my 'human revolution' idea – that sociobiology became a powerful influence in both palaeoanthropology and primatology. The versions of primate politics underlying my original myth were not sociobiological at all. The narratives I had explored had been those of Solly Zuckerman (1932), Sherwood Washburn (1962), Irven DeVore and others for whom primate social structure meant essentially 'Dominance', whilst 'Dominance' meant essentially the political supremacy of *males*.

Haraway (1989: 176–9) has beautifully described how such early primatological fieldworkers who shaped my vision in those years simply failed to 'see' females as active subjects. They saw baboon or chimpanzee females basically as valuables to be fought over by males, whose noteworthy actions alone shaped and structured the entire social field. With equal insight, Haraway has shown how this blindness was served and masked by the functionalist biological paradigms of the period – paradigms which obfuscated analysis at the micro-level of individual motivation by dealing not with individuals but with supposedly functional wholes such as 'troops', 'hordes', 'bachelor bands', 'harems', 'mother–infant dyads' and so on.

The first systematic attempt to apply what was to become known as sociobiological theory to primates – according to Haraway (1989: 176) – was a thesis entitled 'Natural selection and macaque behavior', based on fieldwork on the island of La Cueva, Puerto Rico, in 1970. The author was Barbara Smuts, who as an undergraduate had been strongly influenced by one of sociobiology's founding prophets, Robert Trivers. In her thesis and her subsequent work, Smuts explored the doctrines of Bateman (1948), Williams (1966; 1975) and Trivers (1972) – later developed within primatology by her colleague, Richard Wrangham (1979, 1980) – according to which males and females have radically different genetic interests. Since this is an absolutely key concept, it is worth dwelling on Smuts' and others' use of it here.

Simplifying somewhat, the underlying idea is that males can have virtually limitless offspring and should therefore try to inseminate as many females as they can, whilst females can only produce a small number of babies, and should therefore concentrate not on consorting with one male after another but on ensuring that any offspring born should actually survive (Bateman 1948). Another way of putting this would be to say that, after a period, females should be uninterested in seeking more male sperm. The substance is plentiful, and enough is enough. But males should not have the same attitude towards fertilisable female ova. These are scarce. From a male's genetic point of view, more should always be welcome. If another female *can* be made pregnant, she should be. What 'limits' a male's genetic fitness, therefore, will tend to be the restricted availability of receptive females. What 'limits' a female's genetic fitness, however, is *not* a mirror-image of this. It has little to do with the availability of sperm – and much more to do with such things as food, shelter and other means of keeping existing offspring alive. Primate females, then, should distribute themselves within their environment motivated mainly by 'economic' concerns; males, by contrast, should map themselves in accordance with the search for receptive females.

This new, starkly Darwinian, way of looking at matters immediately introduced *gender* into all attempts to examine how food availability or other ecological constraints affected primate social organisation. The crucial point was that such constraints affected males quite differently from females. Sociobiology had clarified this, and the result was a sudden realisation – exploited by Smuts as well as by other feminist-minded primatologists – that the old primatological fieldwork had left immense blank spaces of ignorance as to how females pursued strategies to ensure the survival of their young. To ask how ecological constraints shaped social organisation, it was now realised, would mean studying female action in its own right. Simply to say that females were herded around 'functionally' by males, incorporated within 'harems' or 'mother–infant dyads', was no longer enough.

It is in this context that Haraway makes one of the most vital points in her entire book. The new explanatory framework, she writes (Haraway 1989: 176), began to revolutionise primatology from top to bottom. The absence of data on female–female interactions and female behavioural ecology began to be remarked upon in the literature, and young graduate students began to plan their field studies to explore such topics. In addition, primate workers began to understand that sociobiological explanatory strategies destabilised the centrality of male behaviour for defining social organisation. 'Female reproductive strategies began to look critical, unknown, and complicated, rather than like dependent (or entirely silent and unformulated) variables in a male drama, she writes.'

Female observers, continues Haraway, pressed these points with their male associate in the field and in informal networks. In general,

> since the men were not taking many data on females, they were not in a position to see the new possibilities first. In general, the women had the higher motivation to rethink what it meant to be female.

During interviews with Haraway, several of the women reported to her that it was the atmosphere of feminism in their own societies which had made it seem personally and culturally legitimate to focus scientifically on females for the first time:

> Men also reported the same sense of legitimation for taking females more seriously, coming from the emerging scientific explanatory framework, from the data and arguments of women scientific peers, from the prominence of feminist ideas in their culture, and from their experience of friendships with women influenced by feminism. (Haraway 1989: 176)

Discussing how Barbara Smuts, Jeanne Altmann, Adrienne Zihlman, Sarah Blaffer Hrdy, Shirley Strum and other western women have recently revolutionised primatology, Haraway concludes that these middle-class feminists

have projected their own political grids in the most fruitful imaginable way
upon the primates they have been studying. These women were hostile to the
notion that 'woman's place is in the home' — *and proceeded to remove all female
primates from the maternally nurturant 'dyad' relationships in which they had
previously been embedded*. As scientific primatologists, they were go-getters,
assertive intruders into a male scientific world, determined to prove that they
were 'as good as' — if not better than — any man. They succeeded — and cast
their female primates as active strategists in an identical mould.

And all this was thanks to late capitalism — or rather, to its highest expression in primatological thought. As Haraway (1989: 178–9) concludes:

> Plainly, sociobiological theory can be, really must be, 'female centered' in
> ways not true for previous paradigms, where the 'mother–infant' unit
> substituted for females.

The 'mother–infant' unit had not been theorised as a rational autonomous
individual; its ideological-scientific functions were different, 'located in the
space called "personal" or "private" in western dualities'. The sociobiological
kind of female-centring, states Haraway,

> remains firmly within western economic and liberal theoretical frames
> and succeeds in reconstructing what it means to be female by a complex
> elimination of this special female sphere. The female becomes the fully
> calculating, maximising machine that had defined males already. The
> 'private' collapses into the 'public'. The female is no longer assigned
> to male-defined 'community' when she is restructured ontologically as a
> fully 'rational' creature, i.e. recoded as 'male' in the traditional explana-
> tory systems of the culture.

The female ceases to be a dependent variable when males *and* females both are
defined as liberal man. The result — notes Haraway — was the construction, in
both human and non-human primate forms, of a liberated 'female male'.

The Class Struggle: Point, Counterpoint

Although I could not have formulated matters so clearly at the time, by the
mid-1980s I was dimly aware of many of these subtleties, which so closely
challenged and yet vindicated my own evolving myth. Although I scarcely
understood its scientific complexities, sociobiology by this stage did not
simply repel me, despite its obvious political roots. Indeed, I warmed to its
ideological excesses. They seemed to promise for the first time a publicly
communicable way of validating my own narrative. If the stockbrokers,
the company directors and the bourgeois feminists could be uninhibited
about projecting their pure political constructs into primatological and
palaeoanthropological debate — then how could they object to a socialist
doing the same? Obviously, it seemed to me, they could not object *on*

principle. The bone of contention could only be the extent to which – if at all – our respective grids worked.

I was happy about seeing *primates* as 'primitive capitalists', not only genetically but to some extent also on a behavioural level. I point-blank refused to see hunter-gatherer *humans* as maximising, competitive calculators within the same mould. It was here that I parted company with sociobiology. Their importation of the constructs of our own culture, it seemed to me, was unfair and one-sided. If you could have calculating, maximising capitalists operating in human origins narratives, why could you not *also* have militant trade-unionists? If you could have profits and dividends, why not also industrial action, pay bargaining and strikes? Our world, I reasoned, was a mixture of conflicting forces and political dynamics, not 'pure' capitalism. If scientists were going to transpose the modern world's constructs on to other cultures, on to nature and on to our own most distant past, why stop half-way? Why just take the selfish, competitive bits? Why not harness the whole of modern industrial culture in its entirety – class struggle, trade unionism, movements for socialism and all?

I felt equally ambivalent about bourgeois feminism. Influenced by friends and comrades who were feminists, I naturally felt feminism of any variety to be a liberating political force. But the currents I felt politically closest to were not those which Haraway in her discussion of primatologists describes. For the women I was closest to (many of them involved in the Greenham Common anti-Cruise missile campaigns of the early 1980s), the construction of 'female males' was not what the struggle was all about, any more than joining the capitalists was the essence of working-class emancipation. The struggle was more about refusing to collaborate with the whole masculinist political set-up, organising autonomously as women, drawing on support for real change from the wider class struggle – and fighting to bring men as allies into a world transformed on women's terms.

The Menstrual Dimension

I was at first unaware that my Labour versus Capital myth could or should have anything to do with menstruation. Although in 1967 I had read Briffault's *The Mothers* (1927), in which traditional beliefs about menstruation and the moon figured prominently, my politically shaped need to vindicate what I saw as the Marxist orthodoxies made me shy away from such themes. Nonetheless, I must have unconsciously absorbed from Briffault an awareness that menstruation can be positively viewed, perhaps internalising a hint that it might once have had something to do with that all-female 'strike action' on which my origins myth relied.

It was in 1977–8, during my first year as an anthropology postgraduate in University College London, that the topic suddenly began seeming more pressing.

Just before going to college, I had become aware of a small women's publishing network, one of whose pamphlets, 'Menstrual Taboos' (Matriarchy Study Group, n.d.), had attracted my attention. The historical and personal accounts by women in its pages made me aware that there were activists in the women's movement who were drawing on Briffault and other writers from an earlier generation in reasserting myths about a 'primitive matriarchy' – myths with at least some potential relationship, as I thought then, to my own evolving narrative. Although my gender, politics and antipathy to religion – even 'Goddess' religion – kept me from close contact with this particular separatist group, the tangential encounter was helpful in strengthening my awareness that women could find menstruation empowering. Menstrual experiences were not necessarily ups and downs to be disguised, suppressed or flattened out with artificial hormones. It seemed to me clear, in any event, that it was only an extremely *masculinist* and *non-periodic* culture which could impose its one-sided constraints so deeply as to make women conclude that it was they – but not men – who would have to suppress and deny their own biology as the condition of feeling liberated. There was a link in my mind between refusing the construct of the 'female male' and determining that cultural liberation *ought* to give women the chance (where they wish to) to validate and derive social pride, status and power from uniquely female experiences such as childbirth and menstruation.

At about the same time, I came across Martha McClintock's (1971) article in *Nature* documenting for the first time that closely associated women tend to synchronise their menstrual cycles. Like most men, I had not known this – had not known what nearly all women, I now realise, take to be an unremarkable fact of life. In my ignorance, I had had problems in integrating menstruation into my palaeoanthropological model of gender-based 'class solidarity' or 'sex strike'. My difficulty had been that women's menstrual cycles, as far as I had known, were necessarily randomised. Effective strike action, by contrast, presupposes joint action on the picket line. How, then, could menstruation coincide with the 'trade unionism' of my treasured origins myth?

The McClintock article solved this particular difficulty for me. Where women have solidarity, their cycles *automatically* tend to synchronise. The logical link between menstruation and strike action was now secure. My myth was vindicating itself and taking on new forms.

Then, during my first year as a diploma student at University College, Mary Douglas gave a lecture on 'male menstruation', citing in particular Hogbin's (1970) book on the Wogeo Islanders, *The Island of Menstruating Men*. The story made a searing impression, as with some gusto Douglas shocked her student audience with vivid descriptions of warriors and hunters preparing themselves for armed action, purifying themselves from weakening 'contamination' with the opposite sex – by gashing their genitals so as to make the blood flow in streams.

I was puzzled to understand why men should want to do this – particularly as I learned with growing astonishment that comparable practices were central to secret male initiation rites over immense areas of Australasia, Melanesia, Africa and the Americas. If menstruation were necessarily emblematic of feminine weakness, why should men want to emulate it? Not satisfied with the various psychoanalytic theories I came across (Bettelheim 1955), I suspected that on some level it was because menstruation had been for women not 'weakness' at all. Menstruation had been culturally constructed as a source (perhaps even *the* symbolic source) of ritual power – power which these 'menstruating men' were now motivated to usurp and appropriate for themselves.

Then, not long after my first excitement at making these discoveries, Peter Redgrove and Penelope Shuttle published *The Wise Wound* (Shuttle and Redgrove 1978). Although I felt not wholly sympathetic with the Jungian, far from Marxist style and tone, as a cultural influence upon me the book's impact was tremendous. Little was said about menstrual collectivity or synchrony – the emphasis was intimate, sexual, personal. Yet it became abundantly clear to me that my own myth now could connect up with massively powerful echoes in both modern and ancient literature, art, ritual and myth. Shuttle and Redgrove's poetic and psychological insights into the menstrual dimensions of the Holy Grail legend and countless other pivotal narratives now seemed not merely astonishingly original but also familiar and inevitable. They were my original Engels myth, Briffault's myth – and now my own evolving origins myth working itself out in my head.

The Language of Blood

In the light of all this I revised my cultural 'initial situation', incorporating – now – the symbolism of blood. It all seemed neat and parsimonious. For babies to be conceived, the sexes had to come together. For efficient hunting to take place, they had to separate. If both successful hunting *and* conceptions were to occur, the sexes had to alternate between conjunction and disjunction. Periods of sex strike and of marital togetherness had to alternate. I assumed that this alternation must have been socially synchronised, rather than a matter for individuals to decide autonomously within couples. It also seemed unlikely that any such alternation – if women had anything to do with it – could have disregarded the menstrual cycle. The default condition. I reasoned, must have been one in which the sexes came together when women were fertile.

This meant disjoining – organising each sex strike – during menstruation. Synchronised cyclicity would have made of this a collective rhythm. Had women required some external standard by which to regulate their synchrony, they could have used the moon. I was not a believer in mystic lunar influences; the moon was just the only appropriate clock. It may also have made sense for men, intermeshing their own rhythms with those of women, to regulate their hunting schedules in accordance with a lunar calendar. In addition to the obvious sexual/reproductive advantages of keeping in tune with women, hunters – particularly when winter daylight lasted only a few hours – may have benefited by maximising their overnight travel and associated exertions when there was sufficient moonlight to significantly lengthen the effective day. I reasoned that this might help explain the explicitly lunar attributes of hunters' deities such as the Greek Artemis and the Roman Diana, in addition to hunting ritual and folklore throughout much of the world, (see Chapter 10).

It was necessary not only for the *sexes* periodically to conjoin and disjoin. The same also applied to relations between *men and game animals*. Hunters had to encounter animals in order to kill them. But they had to be subsequently separated so that others could obtain the meat. In this context, I had been intrigued for some time by certain implications of Lévi-Strauss' *The Raw and the Cooked* (1970; see Chapter 13). I was also fascinated by the work of the French Marxist anthropologist Alain Testart (1978, 1985, 1986), in which he posits as central to culture's initial situation an 'ideology of blood' linking menstruation recurrently with hunting blood. Both Lévi-Strauss' and Testart's findings could be nicely integrated with my model.

Blood had been constructed, during the course of the human revolution, to signal inviolability or 'taboo'. In my narrative there was nothing complicatedly 'symbolic' about this. Women just went on sex strike at the biologically appropriate period – during the time of month when menstruation normally occurred. Any man noticed to be blood-covered might then have been suspected of 'strike-breaking'. Like a rapist or murderer, he would have had 'blood on his hands'. Assuming that men wanted to avoid suspicion, this consideration would have motivated the shunning of menstrual stains. By this route, women's blood as such would have become conceptualised as 'taboo'.

The hunter-gatherer ethnographic record, I knew, was replete with examples of 'hunters' taboos' which seemed to assume magical connections linking women's menstrual condition with men's hunting luck, or women's blood and the blood of raw meat (Testart 1985, 1986; cf. Lévi-Strauss 1970, 1978). To explain all this, I put the finishing touches to my model.

Somehow – I supposed – in the course of evolution it had become established that blood was simply blood. That is, it made no difference where the blood came from: it was conceptually all the same. The blood of rape, murder or strike-breaking, the blood of the hunt, the blood of menstruation or of childbirth: it was all in the final analysis just blood.

However this identification had been arrived at, the important thing was that once the confusion or perceptual merging had been accomplished, an extraordinary result would have been achieved. Given my arguments about menstruation and the theoretically necessary inviolability of women's sex strike, no form of blood could have been equated with menstrual blood without the most potent of consequences in evoking 'respect' or in conveying the notion of 'ritual power'. *Raw meat, after all, could have marked a man with bloodstains just as easily as could contact with a menstruating woman.* The only way to remain above suspicion might have been for men to remain wary of contact with blood of any kind – particularly when women were around. In accordance with this logic, all raw meat may have become in effect labelled 'unavailable' (in ethnographic translations 'taboo', 'totemic', 'sacrificial' and so on) within the vicinity of the camp. It would have stayed taboo for as long as it remained uncooked – just as women remained 'taboo' whilst menstruating.

Sex Strike as 'Elementary Structure'

Having constructed this new version of my model, I treated it rather as Lévi-Strauss planned to treat his long sought after but never actually delineated 'universal structures' of human culture. The model afforded a simple logic from which the more complex cultural constructs could be derived. The logic as such corresponded to culture's 'default condition'. It represented culture's simplest form, its state of rest, its point of departure. Everything started here, and nothing could be understood unless this initial situation were known. Other anthropologists' models of an 'intial situation' – almost all of them based on the supposed centrality of the 'nuclear family' – were not entirely banished, but their significance was now changed. In accordance with my logic, couples in the initial situation naturally conjoined, so that something at least vaguely corresponding to 'the individual family' existed. But they also separated. And it was in ensuring this separation that *culture as such* established its force. Heterosexual bonding naturally occurred, but culture's logic of gender solidarity periodically overrode this. Father-child links could develop, but the logic of the sex strike put blood symbolism and matriliny first. Individualist, self-seeking, profit-maximising tendencies could be tolerated within limits – but community-wide solidarity finally had to prevail.

With this model in place, I saw most aspects of kinship, ritual and mythology in traditional cultures as expressive of its logic. Most hunter-gatherer cultures, as far as I could determine, *did* sustain menstrual avoidances of one kind or another, *did* see prior sexual abstinence as essential to hunting luck, *did* link such abstinence with menstrual avoidances, *did* construct mythological connections between the blood of women and the blood of game animals, *did* draw a sharp conceptual distinction between raw meat and cooked – and so on.

To attempt to isolate invariant cross-cultural uniformities on any level is risky, since 'exceptions' will always be found. Certainly no custom, rule or meaning in one culture is ever really 'the same' as its supposed counterpart in another. But within my narrative – as I had learned from Lévi-Strauss –

'shared structure' had nothing to do with identity on the level of what could be recorded or observed. It meant, on the contrary, precisely a logic of perpetual alternation, opposition, variation, contrast. My structure was a *transformational* template: a set of constraints governing the pattern in accordance with which change and diversification could proceed. Far from blurring distinctions, such a unitary, all-purpose template is like a common standard of measurement: unlike incommensurable standards, it allows one to discern *with precision* just how meanings, rules and customs differ from and are logical transformations of one another. Only a unitary standard can reveal what diversity really means.

I started working on my doctoral thesis to show that Lévi-Strauss' unusually opaque, cumbersome, scarcely read, yet awesomely ambitious *Mythologiques* (1970, 1973, 1978, 1981) could profitably be reinterpreted along these lines. All of his strange stories about 'bird-nesters' alternating perpetually between 'earth' and 'sky' could be seen as accurate expressions of my template. The myths traced in graphic imagery the perpetual alternation of men and women between sex strike (often coded as life in the 'sky') and marital conjunction (renewed contact with 'earth'). When the heroes were in the sky, they lost their wives to male rivals whose 'incestuous' claims had to be challenged at a later stage. When they descended to earth, they got their wives back again. When they were in the sky, they felt 'raw'; once back on earth, they felt, if not always 'cooked', then at least desirable and available to the opposite sex once more. Sky-stranded heroes came into contact with blood, bloodstained faeces or – in one prominent case – celestial wives whose synchronised menstruation regularly caused all the world's women to menstruate at the same time (Lévi-Strauss 1981: 565). None of this kind of thing happened back on earth, where proper food could be eaten and blood-free marital relations enjoyed.

The Rainbow Snake

I took it that the source of these stories was not just my model in the abstract. The myths could hardly be pure 'collective memories' of a cultural initial situation which had long since passed. To have survived, the tales must have had a living point of reference in the present. My menstrual sex strike must have been on some level *still operative* within the cultures which replicated these myths. It seemed clear to me that ritual action was central to the forms this living tradition took.

This was clearest in the case of that category of ritual action most obviously connected with the myths, as well as most indisputably central to social structure in the cultures concerned. I concentrated on initiation rites.

Where hunter-gatherers focused mainly on *female* initiation rites (as was generally the case among the San and some other African groups), then the mythico-ritual structures were not necessarily oppressive of women; the connection with the model tended to be simple and self-evident. When a young woman first menstruated, her blood was taken to be potentially beneficial, immensely powerful – and intimately connected with male hunting success (Lewis-Williams 1981). The flowing of blood set up a structure of sex-excluding gender solidarity. Hunting success depended on this solidarity. That was all. The model was expressed straightforwardly.

But when hunter-gatherers – as in much of Australia – put the major emphasis on *male* initiation ritualism, the situation was more complex. The major structural feature remained gender segregation. Every ritual began with the women and children, as a group, repulsed in some symbolic sense from the space occupied by ritually active men. Marital sex was still for a period prohibited. Blood was still used to signal this segregation and to mark the gender-defined boundaries. There was still the same connection with hunting success. *But the 'menstrual blood' was now that of men.* Boys had to have their flesh cut to allow the blood to flow. This was what initiation was essentially about. It was now large groups of men whose 'menstrual periods', deliberately synchronised, kept women away *and thereby preserved the boundaries of the cultural domain.* And compared with the southern African (San) situation, all this made a vast difference to the whole atmosphere of the rituals, to their politics, to their 'naturalness' or apparent informality – and to all relations between the sexes, between the generations and between those within each gender-segregated group.

Where 'male menstruation' had become the rule, real women's menstruation became feared as a threat to men's supremacy. Men, now, needed to organise their ritual sex strike *at women's political expense*, actively inhibiting women from replying in kind. This meant challenging women's freedom to exploit the symbolic potency of real cyclicity, real life-giving blood, real reproductive labour. The symbols and hence values were all taken over by men, who to ensure their rule strove always to atomise the productive sex *at the point of reproduction.* Like workers denied collective control over their own labour, mothers were prevented from synchronising their cycles or menstrual flows, prevented from benefiting collectively from the potency of their bodily processes. Menstrual seclusion rules were expressive of this, as menstruants – now said to be saturated with immensely *dangerous* ritual power – were hedged around with restrictions and elaborately marginalised. Male menstruation, the associated mythologies never tired of explaining, is positive, magical, empowering and conducive to good hunting luck. Female menstruation is just dangerously polluting and should be treated as far as possible as a private affair despite the cosmos-endangering properties of the blood.

It was in the north-east Arnhem Land classical ethnographies that I found all this most breathtakingly illustrated. Here, as I described in a reanalysis published in the early 1980s (Knight 1983), men 'menstruated' synchronously in the course of their most important rituals. Whilst expressing their power in this way, they did what they could (although not always successfully) to prohibit women from replying in kind. Only by covering themselves and one another in their own 'menstrual blood' whilst excluding women from doing the same could men safeguard their claimed monopoly of ritual power. And as they enveloped themselves in both blood and symbolic potency, men thought of this experience in terms of being 'swallowed' by an immense 'rainbow' or 'snake' – a creature alleged to be of immense *danger* to living women should they ever become too closely involved. Perhaps the most marked feature of this 'snake' was its arousal in the presence of female body odours: 'The rainbow serpent, a good consumer of smells, is associated with female bodily emissions related to reproductive processes . . . ' (Buchler 1978: 129). In being placed in awe of the 'snake' construed as an alien monster, women were made to *fear their own blood-potency*. Their own reproductive powers were being alienated from them – taken from them, turned into their opposite and constructed as a force opposed to all women – in the most dramatic imaginable way.

This 'snake', I realised, could not have been simply a male invention. Not only was it too feminine, too maternal, too wrapped up in the language of women's odours, babies, bodily fluids and associated powers (Buchler 1978). It also corresponded too closely with my own model of the force at culture's roots. The 'snake' was an ancient menstruation-inspired construct which men had taken over for their own use. It was 'blood relations' in masculinized form.

In this connection, the core of the evolving thesis and perhaps the most exciting ethnographic finding to which my model had led me was that what functionalist-minded fieldworkers of an earlier period had thought of as an Aboriginal construct symbolising 'sex', 'weather-change', 'water', 'phallus', 'womb' or some other ready-made category familiar to Europeans – this so-called 'Snake' was nothing of the kind. Its meaning was not a thing. It referred not to something external to the human subject. It was – I decided when the first dawnings of understanding began to hit me – pure subjectivity. It was solidarity. It was my class struggle. It was the picket line, the blood-red flag, the many-headed Dragon of resistance. It was the overthrow of Primate Capitalism – the triumph of the great Sex Strike which had established the cultural domain. It was women in solidarity with 'brothers', not husbands; men in solidarity with 'sisters', not wives. It was women *as women*, one hundred per cent themselves, bringing sons and brothers into their own world. It was the blood of clan solidarity and kinship, flowing, shimmering, sustaining each participant in birth as in life – whilst pulsing on through mothers and daughters beyond death. It was the pulse which had linked us once to the reason of our being – to a primordial class struggle which had finally reached its culture-creating goal, to be at one with the moon, the tides, the seasons and all other fluctuating, living/dying things.

All this had first hit me in a rather heady way during the autumn of 1980, and for a while I just let the reveries flow. Once I had stopped dreaming and resumed academic work, the task was to see what were the usable insights among the various connections I had made.

As, over the next few years, I read all I could find on the woman-loving, terrifying, magical 'rainbow' or 'snake' at the heart of so much Aboriginal cosmology, I admired more and more the myth-makers' precision in describing the rhythmic logic at the root of their world. Rather as Lévi-Strauss had shown in his analyses of Amerindian mythology, it seemed clear to me that these beautifully rich and complicated stories *never made mistakes*.

To begin with, for the storytellers to describe their magic as 'snake-like' made good sense. Solidarity's concrete manifestation in its default state, according to my model, had been menstrual synchrony, and therefore cyclicity. A humanoid, maternally functioning 'snake' was the perfect zoological metaphor here. Not only — I thought — does a snake with its venomous bite inspire respect, just as any effective picket line must! It also has the correct shape. Its parts are egalitarian, its head like its tail, each segment seeming to be the equivalent of any other. Moreover, what creature on earth, as I reasoned, could connote cyclicity more appropriately than this flowing being, coiling itself up in spirals, undulating its way across water or land, sloughing its skins and so seeming to move between one life and the next? Appropriately for a menstrual metaphor, most snakes have a quite extraordinary sense of smell (Buchler 1978: 125, 128–9); it is after smelling the two synchronously bleeding Wawilak Sisters' blood that the great copper-python Yurlunggur, in the best-known of all Aboriginal rainbow-snake myths, incorporates these dancing, synchronised, women into its body (figure 2). The northern Australian zoological water-python most directly associated with the rainbow snake (Worrell 1966: 99), acts by swallowing its victim whole, as if taking it into its immense super-womb — a kind of birth process played backwards. What a perfect way of describing how women's menstrual flows, within the terms of my model, reasserted the primacy of blood links, of maternal solidarity, of involvement in a picket line of interconnected wombs!

That the Aborigines were not thinking primarily of water-pythons seemed, however, equally clear — despite the authoritative zoological identification of the creature as 'Liasis fuscus Peters' (Worrell 1966). I agreed with the Upper Palaeolithic art specialist Alexander Marshack (1985) that 'the Snake', here as in other parts of the world, was a way of describing cyclicity — *especially lunar cyclicity*. It was an elaborate, wonderful, extravagant metaphor — not just a reptile. This was evident from the fact that in descriptions, the Aborigines insisted on adding that 'she' or 'he' or 'it' was not only snake-like but also 'like our Mother' (or like some other senior relative) and immense as no real snake could possibly be. The *myndie* of the Melbourne area 'could

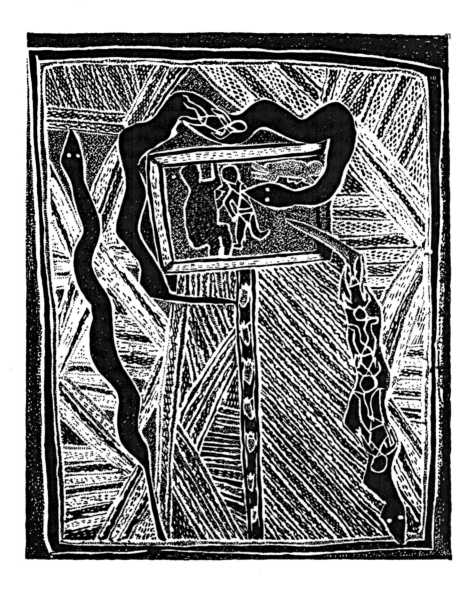

Figure 2 Jurlungur the Rainbow Snake and the Two Wawilak Sisters. The Snake is shown approaching the heroines and their offspring, then swallowing them, and finally departing filled with their flesh. Note the patterning to the left of the vertical path of footprints leading to the women's sacred hut. This symbolises the menstrual blood which aroused the snake. Bark painting. Yolngu, North East Arnhem Land (redrawn by the author from a photograph by Mountford 1978: 77, Fig. 22).

ascend the highest tree and hold onto a branch like a ring-tailed opossum, or he could leave his home and stretch his body across a great forest to reach any tribe, with his tail still in the Bukara-bunnal waterhole' (Mountford 1978: 31–2). Like an expanding picket line incorporating ever more supporters within its ranks, or like a wave of revolutionary militancy rippling across a political landscape, this creature in its various local manifestations 'swallowed' whole communities of humans as no real snake ever could. In Aboriginal conceptions, it also felt aroused by menstrual blood to an extent unknown in zoology, lay behind the birth of *human* babies rather than just snakes – and was decidedly *human* in its 'incestuous' (that is kinship-oriented) matrimonial preferences.

For the Aborigines to say that their world had been created by this magical power – as they did – seemed wholly appropriate within the terms of my own myth. Yes, gender solidarity and synchrony *had* established culture. These stories were, in their own way, good science. By comparison, the interpretations of most pre-structuralist social anthropologists seemed sadly uninformative. I felt immense admiration for the erudition of those early Australian ethnographers such as Spencer and Gillen (1899, 1904, 1927), as well as for marvellous scholars such as W. E. H. Stanner (1966) and W. L. Warner (1957), whose writings shone on every page with respect for all that the Aborigines had achieved. But none of this stopped me from feeling irritated by the condescending scepticism of most of the social-anthropological fraternity, a colonially spawned establishment which had exposed the Aborigines' secrets for my benefit as a library reader in England – only to dismiss the sacred myths as at best functional constructs, at worst incomprehensible irrationality.

It seemed futile to deny the irreversibility of the initial betrayal: no one would suggest burning the monographs which, as part of colonialism's violation of native Australia, had recorded so many details of Aboriginal secret/sacred life. Morally, all participants within the dominant white culture were thereby implicated; there can be no adequate atonement, no easy way out. I am a part of that culture. Yet given colonialism's *fait accompli*, it seemed to me on political grounds that the best attempt at recompense was to vindicate the native narratives within their own terms, showing to the best of my ability their *status as science*.

A refusal to read Warner's (1957), the Berndts' (Berndt and Berndt 1951; Berndt 1951, 1952) or Stanner's (1966) relatively sensitive and wonderfully informative early works on 'the secret life' would have benefited no one. On the other hand, for me to have intruded even vicariously into the Aborigines' secrets and then to have remained silent would have been to collude in the colonialist betrayal, contributing to the initial cruel exposure something perhaps even less forgivable – my own culture's arrogant dismissal of the precious knowledge which these fragile native patterns had the potential to transmit to us all. The Aborigines who had confided their secrets to individual befriended anthropologists, trusting, perhaps, that after colonialism's destruction of much of their culture at least some of its highest accomplishments could have been immortalised safe in our hands – these Aborigines ought surely to be remembered, even if recompense is no longer within anyone's power.

The best we could do, I thought, was to *listen* to what, through their myths, these cultures still have to say to all of us across the planet. Such a course seemed validated by much of Lévi-Strauss' work. I particularly liked his statement (Lévi-Strauss 1968: 351) that 'what we are doing is not building a theory with which to interpret the facts, but rather trying to get back to the older native theory at the origin of the facts we are trying to explain'. For me, of course, the 'native theory' at the origin of these facts was a sexual-political version of my 'class struggle'.

The myths allege that ritual power originally belonged to women. 'We took these things from women', as a learned Aboriginal put it during a performance of the great *Kunapipi* ceremony, referring to the cult's jealously guarded secrets (Berndt 1951: 55). Such storytellers knew the meaning, value and *truth* of their precious narratives, I thought, better than did the puzzled, functionalist-indoctrinated anthropologists who had arrived by boat and plane from a culture cut loose from its roots in its own Dreamtime past. '*White man got no dreaming, Him go 'nother way. White man, him go different, Him got road belong himself*' (Stanner 1956: 51).

As I read through the corpus of traditional, mainly functionalist, anthropological attempts to come to terms with the logic of the rainbow snake, I was struck by the meagreness of the great classical attempts at interpretation. Radcliffe-Brown's (1926) view that the snake represented 'water' seemed unconvincing, as did Warner's (1957) idea that it represented 'the weather', or Berndt's (1951) suggestion that it was a 'phallic symbol'. What seemed unacceptable was these theories' reductionism – their striving to reduce the richness of the Aborigines' own logic to some far simpler construct already familiar at a superficial level to Europeans.

All too apparent was these interpretations' one-sidedness and inadequacy to match the rich detail and complexity of 'the Snake'. What kind of a 'snake' was it if people could *participate in its body by dancing*? Why was this shimmering, rainbow-coloured, male/female creature recurrently described as '*incestuous?*' Why was it depicted as having kangaroo-like prominent *ears*? Why would it so often be a rainbow or rainbow snake which sent floods or thunderbolts as punishment for abuse of the game animals, for attempting to cook meat during menstruation time – or for selfishly consuming one's own kill? Why did humans in need of ritual power have to allow themselves to become '*swallowed*' by this 'snake'? Whence came the persistent associations with life/death alternations, birth and rebirth, the tides, blood-streaked floods, the moon and ancestral dancing women? Such questions were neither answered nor even asked. Above all, I noticed that although one bizarre detail was recurrently stressed by the Aborigines themselves, and usually reported in the ethnographies without comment, no one had attempted to explain it. If this 'snake' was basically a 'phallic symbol' or an emblem for some functional utility such as 'water', why was it always *so thirsty for supplies of real or surrogate human menstrual blood?*

Within the framework of my myth, all this seemed as would be expected. Kinship indeed could not function without blood. Reasserted kinship solidarity was indeed the conjoining of blood with blood, like with like. Blood-marked women with their kin were – within the specifications of my model – very much the guardians of all life-blood, and therefore of game animals protected by blood-encoded rules and taboos. Mother-son and/or brother-sister unity could very appropriately be depicted as 'incestuous' – and as condensable into the image of a 'mother-with-phallus' or 'male-with-womb'. In this context, heterosexual distinctions indeed might be expected to fade away, power during a sex strike being derived not from gender polarity or difference but from the fact that when kinsfolk act in solidarity they can experience themselves 'as one'. Water was – as many early accounts had noted – certainly central to the rainbow snake, but how clear it was from the Aborigines' own accounts that this was not just ordinary water but sacred water, the water of life, womb fluid – the menstrual flow *mingling* in myth and imagination with the surrounding streams and waterholes on which life in reality depended, 'swallowing up' men and women in its synchronising, rhythmic power!

The snake the Aborigines depicted was always rhythmical, tidal, cyclical – synchronised with the changes of moon and season, dark and light, night and day. Cyclicity was absolutely central to her (Maddock 1978b: 115). I noticed that when native artists depicted her/him, they would often use cyclical motifs which *could* be interpreted as waterholes or snake-tracks or yams, breasts, wombs etc. etc. – but that such meanings were never fixed or pinned down (Munn 1973). Almost anything, to the Aborigines, could be part of cyclicity, part of synchrony, part of rainbowness/snakiness. Just as the arch of a rainbow mediates between earth and sky, dry season and wet, sunshine and rain, red colours and violet or blue – so ceremonial life across Australia, it seemed to me, had carried humans in an orderly way from one season or time of month to its opposite, from the 'raw' phase of each ritual cycle to the 'cooked', from blood to fire, kinship connectedness (often coded as 'incest') to marital life. The aim was always to bring humans and nature into rhythmic connectedness and synchrony. Ritual was the endeavour to activate all living beings as vibrant participants within 'the Snake'.

Finally, as if these Aborigines had never heard of functionalist preoccupations with 'the family', their highest divinities were, I noticed, consistently non-heterosexual, blood-empowered, anti-marital. Rainbow snakes always seemed to violate their communities' exogamous laws, conjoining 'incestuously' only with their own blood, their own kin or flesh. She/he/it was said by informants in the various accounts to be not only 'incestuous' (that is, in correct sex-strike fashion, hostile to normal, heterosexual, exogamous marital intercourse) but also 'like a rainbow', 'like our mother', 'like power', 'like metamorphosis', 'like the Dreaming' and like many other shimmering, changing, life-creating or life-devouring things. Moreover, female rainbow snakes seemed 'masculine'; male ones were regularly depicted with female attributes such as 'wombs' or 'breasts'. I wondered how any of this could be reconciled with the views of those seeking in Aboriginal religion evidence for the centrality of heterosexual 'pair-bonding' or the 'nuclear family'. I noticed that in this area, there were simply no functionalist theories at all.

Turke's Model and the End of Sociobiology

In this book I have drawn on Paul Turke's model of ovulatory synchrony to show that – despite my objections to sociobiological attempts to construe hunter-gatherers as primitive bankers, estate agents or property developers – sociobiology itself has arrived at the very threshold of the egalitarian model which is central to my account.

When I first read Turke's 1984 article on ovulatory synchrony, I was as excited as I had been when I had discovered Sahlins' *Origins of Society* almost twenty years earlier. Since it corresponded so closely with my preconceptions, it was not that I was learning anything really very new. But Turke, I realised, was a respected figure in sociobiology. If this school of thought represented intellectual 'late capitalism', then – and here was the really exciting thought – here was that capitalism at last transcending itself. Followed through consistently, Turke had demonstrated, the logic of primatological sociobiology had led to the point at which gender egalitarianism amounting to a kind of communism had been found to lie at the roots of the human condition.

I discovered all this, however, only after my Ph.D. thesis had been completed in 1987. Had I been able to write it all over again, I might have couched it more strongly in Turke's sociobiological terms. I might have been able to make my myth seem rather more respectable – even sociobiologically conventional – had I taken as my starting point his own formulations for describing coalition-building, synchronously cycling females. The theory as such need not have suffered. As far as I can discern, there are no fundamental incompatibilities between Turke's version of the evolutionary role of synchrony and mine. I would certainly have needed to extend and draw out the implications of his model, but this, I think, could easily have been achieved.

In my lighter moments, I have sometimes pictured to myself how events might then have ensued. Obtaining funding from the great United States and other western grant-conferring institutions, I might have written a fully authorised sociobiological theory of human cultural solidarity – of the evolution of matrilineal and other clans, the establishment of menstrual taboos, the emergence of hunting ritual, the invention of initiation rites, the appearance of dance and trance, magic and myth, poetry and song. In tune with the mood of post-1989 capitalist triumph over the world as a whole, I could have assisted sociobiology in its project not only to hegemonise these areas but to redraw the map of all the biological and social sciences, helping it out of its traditional zoological ghetto. The discipline could then have been released from its unfortunate confinement, as it might seem, within the myopic perspectives of wasps, gulls, macaques, chimps or the more chimp-like purposes of human beings – and allowed out at last into the expansive realm of culture, the domain of humans acting *as only we humans can*. In that context, E. O. Wilson's (1975) grandiose dream of abolishing anthropology as a separate discipline and uniting biology with the humanities within the framework of a *single science* might even have been accomplished – although, of course (since at the moment of emancipation the experience of revolution could hardly have been avoided), not in quite the manner he envisaged!

Although I was unable to rewrite the thesis along these lines, following sociobiology's logic even to its self-transcending conclusion, I have been given a new chance to update my story in the writing of *Blood Relations*. I am still not satisfied that I have made sufficient use of this opportunity. The book remains something of a compromise, with some sections taken largely from the thesis while others have been completely rewritten. Improvements could still be made. My patient publishers, however, will not allow me to keep revising indefinitely. Unfinished as it will always be, this is my current version. I am sure you have your own favourite myths. Here for your enjoyment is mine.

Chapter 1
Anthropology and Origins

History itself is a *real* part of *natural history*, of the development of nature into man. Natural science will one day incorporate the science of man, just as the science of man will incorporate natural science; there will be a *single* science.

Karl Marx, *Economic and Philosophic Manuscripts* (1844)

The question of human origins has always held a central place in Marxist theory, and for a good reason. Marx aimed to unite the natural with the social sciences, and was aware that an understanding of our origins was an essential precondition. As 'everything natural must have an origin', he wrote, 'so man too has his process of origin, history, which can, however, be known by him and thus is a conscious process of origin that transcends itself' (Marx 1971a [1844]: 169). By knowing our process of origin, we know what we were, are and must become, and this knowledge 'transcends itself' – that is, enters as a factor in our further development.

Every human tribe or civilisation has its origin-myth, and western society is no exception. Judaeo/Christian mythology held that God made Man and Woman on the Sixth day of Creation, after dividing heaven from earth, light from darkness, land from water and after creating the various celestial bodies, plants and animals on the five previous days. Man's sudden creation, semi-divinity and decisive elevation above the beasts were central features of this myth. Adam and Eve owed their existence to a miracle, and could trace their descent back to God. The cosmos had a meaningful structure and purpose. The earth was the pivot of the material universe, Man was first among mortal creatures, and Woman and all lesser beings existed to fulfil Man's needs and God's plan.

This biblical Genesis was capable of different interpretations and was used in legitimising various social arrangements, but by and large – despite the Copernican revolution in astronomy, despite centuries of social and religious turmoil and despite the slow advance of science – it continued to prevail in

European cultures until the publication in Britain of Charles Darwin's *On the Origin of Species* (1859) and *Descent of Man* (1871). Then, once the initial controversy over apes and angels had died down, a new and very different story came to be believed. It was concluded that our origin (like that of other species) had been a natural one, unconscious, unplanned – the chance product of utterly blind impersonal forces. There had been no miracle, no shattering event, no aim in mind. It was just that upon one particular planet among innumerable dust grains within the universe random events combined with natural selection had produced microscopic marine life, then fish, and eventually the human animal. Humans were simply a zoological species, their mental powers differing in degree, but not in kind, from those of other beasts. Man had begun as an ape, and, at the end of the evolutionary process, he was still essentially an ape – albeit one with peculiar talents and a rather large brain (Darwin 1871).

With firm roots already in social theory, the idea of evolution conquered biology and quickly became the cornerstone of the new science of anthropology as well. The more ardent champions of the new paradigm applied it to human history in uncompromising fashion. All the earliest human institutions were seen as behaviour patterns evolved from the animal world. Earliest human language – far from being the breath of the gods – was made up of animal-like grunts; the first marriage – far from being a God-given sacrament – was in essence indistinguishable from sexual union among apes; the earliest human communities were polygamous ape-like hordes. All this was thought to be confirmed by reports on the animal-like behaviour of 'the savages of today' (Letourneau 1891: xi).

Social and political implications could be derived from the new story. Whereas Christianity had advocated the subordination of the egotistic individual to higher cosmic purposes, popular Darwinism preached 'the survival of the fittest', this concept being borrowed directly from capitalist – specifically Malthusian – economic and social doctrine. In a letter to Engels written in 1862, Karl Marx (n.d. [1862]) noted Darwin's claim to be

> applying the 'Malthusian' theory *also* to plants and animals. . . . It is remarkable how Darwin recognises among beasts and plants his English society with its division of labour, competition, opening up of new markets, 'inventions', and the Malthusian 'struggle for existence'.

Darwin – Marx argued – was transposing the logic of his own society to the natural world, and then deriving from 'nature' a supposed validation of the very cultural logic from which he had set forth.

In *The Dialectics of Nature*, Marx's collaborator, Engels (1964 [1873–86]: 35–6), agreed, adding that Darwin

> did not know what a bitter satire he wrote on mankind, and especially on his countrymen, when he showed that free competition, the struggle

for existence, which the economists celebrate as the highest historical achievement, is the normal state of the animal kingdom.

If Darwin saw no satire in this, it was because he was unaware of an alternative. The possibility of a different principle of human social organisation was simply not present within his conceptual universe. He therefore saw capitalism's logic as an expression of permanent natural necessity, the laws of individualistic competition embracing the entirety of natural and human history alike.

Darwin's case appeared well founded. The parallels between capitalist and zoological laws of competition seemed real enough. Marx himself, after all, had earlier written that capitalist society 'is not a society; it is, as Rousseau says, a desert populated by wild animals' (Marx and Engels 1927, 1, 5: 394; quoted in Kamenka 1962: 36). But like any great prophet exorcising rival gods, Darwin had unconsciously excluded other possibilities, thereby anchoring the values of his own particular culture in the inescapable nature of all life itself. Engels (n.d. [1865]) commented: ' . . . nothing discredits modern bourgeois development so much as the fact that it has not yet got beyond the economic forms of the animal world'.

The Origin Myth of Western Capitalism

'Origin of man now proved.' Darwin wrote these words in his notebook in 1838 (Fox 1975a: 265). He jotted: 'He who understands baboon would do more towards metaphysics than Locke.' The use of non-human primates (apes and monkeys) as models for early human life, and the belief that the problem of human origins had now been 'solved' – in principle if not in detail – were to characterise scientific discussions of human evolution not only for much of the remainder of the nineteenth century, but for most of the twentieth century, too.

Almost every time the question of human origins has been discussed within evolutionary science, it has been within the conceptual framework provided by Darwin. The question has been treated in essentially biological terms – as the problem of determining when and how a certain brain size, configuration of teeth and jaws and other characteristics evolved to produce a creature which could be called human. Even when the evolution of speech and social behaviour has been discussed, it has been assumed that the human stage was reached when social interactions between individual organisms led to the development of 'speech-areas' in the brain, or to the growth of increasingly subtle social instincts or learning skills.

To many, all this may seem natural and even inevitable. In what other way can the question of human origins be discussed? Is it not merely our own conceit which makes us think that we humans are special? Are we not essentially animals like any others, however much we may wish to avoid the fact? And does not a materialist approach compel us to root our behaviour in that most material of realities – our bodies, whose forms have evolved in materialistically comprehensible ways through interaction with one another and with the environment?

Another view, however, is that '. . . the essence of man is not an abstraction inherent in each particular individual. The real nature of man is the totality of social relations' (Marx 1963d [1845]: 83). The attractions of Darwinism are understandable, because unless we grasp the real uniqueness of humanity's social and symbolically constructed essence, we are obliged to treat the problem of origins in a biological way – seeking in the physical individual those 'material' properties responsible for our humanity. To quote Marx (1963d [1845]: 83–4) again, we are forced 'to conceive the nature of man only in terms of a 'genus', as an inner and mute universal quality which unites the many individuals in a purely natural (biological) way'.

As we seek our essence in biology, the importance of language, labour, ideology and consciousness in producing and defining our humanity is simply overlooked. Instead of seeing humans as symbolically constituted persons, our minds formed through childhood socialisation and through collective cultural products such as language, we see only the activities of bodies and brains. Instead of standing back and bringing into focus the evolving collective dimensions of all human life – dimensions such as economic systems, grammatical systems, religions – we view the world as if through a microscope. Increasing the magnification, we shorten our depth of focus, until the only visible realities become physical individuals eating, breathing, copulating and otherwise surviving in their immediate physical environments, their localised interactions filling almost our entire field of vision. Within this myopic perspective, the global, higher-order plane of existence of these physical individuals becomes invisible to us. We are left unaware of the existence of any transpatial plane of collective structure embracing and shaping the biological, localised life processes in which we are all involved. The subject matter of social anthropology – the study of economics, cultural kinship, ritual, language and myth – is not only left unexplained. It is not even seen as a higher-order level of reality in need of being explained.

In the late nineteenth century, many natural scientists, anthropological writers and sociologists within the materialist camp were inspired by Darwin's achievements to such an extent that they saw no other way of looking at human life. They assumed that the laws of competition and selection uncovered by Darwin could be extended to embrace the entirety of the human social sphere. Where origins were concerned, it seemed logical to assume that if humans had inherited their anatomy and physiology from some ape-like ancestor, then they had probably inherited their social institutions, their language and their consciousness in the same way.

As far as social life was concerned, the most basic institution was thought to be 'the family', which was said to have evolved from non-human primate mating systems. Darwin's conception of the origin of marriage was based on the observation that male mammals typically compete with one another sexually, the victors succeeding in monopolising the females. He cited a report on the gorilla, among whom 'but one male is seen in a band; when the young male grows up, a contest takes place for mastery, and the strongest, by killing and driving out the others, establishes himself as the head of the community' (Darwin 1871, 2: 362). In the human case,

> if we look far enough back in the stream of time, . . . judging from the social habits of man as he now exists . . . the most probable view is that primaeval man aboriginally lived in small communities, each with as many wives as he could support and obtain, whom he would have jealously guarded against all other men. (Darwin 1871: 2: 362)

One popular writer concluded that 'primitive marriage' was 'simply the taking possession of one or several women by one man, who holds them by the same title as all other property, and who treats adultery, when unauthorised by himself, strictly as robbery' (Letourneau 1891: 57). This was supposed to be the expression of a universal 'sexual law' – applying equally to humans and animals – termed by Darwin himself 'the law of battle', according to which the males 'dispute with each other for the females, and must triumph over their rivals before obtaining them' (Letourneau 1891: 10–11). For more than a century, cartoon images of 'cavemen' colluded in depicting these as rapacious brutes battling against each other with clubs, each victor dragging home a clump of recently seized, voluptuous cave-females by their hair.

In the sense that the 'law of battle' fits baboon sexual organisation moderately well, Darwin's and Letourneau's views in this context could be called the 'baboon' theory of human origins. This theory did not disappear with the nineteenth century but continued to haunt discussions of origins, figuring centrally in Freud's magnificent myth of the 'Primal Horde'. Freud took the horde-motif directly from Darwin. He assumed that our pre-cultural ape-like male ancestors were ferocious sexual rivals, each pitted in violent conflict against all the others in an attempt to monopolise whole harems of females. In *Totem and Taboo*, however, Freud conceptualised the actual transition to the cultural level not as a simple extension of all this, but as a revolutionary negation achieved when a band of sexually expropriated Sons within a primal horde rose up against their tyrannical Father, killed him, ate him – and collectively outlawed future conflict (Freud 1965 [1913]).

Freud's haunting theory entered subtly into the thinking of many anthropologists, including Malinowski, Róheim, Lévi-Strauss and more recently Robin Fox. Common to the theories of Darwin, Freud, Lévi-Strauss and Fox was an unquestioned, seemingly axiomatic assumption: females are and always have been passive sexual valuables to be fought over, renounced, exchanged or otherwise manipulated by dominant males. In the works of all these thinkers, male dominance is said to have preceded the establishment of human society, and to have continued unbroken and unchallenged throughout humanity's origins and subsequent development.

Throughout the 1960s – when the theoretical premises of the present book were first beginning to take shape – the majority of evolutionist-minded writers accepted the 'baboon' theory in a fairly simple Darwinian form, without bringing Freud's suggestion of revolutionary overturn into the picture. Most experts saw trooping, ground-dwelling monkeys – typically, baboons – as the best model for 'the proto-human horde' (Fox 1967a: 420). It was noted that among baboons, male sexual rivalries tend to be fierce, the victors typically monopolising whole harems of females whilst excluding their rivals completely from the breeding system.

In the 1960s and early 1970s, Fox was the best-known social anthropologist to show an interest in evolutionary theory and in human social origins. Fox (1967a: 420; 1975a: 52–3) took it for granted that earliest 'man' organised his sex life through conflict, the males competing with each other for females. With men as with baboons, 'the status of the male is measured by his control over females' (Fox 1975a: 55). In the case of both species: 'The result of the reproductive struggle is a social system that is profoundly hierarchical and competitive' (Tiger and Fox 1974: 43). And in both human and animal systems: 'Competition for scarce resources – food, nest-sites, mates – is the basis of society and the stuff of politics' (Tiger and Fox 1974: 44).

In Britain and the United States, books such as Desmond Morris' *The Naked Ape* (1967) and Robert Ardrey's *The Territorial Imperative* (1969) elaborated such notions and became overnight bestsellers, being serialised in the popular press and aired repeatedly on radio and television. For the first time in decades, anthropology seemed set to become a popular science! The political implications were seized on with delight. Nicholas Tomalin (1967, quoted in Lewis and Towers 1969: 24) told his socialist readership in the *New Statesman* that the 'new facts' about early human competitiveness 'must make, if not reactionaries, at least revisionists, of us all. Man, and consequently his nature, is immutable. The old adage, "you can't change human nature" becomes true once more.' And Katharine Whitehorn, educating Britain's middle classes through her column in *The Observer* (29 October 1967), expressed gratitude ('I for one feel a lot better for it') for the revelation that the bourgeois world's aggression and violence is 'natural', adding: 'The desire to have and to hold, to screech at the neighbours and say "Mine, all mine" is in our nature too.' Marshall Sahlins (1977: 100) has described all this as 'the origin myth of Western capitalism' – a myth which has decisively pushed Genesis into the shade.

The Culturalist Reaction

But there has always been more to anthropology than Darwinism. The first anthropologists were social philosophers. Hobbes, Rousseau and Comte presented what would nowadays be called 'anthropological' theories of human nature – as did Marx, whose *Economic and Philosophic Manuscripts* (1971a [1844]) and *The German Ideology* (Marx and Engels 1947 [1846]) covered such topics as the nature of labour, the emergence of human language and the origins of the family.

It was a range of interests shared by Lewis Henry Morgan, the American radical business lawyer who is often regarded as the principal founder of kinship studies and of anthropology in its modern sense. In the mid-nineteenth century, Morgan discovered the 'classificatory' system of kinship terminology among the Iroquois Indians, and from this and much other evidence concluded that human society had everywhere evolved from communistic beginnings.

Like Morgan, most nineteenth-century anthropologists used ethnographic findings to throw light on issues such as the origins of human society, the causes of social inequality and the foundations of human morality. 'Grand theory', in other words, was the order of the day. While Morgan's work became central to the thinking of Engels and Marx, the findings of early anthropologists in Australia shaped Durkheim's theories of primitive religion, and Sir James Frazer's *The Golden Bough* – still produced within the Victorian evolutionist tradition – later influenced a generation of poets, writers and thinkers. It is important to remember all this today, when imaginative anthropological theory building has become rare, few publications within the discipline arouse much popular interest, and not many people even know what 'anthropology' means.

More than any other field of knowledge, anthropology taken as a whole spans the chasm which has traditionally divided the natural from the human sciences. Potentially if not always in practice, it therefore occupies a central position among the sciences as a whole. The crucial threads which – if joined – might bind the natural sciences to the humanities would have to run through anthropology more than through any other field. It is here that the ends join – here that the study of nature ends and that of culture begins. At which point on the scale of evolution did biological principles cease to predominate while other, more complex, principles began prevailing in their place? Where exactly is the dividing line between animal and human social life? Is the distinction here one of kind, or merely one of degree? And, in the light of this question, is it really possible to study human phenomena scientifically – with the same detached objectivity as an astronomer can show towards galaxies or a physicist towards subatomic particles?

If this area of *relationships between the sciences* seems to many to be confused, it is only in part because of the real difficulties involved. Science may be rooted at one end in objective reality, but at the other end it is rooted in society and ourselves. It is for ultimately social and ideological reasons that modern science, fragmented and distorted under immense yet largely unacknowledged political pressures, has stumbled upon its greatest problem and its greatest theoretical challenge – to incorporate the humanities and the natural sciences into a single unified science on the basis of an understanding of humanity's evolution and place within the rest of the universe.

Not all anthropologists accept that humanity is 'just another species', that culture is no more than 'an adaptation' or that Darwinism is the best and only necessary framework within which to study the nature or origin of human social life. In fact, most of twentieth-century social anthropology has defined itself as a discipline precisely in opposition to such ideas. In the process of doing so, however, it has accentuated rather than transcended intellectual schism and confusion. Instead of addressing from its own standpoint the problems raised by the evolutionary sciences in relation to human life – cultural anthropology has simply turned its face away. Extraordinarily – as will now be shown – the very idea of research by cultural specialists into the origins of human culture has in effect been tabooed. As a result, *culturally informed* theorising about human origins has been disallowed.

The nineteenth-century evolutionist founders of anthropology almost always regarded 'savages' as on a lower evolutionary rung than themselves, and mixed Darwinian with cultural-evolutionary concepts in illegitimate ways. Their view of evolution tended to be simple and unilinear, each world-historical evolutionary stage being treated as mandatory for all peoples everywhere, and linked in an oversimplified way with some technological advance or other assumed causative factor. Thinkers tended to explain away the more puzzling features of traditional cultures by describing them as anachronistic 'survivals' from some earlier stage – failing to appreciate that unless an institution has some value and meaning in its present context, it is unlikely to 'survive' at all.

Such criticisms could be extended almost indefinitely – and indeed have been, repetitively, for most of this century. But not all the Victorians were equally guilty of such mistakes. Theoreticians such as Tylor, Lubbock and Morgan – or painstaking ethnographers such as the Australianists Spencer and Gillen – were superb scholars, of immense erudition and integrity, making many of today's experts and authorities seem dwarves by compar-

ison. Much twentieth-century criticism of them has been ideologically
motivated, ill informed and unworthy. In any event, at its best, the evolutionist school was united by something of immense value – a passionate
belief in the methods of natural science and in the ultimate reality of
discoverable lawful principles governing human history. Courageously, they
faced even the most daunting questions, refusing to evade issues which
might appear at first sight baffling, inconvenient or too immense to
contemplate.

The war years from 1914 to 1918 were the great intellectual buffers into
which the idea of 'progress' ran. At this point, the Victorians' widespread
optimism and belief in the potentialities of science was decisively repudiated.
Almost simultaneously, in England, France, Germany and the United
States, there arose schools of anthropology which, as Marvin Harris (1969: 2)
has written, 'in one way or another rejected the scientific mandate'. It came
to be widely believed that anthropology could never discover the origins of
institutions or explain their causes. In Britain, 'evolutionism' became not
merely unfashionable but effectively outlawed. In the United States, the
dominant school flatly asserted that there were no historical laws and that
there could not be a science of history.

Despite the presence of continental giants such as Claude Lévi-Strauss,
Britain and the United States have been the two dominant national centres of
world social-anthropological research for most of the twentieth century.
American cultural anthropology was based initially on the study of the
Indians of North America, while British social anthropology was a product of
colonialism, being shaped very largely by the requirements – real or
imagined – of administrators in various parts of the British Empire in the
period 1920–45.

Almost all American anthropologists are the intellectual descendants of
Franz Boas (1858–1942), the German-born founder of the American 'diffusionist' or 'historical particularist' tradition. In a similar way, almost all
British social anthropologists are the descendants of Bronislaw Malinowski
(1884–1942) and A. R. Radcliffe-Brown (1881–1955), founders of the
'functionalist' and 'structural-functionalist' traditions respectively.

In what follows, no attempt will be made to discuss the history of western
anthropological theory as a whole. Indeed, the reader may feel that the
concentration on three English-speaking figures – Boas with his students,
and Malinowski and Radcliffe-Brown with theirs – is a narrow and unrepre-
sentative focus. However, the three are selected because, more than any
others, they succeeded in altering the course of western anthropological
history. In the early decades of the twentieth century they achieved an almost
complete rupture in the traditions of the discipline. Prior to their appearance, social anthropology had been dominated by Morgan and his followers,

evolutionary investigations remaining loosely but ultimately integrated with studies of living traditional cultures. After their work had been done, Morgan was disowned, whereupon cultural studies on the one hand, the evolutionary sciences on the other, went their separate ways. All subsequent anthropological writers and thinkers of any influence in the West, however original or independent, have worked and thought essentially within the parameters established in the course of that rupture. An adequate re-evaluation of twentieth-century western anthropology as a whole would require us to return to the point at which the break was made, retie some of the threads – and make a fresh beginning.

American Diffusionism

To an extent, the Boasian reaction against nineteenth-century evolutionism was understandable – even progressive. Firstly, the untrammelled theorising of many of the nineteenth-century armchair anthropologists had produced innumerable theories to explain the primordial beginnings of marriage, the family, religion and much else, but very few suggestions as to how or why one theory should be selected in preference to another. There were simply too many theories, many of them spun out of thin air, and it began to be felt that an emphasis on fieldwork and a more rigorous, methodical, *fact-finding* approach was required.

Secondly, among social anthropologists early in this century a fierce reaction set in against the view that 'savages' were close to animals, that certain of their customs were 'survivals' from a previous, perhaps ape-like, stage, that biology was the basis of sociology and so on. Actual contact with 'primitive' tribes had been convincing ethnologists that all of this was absurd – that people in all cultures were equally human, that their languages and thought processes were in a formal sense equally complex and 'advanced', that none of their customs showed any signs of being survivals from the apes and that the whole idea of studying simpler cultures to find clues to ultimate origins was a mistake. It became one of the cardinal tenets of anthropologists that, as Franz Boas (1938 [1911]: v) put it, there 'is no fundamental difference in the ways of thinking of primitive and civilized man'. All cultures were equal – and all were therefore equally separated from the animal world. The new anti-evolutionism of Boas, therefore, was to a large extent a campaign against the *biologism* and implicit *racism* of much of the old evolutionist tradition.

The new American anthropologists were fired by hostility to what they saw as grandiose oversimplifications. Nineteenth-century social evolutionary theory, alleged Franz Boas in 1911, had been 'an application to mental phenomena of the theory of biological evolution' (Boas 1938 [1911]: 177). Although there was some truth in the statement, it was one-sided and exaggerated. The best nineteenth-century evolutionist scholars had been quite aware of the need to go beyond Darwin in constructing on an adequate basis the new 'science of man'. But once Morgan, Tylor, Engels and other evolutionists had been lumped together with the real Social Darwinists, the discrediting of their aims and theories – and, indeed, the discrediting of all attempts at 'Grand theory' – became a relatively simple task.

Nothing can ever detract from the inestimable value of Boas' and his students' work in recording myths, recipes, designs and other details of native American cultures. Boas in particular recorded vast amounts of undigested and often indigestible information, and usually did so just in time, a few years before his older native informants were to die and take their irreplaceable store of knowledge with them. It may well have been precisely Boas' lack of interest in theory which enabled him to record so much: it would seem that he simply wrote and wrote, leaving it for later generations to sort the information into some kind of intelligible order. This was an immensely valuable contribution to human knowledge, but it remains the case that his records are often maddeningly unstructured, with vital questions left unasked and unanswered. To attempt to record 'facts' without any guiding theory at all betrays a hopeless misunderstanding of what 'facts' are (Kuhn 1970). And on a broader level – returning, now, to the development of anthropological theory as a whole – a disastrous fragmentation of anthropology as a discipline was one of the costs.

The concept of 'culture' was used as a means of rigidly isolating the study of human social life from evolutionary theory. An impenetrable barrier was set up between the two wings – physical and cultural – of anthropological science. While evolutionary biologists continued – and have continued to this day – developing the methods of Darwin in the study of the human species, the specialists in culture (particularly in the United States) clung to an impassioned belief in the uniqueness, freedom, unpredictability and autonomy of the cultural realm. Although the culturalist reaction had some justification, it has often been argued – plausibly enough – that this new anti-evolutionism was a return to religion in another guise (Fox 1975a: 245–6).

The cultural domain was depicted as in essence an unpredictable and inexplicable mystery – inherently so by virtue of its basis in behaviour which was not genetically inherited but freely and voluntarily learned. Boas' student Kroeber (1917; quoted in Murdock 1965: 71) in a famous passage wrote that two ants can be raised from eggs, in complete isolation from any others of their kind, and will nonetheless soon recreate of their own accord the entirety of their social system. By contrast, two human babies provided for physically but unable to *learn from others* will produce only 'a troop of mutes, without arts, knowledge, fire, without order or religion'. 'Heredity', concluded Kroeber, 'saves for the ant all that she has, from generation to generation. But heredity does not maintain, because it cannot maintain, one particle of the civilization which is the one specifically human thing'.

Kroeber went on to argue that since culture was independent of genetic determinism, history must be entirely free from the evolutionary principles uncovered by Darwin.

Unfortunately, however, the insistence that cultural anthropology was not reducible to biology was then used by Kroeber and other Boasians to argue that culture was 'free' in a more absolute sense: free from all forms of necessity or determinism, and hence free from any constraints or patterns which could be formulated as general principles or scientific laws. Anthropologists, according to Boas (1932: 612), could hope to describe not 'general laws' but only 'individual phenomena'. This was in the nature of 'learned behaviour': a person could learn anything – a myth, a design, a technique – from anywhere, or not learn it, or combine it with anything else which was learned. Since people in any human culture could learn virtually any 'custom' from people in any other culture (cultural traits in this way 'diffusing' across time and space in unpredictable ways), the result – so it was argued – was for each culture to be an arbitrary and utterly unique conglomeration of disparate elements. This was certainly the impression created by Boas' and his students' papers and notes.

In 1920, Boas' student Robert Lowie (1920: 440–1) justified this impression of disorderliness in his *Primitive Society*. No 'necessity or design' appears from the study of culture history, he wrote. 'Cultures develop mainly through the borrowings due to chance contact.' Civilisation is a 'planless hodge-podge' to which we should no longer yield 'superstitious reverence'; it is a 'chaotic jumble'. Although there were soon to be retreats from and reactions against this position – for example in the works of Ruth Benedict, Margaret Mead and the 'culture and personality' school – to a very great extent, twentieth-century American cultural anthropology was founded on the basis of this extraordinary judgement.

The diffusionism of Boas, Kroeber, Lowie and others had political dimensions. The element of anti-racism has been mentioned already. Equally important, however, was opposition to the by no means racist American anthropological tradition established by Lewis Morgan. Morgan's admiration for the egalitarian and matrilineal Iroquois Indians and his vision of worldwide human democratisation had earlier been incorporated into the framework of Marxist theory. By the early years of the twentieth century the socialist movement in the United States was becoming a significant force. When Franz Boas (1938 [1911]: 193) attacked the search for laws of history, he linked Social Darwinism in this respect with the view that 'social structure is determined by economic forms' – an obvious reference to Marxism.

Robert Lowie (1937: 54–5) was politically aware enough to note how Morgan had become identified with Marxism in the eyes of anthropologists of his generation. 'By a freak of fortune' Lowie observed, Morgan 'has achieved the widest international celebrity of all anthropologists'. This was 'naturally' not due to Morgan's solid achievements 'but to a historical accident': his *Ancient Society* (1877) attracted the notice of Marx and Engels, who accepted and popularised its evolutionary doctrines as being in harmony with their own philosophy. As a result, Morgan's work was promptly translated into various European tongues and, continued Lowie, 'German workingmen would sometimes reveal an uncanny familiarity with the Hawaiian and Iroquois mode of designating kin, matters not obviously connected with a proletarian revolution'.

Lowie went on to note that Morgan 'has been officially canonised by the present Russian regime', whose spokesmen declare his work 'of paramount importance for the materialistic analysis of primitive communism'.

The Boasians therefore felt obliged to fight on two fronts. On the one hand, they attacked racist and biological-reductionist theories of evolution and history; on the other, they aimed to demolish key Marxist notions such as that of 'primitive communism', arguing repeatedly – in direct opposition to Engels – that private property, the state and 'the family' were timeless universals of all human existence. 'With Morgan's scheme incorporated into communist doctrine', concludes Marvin Harris (1969: 249), 'the struggling science of anthropology crossed the threshold of the twentieth century with a clear mandate for its own survival and well-being: expose Morgan's scheme and destroy the method on which it was based'.

Harris argues that this consideration was more important than anti-Darwinism, and that virtually the whole of twentieth-century anthropological theory has been shaped by the perceived need to suppress the tradition of Morgan and the influence within anthropology of Engels and Marx.

Despite this, there was something refreshingly honest and uncomplicated about the writings of the American diffusionists. Unlike Britain's functionalists, they had no great pretensions, and apparently few axes to grind. Although they were hostile to Marxism, and in particular to the notion of primitive communism, they were quite able to admit the drawbacks of their own chosen methods and conclusions. When Kroeber reviewed Lowie's *Primitive Society*, he praised the author for his 'chaotic jumble' remarks, identified with his methods – yet admitted that the result was a *basically useless* form of knowledge: 'its products must appear rather sterile. There is little output that can be applied on other sciences. There is scarcely even anything that psychology, which underlies anthropology, can take hold of and utilize.'

Anthropology could only note unique facts, without ever answering the fundamental question: Why? But people, Kroeber went on, do want to know why, and always will. After the absorption of the first shock of interest in the fact that the Iroquois Indians have matrilineal clans and that the Arunta Aborigines have totems, they want to know why some primitive cultures develop clans and totems while others fail to. In answer, all the diffusionists could offer – admitted Kroeber – was the uninspiring information 'that we do not know or that diffusion of an idea did or did not reach a certain area'. Kroeber concluded sadly:

> That branch of science which renounces the hope of contributing at least something to the shaping of life is headed into a blind alley. Therefore, if we cannot present anything that the world can use, it is at least incumbent on us to let this failure burn into our consciousness.

If anthropology was ultimately useless, the best thing to do was to admit the fact (Kroeber 1920: 377–81).

Kroeber's misgivings indicate how far the new anthropology had departed from the spirit of Morgan and the nineteenth-century founders. The earlier writers, whatever their faults, had not questioned the usefulness of what they were doing. To them, science was enlightenment – and enlightenment was not something which had to be justified. Morgan had seen science as inseparable from democracy, just as prejudice and superstition were inseparable from tyranny (Resek 1960: 60, 122–30). To Tylor, civilisation was the fruit of man's intellect; to be human meant to be guided forward by the light of reason (Voget 1975: 49). To men such as these, the anthropological questions they confronted were of immense philosophical importance and intrinsic human interest. Enlightenment was an end in itself; their own new science was an important aspect of the gradually advancing self-awareness of humankind. The idea of debating whether this self-awareness was 'useful' would not have occurred to them. And indeed, it was only after the science of culture had isolated itself from almost all related branches of science and had *ceased to ask itself fundamental questions* that such an idea could have arisen.

British Functionalism

If British social anthropology in its 'Golden Age' was somewhat less troubled and less uncertain of its practical usefulness in the world, it was for a tangible enough reason. To a far greater extent than the North American Indians – whose resistance in most cases had been savagely broken some time before anthropologists began their studies – the inhabitants of Britain's colonies presented a real problem in terms of long-term political control. To the extent that North American ethnology answered a practical need, it was largely that of a salvage operation for writers of history books, involving talking to old Indian informants on reservations in order to recover for posterity some idea of what their cultures had once been like. The 'functionalism' of Britain's Bronislaw Malinowski and the 'structural-functionalism' of Radcliffe-Brown answered more weighty needs.

Functionalist theoretical frameworks were designed to analyse *living* social structures in order to control them from the outside. As Malinowski (quoted in Harris 1969: 558) himself candidly insisted:

> The practical value of such a theory [functionalism] is that it teaches us the relative importance of various customs, how they dovetail into each other, how they have to be handled by missionaries, colonial authorities, and those who economically have to exploit savage trade and savage labour.

Or, as Radcliffe-Brown (1929: 33) put it, anthropology 'has an immediate practical value in connection with the administration and education of backward peoples'. None of Kroeber's fears lest 'we cannot present anything that the world can use' are discernible here.

Britain's functionalists enjoyed poking fun at the notion of culture as a planless hodge-podge. The absurd anti-theoretical stance of the Boasians provided an easy target – and a welcomed one, since without the 'chaotic jumble' idea, the neat and tidy mirror-image theory that cultures are and must always be perfectly functional wholes might have seemed pointless and unnecessary.

According to functionalist dogma, a cultural fact had been explained once its necessary function had been revealed. Once a mythico-religious system had been shown to be useful, that was all that needed to be said. The details, the inner logic, the symbolic connections – these did not need to be subjected to theoretical labour once the functionality of the overall result had been demonstrated. In an early work, Malinowski (1912), for example, 'explained' the complex and elaborate *Intichiuma* ceremonies of the Central Australian Aranda Aborigines by noting that they presupposed the preparation of much food, required strict discipline and synchronised collective effort – and therefore provided excellent stimulus to labour and economic production. From this point of view, precisely what the Aborigines did in their rituals was irrelevant. They could dance or sing in any way they liked: provided the result was to discipline themselves so that they could become adept at physical labour, the function was the same. 'Such conceptual impoverishment', as Marshall Sahlins (1976: 77) much later commented, 'is the functionalist mode of theoretical production'. Fortunately, in his mature, fieldwork-based writings on the Trobriand Islanders, Malinowski allowed his informants to speak for themselves, and gave us some of the most magnificently vivid, rich, detailed and moving ethnographic writing ever to have been penned. No one has surpassed Malinowski as a sensitive observer. The fact remains, however, that Malinowski's theoretical framework – to which he became more and more narrowly committed as the years passed – could only diminish this richness of his output, for it could do no more than harp endlessly on the uninteresting dogma that each 'custom' in each culture must be functional in relation to the whole. Even when we can agree, it is not an idea which does much to enlighten us or to stimulate investigation into the inner logic of the 'customs' themselves.

With its crassly organic analogies, functionalism left no room for conflict, contradiction, dysfunction or clashes between rival interest groups. The idea that different classes or groups could define mutually incompatible 'functions' seems not to have occurred to anthropologists at the time. Societies were supposed to be harmonious and stable systems whose components all functioned for the benefit of the whole – or, as Malinowski himself tended to express matters, for the benefit of the biological individual whose needs mysteriously coincided with those of the whole. There was more than a touch, here, of the administrator's 'law and order' perspective on life: a vision of the world as a pacified, conflict-free system – if only people would behave! This was not accidental. Anthropology's own function within the world provided one of the more convincing confirmations of the model. Functionalism's declared and explicit function was to enable Europeans more effectively to pacify 'savage' societies in the interests of imperialism as a harmonious whole.

Whereas in the United States the attack on evolutionism was well under before the First World War, in Britain events moved more slowly. Writers in the evolutionist tradition – such as W. H. R. Rivers and Sir James Frazer – continued to be influential and it was not until the 1920s that the tide began to turn. When the evolutionist tradition was finally repudiated, it was not so much through philosophical scepticism as out of directly practical political interest. In the dying decades of the British Empire, huge administrative problems were presenting themselves, and an answer had to be found to Radcliffe-Brown's question: 'What sort of anthropological problems are of practical value in connection with such problems of administration?' (Radcliffe-Brown 1929: 33).

With the exception of occasional keen amateurs, the administrators of Britain's colonies felt no reason to interest themselves in the origins of humankind or the past histories of peoples or civilisations. What concerned them were the present and immediate problems involved in controlling particular territories and groups of 'natives'. What they needed – according to both Malinowski and Radcliffe-Brown – was an applied science, a manipulative set of rules, so that 'the natives' could be governed in much the same way that a chemist or physicist can govern and manipulate natural forces. 'To exercise control over any group of phenomena', as Radcliffe-Brown (1929: 35) put it,

> we must know the laws relating to them. It is only when we understand a culture as a functioning system that we can foresee what will be the results of any influence, intentional or unintentional, that we may exert upon it.

If, therefore, anthropological science was 'to give any important help in relation to practical problems of government and education' it had to 'abandon speculative attempts to conjecture the unknown past and . . . devote itself to the functional study of culture'.

Colonialism and Anthropology

In the 1920s, most British colonial administrators still tended to be scornful of the traditional image of the 'anthropologist' – thinking of this figure as something of a crank, perhaps a fraterniser with the natives, and almost certainly someone of an impractical frame of mind, wrapped up in strange antiquarian interests and theories about the origins of the race. Of what conceivable practical value to an administration could an anthropologist of this sort be? (James 1973: 53–4). Malinowski and Radcliffe-Brown were well aware of such official scepticism and were determined to transform their image. Their endlessly repeated denunciations of 'speculations', or of evolutionism, Darwinism, 'Bolshevism' and other 'unsound' or 'dangerous' theories are best seen in this light. Like Darwinism itself in the previous century, anthropological evolutionism had never been altogether respectable. It was necessary to make a clean break and repudiate anthropology's past.

One of the first things to be repudiated was any interest at all in evolutionary origins. In his early book on the family among the Australian Aborigines, Malinowski (1963 [1913]: 89) was already arguing that questions about the past were a problem with which 'we need not concern ourselves . . . '. He later wrote: 'I have grown more and more indifferent to the problems of origins . . . ' (Malinowski 1932: xxiii–xxiv). In a footnote to his *Argonauts of the Western Pacific*, Malinowski declared with some pride that, while he was presenting 'the facts' about native institutions as carefully as he could, it was 'hardly necessary perhaps to make it quite clear that all questions of origins, of development or history of the institutions have been rigorously ruled out of this work' (1922: 100). In introducing *The Sexual Life of Savages* (1932: xxiii–xxiv) he guaranteed 'the complete elimination' from the text of all 'statements about "origins", "primeval states" and other fundamentals of evolutionism', adding that he 'would rather discountenance any speculations about the "origins" of marriage or anything else than contribute to them even indirectly . . . '.

Radcliffe-Brown's attacks on the evolutionist tradition were still more vitriolic. Lecturing on the 'historical bias' of the early anthropology and of 'the false idea of evolution to which it led such writers as Morgan', he complained: 'We have had theories of the origin of totemism, of the origin of exogamy, and even theories of the origin of language, of religion, and of society itself . . . '. One can feel and hear Radcliffe-Brown's merriment and scorn, and the audience's laughter. Radcliffe-Brown was here addressing a white South African audience, to whom problems of 'origins' were hilariously irrelevant in comparison with the need to maintain white supremacy in troubling times. 'In this country', Radcliffe-Brown continued.

> we are faced with a problem of immense difficulty and great complexity. It is the need of finding some way in which two very different races . . . may live together . . . without the loss to the white race of those things in its civilisation that are of the greatest value, and without that increasing unrest and disturbance that seem to threaten us . . . .

This, he continued, was where anthropology could be 'of immense and almost immediate service'. Provided it was not about origins but about detailing the functions of native institutions to facilitate white control, anthropology would greatly help the authorities 'in dealing with the practical problems of the adjustment of the native civilisation to the new conditions that have resulted from our occupation of the country' (1960: 16, 26).

Social anthropology became important to British colonial administration only in the 1930s and 1940s, in the context of retreat from direct rule as difficulties mounted, wasteful and costly blunders were recognised and the need arose to mobilise the colonies behind the war effort (Feuchtwang 1973: 71–100). Malinowski frequently warned that educated African 'agitators' and nationalists should be understood and if possible won over to European aims lest 'by ignoring them and treating them with contempt we drive them into the open arms of world-wide Bolshevism' (quoted in James 1973: 61). He welcomed indirect rule because it involved 'the maintenance of as much as possible of the Native authority instead of its destruction', providing certain compensations for the natives whilst 'leaving the ultimate control in the hands of Europeans'. The object, Malinowski declared, was 'to create in Native authority a devoted and dependable ally, controlled, but strong, wealthy and satisfied' (Malinowski 1945, in Feuchtwang 1973: 91–2).

A fairly typical liberal, his instincts in a libertarian direction did not extend far. In discussing black 'progress' within white African colonies he was adamant: Europeans should 'make quite clear in preaching the gospel of civilisation, that no full identity can be reached' (Malinowski 1945: 160, quoted in Feuchtwang 1973: 92). Whenever Europeans settle in a colony, he insisted, 'segregation and colour bar become inevitable', a fact which

> ought to be remembered by the enthusiastic minority of good-will, who may involuntarily raise high hopes through such doctrines as the brotherhood of Man, the Gospel of Labour, and the possibilities of assimilation through education, dress, manners and morals. (Malinowski 1945, quoted in Harris 1969: 558)

Malinowski's political allegiances were not in any sense with 'the natives'; he simply aimed to make colonialism more efficient through being self-aware. Radcliffe-Brown (1940; quoted in Feuchtwang 1973; 90), voicing a similar aim, put matters well: 'Imperialism is the self-assumed role of controller of other peoples. They will not let this continue indefinitely. In the meantime, let this blind experiment become less blind.'

Until about 1960, it was virtually impossible for anyone to become trained as a social anthropologist without political collusion in all this. Evans-Pritchard (1946: 97) stressed that the anthropologist who was used as a consultant to an administration 'should be a full member of it'. He could not give good advice without knowing the bureaucratic machinery of colonial rule 'from the inside', having full access to all government documents, and meeting the heads of departments around the same conference table as an equal: 'Administrators naturally resent advice from outsiders but will gladly accept it from one who has the same loyalty to the administration as themselves . . .'

From this it followed that those who lacked the necessary 'loyalty' could find it extremely difficult to obtain permission to do fieldwork, whilst those without fieldwork experience were not permitted to contribute to the development of theory at all. In this way, through the allocation of grants and through countless other bureaucratic and administrative means, the 'science of man' was moulded into conformity with the most narrow of political ends.

Conclusion: Anthropology and Origins

In both Britain and the United States, then, twentieth-century social anthropology turned its back upon evolutionary theory and upon all interest in questions of social origins. As late as the 1960s, Evans-Pritchard (1965: 104, 100) was still vigorously repudiating the 'vain pursuit of origins' and theories of evolution, all of which were said to be 'as dead as mutton'. Edmund Leach (1957: 125) spoke for almost all his professional colleagues when he declared that 'whether or not evolutionary doctrine is true, it is certainly quite irrelevant for the understanding of present-day human societies'. France was before long as firmly gripped as Britain or America. The ferocious intolerance of the new consensus expressed itself in the fact that Claude Lévi-Strauss, whose *The Elementary Structures of Kinship* outlined a new theory of human cultural origins, earnestly assured his readers that, on the contrary, 'we have been careful to eliminate all historical speculation, all research into origins, and all attempts to reconstruct a hypothetical order in which institutions succeeded one another' (1969a: 142). The result was a book about origins which was presented as a book about eternal principles or 'structures'. 'We do not know', Lévi-Strauss wrote elsewhere (1969b: 141), 'and never shall know, anything about the first origins of beliefs and customs the roots of which plunge into a distant past'.

The ideological and political motivations involved in all of this have been stressed. The main and overriding aim was to root out Morgan's notion of 'primitive communism' and to discredit Engels' *The Origin of the Family, Private Property and the State*. So much was this the priority, that on both sides of the Atlantic, from the earliest days, diffusionists and functionalists were quite capable of resorting to arguments about 'origins' themselves – usually in throw-away remarks or casual asides – whenever it served their polemical purposes. It was as if they were warning their students and readers not to investigate such questions too closely, yet claiming to be unafraid of the consequences should such warnings be defied – after all, even if research into origins *were* to be carried out, Marx, Morgan and Engels would surely be found to be wrong! Robert Lowie, for example, wrote a book entitled *The Origin of the State* (1962: 2), in which he endorsed the view of Eduard Meyer that the state was the equivalent of the herd among lower animal species, inherited by humankind without break from the primeval past and therefore absolutely universal. This, of course, was a direct riposte to Morgan's and Engels' view that the state was a relatively recent historical invention. And even as he insisted that all interest in 'origins' was unscientific, Malinowski was not above allowing it to be known that he, too, knew in advance what the origins of the family would turn out to be should anyone ever be so foolish as to investigate the matter. In this context, he stated categorically in a BBC radio debate in 1931: 'marriage in single pairs – monogamy in the sense in which Westermarck and I are using it – is primeval . . .' (Malinowski 1956: 28).

It is now possible to sum up the effects of the taboo on culturally informed discussions of origins which has been imposed upon us for most of the twentieth century. When Kroeber declared (1901: 320) that 'all search for origin in anthropology can lead to nothing but false results', and when similar statements were made on both sides of the Atlantic for the next fifty years, the effect was not to prevent people from believing in evolutionary theories. The effect was, rather, to allow the public access only to theories of a particular – culturally uninformed – kind.

By remaining aloof from evolutionary debate, social anthropologists of virtually all schools in the West have allowed this dire situation to come about. From the very beginning, the cultural specialists' abstention did not produce any decline in popular interest in questions of human origins. It simply caused a lack of interest in social anthropology which – on this as on so many other philosophically important issues – seemed to have nothing to say. Every society must have its origin myth, and if it cannot obtain it from one source, it will obtain it from another. Finding the social anthropologists silent, the wider public has turned, for lack of an alternative, to Social Darwinists, neo-Darwinists and most recently sociobiologists – in other words, to people who (to exaggerate only slightly) know nothing about culture at all. In this sense, a division of labour appears to have operated for something like half a century, with both Darwinians and social anthropologists denying our human potentiality for significant change in different ways. On the one hand, unchangeable biological functions have been upheld as the basis of the most important human cultural institutions – institutions such as the family and the state. On the other hand, change has been denied or excluded from view by a diametrically opposite argument: by the insistence that culture simply exists, that cultural principles are not reducible to biological ones, and that ultimate origins can never be known or understood.

Chapter 2
Lévi-Strauss and 'the Mind'

My dialectic method is not only different from the Hegelian, but is its direct opposite. To Hegel, the life-process of the human brain, i.e., the process of thinking, which, under the name of 'the Idea', he even transforms into an independent subject, is the demiurgos of the real world, and the real world is only the external, phenomenal form of 'the Idea.' With me, on the contrary, the ideal is nothing else than the material world reflected by the human mind, and translated into forms of thought.

Karl Marx, *Capital*. Afterword to the second German edition (1873)

Until recently, Claude Lévi-Strauss was the dominant figure in post-war western social anthropology. His contribution was to make imaginative thinking, speculation and theory building respectable once more. His first major work was an ambitious world survey of kinship systems designed to revolutionise our understanding of human culture as a whole. He remains to this day the only eminent cultural anthropologist to have based his analyses upon a theory of how human culture originated.

Lévi-Straussian methodology was to an extreme degree mentalist and idealist. Its most significant findings were restricted to the cognitive level, whilst even these still cry out for further corroboration and in many cases have *not* been confirmed. Nonetheless, Lévi-Strauss cannot be omitted from any discussion on human origins. Too many Darwinian and sociobiological contributions are in cultural terms simply uninformed. They explain various things, but they do not explain *culture*. No theory can do this, unless it is based on a broad, cross-cultural understanding of the kinship systems, rituals, myths and other institutions of hunter-gatherers and other traditionally organised peoples. We need to know in detail what human culture at the most basic level is. Lévi-Strauss did not satisfactorily provide this understanding, but no one nowadays can even approach such a study without drawing on the contributions that he made.

Structuralism became fashionable in the 1960s, when – as the consequences of the post-war colonial revolution worked through the discipline – social anthropology began seeking new reasons for its existence. Seeming to offer intellectual integrity and lofty, planet-embracing objectivity, the new movement addressed its appeal not to colonial administrators but essentially to western intellectuals attempting to redefine the relationship between their own imperialist, nature-denying, nuclear-age industrial mono-culture and the fast disappearing kaleidoscope of non-industrial cultures of the planet. Promising to make anthropological grand theory a respectable pursuit once more, it gained an enthusiastic following within literary circles and among many social anthropologists from about 1960 until the mid-1970s.

Concurrently with those political developments which were to culminate in the French revolutionary upheavals of May 1968, structuralism fostered a widespread atmosphere of intellectual excitement and anticipation, as if humanity were on the edge of some breathtaking advance in scientific self-understanding. Such hopes were short-lived, however. 'The messianic overtones associated with that intellectual movement', in the words of one former participant (Willis 1982: vii),

> which the sibylline pronouncements of Lévi-Strauss himself did much to maintain and promote, are to a considerable extent responsible for the neglect and even obloquy into which structuralism has fallen in more recent years, now that the Promised Land of total human self-understanding seems as far away as ever.

In the bitter aftermath of such disillusionment, structuralist versions of anthropology have now been repudiated almost universally.

Lévi-Strauss published his mature work in three stages. First, in 1949, came *The Elementary Structures of Kinship*, which became and remained for three decades the most reviewed, written about and discussed book in contemporary anthropology. In it, the author presented his theory that 'the exchange of women' – resting upon men's conceptual ability to distinguish between 'sister' and 'wife' – gave rise to human culture. In the light of this theory, Lévi-Strauss undertook an ambitious cross-cultural survey and re-analysis of many of the world's most frequently discussed kinship systems. A revised version of the work was published in English translation in 1969 (Lévi-Strauss 1969a).

Then in 1962 Lévi-Strauss published his *Totemism* and *The Savage Mind*. These short works marked a change of course – a shift of interest away from social processes towards systems of cognition. Lévi-Strauss challenged the notion that the concept, 'totemism' – once considered to be the most primitive form of human ritual and religion – had any practical meaning or consequences at all. In his own words, 'totemism is an artificial unity, existing solely in the mind of the anthropologist, to which nothing specifically corresponds in reality' (1969b: 79). In fact, Lévi-Strauss redefined totemism so as to exclude food taboos and other ritual dimensions from consideration, and described the remaining cognitive aspects as intellectual procedures of classification, in essence no different from those used by people in contemporary western cultures.

Finally – beginning in 1964 – came Lévi-Strauss' *Mythologiques*, which was intended to be the grand consummating achievement of structural anthropology. This four-volume in-depth study of more than 800 American Indian myths was widely expected to reveal, finally, the 'universal mental structures' which structuralism had been promising from the outset.

Mythologiques attempted to prove that the deepest recurrent structures of cultural symbolism are universal because they reflect the genetic constitution and internal organisation of the uniquely human 'mind'. The aim was to reveal what Lévi-Strauss in his *Totemism* had termed 'the least common denominator of all thought' – 'an original logic, a direct expression of the structure of the mind (and behind the mind, probably, of the brain), and not an inert product of the action of the environment on an amorphous consciousness' (1969b: 163).

The first volume, entitled *The Raw and the Cooked*, studied myths which portrayed culinary operations 'as mediatory activities between heaven and earth, life and death, nature and society' (1970: 64–5). The author added a new element to his theory of cultural origins, suggesting that the discovery of cooking fire must have been associated with a conceptual opposition as important as that between 'sister' and 'wife' – the contrast, namely, between raw meat and cooked. Succeeding volumes raised arcane issues such as why, throughout the Americas, noise should have been believed to be antithetical to cooking (1970: 148–9, 287, 294; 1978: 305–6, 322–3, 496–7; 1981: 307), why eclipses should have provoked noisemaking (1970: 287, 295, 300–1) and the overturning of cooking-pots (1970: 298), and why female menstruation should have been linked with moon-spots, incest and cannibalism (1970: 312; 1978: 389; 1981: 219, 268). These were among the findings used to argue that the myths of the Americas were reducible in the final analysis to 'One Myth Only' (1981).

Lévi-Strauss' Anti-evolutionism

The Elementary Structures of Kinship was presented as an exercise in dialectics. Unlike Hegelian dialectics, however, the Lévi-Straussian version excluded the possibility of significant historical change. In this as in other respects, structuralism was about as far removed from both Marxism and classical evolutionism as it is possible to get. Far from viewing things in their change and development through time, Lévi-Strauss sought only static, synchronic consistencies and correlations. Seeking neither origins nor causes but only patterns, structuralism aimed to isolate significance on one level – an assumed plane of ultimate changelessness beneath all appearances of change. A sympathetic critic (Murphy 1972: 197) put it well when he wrote of *The Elementary Structures*: 'It shows a capacity for seeing a universe in a sand speck and all of evolution in a moment'. It is a good description of Lévi-Strauss' work at its best.

'Structure' was conceptualised as a set of ultimate rules for playing life's game – an invariant logic beneath culture's surface variations. This 'logic' or 'structure', whilst never in fact brought to light or specified, was equated by Lévi-Strauss with the supposedly unchanging and unchangeable internal architecture of the human 'mind', subsisting frozen in timeless eternity. Not only was this anti-materialism on a scale rarely attempted since the time of Hegel – it was also anti-evolutionism carried to its most extreme and bizarre twentieth-century conclusion.

Lévi-Strauss, then – like Boas, Malinowski and Radcliffe-Brown – denied any interest in evolution or in the search for ultimate origins. For him, change in human culture was at the deepest level unreal – what really mattered were 'structures', and these were immune to historical change. Nonetheless, structure itself was assumed to have had a beginning, and in *The Elementary Structures of Kinship*, Lévi-Strauss depicted this as some kind of quantum jump which had occurred when the cultural domain had become established. In opposition to the argument that humans are essentially animals, and that all cultural change is ultimately constrained by fixed biological functions characteristic of the species, Lévi-Strauss stressed the nature/culture opposition, depicting human life as emerging from culture's overthrow of nature's reign. But he froze the story of human evolution from this point onwards. Following the decisive moment in which a 'new order' had emerged, the basic structures of culture in this narrative endured eternally unchanged.

The Exchange of Women

Lévi-Strauss' myth of the origins of culture was presented in the opening pages of *The Elementary Structures*. The central focus was 'the incest rule'. The story ran as follows. In the pre-cultural state, groups of males, in seeking sexual partners, had tended to monopolise the females reared in their own group. There was no taboo to inhibit them from this. Boundaries between categories such as 'wife', 'sister' and 'daughter' were non-existent or blurred. Males in this system exhibited sexual selfishness, for 'incest, in the broadest sense of the word, consists in obtaining by oneself, and for oneself, instead of by another, and for another' (Lévi-Strauss 1969a: 489). To the extent that such sexual selfishness prevailed, there were no social relationships of gift-giving or reciprocity between neighbouring groups of males.

At a certain point, however, protohuman males rejected such sexual selfishness. One group of males 'gave' its females to a second, trusting that the recipients would reciprocate in kind. This was the quantum jump in which culture was born. Gift-giving on such a level was the ultimate in generosity, for a woman was the most precious of possible gifts. From this point on, the daughters and sisters reared in each group were valued as potential gifts, to be used by their male kin in order to make social relationships with other groups of men.

Women, according to Lévi-Strauss, were now reared for exchange rather than for selfish direct use. To guarantee exchange, a new order of reality – a cultural rule – emerged. This was the taboo against incest. With its establishment, each male group, unable to enjoy its own women, had to find another group like itself, exchange its females for theirs – and forge a relationship of mutual trust and reciprocity in the process (Lévi-Strauss 1969a: 3–25). Because of the advantages of such mutuality and co-operation, this pattern came to predominate. Unlike selfish, pre-cultural males, those who were sexually generous formed wide alliances which enhanced their ability to survive.

An important conclusion was that, contrary to the views of most anthropologists of Lévi-Strauss' time, the nuclear family cannot be considered the cellular unit of human kinship. If there is an 'atom' of kinship, it is the unit consisting of a woman, her husband, her child – and her brother who gave the woman away in marriage to the husband in the first place (Lévi-Strauss 1977, 1: 46; 2: 82–112). Without the existence of this incest-avoiding brother, nothing could work. To an incestuous man, a woman would be potentially both sister and wife, and he would be both brother and husband. Lacking polarity or complementarity, building-blocks consisting of such indeterminate individuals would not interlock with one another to form extended chains. *No one would need wives, if they already had sisters who could be sexually enjoyed.* For Lévi-Strauss, the bonds which turn natural kinship into cultural interdependence are therefore neither parent–offspring relations nor sexual pair-bonds. If the fabric of human culture is held together by stitches, the basic stitches are those of marital alliance – essentially, bonds between men as woman-exchanging in-laws. It is alliance which enables biological families to transcend their own limitations, forming into chains of interdependency which constitute the essence of the cultural domain.

In *The Elementary Structures*, Lévi-Strauss touched on physical evolution, but only briefly. He noted among monkeys their 'irremediable lack of language and the total incapacity to treat sounds uttered or heard as signs', adding that this was all the more striking in view of the fact that 'there is no anatomical obstacle to a monkey's articulating the sounds of speech' (1969a: 6). But apart from implying that the use of signs and symbols presupposed some radical reorganisation of the primate brain, Lévi-Strauss left evolutionary biology out of his discussion. The symbolic function, he felt, had simply 'arisen', quite suddenly, the precise reasons for this occurrence being of secondary interest: 'Whatever may have been the moment and the circumstances of its appearance in the ascent of animal life, language can only have arisen all at once. Things cannot have begun to signify gradually' (1987 [1950]: 59).

More generally, despite brief mention of attempts to teach chimpanzees to speak (1969a: 6), lessons to be drawn from monkey and ape sexual behaviour (pp. 7–8), and research into the Neanderthals and their lithic industries and burial rites (p. 3), Lévi-Strauss made very little use of others' findings in areas usually considered relevant to the study of human origins.

A modern response to the 'exchange of women' idea would be to ask how such exchange differed from the familiar finding that females are transferred between groups of non-human primates, such as chimpanzees. To the extent that differences could be demonstrated, the need would then be to seek some explanation in terms of changing ecological conditions and foraging strategies. What changing mode of production required and determined the hypothesised changes in the way sexual relations were organised? Lévi-Strauss said nothing of the mode of subsistence associated with the transition from nature to culture. Nothing was said of gathering, or of the evolution of hunting. And just as the mode of production was not specified, neither was the technological level. The notion of 'Man the Tool-maker' – staple of most origins theories of Lévi-Strauss time – was not criticised, but ignored. What was the connection, if any, between technological development and the sexual developments that Lévi-Strauss envisaged? Lévi-Strauss seemed simply uninterested in questions such as these.

A transformation in male sexual strategy as profound as that envisaged by Lévi-Strauss would also have had anatomical and physiological evolutionary consequences. Over time, differing sexual selection pressures would have produced different anatomical and physiological results. Lévi-Strauss excluded from his discussion this dimension, too, offering only a few hints that there must have been internal changes taking place within the brain –. changes resulting in pan-human mental 'structures' helping to shape the patterns of kinship and culture.

To be fair, Lévi-Strauss' anti-evolutionism led him explicitly to deny any attempt to contribute to evolutionary theory. His origins-scenario was presented hesitantly and almost apologetically, emphasising not so much the processes or determinants of the nature/culture transition as the mere fact of the transition itself. As the incest taboo comes into operation,

the whole situation is completely changed. . . . Before it, culture is still non-existent; with it, nature's sovereignty over man is ended. The prohibition of incest is where nature transcends itself. . . . It brings about and is in itself the advent of a new order. (Lévi-Strauss 1969a: 25)

In passages such as this, the contrasting patterns 'before' and 'after' the establishment of the incest taboo are compared, but the details of any evolution from one to the other are left to the imagination.

Lévi-Strauss' theory was certainly an advance on certain others of the time in that it went beyond the idea that biological pair-bonds or 'nuclear families' were sufficient to form the cellular units of culture: it emphasised that some higher-order emergent configuration had to transform the signification of this biological material in order for the realm of culture to be established. It examined the large-scale integrative effects of marriage rules and rules of incest avoidance or exogamy, concentrating not on families but on the higher-order, collective and impersonal domain of relationships between them. But although these were advances, the origins theory was presented in a manner all too reminisent of the conjectures of theorists of the nineteenth century. Few if any predictions were made which archaeologists, primatologists, evolutionary biologists or even social anthropologists could follow up and test – and indeed Lévi-Strauss expressed his disdain for the whole notion of testability by saying: 'Social structure . . . has nothing to do with empirical reality but with models built up after it' (Lévi-Strauss 1977, 1: 279). The theory was largely indeterminate in all but one particular – its stipulation that men must have inaugurated culture through the 'exchange of women'.

For Lévi-Strauss, it hardly needed stressing – because it was indisputable and virtually self-evident – that sexual rather than economic or ecological/foraging relations were primary in the transition to culture; and that males were responsible for the origins of culture, the female sex playing no active or initiating role. Almost the only potentially falsifiable prediction, consequently, was that human kinship systems should turn out to be systems of male-regulated sexual exchange. In *The Elementary Structures of Kinship*, this expectation was elaborately explored and in many instances confirmed, but this was insufficient to confirm the theory as such. Even if many cultures are male-dominated and do exchange women in something like the manner described, we are not obliged to accept the view that culture as such was invented by men who discovered the advantages of man-to-man bride-exchanging alliances! The cultural incest taboo could have evolved in some other way whilst still giving rise to the exchange systems which Lévi-Strauss so exhaustively analysed.

Lévi-Strauss' theory has appealed to cultural anthropologists because it reflects an awareness of the richness and relative autonomy of the symbolic level of culture. But in the eyes of most evolutionary specialists it fails because it does not explain the mechanisms through which biological evolution could have produced such a result.

Why did those previously 'selfish' males suddenly become animated in their sexual lives by the 'spirit of the gift'? Lévi-Strauss suggests a selective advantage (the advantage of being part of an alliance) but provides no evolutionary timescale, no hypothesised ecological context, no theory of foraging behaviour or economics to supplement his theory of sex. Most of his life's work has been devoted to the demonstration that the distinction between 'sister' and 'wife' is a binary distinction of immense symbolic significance in all human cultures, that it emanates from certain basic categorising propensities or 'structures' of the human brain, and that other binary contrasts – such as that between raw meat and cooked – demonstrate the existence of the same 'structures'. But the idea has gained little enduring support, not only because the locus and nature of the supposed 'structures' has seemed mysterious, but also because the theory presupposes these structures without in fact accounting for their origin.

Mythologiques

After writing *The Elementary Structures*, Lévi-Strauss felt dissatisfied with the results. His reservations struck many of his colleagues as strange, however, for they were based, not on a realisation that he might have made certain errors, but on the fact that he had studied 'life' rather than 'thought'. He had concentrated on the analysis of embodied, acted-out, practical forms of social organisation: kinship systems as systems of matrimonial exchange. He now felt that such a study was not the best way to reach a 'pure' picture of the internal architecture of the human brain. For this, the study of myths was required.

The Elementary Structures, he writes, had discerned behind an apparently chaotic mass of seemingly absurd rules governing the question of who could marry whom in various traditional cultures 'a small number of simple principles' thanks to which the entire field could be reduced to an intelligible system. The book had revealed the force of certain inescapable obligations, as coercive as the laws discovered by physicists and chemists in other spheres, to which the world's kinship systems of necessity conformed. 'However', Lévi-Strauss (1970: 10) writes – and in this lies his real criticism – 'there was nothing to indicate that the obligations came from within'. He had not proved that the structures of marital exchange which he had isolated really displayed for our inspection the internal architecture of the human brain.

This was simply because kinship systems – the subject matter of *The Elementary Structures* – are material in their functions and effects. However much they may display a mental or cognitive dimension, they are contaminated through their inevitable involvement in sex, babies, practical affairs, institutionalised social demands, economic necessities, historical contingencies and other 'external' factors. Although Lévi-Strauss wishes he could have claimed that the constraints discovered in his kinship analyses were purely internal, deriving from the inner properties of the human brain, he concedes a point to his opponents on this score: 'Perhaps they were merely the reflection in men's minds of certain social demands that had been objectified in institutions' (1970: 10). In other words, materialists could still claim that it was social life which had determined the structures of human consciousness, rather than the architecture of the human brain which had produced the patterns discernible in social forms.

Impatient to prove that the internal structure of the mind was the source of all structure in culture, he would now focus not on social practice but on cognition. He began to delve into what Leach (1967: 132) memorably termed 'the land of the Lotus Eaters' – the world of mythology considered as the free creation of the human mind 'communing with itself'.

The significance of Lévi-Strauss' *Mythologiques* lay here: the new study would at last demonstrate the independent structure-imparting contribution of the human 'mind'. Unlike kinship systems, as Lévi-Strauss writes in the opening pages (1970: 10), mythology 'has no obvious practical function'. It is 'not directly linked' with more 'objective' kinds of reality which might be considered to constrain it. 'And so', he continues, 'if it were possible to prove in this instance, too, that the apparent arbitrariness of the mind' displays 'the existence of laws operating at a deeper level', we would have to conclude

> that when the mind is left to commune with itself and no longer has to come to terms with objects, it is in a sense reduced to imitating itself as object; and that since the laws governing its operations are not fundamentally different from those it exhibits in its other functions, it shows itself to be of the nature of a thing among things. (1970: 10)

The Problem of Ritual

Now, the project to isolate myths from their social context immediately came up against a problem. Lévi-Strauss' specialist colleagues had long held that myths *do* in fact have ideological and other practical functions, and that ritual action in particular mediates between mythology and life, shaping and constraining the logic of myths. Lévi-Strauss wanted to demonstrate that myths emerge *not* from collective, social action as this structures people's minds, but independently from a 'mind' which lies behind culture and whose 'structures' are already fully formed prior to any influences which might be derived from culture. It was his intransigent insistence on this point which had led to his dissolution of the classically defined concept, 'totemism' (1969b). Similar objectives would now lead to perhaps the most extraordinary characteristic of his later work: his unrelenting campaign either to deny the significance of ritual in general, or – where that proved impossible – to depict ritual as the very antithesis of the 'thought' which is embodied in myths.

It is difficult for non-anthropologists to appreciate the significance of ritual in non-western cultures, because, as Mary Douglas (1982: 34) has written, the belittlement of ritual is central to our European tradition. To us ritual means, as she writes, 'the formal aspect of religion. "Mere ritual", one can say, and "empty ritual", and from there to mumbo jumbo and abracadabra'. Ritual is merely external; Europeans give priority to the internal, 'spiritual' aspects of religion. Ritual is mere form; we give priority to content. Ritual seems like a façade – we want to know what lies behind the façade.

But in non-western cultures, such activities as singing, dancing, healing, rain-making, life crisis ceremonial and public mourning are not façades or masks drawn across life. They are the meaningful stuff of life itself. Without ritual there would be no sociality, no collective power, no sharing of life's central and most meaningful moments. In some of the finest anthropological studies, such as Godfrey Lienhardt's (1961) work on the Dinka of the Sudan, ritual is shown not as a mask or dead crust over the face of living experience, but as that which creates and inspires it. 'It is form indeed,' Mary Douglas (1982: 36) comments, 'but inseparable from content, or rather there could be no content without it. It is appearance, but there is no other reality.' For many people in non-western cultures, ritual *is* culture.

Perhaps the best starting point in attempting to define ritual is to think of it as the collective dimension of intimate, emotionally significant life. It is collective action at those points where this reaches deep into personal, sexual and intimate emotional experience. Hence sexual intercourse is not necessarily a ritual, but if it occurs during a preordained 'honeymoon' following a public marriage ceremony it is. A young woman's first menstruation is not a ritual, but her puberty ceremony makes it so. To eat food is not ritual, but to participate in a public feast is. What turns even the most intimate and physiological of personal experiences into 'ritual' is symbolic behaviour which makes it collectively acknowledged, sanctioned and controlled. And with collective control comes power.

Ritual is *collective* symbolic action which in the most powerful way organises and harmonises emotions. Without this, there could have been no early human language, no 'kinship', no culture. A society which was a mere assemblage of egotistic, competing individuals would have no ritual domain and could not have one. On the other hand – turning to the opposite extreme – let us visualise an imaginary society whose members were unwilling to eat, to make love, to speak, to mourn their dead or to do anything unless they were sure that what they did formed part of a collective act. In such a society, each person would try to *synchronise* her or his behaviour with that of others – with the result that life would seem 'ritualised' to an extreme degree.

This is why 'form' in ritual is so important. It is simply not possible for humans to synchronise their behaviour collectively without reference to recurrent, standardised, memorable patterns. To Westerners, this may make ritual seem insincere or artificial. How can genuine tears – as at a funeral – be brought on to order at a precise moment determined in advance? How can a *chorus* legitimately express joy or love? It is thought that no act which has to be directed or controlled collectively can be as valid as the spontaneous action of an individual. This, however, says much about the individualistic assumptions of western culture. It helps to explain 'the poverty of our rituals, their unconnectedness with each other and with our social purposes and the impossibility of our having again a system of public rituals relating our experiences into some kind of cosmic unity' (Douglas 1982: 38). In general it can be said that societies or groups value ritual to the extent that they value the maintenance of collective solidarity, and disregard it to the extent that individualism becomes the dominant ethic.

Perhaps the most important point, however, is that ritual is inseparable from myth. 'Myth and ritual', as Edmund Leach (1954: 264) put it, 'are one and the same. Both are modes of making statements about structural relationships.'

In certain cases, the identity may be so close that a myth functions in effect as the rule-book for a recurrently staged ritual performance. Hence the many versions of a Northern Australian myth about being swallowed by a Great Snake-Mother were acted out in real life – young men and boys were ritually 'swallowed alive' by older male actors playing the part of 'the Mother'. Until recent decades, the terrifying experience of being thus 'swallowed' and then 'regurgitated' was all part of young men's initiation into adult life. It is true, the great Australianist W. E. H. Stanner (1966: 157) conceded, that some myths in Western Australia were not acted out in any particular ritual. But taken as a whole, the myths made sense only within the total framework of Aboriginal ritually structured experience. If certain myths became detached from rituals, it was because – like stone monuments – magical stories many often survive even when their ritual re-enactments have ceased to be performed. Myths currently disembodied – floating free of any particular ritual tradition – are therefore (writes Stanner) 'as much the memorials of old formations of cult' as are the still-surviving stone circles or other patterns marking out the ritual dance grounds in which performances were once staged.

The classical scholar Fontenrose (1959: 3–4) proposed for this reason that we should really reserve the term 'myth' for stories which act as native scripts for ritual performances; other stories would then be 'legends' or 'folktales'. Robert Graves (in Cohen 1969: 345) made a similar point: 'True myth may be defined as the reduction to narrative shorthand of ritual mime performed on public festivals . . .'

However, if all magico-religious myths refer ultimately to ritually in-duced experiences, there may be no need to draw so sharp a distinction between 'true' myths and mere 'folk-tales' or 'fairy-tales'. Lévi-Strauss' great precursor in structural analysis, Vladimir Propp (1968: 105–7), viewed Russian and European magical 'fairy-tales' as surviving intellectual remnants left over from a time when ritual and myth had been inseparable: 'A way of life and religion die out, while their contents turn into tales.'

The Attack on Ritual

Lévi-Strauss' view of the relationship between myth and ritual, however, was very different from all this.

In 1964, the first volume of *Mythologiques* appeared in French. It had been widely looked forward to, Lévi-Strauss' more eager supporters anticipating an elegant revelation of the simple logic underlying even the most complex categories of cultural phenomena. But as *The Raw and the Cooked* and subsequent volumes appeared, a sense of disappointment set in.

Amongst other criticisms, it was soon noted that while Lévi-Strauss laboriously attempted to explain myths by reference to countless other myths, he seemed unwilling to take the obvious step of interpreting any one myth by reference to its living social context. In particular, he maintained an 'almost complete silence on ritual' (Yalman 1967: 82). In *The Raw and the Cooked*, even the Amazonian Bororo 'key myth' about a bird-nester – a story which referred to the youthful hero's impending initiation ritual in its opening lines (1970: 35) – was not interpreted in the light of this evidently important ritual context.

To the consternation of many of his admirers, Lévi-Strauss' rigidly maintained silence on ritual proved to be sustained throughout the four volumes of *Mythologiques*. It was not until the closing pages of the last volume, *The Naked Man*, that the author at last came to an attempt to justify this stance. He then gave ritual such a dismissive treatment that one former admirer (De Heusch 1975: 371) could only term it 'astounding'. Another sympathetic critic (Willis 1982: ix) described it as 'idiosyncratic and misleading'. Such adjectives are hardly surprising, for Lévi-Strauss (1981: 675–9) summed up the situation as follows: 'On the whole, the opposition between rite and myth is the same as that between living and thinking, and ritual represents a bastardisation of thought, brought about by the constraints of life' (1981: 675). 'Ritual', Lévi-Strauss continued, 'reduces, or rather vainly tries to reduce, the demands of thought to an extreme limit, which can never be reached, since it would involve the actual abolition of thought'.

Ritual, in this view, is not the fertile soil within which myths grow. It is, on the contrary, the 'bastardisation' of mythological thought, aiming at 'the actual abolition of thought'.

It is difficult to sympathise with Lévi-Strauss' reasoning here, but he seems to mean the following (Lévi-Strauss 1981: 679). Life is unstructured sense experience; it is the realm of 'the continuous', in which everything potentially merges into everything else. When 'mythic thought' is superimposed upon life, the latter is put under an intellectual grid: it is segmented by means of artificial 'distinctions, contrasts and oppositions', a process which leads to 'an ever-increasing gap between the intellect and life'. This gap arises because thought's work in fragmenting the world into polar-opposite concepts leads to a loss of concreteness, a loss of sensuous unity with nature, threatening to 'make it impossible to recover contact with the continuity of lived experience'. Unthinking human impulses revolt against this, desiring to get back from the realm of thought to sensuous life, and they express this revolt through ritual. But their irrational revolt cannot be allowed to succeed. Mythic thought represents culture's supremacy over nature, a supremacy which is irrevocable, and so ritual is doomed to impotence, a situation which explains its 'desperate, maniacal aspect'.

What actual evidence does Lévi-Strauss have for such a picture of ritual? In referring to the 'abolition of thought', he apparently has in mind not only ritual's general identification with the physical intimacies of 'life' but also the fact that few recurrent features of ritual in traditional cultures seem to uphold his notion of what 'thought' ought to be. Ritual, he feels, does not seem to single out for special attention men's marital alliances or 'the exchange of women'. Instead, it appears to foster confusion between the categories of 'sister' and 'wife', as also between 'animal' and 'human'. Far from crystallising the observance of marital obligations and the incest taboo, ritual often seems to celebrate sexual licence and symbolic incest. Far from creating the 'axioms underlying social structure and the laws of the moral or natural order', ritual 'endeavours rather, if not to deny them, at least to obliterate, temporarily, the distinctions and oppositions they lay down, by bringing out all sorts of ambiguities, compromises and transitions between them' (1981: 680).

Correspondingly, the shaman or other ritual leader – according to Lévi-Strauss – is often not a normal husband or wife but is bisexual, or a transvestite, or half-animal. 'There are myths', writes Lévi-Strauss (1981: 769),

> which say that, for ritual to be invented, some human being must have abjured the sharp, clear distinctions existing in culture and society; living alongside the animals and having become like them, he must have returned to the state of nature, characterised by the mingling of the sexes and the confusion of degrees of kinship. . . .

Lévi-Strauss deduces from all this that ritual 'moves in the opposite direction' to thought, systematically merging and confusing the very polar-opposite categories which 'the mind' strives continually to differentiate (1981: 679). In short, Lévi-Strauss sees ritual as anti-culture, vainly attempting to drag humanity back from the accomplishments of the intellect, pulling people away from the achievements of the 'mind' and towards animalistic life, or towards undifferentiated unity with nature.

Viewing myth and ritual as 'opposites' – the first upholding culture, the second striving to undermine it – Lévi-Strauss goes on to attack those anthropological colleagues who 'confuse' ritual with myth. Thinkers such as the eminent Africanist and ritual specialist Victor Turner, for example, are accused of taking no account of 'the fact that mythology exists in two clearly different modalities' (1981: 669). They are charged with failing to realise that 'explicit' myths ranking as 'works in their own right' are quite separate from myths which are mere adjuncts of rites, told only in the course of ritual performances. Such anthropologists, Lévi-Strauss continues, fail to draw 'the dividing line' in the correct place – that is, between mythic thought in any form and ritual in any form – and so get everything 'thoroughly confused', treating rituals as if they were inseparable from the myths which in native terms describe, regulate and explain them:

> Having mixed up the two categories inextricably, they find themselves dealing with a hybrid entity about which anything can be said: that it is verbal and non-verbal, that it has a cognitive function and an emotional and conative function, and so on.

Lévi-Strauss' answer here is 'to study ritual in itself and for itself, in order to understand in what sense it exists as an entity separate from mythology'; this can only be done by 'removing from it all the implicit mythology which adheres to it without really being part of it . . . ' (1981: 669).

In practice, for Lévi-Strauss, this meant not studying ritual action at all, on the grounds that it has nothing to do with myth, and nothing to do with culture or thought either.

An alternative view, of course, would be that ritual action in traditional cultures is inseparable from mythic thought, does intelligently follow logic and does uphold social structure, the problem being simply that human culture rests on a basis quite different from that imagined by Lévi-Strauss. Were we to follow up this thought, it might be concluded that only a thinker setting out with an inverted picture of the relationship between thought and social reality, and with an upside-down model of culture's inner logic, could imagine that for millennia, ritual performances throughout the world had consistently run counter to their own associated myths and striven continuously for the overthrow of 'thought' and of the cultural domain.

In Lévi-Strauss' case, it seems that once an inadequate and one-sided origins theory had been embraced, the struggle to defend it involved an increasingly difficult battle against the evidence. This had its own inescapable dynamic. It led to a model of social structure which, since it was clearly not upheld by ritual action in traditional societies themselves, had to be explained as emanating from some other source. In the end, Lévi-Strauss could find no other source but the mind as an entity which stands opposed to the social reality which surrounds it. This led him to deny all continuity between mythic thought and ritual performances of any kind – and ultimately all continuity, indeed, between thought in general and life itself.

Lévi-Strauss in Retrospect

For nearly two decades, Lévi-Straussian structuralism was the most influential anthropological strategy in Western Europe, and this has had an enduring effect. More daringly than anyone before him, Lévi-Strauss rejected the narrowness and parochialism of so much twentieth-century anthropology. He followed Morgan and the classical founders not in all respects, but certainly in striving as a kind of internationalist to reduce the entirety of our planet's cultural domain to some kind of intelligible order.

His grandiose conception of the collective mind as a precisely wired, pan-human, computer-like generator of culture inspired him to reject completely the parochialism of Malinowski's functionalism – its myopic focus on individual 'cultures' and its rejection therefore of cross-cultural comparisons. Although his special area of interest was native America, he was happy to cull evidence from almost anywhere; social anthropology was for him the study of humanity as a whole. His ultimate focus was not individuals, nor cultures, nor even continent-wide culture areas – but a planetary web of cultures viewed as if from a point high above our world.

Lévi-Strauss' methods produced, as we have seen, some disastrous blind spots. But whatever else may be said of them, his procedures at least enabled him to focus upon cognitive details – perhaps most spectacularly and exhaustively, the details of traditional myths. A vast number of such myths had been recorded before Lévi-Strauss appeared on the scene, but few anthropologists had ever thought of anything very useful or interesting to do with them. Rather little theoretical attention had therefore been paid to myths except by folklorists, religious thinkers, mystics, artists and various writers outside the discipline of anthropology.

In his understanding of the internal logic and cross-cultural uniformity of Amerindian (and by implication world) mythology, Lévi-Strauss was in fact far ahead of his time. Frequently in the history of science, intuitive thinkers prematurely perceive significant patterns which current theories cannot account for. In the period before normal science catches up, such patterns – those underlying the periodic table of the elements, for example, or those which were to lead to the theory of continental drift – are dismissed as no more than coincidental. Only a small number of people insist that they are significant, and that they will eventually necessitate a new understanding of how the world works. These thinkers, however, can only assert their findings – they cannot explain them in terms of current materialist theories.

And in the absence of any real explanation, the arena opens wide to a variety of idealist rationalisations which may seem helpful until a genuine explanation is eventually found.

Lévi-Strauss discovered some extraordinary patterns linking myths from far-flung corners of the Americas, patterns to which we will turn in the closing chapters of this book. Myths, Lévi-Strauss has shown us, are surprisingly rigidly determined, virtually identical sequences sometimes revealing themselves in stories from cultures separated by thousands of miles. When he was writing, no one had expected such patterns, and no materialistic scientific paradigm could as yet account for them or find any place for them. In this context, Lévi-Strauss' weakest point was for him paradoxically a strength. His idealist belief in the world-governing supremacy of a logical human 'mind' (which he equated, in his hour of grandeur, with his own mind as it worked on *Mythologiques* – 1970: 6, 13) enabled him to seek and to find meaning and law-governed necessity in even the tiniest details of every myth, ignoring the fact that no currently accepted theory could possibly explain such patterns. His belief gave him the courage to press on regardless, roaming as he pleased, linking any myth from any culture with virtually any other story from anywhere else in the world, carrying the reader along the most convoluted paths, almost any digression whatsoever being justified on the grounds that one and the same human 'mind' must have been responsible for whatever happened to be found. Lévi-Strauss' idealism in this context was a kind of magic carpet, enabling him to skim over all theoretical difficulties and simply keep going.

In the end, Lévi-Strauss' real achievement has been to lead us to suspect *more* intelligibility and significance in the cross-cultural symbolic record than had previously been hoped for:

> To see a World in a Grain of Sand,
>   And Heaven in a Wild Flower,
> Hold Infinity in the palm of your hand,
>   And Eternity in an hour.

Seeing the universe in William Blake's way (Murphy 1972: 197) is not necessarily such a bad thing; it may indicate an awareness that there is probably more intelligibility and meaning to be gleaned from the world around us than we currently understand.

Stated most positively, it is thanks to Lévi-Strauss that we now know the scale of the tasks facing us in understanding what human symbolic culture is. It turns out to be an exceptionally complex planetary entity which we are barely beginning to understand, although we have glimpsed enough to know that it has its own consistent and comprehensible inner logic, involving recurrent patterns and connections many of which were wholly unsuspected before the founder of structuralism drew our attention to them. *Mythologiques* is a vast, unwieldy, shapeless and ultimately confused and confusing work, but no one can carefully read it without suspecting that the order which eluded its author does in fact reside somewhere within this vast storehouse of material, waiting to be brought out.

Some of Lévi-Strauss' earlier findings – for example, the idea that kinship systems are systems of marital exchange – were not entirely new and have become part of the conventional wisdom of kinship studies. But whoever would have thought that an equation linking lunar eclipses with incest, rebellion, ritual noise-making and 'the coloured plumage of birds' (1970: 312) should have been central to the mythological systems of virtually the whole of South America?

And who would have thought that the many different versions of a pan-American myth justifying male dominance should have blamed women for their supposed inability to synchronise correctly their cosmos-regulating menstrual periods, advocating male intervention to control women's blood-flows as the only means to avert universal chaos? In presenting this finding in the third volume of *Mythologiques*, Lévi-Strauss (1978: 221–2) described himself as lifting a veil to reveal the basic secret of 'a vast mythological system common to both South and North America, and in which the subjection of women is the basis of the social order'.

Lévi-Strauss' findings regarding such things have irritated anthropologists who simply do not know what do with them, and certainly few if any sociobiologists or students of human origins have considered them interesting or relevant to their specialist concerns. But if they are true – and some certainly are – then they are important. Anthropologists cannot be simple behaviourists. What native peoples believe, think and mythologise – and what their palaeolithic ancestors may also have thought – is an essential component of their collective being. It would be a point in its favour if a theory of cultural origins and evolution could help account for such findings as these.

Chapter 3
Totemism as Exchange

In so far as man is human and thus in so far as his feelings and so on are human, the affirmation of the object by another person is equally his own enjoyment.

Karl Marx, *The Economic and Philosophic Manuscripts* (1844)

In his *Totemism* and *The Savage Mind*, Lévi-Strauss approached the study of ritual only to dissolve it into a kind of psychology – an investigation into the nature of 'the mind'. In effect, by subsuming most forms of ritual action under the heading, 'totemism' – which he then described as essentially imaginary – he avoided having to construct a theory of ritual action at all. Instead, he simply conjured the problem away.

Lévi-Strauss' finding that 'totemism' is simply 'imaginary' has been widely accepted. For over twenty years, the verdict of many scholars has been that the whole issue is now closed. In this chapter I challenge this consensus, surveying some of the classical literature on totemism in the light of the preceding discussion. Many of the texts to be cited will seem outdated to the modern reader; I draw on them in order to locate Lévi-Strauss' work in its context as one particular contribution to a long-standing and still unresolved debate.

In making his case, Lévi-Strauss devoted much care to the refinement of definitions enabling him to set apart 'sacrifice' as wholly distinct from 'totemism', and 'totemism' as quite unconnected with other beliefs and institutions such as food taboos. Here, by contrast, I aim to show that 'sacrifice' is not a separate 'thing' from 'totemism' or 'food taboos', any more than these are separate 'things' from beliefs in the immortality and super-natural efficacy of animal 'souls'. It is a fruitless endeavour to pull portions of a reality which is continuous into neat and tidy separate bits. If we are to succeed in accurately describing ritual phenomena and cataloguing and classifying them in an intelligible way, more than ingenious definitions and counterpositions will be required. What we need is a grasp of underlying principles – of abstract generative structures. We also need a dynamic model which explains how these structures – not separately but as an integrated, logical totality – came into being.

My argument is a simple one. Culture starts not only with the incest taboo, but also with its economic counterpart in the form of a rule prohibiting hunters from eating their own kills. This second taboo – like strict exogamy – is not always rigidly adhered to. *It is in fact systematically evaded or undermined in a multiplicity of historically determined ways*. It is out of this process that 'totemic' and related phenomena arise.

Before turning to my examples, let me quickly survey the territory which this chapter will cover. I am interested in *methods of getting around the rule that one's own kills are for others to enjoy*. The possibilities are virtually limitless, but it will clarify my argument if I list some of the more obvious potential loopholes in the law here.

Firstly, the 'own-kill' rule can be partially evaded *by applying it only to hunters prior to their reaching a certain age*. Older men can be allowed to escape from its obligations altogether. Related to this can be the argument that a hunter should adhere strictly to the rule until his wife has had her first baby, or until some other risk-laden life crisis is safely over.

Another way to lessen the rule's rigours is to apply it only to 'firsts' – for example, to the first animal a man kills in a given season, or the first he kills of a given species, or in a given place. As in the previously mentioned case, this at least preserves *the principle* of the rule, whose material costs may be thought to be more safely diminished or evaded as a result.

Then come the apologies, atonements and restitutions. A hunter may be allowed to eat his own kills *provided he apologises*. Whether this apology is addressed to a shaman, to one's in-laws, to 'the spirits' or to the animal itself is of less importance than the fact that the speech, perhaps accompanied by a request for forgiveness, enables once again the *principle* of the taboo to be maintained. There is an obvious link between such apologies and claims that the animal is 'not really dead' – its 'life-essence' or 'soul' being claimed to survive unharmed.

Linked to his apologies and as reinforcements of them, the hunter may feel that he can safely eat his own kill provided he *first symbolically offers it to someone else*. This recipient need not be a flesh-and-blood person or social group. It might be an imaginary being – a 'spirit' or 'god'. If it becomes more and more established that the offering is merely a gesture – the recipient being expected to return or decline the gift – then the potential for guilt can still be lessened in various ways. It can be said, for example, that the recipient retains and is empowered by the metaphysical 'essence' or 'life-blood' of the kill, allowing the killer only the baser parts. It may be conceptualised as no more than good fortune that such base, fleshy cuts of meat happen to be precisely those which the hunter's stomach needs! I derive much of the earliest logic of 'sacrifice' from this source.

All of the evasive strategies mentioned here involve segmentation, fragmentation, theological logic-chopping. Debates about the precise age of the hunter, the precise nature or condition of his kill, the precise motives involved in his offerings may now abound. An obvious further way to enrich the debates and evade the rule would be to claim that generosity is obligatory with respect only to certain *parts* of a killed animal – say, to its head, or its blood – the rest being exempted. Alternatively, only certain *species* may be said to come under the gift-giving rule's ambit. 'Totemism' in my view starts here.

Where the aim is to escape as far as possible from the material burdens of the rule, the various species chosen to taboo can be those which are rare, unwanted or virtually inedible – their 'respect' then becomes of purely symbolic significance. On the other hand, if for historical reasons the material consequences of economic generosity seem less burdensome, different criteria for selecting 'totemic' species may be used. For example, it may be said that the own-kill taboo applies only to 'large' animals which it is virtually impossible not to share, 'small' animals not counting. Theological metaphysics may again flower here, as the need arises to decide on definitions of what counts as 'large' or 'small'.

Finally, the segmentation of the world of edible species can be mapped carefully on to the segmentations of the human social world. That is, what is tabooed for one clan or segmentary group can be declared perfectly edible for another. This avoids the problem of resource under-utilisation which might ensue if everyone tabooed the same species. If kangaroos, for example, were said to be subject to the own-kill taboo in a situation where no one wanted to hunt except for their own needs, the upshot might be a total lack of interest in kangaroos! Far better to let one group 'respect' one species whilst others 'respected' others. Then no resource need be wasted, and ritualised exchanges serving to emphasise the 'own-kill' principle could be organised whenever the need or opportunity arose. This, I think, gives us some of the more elaborate forms of what used to be termed 'totemic ritualism'.

Totemism by Elimination

I now turn to my examples. Among the Kaingang in Brazil, when a tapir has been killed and eaten, a short speech is addressed to its soul or *kuplêng* 'in order that succeeding tapirs may stand still and allow themselves to be shot. . . . ' (Henry 1964: 85). The derivation of this might have remained obscure had not the ethnographer clarified a vital point. Under normal circumstances, a man *'must never eat of the tapir he has brought down himself, although he may share the kill of other men'* (1964: 85; my emphasis). Any older hunter who, despite this, does in practice regularly eat his kills, must be doing so through a special privilege, conferred upon him as he reaches a suitable age. He is then deemed to have at last reached the point where, without fear of death from supernatural causes, he may evade the own-kill taboo. The evasion is welcomed, because it implies liberation from an earlier framework of collective accountability and control: 'Previously, not being able to eat the meat of the tapir he had killed, he was dependent on others; no matter how great his prowess, he had to remain in the group or run the risk of starvation.'

Now that the older hunter can eat his own kills, he is more free — although, as we have seen, he is still careful to continue to 'respect' his own kills in other, more symbolic, ways (Henry 1964: 85).

My second South American case is the Bolivian Siriono, who appear to have gone even further in releasing hunters from the 'own-kill' rule. Holmberg (1948: 462) writes as follows in an early brief article on this tribe: 'A hunter is not allowed to eat the meat of a particular animal of certain species that he kills (e.g. the tapir) lest he offend the animal and be unable to hunt another.'

This looks like a very unexceptional hunters' taboo, of a religious kind familiar from countless cross-cultural hunter-gatherer studies. Had no further information been given, we might have had little reason to suspect that a rule of economic exchange lay behind it.

But fortunately, in his major later work on the Siriono, Holmberg (1950: 33) provides sufficient data to make it clear that here as elsewhere the supposed tapir avoidance rule is only a *residue* left when a more substantial rule of exchange (applying in principle to *all* game) is partly relaxed:

> Theoretically, a man is not supposed to eat the flesh of an animal which he kills himself. If a hunter violates this taboo, it is believed that the animal which he has eaten will not return to be hunted by him again. Continued breaches of this taboo are consequently supposed to be followed automatically by the sanction of ill-luck in hunting.

What has this to do with the 'totemic' idea that the tapir is specially to be avoided as food? Holmberg gives us the answer: the own-flesh rule has fallen into disuse, applying to fewer and fewer species until only one or two are left within its ambit. As he puts it, the taboo on eating one's own kill

> may formerly have been an effective mechanism by means of which to force reciprocity in the matter of game distribution, but if so, it has certainly lost its function today, for the disparity between the rule and its practice is very great indeed. Few hunters pay any attention to the rule at all, and when they do it is only with respect to larger animals, such as the tapir and the harpy eagle, that are rarely bagged anyway.

In the case of smaller animals, such as coati and monkeys, Holmberg (1950: 33) reports that he 'never saw hunters show any reluctance to eating those that they had killed themselves'.

The tapir and harpy eagle are special because of their large size, which makes it harder to violate the own-kill taboo in their case. If these species now appear to be especially 'tabooed', in other words, this is only a residue of what was once a much wider rule of exchange applying to all game indiscriminately:

> Embuta, one of my older informants, told me that when he was a boy he never used to eat any of the game that he killed, but that nowadays the custom had changed and that it was no longer possible to expect meat from someone else who hunted.

Property Relations and the 'Own-kill' Taboo

It has long been known that in most hunting traditions, fixed rules exist to define unambiguously to whom a killed animal 'belongs'. The rules vary widely from culture to culture but it seems to matter little, as one writer has put it (Ingold 1980: 158), 'whether a slain animal belongs to the man who first sighted it, chased it, killed it or butchered it, or whether it passes to a recognised leader, a kinsman or affine, or to some passive bystander'. Conflicts at the kill site or distribution point can be avoided 'so long as *some rule exists*, capable of more or less unambiguous application'. What matters is that the issue is decided not just as an outcome of interpersonal interaction but through the application of unalterable 'rule' or 'law'.

Europeans once persistently concluded that such rules of 'ownership' proved the importance of private property among hunters and gatherers. We now know, however, that such rules 'concern only the establishment of prior claims to the kill' (Ingold 1980: 158), often considerably before the consumption phase begins. In other words, 'possession of a kill in a hunting society confers not the right to its consumption, but the privilege of performing its distribution' (Ingold 1980: 158, citing Dowling 1968: 505). Quite often, the 'property rule' seems unmistakably analogous to incest avoidance, in that the hunter cannot enjoy his own produce at all.

Statements on the Hunter's Own-kill Rule in North America

(a) General

Among numerous North American 'own-kill' statements, the following are worth singling out for two reasons. Firstly, the earlier ones in particular show how the norm was conceptualised in the literature through familiar pre-existent religious categories – feast-giving, 'first-fruits ceremonies', 'sacrifice', 'rites of atonement' and so forth. Secondly, the statements illustrate something of the norm's range of variability in form:

> It is the custom among the Delawares that if a hunter shoots down a deer when another person is present, or even accidentally comes by before the

skin is taken off, he presents it to him, saying 'Friend, skin your deer', and immediately walks off. (Heckewelder 1876: 311; Delaware)

According to one informant the man who killed an animal had the least to say about its distribution and generally got the poorest share. (Radin 1923: 113; Winnebago; but other informants state the reverse)

Whenever he hunted with me, he gave me all, or the greater part of what he had killed. (Tanner 1940: 62; Ottawa)

any sharp utensils which you use to eat us with, you shall not have in your hand when you hunt. If you do, you will scare us far away. (Instructions given by the ancestral Deer-people, spiritual 'owners' of all deer, Luckert 1975: 40; Navaho)

When a deer or bear is killed by them, they divide the liver into as many pieces as there are fires, and send a boy to each with a piece, that the men belonging to each fire may burn it. . . . (Romans 1775, 1, 83; Choctaw)

when a young man killed his first game of any sort he did not eat it himself, but distributed the meat among his clansfolk. (Adair 1775: 54; Chickasaw)

(b) California

Statements on California are of special interest within North America because they cover rules which were unusually strict. Hugo Reid (1939: 238) wrote in general terms of the Indians of Los Angeles County that hunters – particularly the younger ones – 'had their peculiar superstitions': 'During a hunt they never tasted food; nor on their return did they partake of what they themselves killed, from an idea that whoever eat of his own game hurt his hunting abilities.' This rule was frequently noted in the region. Among the Juaneno in the south, the regulation that a hunter must not partake of his own game or fish was adhered to tenaciously. 'Infraction brought failure of luck and perhaps sickness' (Kroeber 1925: 643). These Indians in fact used a special verb, *pi'xwaq*, meaning 'to get sick from eating one's own killing' (Harrington 1933: 179), emphasising once again both the *existence* of the rule and the fact that it was by no means always strictly *obeyed*.

The Franciscan missionary, Boscana (1846: 297–8) at an early stage condemned such beliefs as 'ridiculous', commenting that 'the deer hunters could never partake of venison which they, themselves, procured, and only of such as was taken by others, for the reason, that if they did, they would not get any more'. Fishermen possessed the same idea with regard to their fish. 'More singular, however, than this', continued Boscana,

was the custom among the young men, when starting for the woods in search of rabbits, squirrels, rats or other animals. They were obliged to take a companion for the reason, that he who killed the game, could not eat thereof – if he did, in a few days he complained of pains in his limbs, and gradually became emaciated. On this account, two went together, in order to exchange with each other the result of their excursion.

Of the Southern Californian Luiseño, Kroeber (1908: 184) writes that when a man killed a deer, or rabbits, he brought them to the camp:

Then the people ate the meat, but he did not partake of it. If he should eat of the meat of animals he himself had killed, even only very little, he would not be able to kill others. However, if he confessed to the people that he had taken some of the meat, he would again be able to hunt successfully.

Among the Shasta (Northern California), the strict own-kill rule apparently applied only to the younger hunters: 'For a year after he began to hunt a boy never ate any game of his own killing for fear of his luck leaving him permanently. From his very first quarry his entire family refrained' (Kroeber 1925: 295). Alfred Robinson (1846: 233) inferred that own kill prohibitions characterised the Indians of Upper California as a whole, and Bancroft (1875: 1, 418) generalised similarly for the whole state of California, seeing the rule in terms of native 'superstition', fears of 'eclipses' and beliefs in 'all sorts of omens and auguries'.

The Own-kill Rule in Australia

Australian myths often centre upon the misfortunes befalling those foolish enough to violate the own-kill taboo. Very often it is the 'spirit' of the abused animal species – sometimes an ancestral kinsperson connected in some way with the Rainbow – which inflicts the well-deserved punishment.

Berndt and Berndt (1970: 44) report a story from the Gunwinggu of North Australia in which 'one man in a group travelling south near Nimbuwa killed a small rock wallaby and ate it secretly by himself, but its sizzling attracted the Rainbow, who swallowed him and his companions as well'. In a myth of another Arnhem Land tribe, the Birrikilli (Robinson 1966: 117–20), a man and his son keep killing and eating turtles, cooking the flesh on a fire of their own on the beach. However, the spirit of Garun the Turtle awaits revenge. The myth ends with the cooking of the two men as the Great Mother of Turtles tells them: 'You came here to kill my spirit. My spirit has killed you now.' An equally appropriate punishment features in a myth of the Kuppapoingo, who tell the story of a man called Kunji, who used to eat his own fish. His punishment was to be speared from behind, the spear-tip running through his body and protruding from his mouth, transforming him through death into a jabiroo bird with a long bill, enabling him to spear and eat fish to his heart's content (Robinson 1966: 162–3). Often, a man who eats his own kills is regarded as incapable of self-control – and, in particular, as having an uncontrollable and ridiculous penis. In an Aranda myth (Róheim 1974: 233–4) a man uses his penis to spear rats for him, which he then eats himself. One day his penis is searching for meat in a hole in the ground when it is mortally bitten by snakes.

An early Australian report (Taplin 1879: 52) stated that when the Narrinyeri cook an emu 'they recite incantations, and perform a variety of genuflections over it.' Among the Wongaibon (Mathews 1904: 358; cited in Blows 1975: 31–2), young men could kill emus but were prohibited from eating any of the flesh themselves, although they could eat some if presented a piece by an old man or if they had been released from the taboo by singing a special song for the bird.

Among the Wuradjeri (Berndt 1947: 353) a man who ate his own emu flesh was made ill 'by the emu feathers and nails, said to have entered the eater with the meat'. In this region, the emu was kin – identified with the ancestral All-mother, Kurikuta (Berndt 1947: 77). Beckett (cited in Blows 1975: 42n) 'reports the tradition that if someone griddled emu in the bush instead of bringing it back to camp to be roasted, Kurikuta would come down in a thunder cloud to punish him'.

In South West Victoria there were 'strict rules' regulating the distribution of food:

> When a hunter brings game to the camp he gives up all claim to it, and must stand aside and allow the best portions to be given away, and content himself with the worst. If he has a brother present, the brother is treated in the same way, and helps the killer of the game to eat the poor pieces, which are thrown to them, such as the forequarters and ribs of the kangaroos, opossums, and small quadrupeds, and the backbones of birds. (Dawson 1881: 22–3)

Interestingly, the Aborigines consciously formulated this as a rule of exchange:

> The narrator of this custom mentioned that when he was very young he used to grumble because his father gave away all the best pieces of birds and quadrupeds, and the finest eels, but he was told that it was a rule and must be observed. This custom is called yuurka baawhaar, meaning 'exchange' . . . .

To 'show the strict observance of it, and the punishment for its infringement', continues Dawson (1881: 22–3),

> they tell a story of a mean fellow named Wirtpa Mit, signifying 'selfish', who lived on kangaroos, which were very scarce in those days. When he killed one he ate it all himself, and would not give away a morsel. This conduct so displeased his friends that they resolved to punish him, but as it was difficult to do so without infringing the laws of the tribe, they dug a deep pit and covered it over with branches and grass. . . .

There follows a lengthy account of the killing of Wirtpa Mit, who ate his own kangaroos until, appropriately, he was himself caught in a kangaroo trap.

One of the better-known myth analyses in classical social anthropology is Radcliffe-Brown's treatment of a Western Australian myth about Eaglehawk and Crow:

> Eaglehawk told his nephew to go and hunt wallaby. Crow, having killed a wallaby, ate it himself, an extremely reprehensible action in terms of native morality. On his return to the camp his uncle asked him what he had brought, and Crow, being a liar, said that he had succeeded in getting nothing. (Radcliffe-Brown 1960: 96)

Crow is forced to regurgitate the meat as Eaglehawk tickles his throat. It is worth nothing that 'Eaglehawk and Crow' myths, hundreds of which have been recorded, cannot be understood without knowing that, to the Aborigines, ravens or crows are distinguished by the fact that they follow eagles, mob them and take their kills, a kind of 'forced exchange' of game between the two birds being the result (Blows 1975: 26–7).

Turning now from ritual and mythology to everyday life, Fison and Howitt (1880: 261–3) long ago summarised the rules according to which Kurnai hunters had to distribute their catch:

> *Kangaroo*. The only parts which the hunter and his companions may cook and eat on the spot are the entrails. If the hunter has nothing to eat, he may keep a little, or receive some back from his wife's parents the following day.
> *Black Wallaby*. The hunter keeps nothing.
> *Wombat*. 'All of the animal is sent to the wife's parents, being regarded as the best of food. The wife's father distributes it to the whole camp, but he does not give any to the hunter, who is supposed to have eaten of the entrails in the bush, and therefore not to be hungry.'
> *Swan*. If one or two are killed, they are given to the two sets of parents, the wife's parents being put first. Only if several have been killed may the hunter himself keep some.
> *Conger Eel*. All given to the wife's parents.

'In all cases', as Fison and Howitt (1880: 261–3) remark, 'the largest and the best of the food is sent to the wife's parents'.

In a slightly different vein, Warner (1957: 128) found a form of the own-kill rule among the Murngin. His description concerns, in principle, 'all the animals a male kills until he has a baby':

> The bones of the animal or bird are painted with red ocher. If a boy kills a turkey or other large bird, he does not pick it up but leaves it, returns to the camp and tells some old man. . . . If a young man finds a porcupine

(echidna), he will not kill it but goes to tell an old man of his find. If it is killed, he cannot eat it.

Among the Tiwi, it is 'against custom for the hunter to cook what he has obtained; he must give it to another'. In this way, 'the very act of cooking distributes the food to others beside the hunter and his or her spouse'. When an animal is caught, the first to call out must always cook the food. The second to call claims the head, the third, a leg. 'This order is invariable.' Even this, however, is only a preliminary distribution. Once each man has gained his piece, he still cannot just eat it. He must share it with a series of persons in an invariant order defined by their relationships within the kinship system (Goodale 1959: 122–3).

To turn to some more recent reports, Myers (1986: 75) writes of the Pintupi that 'a hunter gives the kangaroo he kills to others for preparation', keeping only the head for himself. In the eastern Western Desert, 'the preparation and distribution of game is wholly collective. The hunter never cooks and distributes what he has caught' (Hamilton 1980: 10). Gould (1981: 435), likewise, writing in general of the Western Desert Aborigines, notes that 'food-sharing relationships are too important to be left to whim or sentiment'. When a group hunts a kangaroo or other large animal, the man who kills it is the last to share, sometimes receiving only the innards. Gould (1969: 17) comments that although at first glance 'this system of sharing seems unfair to the hunter', such unfairness is illusory. The hunter is recompensed (a) by the prestige which his gift-giving creates and (b) by his own obtaining of meat 'when, according to the same set of rules, he takes *his* share from someone else's catch'.

There is a strongly socialist, redistributive, logic in all this. Yengoyan (1972: 91) writes of the Pitjandjara that the least productive individuals – old men, old women, nursing mothers, pregnant females, young children – 'always have access to the full range of foods', whilst it is the most able hunters who are cut out:

> Thus, for example, when a male gets a kangaroo and brings it in, the animal, after it has been cooked is divided out to all according to kinship ties, and the oldest males get the best parts, etc. What you commonly find is that the hunter gets virtually nothing.

Similar rules enforcing redistribution were, in fact, almost certainly universal in Australia up until European contact. Alain Testart (1988: 10) concludes that 'the principle of intelligibility' of Australian society as a whole is a single, all-embracing law stating that 'one may not dispose of what is one's own'. One's initial 'closeness' to any valuable precludes keeping it for oneself: 'Contiguity (between hunter and game, between totemist and totemic species, between brother and sister) always translates as an advantage for others.'

In this light, exogamy, totemism and the own-kill rule appear as so many differing expressions of one and the same fundamental principle of exchange.

Australian Totemism as Exchange

Prominent in the classical literature on Australia is a form of totemism which explicitly centres on exchange. The exchange occurs between ritually defined collective partners, one group refusing to eat certain edible species so that another may enjoy them more plentifully, this group reciprocally 'producing' species for consumption by others. Lévi-Strauss refers to exchanges of this kind in *The Savage Mind* (1966 [1962]: 226), referring particularly to the *Intichiuma* ceremonies of the Aranda and other Central Australians. The ceremonies, in his view, are a 'game' in which human groups and natural species arrange themselves in complementary pairs, 'species nourishing the men who do not "produce" them, and men producing the species which are forbidden to eat'.

In *The Native Tribes of Central Australia* – Lévi-Strauss' main source – Spencer and Gillen (1899) show how, among the Aranda, witchetty grubs are gathered (as they come into season) by men who do *not* belong to the witchetty grub totemic group. The collected grubs are then ceremonially presented to an assembly of witchetty grub men. These grind up the food and taste just a little, as if to assert their peculiar rights in it. They then make a point of renouncing the bulk of the grubs, handing them to men of other totems to eat (p. 204). A similar ritual is played out in relation to the *Idnimata* (grub of a large beetle) totem. In the case of the Bandicoot, men *not* of this totem kill a bandicoot. They then put fat from the animal into the mouths of men of the totem, who may then eat the animal sparingly (pp. 205–6).

There are many variations. Sometimes the killers of an animal eat none of it themselves; sometimes they assert their right to eat it by tasting some, in order (it seems) to emphasise the act of renunciation which follows; at other times, the 'producers' feel at liberty to eat a portion of their own produce, but not until *after* the bulk of it has been handed to others as a gift. In all cases, though, two things stand out. First, a boundary is drawn between those with the right to kill (or gather) a species and those entitled to eat it. Second, the 'taboos' – which, where they concern animals, are rules against eating one's own kill – are more than mere negative rules of avoidance. They give expression to a positive principle of gift-giving or exchange.

What ensures this exchange is the separation of *killing* rights from rights to *eat*. With regard to any one species, the two kinds of rights are vested in opposed 'kinds' of men: (a) members of the totem and (b) non-members.

This binarism is not limited to the Aranda, but was widespread in Central Australia. A Warramunga man, for example, 'will not hesitate, under certain conditions, to kill his totem animal, but he hands it over to men who do not belong to the same totemic group, and will not think of eating it himself'. Or to take the case of the Urabunna, no member of any totemic group eats the totem animal or plant, 'but there is no objection to his killing it and handing it over to be eaten by men who do not belong to the totemic group'. 'The fundamental idea', as Spencer and Gillen (1904: 327) summarise matters,

> is that men of any totemic group are responsible for the maintenance of the supply of the animal or plant which gives its name to the group. . . . If I am a kangaroo man, then I provide kangaroo flesh for emu men, and in return I expect them to provide me with a supply of emu flesh and eggs, and so on right through all of the totems.

The Own-kill Rule in Papua New Guinea

Turning to Papua New Guinea, among the Mundugumor 'A hunter may not eat his own kill or it will spoil his magic' (Mead 1947: 218n). The Gnau refuse their kills because each hunter automatically projects 'his own blood' into the meat, a basic rule being that people 'should never eat their own blood' (Lewis 1980: 174). The Umeda hunter 'cannot eat any part of the animal he has killed – a kind of incest taboo on meat' (Gell 1975: 109). Gell (1975: 117) gives a good story highlighting woman's role in enforcing this rule:

> The myth . . . concerns a man who hunts in the forest killing a pig, but instead of taking it home to his wife, he eats it by himself in the forest (hubris). The wife finds out her husband's crime and turns herself and her children into pigs (by donning pig tusk nose ornaments) and eventually gores her husband to death (nemesis).

The abused pig-flesh, then, takes vengeance in the form of the hunter's own wife. Among the Siane, the idea of eating one's own pig 'is treated with the same distaste and horror as is expressed at the idea of cannibalism' (Salisbury 1962: 65). In the Tor Territory, the hunter who has killed a boar 'must divide it amongst the villagers, but he is not allowed to eat any of it' (Rubel and Rosman 1978: 13, citing Oosterwal 1961: 65). In the case of the Iatmul: 'One cannot eat one's own pig, or cassowary and wild pig caught in the bush' (Rubel and Rosman 1978: 45). The same applies to the Northern Abelam (Rubel and Rosman 1978: 61).

The rule about pigs also applies to the Wogeo, Keraki, Banaro and many other groups. Rubel and Rosman (1978: 287) make the 'own produce' rule central to their analysis of social structure in the area. They argue persuasively that 'own sister' and 'own pig' rules in Papua New Guinea represent merely two aspects of a unitary principle of give-and-take whose institutional outcome is 'a dual organization in which like is exchanged for like'. In the case of the Arapesh, Mead (1935: 29) writes:

> The ideal distribution of food is for each person to eat food grown by another, eat game killed by another, eat pork from pigs that not only are not his own but have been fed by people at such a distance that their very names are unknown. . . . The lowest man in the community, the man who is believed to be so far outside the moral pale that there is no use reasoning with him, is the man who eats his own kill – even though that kill be a tiny bird, hardly a mouthful in all.

For a man even to eat game which he had *seen* alive would be to risk losing his hunting luck (Mead 1941: 449). Nor must one 'eat the animal for whose capture or growth one knows the magic' (1941: 412).

In Arapesh culture, '*the taboo upon eating one's own kill is equated with incest*' (1941: 352; my emphasis). Own kin and own produce are equally for others to enjoy. 'The native line of thought', as Mead (1935: 83–4) explains, 'is that you teach people how to behave about yams and pigs by referring to the way that they know they behave about their female relatives'. And these *relations with female relatives* are explicitly thought to express the spirit of gift-giving and exchange:

> To questions about incest I did not receive the answer that I had received in all other native societies in which I had worked, violent condemnation of the practice combined with scandalous revelations of a case of incest in a neighbouring village. Instead both the emphatic condemnation and the accusations were lacking. 'No, we don't sleep with our sisters. We give our sisters to other men and other men give us their sisters'. Obviously. It was as simple as that. Why did I press the point? (Mead 1935: 84)

The Own-kill Rule in Africa

Young San (southern African) hunters say that their elders 'do not allow us to take hold of springbok's meat with our hands, because our hands, with which we held the bow and the arrow, are those with which we are taking hold of the thing's flesh . . . ' (Bleek and Lloyd 1911: 274–5). The man who has killed an animal is not allowed to carry it; he must also sit at a distance during the butchery 'because he fears lest he should smell the scent of the springbok's viscera . . . '.

Still in southern Africa, a Khoekhoe hunter could not eat his own kill of an elephant, rhinoceros, or hippopotamus: if he wanted meat following a killing, it had to be that of a sheep or goat (Schapera 1930: 306). The Heikum hunter was permitted a few strictly specified parts of the animal he shot with a poison arrow, but the rest was tabooed on pain of his losing his luck (Schapera 1930: 98–9). Comparable rules are reported of the !Kung, whose society 'seems to want to extinguish in every way possible the concept of the meat belonging to the hunter' (Marshall 1961: 238). Strict 'own-kill' rules apply, however, only to big game animals which the !Kung deliberately hunt in organised parties. A man who picks up a small animal may keep it for himself and his immediate family (Marshall 1961: 236–7).

To select a few interesting statements from elsewhere in the continent, Evans-Pritchard (1974: 58) cites a Central African (Azande) anecdote concerning a furious woman who complains of her husband: 'That man, that man, he is not a human being, he behaves just like a dog . . . – he goes and kills a beast and keeps it entirely for himself'. Among the Zambian Ndembu, a hunter who eats his kills is likened to a cannibal, suspected of incest and believed to be quite capable of killing his own human kin by sorcery to consume their 'meat' or 'flesh' (Turner 1957: 141, 252). Finally, among the West African Ashanti, many game animals had a dangerous *sasa* or soul; a 'hunter who kills a *sasa* animal may not himself eat its meat' (Rattray 1927: 184). The Ashanti material additionally suggests a native conceptual link between the own-kill rule and the local rule of matrilineal clan exogamy – defined as the prohibition against 'the eating up of one's own blood' (Rattray 1929: 303).

The Own-kill Rule in South America

The 'custom of the hunter's not eating the game he kills' prevailed in eastern and southern Brazil in several tribes 'with a typical hunter culture' (Baldus 1952). In seeking an explanation, Baldus (1952: 197) notes the Kraho belief in a supernatural relationship between the hunter and his prey. The 'strength' of the hunter is said to be transmitted through the arrow or spear

> like his 'blood' entering the animal. This would cause such weakness in a young person that the spirit of the animal could easily take possession of the spirit of the hunter and destroy it if the abstention from eating the meat and ritualistic treatment were not applied to the killer.

Eating one's own kill, then, would in effect involve eating one's own 'blood'.

The Guayaki of eastern Paraguay, writes Clastres (1972: 168–70), are 'hunters par excellence'. They observe 'a food taboo which dictates that a hunter cannot eat his own take from the hunt. Neither he nor his parents are allowed to eat the meat he brings into camp . . . '. If a hunter were to eat his own kill, his luck would leave him, a condition known as *pané*. Because women reject husbands or lovers who lack hunting luck, loss of *pané* amounts to sexual impotence. The fear in this context 'is a veritable anguish', writes Clastres, and every man scrupulously avoids taking any risk that might cause it. As if to ward off the always possible evil, each gives away as much meat as he can, and unceasingly dwells on his hunting exploits and good hunting luck. Every young boy aspires to become a great hunter, a virile lover – a man of good luck. The taboo against eating one's own kill is therefore powerfully motivated, and is indeed the most important rule on which the whole culture is based. The social life of the Guayaki, as Clastres puts it, 'is organized around this taboo. . . . ' In a conclusion clearly modelled on Lévi-Strauss's (1969a) treatment of the incest taboo, Clastres concludes his discussion by describing the rule as the 'fundamental law' of Guayaki society.

The own-kill norm in South America is in fact widespread, indicating its universality as a point of departure from which varying totemic and other traditions have been derived.

We may begin a more general survey in the Amazonian rain forest, with the Yanomami. Here, generosity is an essential prerequisite of hunting success:

> Hunters do not eat the meat of game they have killed themselves, for any man who does so will, the Yanomami believe, be deserted by the hawk spirit which must enter him if he is to thrive in the chase. (Hanbury-Tenison 1982: 95)

If hunting with other men, the killer will not even carry his catch back to the communal house, but surrenders everything at once. At home, the recipient will then distribute the meat to his own network of relatives. The original hunter will not go hungry, however, 'for the man to whom he gave his kill will generally reciprocate by offering in return his own bag' (Hanbury-Tenison 1982: 95).

In the case of the Bororo of central Brazil:

> the hunter never roasts the meat he has shot himself, but gets someone else to do it for him. Failure to observe this taboo, as well as failure to carry out the propitiatory ceremony (the so-called 'blessing'), causes the vengeful animal spirit to send sickness and death to the hunter and all those who eat of its flesh. (Zerries 1968: 272, citing Steinen 1894: 491)

Lévi-Strauss (1977, 1: 109) notes that before a large animal could be eaten, the Bororo shaman had to consecrate it with a special ritual of biting and shrieking lasting several hours. Should anyone touch unconsecrated meat, he and his entire tribe would perish. A connection between the Bororo own-kill rule and matrilineal moiety exogamy is suggested by Crocker (1985: 166), who comments that the meat transactions which follow from a collective hunt may be regarded 'as an elaborate metaphoric parallel to the exchange of feminine sexuality between the moieties'.

Among the Urubu (at the south-eastern limit of the Amazonian basin), 'the man who kills an animal leaves the cutting up to one of his companions . . . '. He keeps for himself only the head and spine. The best pieces he gives to relatives such as his brothers-in-law, whilst if there is anything left over the others in the village get it (Huxley 1957: 78, 85–6). The man who kills a deer may not bring it into the village himself. He lays down the meat at the edge of the clearing 'and sends his wife to get it or, if he has no wife, another woman, or even a man who has not been hunting that day'. A hunter who brought his own game into the village would be punished with a terrible fever and become *kaú*, crazy (Huxley 1957: 83–4).

Rules of this kind – taboos preventing a man from fetching his kills beyond a certain point – illustrate how sexual boundaries mapped out spatially can function in support of the own-kill norm. The Desana (of the Columbian North-west Amazon) provide a further example:

> When returning from the forest, the hunter deposits the dead animal near the entrance of the maloca, and it is then taken in by the women; if the hunt took place in a site accessible only by river, he leaves the dead animal in his canoe at the landing and goes to the maloca to tell the women.

In no circumstances should the man carry the animal into the maloca, whether this is represented by the door of the dwelling or the canoe at the landing: both form a threshold, a limit between two spheres of activities, that must be very strictly observed: 'To this point, but no further, can the hunter act; once this threshold is crossed, the prey enters the feminine sphere where it will be transformed into food' (Reichel-Dolmatoff 1968: 231).

The Desana explicitly link incest/exogamy with hunting taboos. 'It can be said', according to Reichel-Dolmatoff (1968: 67), 'that the law of exogamy refers not only to society but also to its symbolic complement, the animals'.

Among the Trio of northern Brazil and southern Surinam a married man does not keep the game he brings home but gives it to his wife who, in turn, hands it over to her kin. 'Normally, at a communal meal, a man does not eat meat which he himself has killed.' The initial transfer of meat is almost always between affines (Rivière 1969: 214, 214n, 220). In the case of the Waiwai, along the frontiers of Guiana and Brazil, an informant told Fock (1963: 121) that when he was a young man he never ate any meat (apart from tapir flesh) that he himself had killed, believing 'that he would lose his aim if he consumed his own bag'. Finally, we can end our brief world survey of assorted statements with a note on the Kraho of the eastern highlands of Brazil. Here, the mythical culture hero Kenkunan teaches respect for the taboos on which a successful hunt depends:

> The hunter must not eat the game he himself has killed or, if he eats it, he must at least postpone the act of consumption in two ways which are complementary to each other: in time, by allowing the meat to become cold; and in space, by taking care not to grasp it with his naked hands, but to pick it up on the pointed end of a stick. (Lévi-Strauss 1973: 145, citing Schultz 1950: 108)

'Totemism' and Anthropology

We have glimpsed 'totemism' as something inseparable from that 'spirit of the gift' which animates economic life in all hunter-gatherer and other pre-'civilised' cultural traditions (Mauss 1954). Unfortunately, in the classical literature, totemism was not looked upon in such terms. It was not seen as the cognitive and social outcome of a very practical principle of *ritualised gift-giving and exchange*. Instead, assumptions about private property were made, whilst hunters' rules of 'respect' or 'avoidance' were interpreted in terms of western concepts of religious 'worship' or 'spirituality', eventually to become dissolved into Lévi-Strauss' mystical concept of an anonymous and impersonal universal human 'mind'.

Totemism was put on the scientific map for the first time when J. F. McLellan (1869) published two short articles entitled 'The worship of animals and plants'. McLellan proposed that primitive peoples believe in the sanctity and mystical powers of animals and plants, and that 'there is no race of men that has not come through this primitive stage of speculative belief' (1869: 423). Over the next few decades, this view came to dominate most European and American social anthropology, and was developed into an elaborate scheme linking (a) mythological beliefs, (b) food prohibitions, (c) exogamy and (d) 'the matriarchal stage of culture' (Haddon 1902: 7n). One of the most ambitious and influential works in this spirit was Durkheim's (1965 [1912]) *The Elementary Forms of the Religious Life* which treated totemism as humanity's most primitive form of religion.

Modern studies of totemism, however, date from an article in the *Journal of American Folklore* by Boas' student, Goldenweiser (1910). This author concluded that 'the group of phenomena which in various areas have been termed "totemic"' are in fact 'conglomerates of essentially independent features' (p. 266). The exogamy rule had no necessary connection with seemingly associated food taboos. On the one hand, 'taboos, whether totemic or not, permit of a great variety of origins' (p. 258), while on the other, the 'conditions under which exogamy may develop are practically innumerable' (p. 265). Instead of an integral totemic logic operating on different levels at once, Goldenweiser saw only isolated fragments thrown together by history and chance. The essay caught the mood of the times. Lévi-Strauss (1969b: 73) points out that 'in the end Goldenweiser's 110 pages were to exercise a more lasting theoretical influence than the 2,000 pages in Frazer's four volumes' on totemism which were published in the same year.

Defining an Illusion

Lévi-Strauss' *Totemism* (English edition, 1969b) was published in France in 1962, as was *The Savage Mind* (English edition, 1966). The two books were essentially two volumes of a single work, their joint purpose being – on the surface, at least – to endorse Goldenweiser's findings and deliver the *coup de grâce* to 'totemism' as a subject of study. It can be seen, however, that what Lévi-Strauss really set out to achieve was a more subtle victory. His aim was to justify his own reluctance to develop a theoretical framework specifically to analyse the ritual domain.

In the two volumes, Lévi-Strauss does two things. Firstly, he describes totemism as an arbitrary category invented by nineteenth-century thinkers – 'an artificial unity, existing solely in the mind of the anthropologist, to which nothing specifically corresponds in reality' (1969b: 79). Secondly, treating totemism as cognition or thought, he defines it as a mode of classification, qualifying this immediately by terming it 'not even a mode of classification, but an aspect or moment of it' (1966: 218).

In relation to this second point, he claims that totemic classifications are really no different from other forms of classification (1966: 162–3). All human beings classify things in essentially similar ways, conceptualising similarities and differences in binary terms and by reference to familiar categories drawn from various spheres of experience (1966: 135). When people in traditional cultures identify hunted animals as 'kin' – or (to put this another way) identify their clans or exogamous groups with various species of animals – they are doing no more than that. They have simply found a convenient way of using the differences between animal species as a way of conceptualising the distinctions between human social groups. From totemism we can learn nothing about the past of humankind, for even to the extent that totemism is real, 'there is nothing archaic or remote about it' (1969b: 177). We are all using totemic modes of thought all the time – or, alternatively, it could be said that to define thought as 'totemic' means nothing at all. Lévi-Strauss in this way dissolves into thin air the study of most of the ritual distinctions, taboos and observances previously linked together as 'totemic'. As Edmund Leach (1965: 24) put it,

> In its new guise 'totemism', as such, really disappears; it becomes just one specialised variety of a universal human activity, the classification of social phenomena by means of categories derived from the non-social human environment.

Now, if Lévi-Strauss were simply suggesting a helpful redefinition of 'totemism' as a category – restricting it henceforward to the mental activity of allocating names to social groups – the usefulness or otherwise of this new definition could perhaps profitably be debated. Unfortunately, Lévi-Strauss never tells us that he is simply redefining 'totemism' as a term. Following Goldenweiser, he argues instead that 'the facts' themselves indicate the lack of any internal connection between the previously linked phenomena.

Most importantly, Lévi-Strauss insists that in the ethnographic record itself there is no sign of any intrinsic connection between kinship-linked 'naming systems' and 'food taboos'. Naming systems (he asserts) are 'mental': in them, animal species are chosen, not because they are 'good to eat' or 'good to prohibit' but because they are 'good to think', the differences between one species and another providing the human intellect with a useful model through which to conceptualise distinctions between human categories of kin. Entirely separate are 'food taboos', which revolve around the natural and/or cultural edibility of different species of animals and plants. It was a profound mistake of earlier generations of anthropologists, alleges Lévi-Strauss, to have confused the two.

In arguing this point, *Totemism* begins with a discussion of the Ojibwa Indians, as most treatises on 'totemism' do (*ototeman* being an Ojibwa word). We are told almost immediately that 'all the food tabus reported from the Ojibway derive from the *manido* system', which is 'entirely distinct from the system of totemic names' (1969b: 90). In other words, the fact that a man belongs, say, to the Bear 'totem' need in no way make him feel guilty about hunting and eating bears. Although this statement is directly contradicted by Long (1791: 86), whose account of Chippewa and Ojibwa 'superstition' first brought the expression 'totamism' into print, Lévi-Strauss disposes of this problem without difficulty. Long was obviously 'confused' (Lévi-Strauss 1969b: 92).

Turning to Tikopia, the author enumerates a list of food taboos which most previous writers had been content to label 'totemic'. But Lévi-Strauss will not allow food prohibitions to be in any way 'confused' with totemic naming systems. He states – as if this were a matter of simple fact, rather than of definition – that the prohibitions are 'not . . . of a totemic character'.

As evidence, he offers the fact that among the Tikopia the food prohibitions seem to give expression to a principle of exchange. For example, when a dolphin is stranded on the beach, members of its affiliated lineage make it a *putu* or 'offering on the grave of a person recently deceased'. The meat is then cooked and everyone joins in eating it, 'with the exception of the kin group in question, for which it is *tapu* because the dolphin is the preferred form of incarnation of their *atua* [spirit]' (1969b: 97).

This presents a problem for Lévi-Strauss. A totemic kinship identification or affiliation is here indisputably *linked with a food taboo*. Those who avoid eating dolphin flesh do so *because* they identify, in kinship terms, with the dolphin. People are not willing to eat what is, in some sense, 'their own flesh'.

The Tikopia ethnography is rich in examples of this kind. But after discussing some taboos against eating various fish, birds and bats, Lévi-Strauss declares that the solution is simple:

These prohibitions, which may be either general or limited to a clan or lineage, are not, however, of a totemic character: the pigeon, which is closely connected with Taumako clan, is not eaten, but there are no scruples against killing it, because it plunders the gardens. Moreover, the prohibition is restricted to the first-born. (1969b: 96)

It is difficult to know how to respond to this. We are here introduced, quite without prior warning, to two new rules by means of which food prohibitions can be declared to be 'not . . . of a totemic character'. They are not of a totemic character when people are allowed to kill an animal which they nevertheless will not eat; and the eating taboos are not of a totemic character when they are 'restricted to the first-born'. What possible grounds can there be for such seemingly arbitrary pronouncements?

There is no need to follow Lévi-Strauss as he surveys the world, carefully excluding peoples' food avoidances from what he calls their 'totemism' – and attacking all previous writers who had 'confused' matters by linking food taboos with kinship names and rules. The real question is not whether we should define food taboos or avoidances as 'totemic'. What matters is whether the earlier writers were correct to perceive some unity of principle linking (a) the identification of oneself or one's clan with a natural species which is thought of as 'kin' and (b) the idea that a creature defined as 'kin' – as one's own flesh or substance – is not to be selfishly appropriated or consumed. It is here argued that there is a profound internal logic – as universal in its way as the 'incest rule' – connecting these two. Lévi-Strauss' argument is that we have no reason to suppose any such connection at all.

To speak of someone as 'my own flesh' means, in many languages of the world, that the person concerned is a close relative, usually by 'blood'. The Peruvian Sharanahua say 'my kin, my flesh' (Siskind 1973a: 54). Both in Hebrew and in Arabic, 'flesh' was traditionally synonymous with 'clan' or kindred group; kinship meant 'participation in a common mass of flesh, blood and bones . . . ' (Robertson-Smith 1914: 274). Among the Trobriand Islanders (Malinowski 1922: 191), matrilineal kinship means collective 'identity of flesh'. When Trobriand men learn that a sister has just had a child, they feel that an addition to their own bodies has been made: 'The kinsmen rejoice, for their bodies become stronger when one of their sisters or nieces has plenty of children.' Malinowski (1932: 170) comments that the wording of this statement 'expresses the interesting conception of collective clan unity, of the members being not only of the same flesh, but almost forming one body'.

It is significant that among the Trobrianders, the concept of *bomala*, 'taboo', is likewise identified with the very body or kindred of the person observing the taboo. Writes Malinowski (1932: 388–9; quoted in Fortes 1966: 18):

This noun takes the pronominal suffixes of nearest possession . . . . which signifies that a man's taboo, the things which he must not eat or touch or do, is linguistically bound up with his person; parts of his body, his kindred, and such personal qualities as his mind (*nanala*), his will (*magi'la*) and his inside (*lopoula*). Thus *bomala*, those things from which a man must keep away, is an integral part of his personality, something which enters his moral make-up.

A man must 'keep away' from a whole series of female relatives – his 'flesh' – and also from certain kinds of food. In either case, he is 'keeping away' from something which is 'his own' – as if it were a part of himself.

Turning to Australia, according to Elkin (1933: 118n), 'the usual word for totem in north-eastern South Australia means flesh'. Among the Wotjobaluk of south-east Australia, Howitt (1904: 145) found that 'the group totem is called by the terms *Mir, Ngirabul*, and *Yauruk*, the latter word meaning flesh, frequently expanded into *Yauruk-gologeitch*, that is, "flesh-of-all"'. Among the Buandik, according to the same author (p. 146):

> A man would not kill or use for food any of the animals of the same subdivision with himself, excepting when compelled by hunger, and then he expresses sorrow for having to eat his *Wingong* (friend), or *Tumung* (his flesh). When using the latter word, the Buandik touch their breasts to indicate close relationship, meaning almost a part of themselves.

Elkin (1933: 136–7) likewise writes of what he terms 'matrilineal social clan totemism', which he identifies in most of Queensland, New South Wales, Western Victoria and eastern South Australia. Over this vast area, one's matrilineal clan relatives 'are one flesh, for all have ultimately received their body, their means of incarnation, from and through the womb of the same matrilineal ancestress'. Further, continues Elkin, because the totem – identified with the matrilineal ancestress – is also one's flesh, in many tribes it is neither injured, killed nor eaten, except on very rare occasions of hunger and after regret and sorrow have been expressed. A person respects the symbol, the 'flesh' of his mother's line. Elkin immediately adds:

> Likewise, the exogamy of the matrilineal social totemic clan is observed, for it is based on the fundamental aboriginal incest laws, which forbid marriage with sister or mother, and all who belong to the one totem, being one flesh, are brothers and sisters, or children and mothers.

Avoidance of totemic meat and avoidance of female relatives are, then, equally the avoidance of 'one's own flesh'.

In fact, the evidence suggests a cross-cultural pattern in which totemic food avoidances are in some sense avoidances of the self. If one's 'taboo' or 'totem' is not one's 'meat' or 'blood' or 'flesh' in the most literal sense, it is at least one's 'spirit', 'substance' or 'essence'. And the crucial point is that the 'self', however conceived, is not to be appropriated by the self. It is for others to enjoy.

According to this logic, a man's sisters are inseparable from himself and, sexually, they are therefore for others to take as sexual partners. A man's hunting products – the game animals which he kills – are likewise inseparable from himself, and are his own flesh, his own blood, or his own essence which he is not allowed to eat. Not two rules are in force but only one: the rule against 'eating one's own flesh'. This conceptual simplification has obviously been achieved by countless traditional cultures, for again and again we find the two kinds of prohibition – dietary and sexual – simply equated. A woman who 'ate', sexually, her own son or younger brother, would be doing the same thing, in principle, as a man who ate his own totem or the game animals he killed himself. Both would be 'eating their own flesh'. They would be appropriating their own produce – conceived as a part of themselves – for their own private use.

At a deep level, then, in many traditional cultures, there are not two or several conceptualised rules of exchange but only one: the rule against 'eating one's own blood' or 'eating one's own flesh' or 'self'. There is no separate thing called 'totemism'. There is not even any special term for what Europeans have labelled a 'totem'. In the native languages, the term for 'totem' is simply the term for 'meat' or 'flesh' – or perhaps some other aspect of the social or collective 'self'. In this connection it is worth remembering that our very word 'totemism' is derived from an Ojibwa expression which means nothing exotic at all, but simply 'uterine kin':

> *Totem*: irregularly derived from the term *ototeman* of the Chippewa and other cognate Algonquian dialects, signifying, generically, 'his brother-sister kin', of which *ote* is the grammatic stem signifying (1) the consanguine kinship existing between a propositus and a uterine elder sister or elder brother; and (2) the consanguine kinship existing between uterine brothers and sisters. (Hewitt in Hodge 1910: 2, 787–8)

Would it, then, clear away much confusion if we were to cease to speak of 'totemism' at all, and to refer instead to the 'own-flesh' rule? In the light of many ethnographies, the temptation to do this becomes strong.

Let us take, for example, Margaret Mead's set of aphorisms obtained from the Arapesh, to which Lévi-Strauss gives prominence in *The Elementary Structures of Kinship* (1969a: 27, citing Mead 1935: 83):

Your own mother,
Your own sister,
Your own pigs,
Your own yams that you have piled up,
You may not eat.
Other people's mothers,
Other people's sisters,
Other people's pigs,

Other people's yams that they have piled up,
You may eat.

It would seem unnecessarily confusing to refer to this as a form of 'totemism'. Admittedly, contained here are virtually all the usual 'features' of totemism, for we have (1) a set of sexual taboos, (2) a linked set of food taboos, (3) a system of classification of the social universe matched precisely by (4) a system of classification of edible parts of the natural universe. Finally, there are contained here, at least implicitly, (5) the idea of a man's intimate connection with his 'mothers' and 'sisters' matched by (6) belief in his equally intimate connection with the animals he has killed, the pigs he owns or the foods he has otherwise produced. Yet it seems unnecessarily laborious to describe this as a set of various *different* rules and concepts corresponding more or less closely to what anthropologists once described as 'totemism'. It is crystal clear that to the Arapesh, there is only one rule involved, not an assemblage of different ones, and that the simple point is that one's own 'flesh' (in the sense already defined here) is for others to consume or enjoy.

The unity of principle involved here – the equation of own kin with own produce, so that one's own produce 'is' one's kin – is so widespread that it is acknowledged as a virtual universal by Lévi-Strauss himself. He refers to Australia as a place 'where food prohibitions and rules of exogamy reinforce one another' (1966: 111), and treats both kinds of rules as exchange rules with similar functions: 'Both the exchange of women and the exchange of food are means of securing or of displaying the interlocking of social groups with one another' (1966: 109). In a more general context, in *The Elementary Structures of Kinship* (1969a: 32–3), he writes that marriage prohibitions represent only a particular application, within a given field, of principles and methods encountered whenever the physical or spiritual existence of the group is at stake. The group controls the distribution not only of women, but of a whole collection of valuables:

> Food, the most easily observed of these, is more than just the most vital commodity it really is, for between it and women there is a whole system of real and symbolic relationships, whose true nature is only gradually emerging, but which, when even superficially understood, are enough to establish this connection.

He observes that there 'is an analogy between sexual relations and eating in all societies' (1966: 130). And writing of 'certain Burmese peoples', Lévi-Strauss (1969a: 33) comments on 'the extent to which the native mind sees matrimonial and economic exchanges as forming an integral part of a basic system of reciprocity', adding that the 'methods for distributing meat in this part of the world are no less ingenious than for the distribution of women'.

Lévi-Strauss' statement that between culinary exchanges and sexual ones 'there is a whole system of real and symbolic relationships, whose true nature is only gradually emerging' suggests that he felt the temptation to analyse totemic food taboos as exchange rules, following the method he was demonstrating so effectively in *The Elementary Structures of Kinship*. Yet when, after a long pause, he came to his study of totemism, Lévi-Strauss chose not to take this course. While he admitted that food taboos and rules of exogamy were connected, he insisted: 'The connection between them is not causal but metaphorical' (1966: 105). He insisted that 'food prohibitions are not a distinctive feature of totemism' (1966: 129), and argued that all exchanges on the model of the Australian *Intichiuma* rituals pertained only to metaphor and the realms of the mind. As he put it:

> marriage exchanges always have real substance, and they are alone in this. The exchange of food is a different matter. Aranda women really bear children. But Aranda men confine themselves to imagining that their rites result in the increase of totemic species. In the former . . . what is in question is primarily a way of doing something. In the latter it is only a way of saying something. (1966: 110)

In this passage Lévi-Strauss seems to be unequivocal in stating that food exchanges, unlike marital ones, are unreal. Yet he cannot have been unaware of the fact that in hunter-gatherer cultures at least, the universality of bride-service renders meaningless any attempt to disentangle 'exchanges of women' from economic exchanges such as those of meat or other food.

Lévi-Strauss can give plausibility to his case only by concentrating on the theme of erroneous belief. Hence, for Lévi-Strauss, totemism represents only a 'purported reciprocity' (1966: 125). In rituals such as the Australian *Intichiuma*, each totemic group 'imagines itself to have magical power over a species, but as this illusion has no foundation it is in fact no more than an empty form . . .' (1966: 125). Or, even more caustically:

> Totemic groups certainly give an imitation of gift-giving which has a function. But, apart from the fact that it remains imaginary, it is not cultural either since it must be classed, not among the arts of civilization, but as a fake usurpation of natural capacities which man as a biological species lacks. (1966: 126)

Totemism, according to Lévi-Strauss, may look superficially like a system of economic division of labour, as in a caste system. But the appearance of functional value is purely illusory. Each totemic group in an Aranda *Intichiuma* ceremony claims to make available supplies of its totem species for other groups, just as each caste in a caste system practises 'a distinctive activity, indispensable to the life and well-being of the whole group'. However, 'a caste of potters really makes pots, a caste of launderers really washes clothes, a caste of barbers really shaves people, while the magical powers of Australian totemic groups are of an imaginary kind' (1966: 122). Lévi-Strauss hangs his case on the fact that, while women really produce babies, groups of men in totemic rituals do not really produce game animals. *Therefore* the only 'true reciprocity' is the sexual and procreative kind. The meat-producing reciprocity is only a 'fake usurpation' *because the magic does not really work.*

By means such as these, Lévi-Strauss manages to destroy altogether the unity of principle underlying the various aspects of Australian totemic and matrimonial exchanges. It is a sleight-of-hand allowing him to dismiss bride-service exchanges, marriage gifts, feasts and so on as related only in a 'metaphorical' way to the 'exchange of women', which alone has 'real substance'. The entire field of human social existence is bisected into 'ways of doing things' and 'ways of saying things'. As far as 'ways of doing things' are concerned, exchange is said to be reducible to the sexual aspects of exogamy, which provide the 'basis' for all other forms of culture and exchange. *The Elementary Structures of Kinship*, the implication runs, has said in principle everything that needs to be said on that subject. If Lévi-Strauss is to say any more about anything, therefore, he must turn to 'ways of saying things'. And if this is to be done, it is best to leave ritual aside and go straight to the heart of matters. Leaving all his earlier work behind him, Lévi-Strauss turns to myths and the world of the mind.

In effect, this meant the abandonment of Lévi-Strauss' most powerful earlier arguments – those stressing that exchange as such was the essence of human social life. It was a damaging blow to our understanding of culture. Had Lévi-Strauss chosen to link his 'exchange of women' concept in a materialistic way with the realities of economic circulation and exchange, a unified theory might have been produced. So-called 'totemism' could then have been interpreted as an expression of exchange. Once it had been realised that 'incest taboos' could be applied to meat or other food, the logic of treating natural species as 'kin' – the essence of 'totemism' – would no longer have seemed either mysterious or illusory. Kinship, ritual and mythology could all have been treated as expressions of exchange of one and the same kind, albeit manifested on different levels and in different ways according to circumstances. Instead of a complete rupture between the study of kinship and the study of myths – the study of 'life' and the study of 'thought' – there might then have been some real inner unity and coherence to Lévi-Strauss' life's work as a whole.

Why did not Lévi-Strauss follow such a course? The problem is tantalizing because evidently the founder of structuralism appreciated that *The Elementary Structures* had been well received precisely because it promised such unity. It is clear that Lévi-Strauss glimpsed the reality of the 'own-flesh' rule, and glimpsed the possibility of treating this rule, as he had treated the incest rule, as the expression of an exchange principle through which an immense mass of seemingly irrational 'taboos' and 'customs' could be reduced to an intelligible system. So why did he fail to take advantage of this clue, fail to follow up the logic that he himself had revealed and fail to link his studies of myths with the study of kinship systems that he had already begun? Why did he have to violate so insistently not only the unity of the evidence of ethnology itself but also the conceptual unity at first promised by *The Elementary Structures*?

The answer seems clear, and takes us back to our discussion in the previous chapter. Had this course not been taken, the study of mythological beliefs would have been tied in inextricably with the study of structures of ritual, economic and sexual exchange. The whole of Lévi-Strauss' argument about the existence of a general human 'mind' acting independently and determining, godlike, the structures discernible beneath human beliefs, customs and institutions – this whole argument might have risked seeming unnecessary or even absurd. For once it had been conceded that kinship systems were explicable without recourse to such a 'mind', then any admission that ritual and mythological systems were explicable in similar terms would have posed a threat. If practical, material social life – exchange as something tangible, institutional and real – could be seen to produce structuralism's 'binary oppositions' on all levels, economic as well as sexual, ritual as well as mythological, then what remaining role could have been found for the Lévi-Straussian 'mind'?

The Phoenix 'Totemism'

Goldenweiser's 1910 complaint about 'totemism' was that it was an artificial construct:

> On the basis of material furnished by some one area or a number of areas, a definite group of features is called 'totemism'. Another totemic area is discovered where an additional feature is found, or where one of the old ones is missing. Immediately the questions arise (and here we are on historical ground), Is *this* totemism? or Was *that* totemism? or Is *this* true totemism and *that* was *incompletely developed*, totemism *im Werden*? or Was *that* true totemism and *this* is a *later development*? In the light of the foregoing discussion, any definite answer to these questions must needs be arbitrary. (Goldenweiser 1910: 267–8)

If totemism includes, 'roughly speaking, everything' (Goldenweiser continued), is totemism itself anything in particular? Is there anything specific in this phenomenon, or has the name 'totemism' simply been applied to one set of features here, to another set there, and still elsewhere perhaps to both sets combined? (p. 267).

It is easy to appreciate how valuable this scepticism later appeared to Lévi-Strauss when – on the verge of embarking upon his *Mythologiques* – he was seeking theoretical justification for his decision to avoid analysing (to use Goldenweiser's words) 'roughly speaking, everything' intermediary between kinship systems and myths. If the unity of principle underlying the entire spectrum of 'totemic' phenomena could be declared an illusion, then Lévi-Strauss could feel justified in denying any need to discuss this unity or account for it. He could proceed without further ado from the study of kinship systems to the study of myths. 'Roughly speaking, everything' in between could be equated with 'totemism', and this in turn – thanks to Goldenweiser – could be treated as an illusory phenomenon.

In Lévi-Strauss' work, the attack on totemism is so emotionally charged as to indicate extraordinary depths of feeling on the issue – feelings which the surface problematic of *Totemism* in no way equips the reader to expect. He tells us that totemism is not only a 'fake usurpation'; it is also 'like hysteria', in that it is an invention of bigots aiming to contrast themselves with 'savages' just as late nineteenth-century doctors and psychologists contrasted themselves with the 'insane' (1969b: 69). Such is his hostility that he cautions against even mentioning the subject without due precautions being taken:

> To accept as a theme for discussion a category that one believes to be false always entails the risk, simply by the attention that is paid to it, of entertaining some illusion about its reality . . . for in attacking an ill-founded theory the critic begins by paying it a kind of respect. The phantom which is imprudently summoned up, in the hope of exorcising it for good, vanishes only to reappear, and closer than one imagines to the place where it was at first. (p. 83)

Such anxieties indicate the real significance of Lévi-Strauss' encounter with the totemic problem. 'Totemism' simply *had* to be eliminated or at least neutralised ('exorcised'). Lévi-Strauss' impending mythological project depended upon it. It was absolutely essential that the unity underlying totemic phenomena was broken into fragments, leaving as a common residue only the fact that all systems of human belief and ritual are in some sense products of one and the same kind of human brain. The demolition job was conducted with energy. Yet the very vigour of this 'exorcism' indicates just how much damage would be done to Lévi-Strauss' entire system if, after all, it could be shown that the unity of principle against which he was struggling had some life and force in it still. If it could be demonstrated that a few simple principles or rules in fact suffice to generate the worldwide totality of possible kinship structures, ritual structures and myth structures alike, then the genuinely bogus 'phantom' in all this might at last have been laid to rest. The illusion of the human mind as an independent, world-governing force, its patterns of motion emanating directly from the arrangement of cells and connections given genetically in the brain – this most bizarre of delusions might no longer seem required.

I would concede at once: Goldenweiser was correct. It is impossible to classify the varieties of ritual action in a satisfactory way by assuming that there is a 'thing' called 'totemism', another 'thing' called, say, 'sacrifice', another called 'rituals of atonement', and so on. The borderlines between these supposedly distinct phenomena will always be confused. To take a particular form of ritual prohibition and try to decide whether it constitutes 'totemism' or not (which is, ironically, precisely what Lévi-Strauss does when he declares certain food prohibitions to be 'not of a totemic character') is an exercise of limited value. Is *this* totemism, or is *that* totemism? – the question, as Goldenweiser understood, will usually admit of no very satisfactory answer. But this is not because there is no unity of principle underlying the dimensions of variability of totemic ritual in traditional cultures. It is, on the contrary, because the unity of principle is far more fundamental and universal than can possibly be consistent with the various arbitrarily drawn distinctions between what is 'totemism' and what is not, what is 'sacrifice' and what is not, what is an 'atonement ritual' and what is something else.

The Nuer, Sacrifice and the Own-kill Rule

In *The Savage Mind*, Lévi-Strauss (1966: 224) goes to great lengths to explain the 'fundamental differences between the system of totemism and that of sacrifice'. He is adamant that 'the two systems are mutually exclusive' (p. 223). He is insistent that while 'totemism' is only an illusion, 'sacrifice' is an 'institution' and perfectly real (p. 223). I now want to show, on the contrary, that rituals of sacrifice constitute not a separate 'system' characteristic of countless cultures and religions but only so many *other* ways of expressing the principle that one's own 'flesh' is for others to consume or enjoy. They constitute only one portion of a continuous spectrum of rituals relating to animal or human 'meat' or 'flesh', other portions of this spectrum corresponding to 'totemism', 'atonement rituals', 'hunters' taboos', 'increase rites', blood avoidances, 'menstrual taboos', cooking rules, 'the couvade', 'male initiation rites' – and so on almost indefinitely. 'Totemism' is not an institution – any more than 'sacrifice' is. Both concepts correspond to realities embodied in almost countless religious and cultural institutions which grade into each other smoothly when properly analysed.

The Nuer of the Sudan abide rigidly by the 'own-flesh' rule. That is, they will not kill cattle in order to eat the meat themselves. Evans-Pritchard writes, in fact, that 'an ox slain simply from desire for meat may *cien*, take ghostly vengeance on, its slayer . . . ' (1956: 265). Life is taken only when it is really necessary, and then the reason is explained carefully not only to God but often to the ox itself. The Nuer 'address the ox and tell it why it is being killed – not that they think it understands. They are justifying themselves in taking its life' (p. 266).

To take life for *oneself* is not a sufficient reason. The life-taking must be for a higher good. When the Nuer are compelled to kill their cattle in times of famine, they make an invocation over the animals asking God that 'the meat may be soft in their stomachs and not bring them sickness'. Evans-Pritchard writes that this is not exactly sacrifice – the people are, after all, killing for the meat – 'but it shows that there is a feeling of guilt about killing animals for food even when hunger compels it' (p. 266). The taboo here is not merely against killing. It is a rule or feeling against killing-and-eating, or killing-to-eat. Killing in itself is perfectly moral, provided it is for the higher good. In fact, life-taking or life exchange is absolutely essential as a means of partaking in this higher good. Cattle are 'reserved for sacrifice' – which means that they are in a special way reserved to be killed – provided only that the killing involves self-sacrifice, renunciation and exchange (pp. 223–4; 266–9). Moreover, there is nothing wrong with eating the meat of the sacrificial victims: 'People show their desire for meat without reserve and it is the festal character of sacrifices which gives them much of their significance in the life of the Nuer.' In an aside indicating once more the reality of the own-flesh rule, Evans-Pritchard immediately adds: 'This is perhaps most noticeable at weddings, when, moreover, those who get the flesh are not those who sacrifice the animal' (p. 263). There is nothing wrong, then, with eating following a killing. The stipulation is simply that an exchange should first occur. The flesh should be consumed only *after* the 'life' of the animal has been received by God, and only on condition that those involved in the killing were acting upon motives transcending mere self-interest or desire for meat.

In the spirit of his times, the theologically motivated Evans-Pritchard goes out of his way to deny significant parallels between Nuer 'sacrifice' (with its apparent resonances in Judaeo-Christian belief) and the all-too-pagan 'totemism' of the same people. For him, Nuer 'sacrifice' is a very definitely demarcated thing, a basic ritual of the Nuer and 'an enactment of their most fundamental religious conceptions' (Evans-Pritchard 1956: 197). Other forms of flesh-giving or renunciation among the Nuer have nothing to do with it.

The Nuer, when no ox is available for sacrifice, sometimes treat a cucumber as if it were an ox, and 'sacrifice' that. This, according to Evans-Pritchard's definition of the term, *is* 'sacrifice'. But the Nuer also cast away lumps of tobacco, beads and other small pieces of property in minor troubles 'when there is a sudden danger for which immediate action is to be taken and there is no time for formalities, or when a man is in the bush and cannot lay his hands on a beast or even a cucumber' (p. 197). This is *not* 'sacrifice', although the intention is evidently similar (the suppliant 'asks God to take the offering and spare him') and although it is only for lack of an animal or cucumber that substitutes have to be found. Evans-Pritchard continues:

I exclude also the offering of beer or milk, poured in libation, often at the foot of a tethering peg to which a beast dedicated to some spirit is tied, by a very poor person who cannot afford animal sacrifices. (p. 197)

So when a person is too poor to afford an animal and has to make an offering of something cheaper instead – in association with an animal – this still does not count as 'sacrifice', even though clearly the poverty-stricken suppliant hopes or imagines that it does!

'The flesh of this animal is as my flesh, and its blood is the same as my blood', says a Shilluk king in making a sacrifice (Evans-Pritchard 1956: 280). In his work on Nuer religion, Evans-Pritchard (1956: 279) notes that there is something universal about this logic: 'All gifts are symbols of inner states, and in this sense one can only give oneself; there is no other kind of giving.' It is a concept, he continues, which has often been expressed:

> But the idea is a very complex one. When Nuer give their cattle in sacrifice they are very much, and in a very intimate way, giving part of themselves. What they surrender are living creatures, gifts more express-ive of the self and with a closer resemblance to it than inanimate things, and these living creatures are the most precious of their possessions, so much so that they can be said to participate in them to the point of identification.

Why, following Evans-Pritchard, Lévi-Strauss (1966: 223) should consider this kind of identification and principle of 'self-giving' to be 'contrasting and incompatible' with identifications of a 'totemic' kind is difficult to under-stand. In each of the two cases – 'totemic' and 'sacrificial' – we have a renunciation of a certain kind of 'flesh' which is identified as in some sense 'one's own'. In each case, a principle of exchange is involved, displayed or concealed ('sacrifice' being, of course, an exchange with the gods). And in each case, the 'flesh' which is exchanged, respected or avoided by ordinary mortals acquires, in being so treated, the characteristics of something 'set apart', 'sacred' or 'divine'.

The Ojibwa Revisited

As mentioned earlier (see above, p. 106), Lévi-Strauss in his discussions on totemism frequently referred to the original account by James Long (1791: 86–7) in which the term 'totamism' first appeared in print. An Ojibwa Indian whose 'totam' was a Bear (according to Long) 'accidentally' killed a bear while on a hunting trip. He was later (according to the Indian's own account) accosted and scratched by an avenging bear who knocked him down and demanded an explanation for the crime. The bear accepted the explanation, promising that the Master of Life would not be angry with either the hunter or his tribe. But the Indian himself, on returning home, was filled with remorse and anxiety. He told Long: 'Beaver, my faith is lost, my *totam* is angry, I shall never be able to hunt any more.'

Tylor (1899: 140) and Frazer (1910, 3: 52) accused the unsophisticated interpreter and trader, Long, of having naively confused together two quite separate 'things', *and Lévi-Strauss (1969b: 90–2) follows them in this accusation.* Lévi-Strauss, accordingly, insists strenuously that the Ojibwa 'system of totemic names' must have been 'entirely distinct' from the system of guardian spirits of individuals – the '*manido* system.' This enables him to make his crucial point: 'All the food tabus reported from the Ojibwa derive from the *manido* system', not the totemic system. In other words, it was only a man's guardian spirit (*manido*) – something entirely distinct from a 'totem' – which he was forbidden to kill or eat. Contrary to Long's story, there was nothing to prevent a man of the Bear totem from killing and eating a bear.

Such is Lévi-Strauss' assertion. Yet despite his attack on 'the confusion between the totem and guardian spirit into which Long fell' (1969b: 92), Lévi-Strauss himself lets slip enough information to confirm the substance of Long's position. If we ignore the *emphasis* in the following sentence and simply concentrate on the facts, it can be seen that hunters had to be somewhat careful about killing and eating their totems. Lévi-Strauss (1969b: 89; citing Landes 1937) writes: 'The totem was freely killed and eaten, with certain ritual precautions, viz., that permission had first to be asked of the animal, and apologies to be made to it afterwards.'

Now, to say that a man can kill and eat his totem 'freely', and also to say that *he can only do so if he asks permission beforehand and apologises afterwards*, is to say two opposite and mutually exclusive things at the same time. If 'certain ritual precautions' were required before killing and eating a totem, then the statement: 'All the food tabus reported from the Ojibwa derive from the *manido* system' is simply not true.

In a eulogistic introduction to the English edition of Lévi-Strauss' *Totemism*, Roger Poole (1969b: 17–18) once again cites Tylor and Frazer in support of the accusation that Long had made a disastrous analytic blunder. Long had written that 'the Ojibwa refrain from killing their totems, when in fact what he should have said was that they refrained from killing their *manitoo*'. Yet, somewhat inconsistently, he continues:

The interesting thing to notice, however, is that both Tylor and Frazer are so *sure* about what 'totemism' is: they can even correct direct observers like Long from the wisdom of their researches. If Long gave a unitary version of what 'totemism' is, and if Tylor and Frazer pulled his single definition into two separate bits, it does not exonerate Tylor and Frazer from holding to another unitary conception of totemism themselves!

The difficulty for Poole, of course, is that if this pointed criticism applies to Tylor and Frazer, it must equally apply to Lévi-Strauss himself. Poole does not pursue this thought.

Conclusion: Totemism and Sacrifice

I want to turn, finally, to two more frequently cited cases from the classical literature. They are part-totemic, part-sacrificial, part-atonement rite. One case is from the Aino of north-east Asia and Japan, the other from the Australian Aranda.

'The Aino of Saghalien', writes Frazer (1926–36, 5, 2: 188–9; citing Labbe 1903: 227–58), 'rear bear cubs and kill them with . . . ceremonies'. The animal is kept for about two years in a cage, and then killed at a festival which always takes place in winter and at night. The day preceding the sacrifice is devoted to lamentation, old women taking turns in the duty of weeping and groaning in front of the bear's cage. Then in the middle of the night an orator makes a long speech to the beast, reminding him how they have taken care of him, and fed him well, and bathed him in the river, and made him warm and comfortable:

> 'Now', he proceeds, 'we are holding a great festival in your honour. Be not afraid. We will not hurt you. We will only kill you and send you to the god of the forest who loves you. We are about to offer you a good dinner, the best you have ever eaten among us, and we will all weep for you together. The Aino who will kill you is the best shot among us. There he is, he weeps and asks for your forgiveness; you will feel almost nothing, it will be done so quickly. . . . Remember', he cries, 'remember! I remind you of your whole life and of the services we have rendered you . . . tell the gods to give us riches, that our hunters may return from the forest laden with rare furs and animals good to eat; that our fishers may find troops of seals on the shore and in the sea, and that their nets may crack under the weight of the fish. . . . We have given you food and joy and health; now we kill you in order that you may in return send riches to us and to our children.

The basic principles of 'sacrifice' – of communion with the gods through the taking of life, of gift-giving to the divine powers in expectation of blessings in return – are here being expressed as clearly as among the cattle-owning Nuer.

The same can be said of the Australian Aranda attitude towards the *inarlinga* or spiny anteater. Reserved especially for the pleasure of the old men, it had to be killed considerately: if its nose bled, a short request for forgiveness had to be addressed to it, otherwise its soul 'would tell the stones of the hills to make the hunter's toenail come off and cause him to fall when he next hunted the euro' (Róheim 1974: 43–4). Likewise – to take an example more clearly 'totemic' in character – an Aranda hunter 'may kill his totem, but in doing so he must proceed humanely: a kangaroo man must not brutally attack the kangaroo "so that the blood gushes out", but is only permitted to hit it on the neck' (Goldenweiser 1910: 196–7). Equally significantly, we are told that having thus killed the animal, the hunter in this situation may eat its head, feet and liver: *the rest he must leave to his friends*. Once again, then, the need for meat-renouncing generosity towards others has become merged with and projected into a kind of 'respect' for the animal itself. Such examples may not be of 'sacrifice' in a strict sense (cf. Maddock 1985). But in all this, a man's 'respect' for his totemic species appears clearly as a self-denying ordinance limiting his right uninhibitedly to *kill and eat*.

It is true, as Lévi-Strauss stresses, that to identify an animal species as 'one's own flesh' is a cognitive act. But in this chapter we have seen that a moral and economic dimension is equally unmistakable. Moreover, in discussing materials of this kind, it seems impossible to decide exactly where 'sacrifice' ends and 'totemism' begins. In every case examined here, there are certain species to which certain rules apply. These rules imply gift-giving. They involve an offering up of 'one's own flesh' – flesh one has made one's own through an intimate act of identification – the gift flowing in some cases to animal souls, in others to the gods, in others to in-laws or other 'respected' social powers. Blessings of one kind or another are expected in return. The common core concept is that you may kill animals of the species concerned (or allow others to kill them), but not greedily, not without a conscience, and not merely to eat the meat yourself. To violate such an ethic is to invite fearsome retribution from the spirits and powers, however these may be conceived.

When Rodney Needham (1974: 42) resoundingly declared 'there is no such thing as kinship; and it follows that there can be no such thing as kinship theory', he was making a statement very like that of Lévi-Strauss in denying the reality of 'totemism'. But kinship studies did not thereupon come to a halt. We were simply invited to question the usefulness or otherwise of the term, 'kinship', along with some other seemingly basic anthropological terms and categories which we habitually and sometimes unthinkingly use. 'Totemism' in this light is only one of a number of partial, inadequate and misleading concepts which were coined by the nineteenth-century founders of anthropology. Like all of these concepts, it corresponds only in the most crude and clumsy way to anything which exists or has ever existed in the real world. In that sense, rather like 'kinship', 'marriage' or 'descent' (Needham 1974: 16, 42–3), totemism is an illusion which once existed and to some extent still exists in our heads. But 'totemism' is by no means the worst of these concepts, or the most misleading. And the fact that it creates certain illusions does not mean that behind and beyond its limitations nothing more substantial is there. Lévi-Strauss may well be correct in criticising a feature of anthropology's history as a discipline: the nineteenth-century inventors of 'totemism' were indeed – as he alleges – for the most part ethnocentric bigots. These thinkers delighted in presenting examples of the irrationality of the 'uncivilised' mind. They were mistaken – at least if it was implied that 'savages' are any more irrational than ourselves. But this does not mean that the founders of anthropology were mistaken to suspect a unity of principle underlying the various phenomena they took to be 'totemic'. Quite the reverse: the unity of principle underlying 'totemic' phenomena is *more* real, *more* astonishing and *more* significant than even the most ardent champions of totemism in the nineteenth century could ever have known.

'The hunter kills, other people have', say the Siberian Yukaghir, among whom the 'selfish' hunter risks losing his luck by angering the 'spirit-protector of the animals' (Jochelson 1926: 124–5). 'The society seems to want to extinguish in every way possible the concept of the meat belonging to the hunter', writes Marshall (1961: 238) of the !Kung Bushmen. Hayden (1981: 386), Dowling (1968), Sahlins (1974: 149–275), Ingold (1980: 158), Gould (1981: 435), Testart (1988: 10) and many others have likewise commented on the cross-cultural significance of such norms. The 'own-flesh' rule is not just a way of thinking or a magical belief: it points to a way of life pursued by humanity for millennia before the concept of private property was permitted to gain a hold. The unity of principle underlying 'totemism' links sex with food, kinship with economics, ritual with myth and thought with life with a simplicity too stunning to be attributed to chance or the random coming together of separate 'features'. And, when all is said and done, the old-fashioned word, 'totemism', with all the connotations, meanings and ambiguities which have been lent it by literary or anthropological usage over the years, still evokes this unity more tellingly than any other of the traditional expressions we have. The 'phantom' which Lévi-Strauss (1969b: 83) feared his own work might, despite himself, reawaken to life may indeed be impossible to exorcise. Von Brandenstein (1972) likened totemism to 'the old Egyptian Bennu bird which burned itself to death only to emerge from the ashes in the old form but with a new life essence'.

Chapter 4
The Sex Strike

The history of all hitherto existing society is the history of class struggles. Freeman and slave, patrician and plebeian, lord and serf, guild-master and journeyman, in a word, oppressor and oppressed, stood in constant opposition to one another, carried on an interrupted, now hidden, now open fight, a fight that each time ended either in a revolutionary reconstitution of society at large, or in the common ruin of the contending classes.

Karl Marx, The Communist Manifesto (1848)

The first class antagonism which appears in history coincides with the development of the antagonism between man and woman in monogamian marriage, and the first class oppression with that of the female sex by the male.

Friedrich Engels, The Origin of the Family, Private Property
and the State (1884)

I now want to address a question which Chapter 3 implicitly posed but left unanswered. Granted that 'totemism', 'sacrifice' and other rituals seem to have emerged through a historical process of transformation of the hunters' 'own-kill' rule — *where did this rule itself ultimately come from?*

Rather than keep my reader guessing, let me anticipate the conclusion and then set out my reasons for arriving at it. My answer is not difficult to state. Since mothers and their offspring must always have been the main beneficiaries of the 'own-kill' taboo, since men probably had no 'natural' (as opposed to cultural) inclination to abide by it, and since men's rewards for compliance appear to have been overwhelmingly marital and sexual — avoiding one's own kill must in some sense have been *motivated and established by women*. I will leave to future chapters the problem of how women could ever have had sufficient motivation or power to do this.

Lévi-Strauss holds men to have created culture. Where conscious, creative action is concerned, he sees not mixed human social groups but groups of men alone. These male groups establish the incest rule through an act of trust and generosity toward one another. Imposing upon themselves a sexual taboo, the men in each group surrender to others 'their own' women (sisters and daughters), hoping and trusting to receive back other women in return.

Lévi-Strauss is at pains to emphasise in this context what he terms 'a universal fact, that the relationship of reciprocity which is the basis of marriage is not established between men and women, but between men by means of women, who are merely the occasion of this relationship' (1969a: 116). Women, in other words, have no active role to play. Lévi-Strauss richly illustrates this model with examples from every continent, and declares it to lie at the basis of all culture.

Lévi-Strauss' 'exchange of women' model of cultural origins inspired a book which remains (despite all the criticisms) the most comprehensive and coherent cross-cultural analysis of kinship systems that social anthropology has achieved. Beginning with the simplest conceivable system of 'restricted exchange' – a system in which two groups of men exchange their sisters and/or daughters between themselves – Lévi-Strauss' *The Elementary Structures* showed how an immense variety of more elaborate systems can be conceptualised as systematic permutations and transformations worked upon this model.

The novelty of Lévi-Strauss' approach was that instead of merely examining the internal structure of descent groups, he visualised streams and currents of precious valuables – above all, women – flowing between groups in often immense cycles. A current of women would flow in one direction whilst, typically, another current of bride-wealth valuables (treated by Lévi-Strauss as less essential or merely symbolic) flowed in reverse. In the more open-ended, 'generalised' structures of sexual exchange, an extraordinary amount of inter-male trust was involved, as men in one group surrendered their most precious sexual and reproductive assets to another or several other groups in an extended chain, knowing or hoping that some time, some day, the system of reciprocity would ensure repayment in kind and the restoration of the temporarily forfeited imbalance. The participants' point of departure was a collective understanding that eventually – after in some cases many generations – the wheel should have turned full circle, with 'wife-givers' and 'wife-takers' having settled accounts. Where the number of male groups linked in each cycle was large, the streams of women functioned as continuous threads binding together into one coherent fabric groups of men dispersed widely over the landscape and stretched across several generations.

I have no wish to survey here the numerous criticisms which have been levelled at Lévi-Strauss' work on kinship. At this point I will simply return to Lévi-Strauss' point of departure – his 'exchange of women' model – and ask some questions posed by our previous discussion.

The 'value of exchange', writes Lévi-Strauss (1969a: 480),

> is not simply that of the goods exchanged. Exchange — and consequently
> the rule of exogamy which expresses it — has in itself a social value. It
> provides the means of binding men together, and of superimposing upon
> the natural links of kinship the henceforth artificial links — artificial in the
> sense that they are removed from chance encounters or the promiscuity of
> family life — of alliance governed by rule.

It is by means of exchange, then, that the 'natural' bonds of kinship are
overridden by the 'artificial' — that is, cultural — bonds of marriage.

A number of features characterise this model. Firstly, it is assumed that
links of 'blood' or kinship are 'natural'; it is only marital alliances which
establish the realm of culture. Culture is based neither on the biological
family, nor on links — however extended — through brothers, sisters or
parents and offspring. It arises exclusively out of the 'artificial' marriage links
forged between biological units — links which are produced by the incest
taboo and consequent need for each male-dominated family to exchange its
sisters and daughters.

Secondly, each marital union, once produced, remains intact as the basis
of social order: there is little room in the model for divorce, remarriage,
promiscuity or extra-marital liaisons. While Lévi-Strauss does not assume
monogamy (1969a: 37), his view is that marriage, whether polygamous or
not, is in principle a permanent bond: a woman, once yielded by a 'wife-
giving' group, remains normatively with her husband's group for life.

Thirdly, whether a woman is sexually available or non-available is,
according to Lévi-Strauss, a matter decided by the application or non-
application to her of male-imposed rules of exogamy or incest avoidance. In
all this, there is little room for decision-making by women themselves.

How does all this correspond with the evidence of ethnography?

The model fits reasonably well with an image of patrilocal, patrilineal
bands or lineages, each organised around a male core of kinsmen who bring
in wives from other similar groups. It is less able to cope with alternative
arrangements, especially where (as in most hunter-gatherer cultures) residence patterns are flexible and/or 'marriage' is established tenuously with a
long period of bride-service and initial uxorilocality. Neither does the model
fit at all easily with a matrilineal and/or matrilocal bias, which may be
pronounced in some systems and a dimension or component in many others.
In Lévi-Strauss' eyes, indeed, a 'matrilineal society, even though patrilocal',
has 'peculiar problems to resolve' because of the difficulties of cementing the
marital union and incorporating the wife firmly in her husband's group
(1969a: 116–17). Yet his account of the development of 'generalised'
exchange posits a dynamic in which 'disharmonic' régimes are superseded
by 'harmonic' ones, usually patrilineal; in the less integrative mixed systems, either the descent rule was matrilineal or the residence rule matrilocal

(1969a: 265–91, 438–55). Given Lévi-Strauss' point of departure – masculine primacy and the centrality of male marital control – it is unclear how such rules could have come to establish their force. Why should either matrilineal descent or matrilocal residence, both treated by Lévi-Strauss as inconvenient to males, have arisen if men from the beginning had always decided on such matters themselves?

A further technical difficulty is that the model gives enormous prominence to incest/exogamy rules as the basic factors constraining women's sexual availability, whilst very little is said about other kinds of sexual taboos. In particular, *periodic* taboos – on sex during menstruation, before and after childbirth, whilst meat is cooking, while preparing a trap, making hunting nets or organising a collective hunting expedition – these and comparable restrictions are not accounted for by the theory. Indeed, given an underlying assumption that sexual availability is a married woman's normal and permanent state, such things inevitably appear as anomalies.

Even more anomalous-seeming are institutionalised elements of marital instability, whether or not these are associated with a matrilineal and/or matrilocal bias. Lévi-Strauss (1969a: 116) insists that for human culture generally, 'patrilineal institutions' have 'absolute priority' over matrilineal ones. Furthermore,

> it is because political authority, or simply social authority, always belongs to men, and because this masculine priority appears constant, that it adapts itself to a bilineal or matrilineal form of descent in most primitive societies, or imposes its model on all aspects of social life, as is the case in more developed groups. (1969a: 177)

In this context, the model's emphasis on the absolute cultural primacy of marital alliance would make factors such as female-initiated separation or divorce appear anomalous in the extreme. The implication is that marriage is final and permanent. Women with their kin can have no say in restricting or terminating sexual access to a spouse *after* marriage.

We have seen that in Lévi-Strauss' model there is no room for women who can indicate 'yes' or 'no' in sexual terms themselves. Women are spoken for in this respect by men. While this may to an extent reflect what happens in numerous male-dominated societies, as a model of the 'norm' – against which to measure elements of female autonomy as 'deviations' or 'anomalies' – it simply does not work. Simplicity in a model may be a virtue, and Lévi-Strauss' model of culture's 'initial situation' certainly excels in this respect. But the advantages are lost if the outcome is that a vast range of 'anomalous' findings remain unaccounted for, leading to the need for various additional models and theories which may serve their own purposes but meanwhile complicate the field. In this connection, we need only mention that Lévi-Strauss' model of incest avoidance attributes the taboo's origin not in part to mothers and sisters but exclusively to the altruistic self-denial of fathers and brothers; it is men in positions of responsibility, not humans of both sexes, who are attributed with the power to say 'no'. The extraordinary cross-cultural strength of the mother-son incest taboo as compared with the notoriously poor record of older or 'responsible' males in keeping away from their daughters/younger sisters (Herman 1981) seems in this light anomalous; it is not discussed by Lévi-Strauss.

Finally, although it claims to present an image of the origins of human culture as such, Lévi-Strauss' model is in fact much more restricted. Despite the wider claims of structuralism generally, the 'exchange of women' has implications only for kinship studies in a somewhat narrowly defined sense. Culture is many things besides formal kinship, and a theory of its origins ought therefore to be testable in the light of cross-cultural economic, ritual, political, ideological and mythological findings – in addition to the kinship evidence on which Lévi-Strauss in *The Elementary Structures* relies. Lévi-Strauss of course turned to some of these other topics in his later works, but by this time – as we noted in Chapters 2 and 3 – he had lost his earlier thread, and was no longer focusing on the incest rule or upon material processes of exchange.

If we take as our starting point, not 'the exchange of women' but gender solidarity and an exchange of services *between* women and men, a model can be produced which enables us to overcome most of these problems. We can retain Lévi-Strauss' insight that in the process of cultural origins a vital step must have been the establishment of sexual taboos. But in this and the following chapters, we will take it that women themselves had a role to play in determining whether they were sexually available or not. A model will be presented within which the 'incest taboo' arises as an aspect of a more basic reality: the capacity of the evolving protohuman female to say 'yes' – and her equal capacity to give a firm 'no'.

Human culture is based on solidarity. What precisely is involved in this will become clearer as we proceed, but at the outset it may safely be supposed that without some capacity for community-wide collective agreement, there could be no language, no rules, no sexual or other morality – and indeed, no 'society' at all. Lévi-Strauss is only one among many to have emphasised this point, even though in his case what is envisaged is exclusively solidarity between men (1969a).

We may accept another aspect of Lévi-Strauss' thesis without difficulty. Human cultural solidarity in its earliest stages must have found a way of surviving in the face of what must have been its most difficult test – sex. In primate societies, coalitions do emerge and play an important role, but the ever-present threat of sexual conflict places severe limitations on what such coalitions can achieve. Outbreaks of sexually motivated inter-male fighting are the stuff of politics among monkeys and apes, as are female sexual rivalries. Where collectively sanctioned sexual and other regulations and taboos are unknown, the disruptive effects of sex can be enormous. Somehow, in the course of human evolution, this problem must have been overcome. As Marshall Sahlins (1960: 80) some years ago put it, writing of human cultural origins: 'Among subhuman primates sex had organized society; the customs of hunters and gatherers testify eloquently that now society was to organize sex . . . '.

But while accepting all this, this book is based on a third assumption which takes us beyond Lévi-Strauss' frame of reference. The forms of human solidarity underpinning the transition to culture must have had sexual dimensions, and could not have been all-male. In fact, I will show that had not females been involved in asserting their own forms of sexual solidarity at crucial moments, our ancestors could not have achieved the profound sexual changes necessary if they were to transcend the limitations of primate sexuality and sociability.

The remainder of this chapter will focus not on solidarity in the abstract but on *gender solidarity*, which will be viewed, using Marxist concepts, as the outcome of various forms of struggle between the sexes – a struggle transcending the boundaries between nature and culture. I will examine gender solidarity (1) among primates and (2) among members of non-western – and particularly hunter-gatherer – societies.

PRIMATES

Primate Politics

Modern primatology is explicitly concerned with the *politics* of ape and monkey social life (de Waal 1983; Dunbar 1988). Whereas twenty years ago, the term 'politics' would not have been used, nowadays this and other terms derived from lay language are increasingly being drawn upon by primatologists, some of whom allow themselves to empathise with the animals almost as if they were human subjects. Supposedly 'clinical' terms such as 'agonistic interaction' – meaning an argument or fight – are going out of fashion. Primates are extremely intelligent animals whose actions cannot be understood in purely mechanistic, behavioural terms. What the animals are *trying* to do, it is now realised, is essential to grasp if what they *actually* do is to be understood (Dunbar 1988: 324).

It is now recognised that chimpanzees, gorillas, gelada baboons and other primates are rational beings able to set themselves goals, work out long-term strategies, memorise the essentials of complex social relationships over periods of time, display distinctive personalities, co-operate, argue amongst themselves, engage in deception, exploit subordinates, organise political alliances, overthrow their 'rulers' – and indeed, on a certain level and in a limited way, do most of the things which we humans do in our localised, small-scale interactions with one another.

Robin Dunbar (1988) is a rigorous materialist and an inventor of ingenious tests for selecting between rival primatological theories. In his published writings he takes great pains to prevent subjective impressions from distorting his findings. Yet he confidently describes his subjects as displaying 'trust', 'opportunism', 'psychological cunning' and similar characteristics, and as 'reneging' on joint understandings, 'retaliating' against those who renege – and even 'voting' on issues of communal concern.

Likewise, the Dutch primatologist de Waal (1983) has described chimpanzee 'power politics' in almost human terms, writing of 'political ambition', 'collective leadership', 'conspiracy' and so on, and portraying the individual personalities of his chimpanzee subjects in Arnhem Zoo with a novelist's attention to detail.

Provided it is constrained by the use of proven techniques of sampling, statistical analysis and the rigorous testing of hypotheses, all this can be validated as good scientific methodology. It is now realised that the esoteric, impoverished and cumbersome clinical terminology of the earlier functionalist and behaviourist studies – studies which avoided the rich resources of lay language for fear of lapsing into 'anthropomorphism' – actually obstructed our understanding of primates, these most intelligent of creatures whose mental capacities so obviously approximate to our own.

Dunbar spent many years studying wild gelada baboons in Ethiopia, and has done as much as anyone to synthesise modern primatological knowledge into a comprehensive overall picture. He argues that the components of primate social systems 'are essentially alliances of a political nature aimed at enabling the animals concerned to achieve more effective solutions to particular problems of survival and reproduction' (Dunbar 1988: 14). Primate societies are in essence 'multi-layered sets of coalitions' (p. 106). Although physical fights are the ultimate tests of status and the basic means of deciding contentious issues, the social mobilisation of allies in such conflicts often decides matters and requires other than purely physical skills.

Instead of simply relying on their own physical powers, individuals pursue their social objectives by attempting to find allies against social rivals and competitors. For example, when two male chimpanzees are aggressively confronting one another – in a quarrel over a female, perhaps, or over food – one of them may hold out his hand and beckon, trying to draw a nearby onlooker into the conflict on his own side. If the onlooker is influential and sympathetic, that may decide the outcome. De Waal (1983: 36) describes the 'aggressive alliance' or 'coalition' among chimpanzees as 'the political instrument par excellence'.

The manipulation and use of coalitions demands sophisticated intelligence. It is even possible (although unusual) for a relatively poor fighter to dominate more muscular rivals if he or she is better able to mobilise popular support. The factor militating against this is that most individuals want to be on the winning side, so a good fighter is also likely to be popular as a focus of successful coalitions, whereas a consistent loser may be shunned by the strong and the weak alike.

In any event, brawn without brain is inadequate, and it is now thought that the considerable brain-power displayed by most of the higher primates functions not only to ensure the individual's survival in a direct relationship with the physical environment but more importantly to aid success in the many 'political' calculations which have to be made within society itself (Chance and Mead 1953; Jolly 1966; Kummer 1967, 1982; Humphrey 1976; Cheney and Seyfarth 1985; Dunbar 1988; Byrne and Whiten 1988). Applying this to human evolution, most authoritative statements have stressed that it was not foraging or tool use as such that generated human levels of intelligence but rather the associated social, behavioural and cultural processes required to direct and organise such activities (Reynolds 1976; Lovejoy 1981; Holloway 1981; Wynn 1988).

Elements of Female Solidarity Within Primate Societies

In the 1950s and 1960s, when field studies of primates were just beginning, specialists tended to think of each species of primate as having its own characteristic form of social organisation, regardless of immediate geographical or ecological conditions.

Moreover, investigators focused almost entirely upon primate males. Hamadryas baboons in Ethiopia seemed to be organised in markedly male-dominated social systems. The males were 'the active sex', fighting among themselves for females, the victors organising their seized or kidnapped females into compact harems which could be efficiently supervised and controlled from above. A straying, wayward female would be brought back into line by means of a bite on the neck – a bite so hard that it sometimes lifted the female off the ground (Kummer 1968: 36–7). The female would follow her overlord closely from then on. There were no successful female rebellions or revolutions. For primatologists, there seemed to be little point in concentrating attention upon what the females were feeling or trying to achieve.

This picture was not decisively modified when, in the late 1960s and early 1970s, attention began to be redirected from baboons to wild chimpanzees. Although chimpanzees seemed to be more easygoing, the males being sexually more tolerant of each other, it was still found that males were the dominant sex. Many accounts concentrated on the degree to which male chimps were prepared to tolerate other males within their ranges and to 'share' their female sexual partners – a pattern which was contrasted with the hamadryas baboon norm of pronounced inter-male sexual intolerance (Reynolds 1966, Sugiyama 1972).

The contrast between baboons and chimpanzees became deeply embedded in almost all primatological thinking. Primate 'family' units were divided between two contrasting categories – 'one-male units' on the one hand,

'multi-male units' on the other. Intolerant ('hamadryas-like') males produced
the first kind of unit; more tolerant ('chimpanzee-like') males formed the
second kind. No one referred to 'one-female units' or 'multi-female units'.
The presence of females with their offspring was taken for granted, the only
question being whether a group of females attached itself sexually to one
adult male or to several.

Inseparable from all this was what is now called a 'priority of access' model
of sexual relations. Females were though of as passive creatures waiting to be
kidnapped, snatched, stolen or conquered by males. The males were seen to
fight one another for priority of access to the females, and, basically, the
possible outcomes were these: either (a) an individual victorious male
exclusively controlled a whole 'harem' of females-with-young or (b) a group
of two or more successful males chose to compromise with one another,
collectively defending and sharing access to a group of females. The first
outcome was popularly conceptualised as a 'Cyclopean' system more or less
corresponding to Freud's 'Primal Horde'; the second was seen, at least by
some writers, as a form of 'group-marriage' (Fox 1975b: 12, 16).

In either case, the object of a male sexual fight was simply to defeat one's
opponent(s) and seize or win over his (or their) females. Noting the mental
demands placed upon males, one of the great founders of modern primatology, M. R. A. Chance (1962: 31), hypothesised that the human brain
may have become enlarged in the course of evolution precisely to deal with
such taxing and risk-laden situations. The protohuman male, in other words,
was thought to have needed a large brain in order to work out when to
attack, when to ingratiate himself with a more dominant rival, when to run
away, when to bluff – and also when and how to express his emotions so as to
convey signals to his own advantage. In developing this theme, Robin Fox
(1966; 1967a) argued that the 'whole process of enlarging the neo-cortex to
take-off point' was based on 'a competition between the dominant and sub-
dominant males', those surviving being 'those best able to control and
inhibit, and hence time, their responses'. He concluded: 'Here then are the
beginnings of deferred gratification, conscience and guilt, spontaneous
inhibition of drives, and many other features of a truly human state.'

Chance himself (1962: 32) cautioned that all this need only have been 'a
phase in man's development', antedating the period of maximum cortical
expansion. Nonetheless, his support for the view that male brain-power
evolved in the context of sexual fighting gave new respectability to a
widespread popular origins myth (see Chapter 1).

But how and why did hominid females develop their brains along with
males? And how might our protohuman female ancestors have responded to
the males supposedly fighting around them all the time? Such questions were
not usually thought to be an issue. Until the impact of sociobiology bacame
felt, an influential view among primatologists was that female behaviour did
not really matter, because it had little bearing on overall social structure. As

one specialist put it: 'the number of adult males and their reciprocal relationships determine the social structure of the group as well as the group behavior as a whole' (Vogel 1973: 363).

It is now widely recognised that all this presented a distorted picture of reality. The defects can be discussed under several headings.

Female Dominance in Primates

Firstly, it is in part coincidental that male dominance came to be assumed to be the 'natural' or 'default' condition for primates. Had primatologists begun their field studies among lemurs in Madagascar instead of among baboons in the Sudan or Ethiopia, a very different picture might have become fixed in the popular mind.

Prosimians are sometimes thought of as the most 'primitive' of living primates (Hrdy 1981: 60). They exhibit pronounced 'matriarchal' tendencies. Ring-tailed lemurs, brown lemurs, white sifakas, ruffed lemurs, black lemurs, diademed sifakas, indris – these and many other Madagascan species are characterised by female dominance as the norm. Alison Jolly (1972: 185) studied ring-tailed lemurs in southern Madagascar and reported that despite male swaggering 'females were dominant over males, both in threats and in priority for food. Females at times bounced up to the dominant male and snatched a tamarind pod from his hand, cuffing him over the ear in the process.'

Admittedly, the prosimians represent only one suborder within the general order of primates. Most primate species *are* male-dominated, in the sense that a dominant male will displace any female from her position if he wants to. But this says nothing at all about 'natural' or 'original' states. As Hrdy (1981: 59) points out, by focusing on baboons, langurs and orangutans, one can 'demonstrate' that male dominance is the natural condition for primates. By concentrating on prosimians, one can argue that female dominance is the primitive and basic condition, for among all the social lemurs ever studied, this is so.

Female Determinance of Social Structure

More interesting than this, however, is the modern sociobiologically inspired finding that among primates generally it is the strategies pursued by the female sex which ultimately determine the overall social structure.

Females and males have different priorities. To a large extent, this stems from the basic fact that, in all mammals, a male can in principle father an almost limitless number of offspring, whereas there are strict limits to the number a female can produce.

Male primates (with some exceptions) are not equippped to do much to ensure the survival of their offspring once these have been conceived. Except

for a few functions such as defence against predators, offspring can gain little
benefit from their 'fathers', who are in no primate species inclined or able to
provide their partners or young with food. In perpetuating their genes,
therefore, it usually makes better sense for males to abandon their mates soon
after conception and attempt to inseminate more females (a general fact of
mammalian biology which may help to explain why only about 4 per cent
of mammal species are monogamous – Hrdy 1981: 35). By contrast, once
they are pregnant or are nurturing offspring, female primates, like most
mammals, have little to gain (in terms of the replication of their genes) by
getting inseminated again and again. What matters is that their existing
offspring survive. This means feeding them, and this in turn means that
females tend to be more interested in 'economics' than sex – or in any event,
tend to prioritise this aspect more than do males.

These differences have spatial correlates and consequences. Female primates, who are burdened with the task of producing and provisioning their
offspring, distribute themselves in space according to their needs and
preferences for shelter, comfort, safety and – most importantly – for
particular types of food. Instead of endlessly searching for males, they
prioritise such on-going, day-to-day 'economic' concerns. Males, on the
other hand, are primarily interested in securing access to oestrus females.
Foraging activities are subordinated to this overriding sexual quest. The
result is that while females distribute themselves according to their own
foraging and nurturing requirements, males note how the females have
arranged themselves in space and then decide how to map themselves on to
this pattern so as to maximise their mating opportunities.

The extent to which the males fight or co-operate, form large or small
groups, define 'closed' or 'open' systems – all this depends on what the
females have set about doing in the first instance. The extent to which the
males are 'tolerant' or 'intolerant' depends not just on genes but on the
immediate social situation, and this is at root female-defined. It is in this
sense that the female pattern is 'basic' (Wrangham 1979; Hrdy 1981:
123–4; Rodman 1984). In Marxist terms, one might say that the female
distribution pattern is to the male sexual-political pattern as 'economic
infrastructure' is to 'political superstructure'. To change the whole system in
any fundamental sense, the underlying 'economic' pattern of female ecological relationships would have to be changed first.

How the females arrange themselves in space depends (a) upon immediate
geographical and ecological conditions and (b) upon the females' genetically
determined preferences and abilities to make use of what the environment
has to offer. For example, chimpanzees have digestive systems rendering
them dependent on ripe fruit, which require much travelling and searching
to find. Quite different are gorillas, which can munch almost anything,
including leaves, and so can usually feed on what is immediately to hand
without moving much at all. Most monkeys fall somewhere between these

two extremes, combining leaf-eating with a preference for ripe fruit when these are available (Hrdy 1981: 123–4).

Where food is hard to find and widely spaced, females may have to travel fast and far in order to eat; if food is available almost everywhere, little movement may be required. If the food is scarce – in the form, for example, of an occasional small bush or tree transiently laden with fruit – the females may not want to be accompanied by others but would prefer to be alone so as to monopolise what they have found for themselves. If the food is abundant, and/or if there are other considerations – such as defence against predators – making group life advantageous, they may prefer to cluster in groups. The variations and permutations are numerous, but the basic result is that females arrange themselves across the landscape in characteristic patterns – grouped or isolated, fast-moving or slow, in trees or on the ground – and the males in pursuing their sexual goals adopt strategies which take account of the situation which the females have defined.

How do the males 'map' themselves on to the pre-existent female distribution pattern? It all depends on the circumstances. If the females are clustered in manageable or defensible groups, a male may realistically attempt to monopolise a whole harem all to himself. If the females are very isolated and scattered, however, any one male may only be capable of monopolising one female at a time. If the females are clustered quite closely, but move too independently, are too assertive or are in groups too large to be fenced off and defended by single males, those patrolling or defending their ranges may find it best to collaborate, particularly if they are close kin, the result being what Robin Fox (1975b: 16) calls 'group marriage' – a pattern in which two or more brother-males collectively defend the joint ranges of several females. This happens among chimpanzees (for a theoretical explanation see Rodman 1984).

The situation can be summed up by saying that in all cases, the basic pattern is that primates, male and female, compete for resource-filled space. Sleeping or nesting space, feeding space, grooming space – the whole of life is, in a real sense, about space and the competition to monopolise portions of it for certain periods. But whereas females in the first instance compete among themselves for foraging space, which may well be 'uninhabited' at the outset, what males compete for is *space already occupied by the opposite sex, the females themselves being the main 'valuables' within it*. It is true that subsequently – once males have established their domain – females may compete among themselves in order to get closest to the dominant male, who may confer various competitive 'privileges' upon his temporary or permanent 'favourites'. For example, when many geladas in a group arrive simultaneously at the same waterhole, the male and dominant females drink first and perhaps wallow in the water; subordinate animals wait their turn – and may even miss their turn altogether if the dominant animals move on whilst jostling around the water remains intense (Hrdy 1981: 106). It makes sense, then, for females to compete for privileged space close to the dominant males. But the male arrangement that ultimately emerges depends fundamentally on the nature of the female-defined space for which males initially compete among themselves.

Female 'Voting' to Confirm or Repudiate Male Status

Most primate systems are male-dominated. That is, once a male has gained control over a space with one or more females ranging within it, he may from time to time choose to displace a particular female from her feeding position in order to eat the food which she has found. If she cannot use her sexual attractions to alter his intentions she may try to resist, in which case the male may use physical force. The literature is replete with examples of dominant males casually stealing food from 'their' females or offspring – in the case of some macaques species, even to the point of nonchalantly raiding the inside of females' mouths (Hrdy 1981: 114–15). Whether in such extreme forms or in milder ones, this kind of thing is really what 'dominance' – the basic organising principle of all primate societies – is about.

But this does not mean that the females are always passive or inactive. On the contrary, they can often determine which male is to be their 'overlord', or which males collectively are to patrol over their ranges.

For example, when a male gelada sets out to attack a previously dominant rival so as to take over his harem, the females concerned may insist on their own say in the outcome. At various stages during the fighting, the females may 'vote' among themselves on whether to accept the provisional outcome. There may be real internal arguments, with some females wanting to restore the old overlord whilst others welcome the newcomer. As Dunbar (1988: 166) in his fascinating account puts it: 'During the process of this "voting" procedure, the females are involved in a great deal of fighting amongst themselves as those who do not want to change males attempt to prevent those that do from interacting with the new male.' The traditionalists, in this account, are clearly attempting to impose a collective sexual boycott upon the unwanted newcomer male. These females are likely to be those who had held a satisfactory status within the harem under the old order. The more 'radical' females – those wanting a change – are likely to be those who were previously discriminated against within the harem; their hope is for a better deal under new management. Voting is simple – 'no' is signalled by refusing to groom the newcomer; 'yes' is signalled by going up to him and grooming him.

Dunbar (personal communication) adds that the females do not make their decisions as such until some time into the fighting. It is as if they were waiting to see how the two males initially shape up before beginning to decide one way or the other. Although the females continue to bicker amongst themselves long after the males have stopped fighting, the struggle effectively ends once a majority of females have 'voted' for or against the new male. Dunbar (1988: 166, 167, 243) writes that the ultimate outcome of an inter-male 'sexual fight' always depends in this way on the female 'votes', although he does not infer that there is any very accurate electoral 'count'!

In some higher primate species, such as hamadryas baboons and gorillas, there is little sisterly solidarity, as a result of which 'females are abjectly subordinate to a male leader' (Hrdy 1981: 162). In the case of geladas, however – despite a rather precarious and superficial male 'dominance' – female solidarity within the harem may confer considerable power. Hrdy (1981: 104) cites an incident in which an overlord male rushed aggressively towards a 'straying' female. Had she been a hamadryas, no sister would have supported her: she would have cringed, received her punishment and got back into line. But the gelada female did no such thing. She snarled and lunged back, whereupon three other females from her own harem joined her and stood their ground beside her until the male, who was supposed to be their 'leader', was chased off!

Among hanuman langurs, when a new male overlord from an external troop wins a harem, his first concern is to bite and kill the young infants so that their mothers stop lactating and so come back into oestrus more quickly, conceiving and bearing offspring by the new male (Hrdy 1981: 82). It is unclear why the females in this species have not evolved counter-measures to resist this. However logical the behaviour may be in terms of the male's calculations of genetic benefit, such wastage of maternal investment is certainly not in the mothers' own reproductive interests (Hrdy 1981: 92). Among savanna baboons and squirrel monkeys, it is quite common to see a group of females collectively 'mobbing' a male who had attempted to molest an infant (Hrdy 1981: 96). However, it must be admitted that successful infanticide is fairly common among primates, including chimpanzees, and that although males may be the worst offenders, rival females are also sometimes guilty (Goodall 1977: 259–82). There is an obvious contrast here with human hunter-gatherer societies, which never tolerate infanticide for these kinds of reason.

In the case of many primate species, if a new male overlord makes a serious political 'mistake' – killing, eating or threatening an infant might be an example – he may antagonise the females so much that they collectively make it impossible for him to maintain his position (Dunbar 1988: 165, 243–4, 261). For one reason or another, his unpopularity may be such as to provoke a 'sex strike' – in the sense that a group of females may simply refuse to turn their attentions to a particular male, even when he has supposedly or provisionally 'won' them in a fight (Dunbar 1988: 165, 167, citing Herbert 1968, Michael et al. 1978).

Finally, among chimpanzees, an intriguing phenomenon is what de Waal (1983: 38) calls 'confiscation'. A ferocious adult male may be 'displaying' aggressively towards a rival, his hair all erect, his body swaying from side to

side – and brandishing a stone in one hand. An adult female 'calmly walks up
to the displaying male, loosens his fingers from around the stone and walks
away with it'. De Waal writes that the male may try to pick up another
weapon – only for the female to take away that one too. On one occasion, a
female confiscated no fewer than six objects in a row!

This female confiscation sequence was a recurrent pattern among de
Waal's chimpanzees. 'In such a situation', writes de Waal, 'the male has
never been known to react aggressively towards the female'. After millennia
during which evolving hominids may have been tempted to fight each other
using hand-axes – lethal conflicts probably occurring from time to time
(Chapter 8) – comparable female-inspired disarmament may eventually have
played an important violence-transcending, culture-creating role.

Matrilineages

A further fascinating finding is that although the females of many species
enter into fewer relationships than do males, the bonds they do forge tend to
be more enduring and play a much bigger role in determining the overall
kinship structure.

This is not a new finding. As J. H. Crook (1972: 89) put it, females form
the more cohesive elements of primate groups and, as a consequence of their
solidarity, tend to play a considerable role in determining who emerges as
their 'overlord' or 'control': 'Males by contrast . . . are the more mobile
animals, transferring themselves, as recent research shows, quite frequently
from one group to another.' Males, being often bigger and stronger than
females, seem to need their relationships less; they are more likely to rely on
their own muscular strength, to wander off on their own, or to visit other
groups. Moreover, in negotiating their way through the political landscape
within any particular group, they tend to switch allegiances more often,
prompted by immediate calculations of transient self-interest.

Except in the case of a few species, such as the monogamous gibbons, it is
the males, therefore, who are the more exploratory sex, tending to establish quite extensive ranges, each overlapping the smaller ranges of several
females. Females, by contrast, choose their partners and their localities
carefully and invest in them more heavily – for each needs to prepare a long-
term protective ecological and social niche for herself and her offspring.

Since males move around and change their relationships, while females
tend to retain theirs throughout life, the result is something like a matrilineal descent system. A concise and emphatic statement on this point was
made by a pioneering authority on hamadryas baboons in 1971: 'Nonhuman
primates', he wrote, 'recognise only matrilineal kinship' (Kummer 1971:
34).

Although it would seem to be a theoretically possible arrangement, in
no known case do females live together in a territory, occasionally receiving
visits from a transient male, whom they drive away once impregnated.

Females always appear to appreciate a degree of continuing male commitment to them and to their offspring, particularly in the form of protection against predators or stranger males. Although non-monogamous male primates may not show any particular long-term commitment to any one female within their domain, their commitment to the defence of this domain as such – and hence to the defence fo their own genetic offspring within it – is strong and of value to the mothers. Genetic calculations suggest that a father should risk his life for the defence of his own offspring more readily even than should a mother's sister (Hrdy 1981: 56).

Nevertheless, within their male-patrolled ranges, primate females of all species tend to choose other females, not males, as their immediate foraging companions (Dunbar 1988: 138). Why this is so is not quite clear, but many intriguing suggestions have been made. It may be simply because of the differences in priorities mentioned earlier. To any female, her male partner is likely to be somewhat unreliable – likely to abandon her for some other female should a good mating opportunity arise. For a mother interested in feeding herself and her offspring, a male constantly on the look out for new mating opportunities could be quite a nuisance: he would keep trying to steer the family in directions quite irrelevant to its search for food. Moreover, even when a female had found food, her dominant male partner would be quite likely to displace her should he feel hungry – and eat the food himself (Ghiglieri 1984: 189). On the other hand, among many species, males and females have somewhat different diets, and so would choose to go in different directions in search of food (Dunbar 1988: 138). Another factor may be the reluctance of females to become involved in inter-male sexual fights; much better to let the males get on with their fighting at safe distance, so that the offspring do not get hurt! More positively, females may appreciate the presence of nearby sisters or non-dominant companions to lighten the load of caring for offspring, or to enable the young of several mothers to benefit from playing among themselves (Ghiglieri 1984: 188–9).

The fact that related females bond with each other, often more enduringly than males, in some cases leads to the formation of 'matrilineages'. Japanese and Indian macaques are an example. They arrange themselves into matrilineal extended lineages or 'clans'. Certain whole clans are dominant over others within a troop, and individuals are ranked within each clan. At the top of each matrilineal hierarchy is the founding female. Clusters of these clans form troops, each associated with a group of males who may not be related, and these males may outrank the top-ranking matriarch of each clan. But despite this male dominance, each male's rank still depends on female support, and derives in large measure from the rank held by his mother from the moment he was born. A high-ranking mother will have high-ranking daughters and sons, while a low-ranking mother's offspring will inherit her lowly status. This is a kind of matrilineal 'feudalism', in the sense that 'individuals inherit unequal lifetime benefits according to the happenstances of birth' (Hrdy 1981: 112). Low-ranking individuals are harassed by others, eat less well, sleep less well and produce fewer surviving offspring (Hrdy 1981: 114–22).

In the case of these macaques, while dominant males associated with a lineage come and go, each male's relationship to the troop being transient, female power is much more enduring. Among Japanese macaques, males move out of their natal troop when they are only two or three years old, and eventually establish sexual relations with other females who remain with their kin. Females remain in the same troop for a lifetime, whereas males transfer out after a few years. This, then, is a kind of 'matrilineal' and 'matrilocal' system (although I hasten to add that what primatologists mean by 'matriliny' and what social anthropologists mean are rather different things!).

Although the 'matrilineages' may not always be so extended or so stable, it is a fact that most primates have some such system. That is – in contrast with Lévi-Strauss' model of human origins – it is usually the males who are 'exchanged' between groups, not the females. Among macaques, baboons, geladas and vervet monkeys, this is certainly the case. Wherever it is the females who stay in their natal group whilst males transfer out, 'matrilineages' tend to evolve as the basic embodiments of solidarity. Only in a few exceptional cases – forest-dwelling chimpanzees being the main example – do primate males remain in their natal groups while females emigrate. Among gorillas and red colobus monkeys, both sexes change groups with more or less equal frequency (Dunbar 1988: 80–1).

Perhaps most interesting of all is the suggestion that life in the more open and exposed, relatively impoverished environments seems to produce 'matrilineal/matrilocal' systems. This has obvious potential relevance to human social evolution and will be returned to later (Chapter 6).

According to Dunbar (1988: 81), where danger from predators is severe, females tend not to leave their own natal group but stay with their kin. Among primates, danger from predators tends to increase with distance from the safety of trees to climb up into, and Dunbar's finding is that among primates in general, there is in fact a good correlation between medium to large group size, low female migration rates, long-term kin-based female coalitions and a terrestrial or semi-terrestrial way of life (1988: 297–305).

In explaining this finding, Dunbar suggests a dialectical sequence of reciprocal causes and effects spurring the formation of extended 'matrilineal' coalitions as groups are compelled to forgo the relative safety afforded by trees. In this view, movement into more open territory increases the risk from external predators, motivating the females to be particularly cautious and compelling the animals generally to seek safety in numbers. However, this aggregation creates a new problem of its own. As large numbers of animals forage together in compact groups, internal conflicts over food, space and sexual partners tend to intensify. Females of low status tend to be harassed by other females and displaced from the best feeding spots and may also find themselves marginalised within their harems and relatively ignored by their male overlords. Such females might have low prospects of reproducing and passing on their genes.

The only way out is for the oppressed females to seek coalition partners – sometimes males who can afford protection, sometimes other females. Dunbar argues that the rather extensive female coalitions and matrilineal kinship networks of the more terrestrial primates evolve through some such logic. Related females support one another to avoid being harassed and marginalised. This then has further consequences. Once a female has become part of a coalition, it becomes very difficult for her to 'emigrate' or move between groups, since any female intruding into a new group would place herself in conflict with the resident females and would have no sisters on whom to rely for support. The upshot is that whereas predation risks as such would only necessitate temporary external aggregations – 'safety in numbers' – the social consequences of crowding combine to bring about a new form of matrilineal internal cohesion, with considerable endurance and internal stability.

Dunbar suggests that if chimpanzees – or protohumans – were to venture right out into the open savanna, this logic would prevail. The females, that is, would form cohesive groups with their own internal solidarity. Dunbar argues that this would initially lead towards a system in which dominant males, faced with relatively coherent female groups, would attempt to monopolise whole harems of females for themselves. These related females, however, would have their own strength derived from solidarity. 'This clearly has implications', Dunbar (1988: 319–20) concludes, 'for the evolution of hominid social systems'.

HUMANS

Female Sexual Solidarity in Cultural Contexts

This chapter began with a discussion of Lévi-Strauss' views on male gender solidarity as the point of departure for human culture. It was then seen that primate studies provide evidence of a struggle between the sexes, males and females having different priorities and forming distinctive patterns of solidarity according to material circumstances. Before turning to consider how human culture might have arisen, we may conclude this discussion by re-examining Lévi-Strauss' views in the light of some evidence for comparably complex patterns in traditional human cultures.

The existence of female power in male-dominated societies has been documented in numerous studies of gender relations (Holy 1985: 186). Such power as women have may be the embodiment of a definite strategy to subvert patriarchal relationships; alternatively, the forms of female solidarity may constitute less conscious defence reflexes against male dominance (see Cronin 1977; Ullrich 1977). In particular, women's refusal to cook or to cohabit sexually with their husbands has been described as 'a usual strategy to which women resort to gain their way in the face of men's dominance or as a sanction against men's actions or conduct which they consider inappropriate' (Holy 1985: 186, citing Paulme 1963; Cohen 1971; Strathern 1972; 27, 45–6; Rosaldo 1974: 37; Lamphere 1974: 99). Holy (1985: 186) writes that in the case of the Berti (Northern Darfur Province, Sudan), 'The woman's favourite stratagem in the case of a dispute with her husband or when she feels that she has been maltreated by him is to refuse him sexual access and to refuse to cook for him.'

In a more full-blooded way, Amadiume (1987: 66–7) describes the Inyom Nnobi (the 'Women of Nnobi') – a traditional all-female council among one group of the Nigerian Igbo. A kind of women's trade union, it was headed by the Agba Ekwe, 'the favoured one of the goddess Idemili and her earthly manifestation'. She carried her staff of authority and had the final word in public gatherings and assemblies. Central among her tasks was to ensure men's strict observance of woman-protective taboos – for example, the two-year ban on sexual intercourse with a nursing mother. She was equally alert to reports of sexual harassment of young girls when travelling along bush-paths. In this rather male-dominated society, the community of women were aware of their strong communications network, and took full advantage of it. 'What the men feared most', the ethnographer adds (p. 67), 'was the Council's power of strike action':

> The strongest weapon the Council had and used against the men was the right to order mass strikes and demonstrations by all women. When ordered to strike, women refused to perform their expected duties and roles, including all domestic, sexual and maternal services. They would leave the town *en masse*, carrying only suckling babies. If angry enough, they were known to attack any men they met.

Idemili, the goddess in whose name such action was always taken, was a 'water-spirit' who sometimes appeared in dreams as a python (Amadiume 1987: 100, 102). Some decades ago, when a male Christian convert deliberately killed a python – totemic symbol of Idemili's worshippers – the women from all around marched half-naked to the provincial headquarters to besiege the resident's office with their complaints. Gaining no satisfaction, they returned to their own locality, went straight to the Christian offender's house and razed it to the ground – a particularly severe method of withdrawing domestic services (Amadiume 1987: 122)! Deprived of his home, the man reportedly died two weeks later. In Chapter 13 we will examine the symbolic logic by virtue of which, on a worldwide basis, female punitive 'class action' of this fearsome kind is traditionally associated with an immense 'All-mother' or goddess-like 'snake'.

The ethnographic record provides a mixed picture of relations between the sexes. Although male dominance may be universal or nearly so, it is offset by numerous factors in different cultures to a greater or lesser extent. Lévi-Strauss' 'exchange of women' models notwithstanding, women after marriage are not necessarily detached in any permanent sense from their own kin, fully incorporated into their husband's group, totally lacking in autonomy or deprived collectively of a sphere of power of their own. Where decisions on sexual availability are concerned – to take only one aspect of decision-making – they often have some say themselves (Amadiume 1987). Within the intimate sphere of marital relations, this is surely no less 'normal' (on any definition) than the situation in which a wife must always be sexually ready for her husband.

But it is not only private intimacies which are at issue. Where – as in most hunter-gatherer societies – a man's marriage for many years gives him no absolute or unconditional sexual rights in his spouse, a woman can draw on the support of her mother, sister, brothers or other kin as a lever to secure advantages for herself within the relationship. Whereas 'a man whose marriage is secure need obey no other' (Collier and Rosaldo 1981: 317), an element of marital insecurity obliges a man to listen to his wife and her kin. An unsatisfactory husband or lover (particularly if he is not well established or is a lazy, inept or selfish hunter) may be unceremoniously told to go. Landes (1938: 131) writes of the Ojibwa of Western Ontario:

> A married man who is too lazy to hunt can be supported by his wife for a time, but her tolerance will be changed for scorn, then to indifference, and finally she will desert him. A man who is unsuccessful on the hunt, and who goes with his wife to her parents' wigwam, can expect to be rejected and left to die of starvation. In one case the parents' scorn was so great that they took their daughter in to feed and lodge her, but refused their son-in-law. Folk-tales are concerned with the same theme.

Sex and economics are here intertwined – no meat means, in effect, no sex and, eventually, complete annulment of the man's marital status. 'If a man does not hunt', writes Richard Lee (1988: 266) of the !Kung San of the Kalahari, 'his wife will make pointed comments about his sexual prowess. And vice versa: if he is no good in bed, he cannot hunt.'

In fairy-tales throughout the world, the theme of suitors' trials refers to the same basic relationship, storytellers often delighting in depicting the hero as overcoming the most extraordinary obstacles to win the hand of his chosen bride. Although reality may be less romantic, prospective bride-grooms often have to prove their worth in difficult trials. Lowie (1920: 22–3) writes that in South America, among the Arawak Indians of Guiana, 'the prospective husband was obliged to prove his marksmanship by, among other tests, shooting an arrow into a woodpecker's nest from a moving boat'. Similar motifs occur 'as a constant refrain in the utterances of North

American Indians, where the skilful hunter figures as the ideal son-in-law'
(Lowie 1920: 22–3). Among hunter-gatherers generally, some such pattern
was certainly the norm rather than the exception (Collier and Rosaldo 1981).

Among most hunters and gatherers, a man's wife was never simply 'won'.
She was not suddenly transferred, in a single, once-for-all transaction called
'marriage'. She had to be earned over a period of years or even decades, in a
process known as 'bride-service'.

Phyllis Kaberry (1939) encountered this pattern among the Aborigines of
Western Australia, describing the passage of gifts from a man to his wife's
kin as 'a constant drain on a man's resources throughout his lifetime'. All this
investment and effort, she went on, constituted 'a definite recognition of the
value of the woman as his sexual and economic partner'. Here as in other
cultures, the man's gifts were mainly of meat which he had hunted himself.
The reader will recall similar Australian and other instances from the
previous chapter, in which men's constant yielding of meat to their wives'
kin was discussed in connection with the 'own-kill' rule.

One interpretation might be that the bride herself in such situations was a
mere pawn, used by her kin to extract labour-service from the in-marrying
husband. But would such a verdict be fair?

It seems probable that in most cultures the authority figures most feared
or 'respected' by the bridegroom were indeed the bride's mother, father,
brothers or other older relatives, rather than the young woman herself.
Nevertheless, usually, the effect was to secure meat for the wife. In
Australia, among the Walbiri Aborigines, a man's wife's brothers or other
kin may

> upbraid and sometimes attack him physically if he refuses to give meat to
> his wife. Other members of the community approve as legitimate their
> attempts to force him to adhere to the law. Moreover, the meat should
> come from game he has hunted himself. . . . (Meggitt 1965: 252)

Among the Siberian Yukaghir, the picture we are given is that of a young
man taken into his in-laws' house where he must 'serve' for his wife for 'as
long as any members of the family older than herself are alive'. His position
is strictly subordinate:

> He must neither look at nor speak to the parents and older relatives of his
> wife. He must obey all the orders given by these relatives. The products of
> his hunting and fishing are under the control of his mother-in-law.
> (Jochelson 1926: 91)

In these and countless other cases, it is the wife's older kin who most clearly
impress the husband as powers to be reckoned with.

However, the evidence is that women who remained with their kin and received visits from their spouses in the early years of marriage – the norm among hunter-gatherers almost throughout the world (Collier and Rosaldo 1981) – were not just 'used' by their kin groups. They positively welcomed the support and protection afforded by their kin, and were involved with them in upholding the value which their sexuality represented for their kin group as a whole.

A Californian myth tells of Seven Sisters who used their collective sexual solidarity as a weapon against husbands who refused to provide them with game. The myth was recorded in Los Angeles County early in the nineteenth century:

The Seven Sisters

There were seven brothers married to seven sisters, who lived in a large hut together. The men went daily to hunt rabbits and the women to gather roots of flags for food. The husbands invariably reported 'bad luck' in their hunt, with the exception of the youngest, who, without fail, handed his wife a rabbit.

This continued every day until the females held a conference and became convinced that they were being cheated by their partners. They agreed that the youngest sister should remain at home the next day, under pretext of having a pain in her jaw, and so watch the return of the party. Next day the men as usual took their bows and arrows and set forth. The six sisters then departed, leaving the other concealed among the flags and rushes at the back of the hut in a position from which she could see all that happened inside.

Several hours before sunset the hunting party returned laden with rabbits which they commenced roasting and eating, except one which the youngest set apart. The others called him a fool and bade him eat the remaining one, which he refused to do, saying he still had some affection for his wife and always intended to reserve one for her. More fool you, said the others; we care more for ourselves than for these root-diggers. When they had finished, they carefully hid all the evidence of their feast.

When all this was later reported to the sisters, they cried a great deal and talked over what they should do. Let us turn into water, said the eldest. That would never do, responded the rest, for in that case our husbands would drink us. The second proposed being turned into stones, which was rejected on the ground of being trodden upon by the fraternity. The third wanted them to turn themselves into trees, which was not accepted because they would be used for firewood. Everything proposed was put aside until it came to the turn of the youngest. Her proposition to change themselves into stars was objected to on account of being seen, but overruled as they would be out of reach.

They proceeded to the lagoon, where they daily collected flag roots and constructed a machine (impossible to describe) out of reeds, and ascended to heaven and located themselves at the *Pleiades*. These seven stars still retain the names of the originals. (Reid 1939: 246–8; slightly adapted and abridged)

With its emphasis on the sisters' not wanting their husbands to use or enjoy them – to 'drink', 'tread on' or 'burn' them – this myth suggests that 'becoming stars', tantalisingly visible but out of reach in the sky, is a metaphor for collective sexual withdrawal. The reader who follows this book to the end will link this in turn with actual or pretended menstruation as a pretext for seclusion in 'another world'. This would make the 'machine' which is 'impossible to describe', and which is associated with female collectivity around a 'lagoon', a code term for female synchronised menstruation (see Chapters 11–14).

In real life, in most of the world, it may have been unusual for sisters as such, without support from their mothers or from male kin, to rely solely on one another in the manner portrayed in this myth. Yet the story encapsulates an important aspect of the logic widely at work. In their own economic interests vis-à-vis their spouses, women relied on one another to uphold their security and sexual status, retaining at all times the ultimate right to withdraw.

Throughout the world, married women have appreciated the availability of female kin on whom to rely in time of need. By the same token, husbands almost everywhere – at least until very recently – have known that a wife is someone with her own independent support system. The following extract from a case-study exemplifies this point:

> wives could not rely upon their husbands to stand by them while they reared their children. . . . So the wife had to cling to the family into which she was born, and in particular to her mother, as the only other means of ensuring herself against isolation. One or other member of her family would, if need be, relieve her distress . . . or share to some degree in the responsibility for her children. The extended family was her trade union, organised in the main by women and for women, its solidarity her protection against being alone.

The notion of such an all-women's 'trade union' will be encountered frequently in later chapters of this book. Although in the above passage they were writing of the traditional extended family in London's East End, Willmott and Young (1957: 189) were conscious of describing a widespread cross-cultural logic. 'It is, to judge by anthropology', as they put it (p. 189), 'almost a universal rule that when married life is insecure, the wife turns for support to her family of origin, so that a weak marriage tie produces a strong blood tie'. As feminists are well aware, this can be put the other way around: if sisterhood is to be prioritised, marriage bonds must be kept relatively weak.

The Mother-In-Law

A woman's 'trade union' would be of little use if her husband could ignore or abuse her mother. This relative's authority has always been, indeed, the minimum condition for a wife's relative autonomy within marriage. Certainly, a wife in most cultures woud tend to seek contact with her mother more frequently during married life than any other authority figure amongst her kin. This may help to explain why, in so many traditional cultures, the figure of the mother-in-law was invested – in husbands' eyes – with awesome supernatural power. Although male relatives were also involved, it was to an important extent she who had 'given' her daughter, and she who – if offended – could take her back. Moreover, unlike male in-laws, the mother-in-law was particularly in need of ritual defences against the merest hint of sexual oppression or abuse. No mother could defend her daughter within marriage unless her own sexual non-availability and social dominance had been established beyond question in her son-in-law's eyes.

Sometimes a man was not allowed even to see his mother-in-law, let alone act disrespectfully towards her, and had to run or hide when she came near. The 'commonest sounds' to be heard in a camp of Navaho Indians, according to an early authority (Stephen 1893: 358), 'are the friendly shouts, warning these relatives apart'. So tabooed was a man's mother-in-law, and so fearsome in his eyes, that in some cases at least this figure seems to have succumbed to the temptation to 'abuse' her own power! Róheim (1974: 29) writes of a case among the Aranda Aborigines of Central Australia: 'I was told of one old woman who would often appear suddenly when her son-in-law was eating. When he ran away, she would sit down and eat the food he had left.'

But the status of the mother-in-law cannot be understood in isolation. It is only one aspect of the fact that in almost all human cultures, no matter how male-dominated, elements of blood solidarity are to be found as a check on husbands' rights in their wives, this being a feature absolutely central to social structure. In this context, whether a wife calls for support upon her mother, upon some other female relative or upon male kin is less important than the fact that she is not alone.

Sex for Meat

Among the Australian Yir-Yiront Aborigines of Cape York Peninsula (Sharp 1933: 418), a man feels constantly in debt to his in-laws. He says: 'I get my wife from that mother's brother's group; I avoid them, give them presents, and take care of them when they are old.' Here as elsewhere, it is quite clear that the husband is repaying his wife's kin for the privilege of being allowed sexual access to her. In the case of this particular community, moreover – and again the pattern is not unusual – a man may have several wives who will all be related to one another as real or classificatory 'sisters'. It might be supposed that these women would all be divided among themselves, but not so. In fact (reminding us, perhaps, of the Seven Sisters in the Californian myth discussed earlier), solidarity in the form of a 'sex strike' is a weapon which the women can fall back upon if need be:

> the solidarity between the wives of a polygynous family gives them considerable influence over the husband. In cases of extreme mistreatment of one of them by the husband, they may institute a *Lysistrata régime*, an economic and sexual boycott in which they may enlist their other sisters in the community. Since a man normally will not have sexual relations outside the conventional limits of those he calls wife, such a programme may prove extremely effective. (Sharp 1933: 430)

All over the world, wherever hunting was part of the traditional way of life, women treated marriage as an economic-and-sexual relationship, claiming for themselves the meat which their spouses obtained. Indeed, contrary to the views of Lévi-Strauss, this was everywhere what marital alliances were largely about. They were not just means to enable male in-laws to form social relationships among themselves. They had an *economic* content which was absolutely central. Marital relations (in contradistinction to mere 'sexual relations') were the means by which women, supported by their kin, achieved something that no primate females ever achieved. They were the means by which they secured for themselves and their offspring the continuous *economic* services of the opposite sex.

Among the Brazilian Shavante Indians, women receive an unsuccessful hunter 'with a marked coldness', while a successful hunter 'flings down his game for the women to prepare' and basks in the resulting glory (Maybury-Lewis 1967: 36). In the case of the Mundurucu, again in Brazil, 'The man brings his kill to his wife . . . and she and her housemates butcher it. They send pieces to other houses, but they determine who gets which parts' (Murphy and Murphy 1974: 132).

Among the Ache, hunter-gatherers of eastern Paraguay, 'men consume very little meat from game items that they themselves killed'. All game caught each morning is taken to the women's group, so that the hunters can continue unencumbered; the meat is shared not just within small family units but throughout the foraging band. Game caught at other times is also distributed widely throughout the band – always by a man other than the hunter himself. Nonetheless, in each case, people know very well who hunted the animal whose meat they receive. There is a strong suggestion that women are sexually attracted to good hunters; certainly, the more successful and generous hunters are most often cited by women as lovers in extra-marital relationships (Hill and Kaplan 1988: 277–89).

Among the Peruvian Sharanahua, to whom we will turn in the next section:

> Both the pleasures and the pains of hunting are related not only to the actual activity but to the implication that a good hunter is a virile man . . . .
> Virility implies a positive response from women. Further, the culturally structured idea that a successful hunter is a virile man carries a sting: the unsuccessful hunter is by social definition not virile. (Siskind 1973b: 232)

Almost universally, similar ideas prevailed, women feeling sexual desire not in isolation but in a situation-dependent way, according to whether their menfolk were proving themselves or not. 'Women expect meat from lovers', as Collier and Rosaldo (1981: 314) put it, referring to 'bride-service societies' throughout the world. Far from being unusual, men's need to ply their wives and/or in-laws with meat as the test of their virility and the condition of the marital tie may indeed be regarded as the norm – certainly among hunters and gatherers and probably much more widely.

A Case Study: the Sharanahua

We will now turn in greater detail to a particular example of this whole complex. We will examine a society in which women themselves, autonomously and as a gender group, use collective control over their sexuality as a means to induce their menfolk to hunt for them. It is worth dwelling on this case at some length, since it will be argued later in this book that a comparable logic of sexual and economic exchange must have been central to the origins of human culture.

Much of the literature on sexual politics in bride-service societies (Collier and Rosaldo 1981) indicates a complex interplay of male influences and female ones, as well as a subtle dialectic between economics and sex. In this connection, one of the most sensitive pictures is Janet Siskind's (1973a, 1973b) account of life in the village of Marcos, among the Sharanahua of Peru (located on the Upper Purús River just west of the Brazilian border). Their cultural heritage is that of interfluvial hunters, and their society is still strongly focused on meat, although the women's contribution through gathering is substantial and they have for generations augmented the proceeds of foraging with small-scale horticultural activities. Residence is matrilocal, a son-in-law contributing meat to his wife's kin. The special value of Siskind's account is that it shows us a mechanism of exchange through which women can gain strength in a hunting context – even though here as almost everywhere, it is the men who kill the animals.

The Sharanahua have two basic patterns of hunting. In the first, each man decides for himself whether or not to go hunting. He usually hunts alone and brings the game back to his own household. But men in this mode are

'reluctant and unenthusiastic', since the relative privacy makes it difficult for
even a good hunter to gain the widespread female acclaim and sexual prestige
for which every man yearns. 'At times', however, when there has been no
meat in the village for three or four days, the women decide to send the
men on a special hunt. They talk together and complain that there is no meat
and the men are lazy (Siskind 1973a: 96). In contrast to the first pattern,
during a 'special hunt' (the second pattern) the young men go hunting as a
group:

> The special hunt is started by the women. Early in the evening, all the
> young women go from house to house singing to every man. Each woman
> chooses a man to hunt for her, a man who is not her husband nor of her
> kin group, though he may be her cross-cousin, her husband's brother, or a
> stranger. The men leave the following day and are met on their return by a
> line-up of all the women of the village, painted and beaded and wearing
> their best dresses. Even the older men will not face this line without
> game, but, if unsuccessful, they beach their canoes and slink to their
> households by a back trail. The choice of partners is usually a choice of
> lovers, and many partnerships are maintained for years. (1973b: 233–4)

There is, then, a collective hunt, initiated by the women, at the conclusion
of which the face-painted women form a kind of 'picket line' at the entrance
to the village, warmly welcoming the hunters if they carry meat but
rejecting and shaming them if they have been unsuccessful.

In motivating the men to go on such a hunt, the women use a mixture of
sexual enticement, teasing and potential threat. While the men are away, the
women talk and laugh among themselves about which of the men each is
'waiting for'. A short time before the men are expected to return, the
younger women pick *nawawakusi* (stinging nettles) 'ready for later use
against the men'. The men can be heard coming upriver when they are still
half an hour from the village, and all the women 'who are taking part in the
special hunt' line up in front of the main house. Assuming a successful hunt,
it is at this point that the women take the game animals from the men:

> The men walk solemnly up from the port, and silently each man drops the
> game he has shot on the ground before the waiting women and walks to
> his own house. Each woman picks up the animal that her partner has
> dropped and takes it to her own house and begins to prepare it. (1973a:
> 96–8)

The meat is skinned, cut up and put to boil by the women, and then eaten in
a general process of feasting and reciprocal visiting. Siskind continues:

> Everyone has barely finished eating when the young women burst into
> action with stalks of *nawawakusi* in their hands, trying to corner a young
> man. The men laugh, but they run, staying out of reach, hiding behind a

house, until they are caught. Then they stand still, letting the girls triumphantly rub their chests, necks, and arms with the stinging nettle, which is said to give strength. The men finally seize some *nawawakusi* from the women and the chase becomes two sided with small groups of men and women in pursuit and retreat, laughing and shouting. (1973a: 98–100)

It is clear that in this society sex is one of the economic forces of production – it is the major factor motivating men to hunt. It is equally clear that the solidarity of the women – expressed in their periodic teasing of the men, their sexual inducements and their implied collective sexual threat – is not a mere superstructural feature, but is central to the economic infrastructure of society. If this underpinning of the social order were to change, the whole economic, social and sexual system would turn on its axis.

For Sharanahua men, the threat of female ridicule and withdrawal is very real. A woman wants to 'eat' a man; but she finds male flesh unaccompanied by the requisite animal flesh simply unexciting:

The prestige system carries a sting: The good hunter is the virile man, but the hunter with little skill or bad luck does not find sympathy. When children scream at their mothers, 'Nami pipai!', 'I want to eat meat!' their mothers' reply, 'Nami yamai', 'There is no more meat', is a goad that women aim at their husbands, provoking them to hunt again, implying that they are less than men since there is no more meat.

A man may spend hours in the forest. One day Basta returned empty handed, tired, muddy from wading through swampy ground and picking ticks off his body. No words of sympathy were forthcoming, and I asked Yawandi why she and Bashkondi were painting their faces. She replied in a voice that carried to the hammock where Basta rested alone, 'We want to paint, there's no meat, let's eat penises!' On other days as well I have suspected that women paint their faces as an unspoken challenge to the men. . . . (1973a: 105)

The special hunt usually results in more meat in the village than a normal day's hunt. The social pressure of the special hunt, the line of women painted and waiting, makes young men try hard to succeed.

And this kind of hunt breaks across any tendency of society to fragment into isolated, self-interested, monogamous 'family' groups – a tendency which would be very risky given the chancy nature of hunting. Referring to hunting generally, Siskind (1973a: 88) writes that a system involving many men, and in which meat is widely shared, 'provides some insurance against the bad luck, illness, or lack of skill of a single hunter providing for a single family' (1973a: 88).

Meat from a special hunt is not just brought by a hunter to his wife, mother-in-law or other relative within the household but to a variety of households depending on the choice of partner on each occasion. The women in each household, receiving meat from their chosen lovers, then issue invitations to eat to their sisters and cousins in addition to many others. And since a basic requirement of the special hunt is female solidarity against men, in which as far as possible none of the women allows marriage or a lover to come between them, the result is an extended network of relationships and households. As Siskind (1973a: 109) puts it, the 'combination of same sex solidarity and antagonism to the other sex prevents the households from becoming tightly closed units'.

The teasing and the provocation of the special hunt games are symbolically sexual, coinciding with the partnerships formed by the hunt:

> Neither husbands nor wives are supposed to be jealous of the love affairs involved in the special hunt. In general, jealousy is considered to be a bad trait in a wife or a husband, and I have heard both men and women complain that they are unlucky to have a jealous spouse. . . . (1973a: 105)

Put at its crudest, comments Siskind,

> the special hunt symbolizes an economic structure in which meat is exchanged for sex. This is neither a 'natural' nor 'rational' exchange since women produce at least as much of the food supply at Marcos, and a rational exchange would consist of viewing the economy as an exchange of women's production for men's. Certainly there is no evidence that women are naturally less interested in sex or more interested in meat than men are. This is a culturally produced socio-economic system in which sex is the incentive for hunting, and a man who is known to be a good hunter has a better chance of gaining wives or mistresses. . . . The special hunt gives an opportunity for men to demonstrate their hunting skill to women other than their wives. It is a dramatic portrayal of the exchange between the sexes, which structures daily interactions between men and women. (1973a: 103–4)

Siskind (1973b: 234) sees all this as a point along a continuum among South American tropical forest peoples:

> One can see variations on a single theme from the crude gift of meat 'to seduce a potential wife' among the Siriono (Holmberg 1950: 166); the elaboration of the special hunt among the Sharanahua; to the young Shavante's provisioning his father-in-law with game after the consummation of his marriage. . . . (Maybury-Lewis 1967: 92). Whether men prove their virility by hunting and thus gain wives or offer meat to seduce a woman, the theme is an exchange of meat for sex.

Finally, it is worth adding that Siskind sees a connection between gardening among the Sharanahua and the development of more stable marital relationships. Agriculture, she writes (1973a: 116–17), demands a synchronisation of the work of men and women. In addition, agricultural work is an investment of time and effort; a man will not work hard for two months clearing land without the security of knowing that women will harvest and prepare the food:

> The sexual incentive for hunting is logical since hunting is a brief but recurring task as sex is a brief but recurring need. The ease with which marriages are established and broken at Marcos fits well with the basic economy, but a more stable relationship is essential for the responsibilities of agriculture.

Relatively weak marital ties – if this interpretation had wider validity – would then be an intrinsic feature of 'the hunter-gatherer mode of production', contrasting with the more tightly secured marriages required when this way of life begins to break down.

Unconditional Marriage as Anomaly

It was noted earlier that Lévi-Strauss' 'exchange of women' model, resting as it does on the absolute primacy of marriage, produces some serious theoretical problems. It precludes female solidarity and fails to explain the patterns actually found in traditionally organised – particularly hunter-gatherer – cultures.

Culture's 'initial situation' cannot be dogmatically asserted, but we can be fairly certain that it bore little relation to Lévi-Strauss' picture of women as ever-available, passive pawns in the political schemes of men. It would seem more likely that women, in the course of cultural origins, could give themselves sexually because they had something to give – their bodies were not completely owned or spoken for by the other sex in advance.

Viewing the same feature in the context of the development of hunting and gathering, we may take it that although women did not usually hunt, they could use a measure of control over their own sexual availability to induce men to hunt for them. An implication is that women (supported by kin) had the capacity to withdraw themselves sexually. In effect – like some female primates but in much more conscious and organised ways – they could go 'on strike'.

Naturally, this does not imply that women did not enjoy sex or that sex seldom happened. It simply means that when sex occurred, it took place as a release from the basic cultural constraints – not in obedience to them. In this sense, no matter how joyfully celebrated and woven into the meanings and symbols of all cultural life, sexual gratification from culture's very beginnings has been delayed, sublimated and harnessed to economic and other ends, its actual consummation always taking place just beyond, behind and in a sense 'in spite of' culture. The bonding involved in love-making, as something tending to undermine wider forms of solidarity, has always been for the public cultural domain something of an embarrassment – in a sense, it 'should not' occur. This, of course, has always been an aspect of the excitement of sex, for lovers can relish their rebellion against rules of behaviour which can be shed like clothes for the occasion – constraints which, for the moment, seem to belong to some other, duller, world. When sexual intercourse is actually taking place, the public, collective assembly either dissolves temporarily and happily for the occasion, or – if it remains in session throughout – it turns to one side, allowing the couple their privacy, as if pretending not to know.

Of course, there is all the difference in the world between sexually relaxed cultures and more repressive ones in these respects, but in no human social context are people simply uninhibited or unembarrassed in public in the manner of monkeys and apes. In any event, the prioritising of sex has never been allowed to last for long or to threaten society's fundamental economic goals.

In what follows, inverting the usual assumptions, the situation in which a man's marriage gives him absolute rights of access to his wife will be treated as anomalous. It may occur, but it has nothing to do with the initial situation for human culture as such. Many of the staple topics of ethnography – features such as menstrual and postpartum taboos, in-law avoidances, taboos on sex prior to hunting, the separation of spouses at meals, 'totemism', the 'ritualisation of male solidarity in antagonism to female solidarity' (Siskind 1973a: 109) etc. etc. – will now appear in a new light. They will present themselves no longer as peculiar anomalies to be explained, but as residual expressions of a common underlying norm according to which wives are as a matter of course set apart ritually and in other ways from their husbands, simply because they belong in the opposite gender camp.

In later chapters, as we follow through the implications of this model, it will be seen that women's normative state of relative autonomy, in limiting men's rights in their wives, simultaneously and by the same token limits hunters' rights in their kills. In western South Australia, 'the man's gift (or obligation) of meat to his wife's parents (tabu to him) is taken by the woman herself'. She then passes it on to her mother, who is particulaly to be avoided by the hunter (Berndt and Berndt 1945: 224). In Central Australia, among the Aranda, a hunter was (a) obliged to surrender his kills to his wife's relatives and (b) was prohibited from eating with these people himself. If a man were to be seen by his wife's kin eating with them 'the food would disagree with him, and he would sicken and suffer severely' (Spencer and Gillen 1899: 469–71). To the Wik-Mungkan Aborigines of Cape York Peninsula, any meat 'stepped over' by a man's mother-in-law becomes 'ngaintja' (tabooed) to him, the blood in the meat becoming powerfully dangerous in a manner suggestive of menstrual blood (McKnight 1975: 77, 85).

In contexts such as these, the forces which 'supernaturally' protect women and those which impose taboos on meat food are seen to converge. Sexual respect rules and food avoidances turn out to be the same thing. The logic, the mechanisms and even the symbolic conceptualisations are at a deep level identical. Backed by each other and by their kin, women periodically reassert sufficient control over their own sexuality to clarify that men cannot take their availability for granted. In this way they make it clear that men as hunters must 'earn their keep' by regularly surrendering their kills.

This is the basic argument of this book. Women, from the beginning, have held the future in their hands. Their responsibilities for offspring have often compelled them to resist men's advances, subordinating short-term sexual to longer-term economic goals. Thanks mainly to female insistence, backed by the imperatives of reproductive survival, culture from its earliest stages held male sexual dominance in check – not always completely annihilating it, but at least preventing it from holding undisputed sway. As the process of 'becoming human' (Tanner 1981) proceeded, women (usually with some backing from their male offspring and kin) resisted and even repressed the raw expression of primate male sexuality, eventually replacing it with something more acceptable. 'The development of culture', as Marshall Sahlins writes,

> did not simply give expression to man's primate nature, it replaced that nature as the direct determinant of social behaviour, and in so doing, channeled it – at times repressed it completely. The most significant transformation effected by cultural society was the subordination of the search for mates – the primary determinant of subhuman primate sociability – to the search for food. In the process also, economic cooperation replaced competition, and kinship replaced conflict as the principal mechanism of organization. (1972: 14)

We begin, then, not with the supposed sudden emergence of male sexual generosity and self-restraint – as in the origins models of Freud (1965 [1913]) and Lévi-Strauss (1969a) – but with something rather more believable. We begin with *female* child-rearing and economic priorities, *female* ultimate determination of social structure and *female* sexual self-restraint in women's own direct material interests. From this, the incest taboo, food taboos and the other basic features of the human cultural configuration will be derived.

Chapter 5
Origins Theories in the 1980s

We must begin by stating the first presupposition of all human existence, and therefore of all history, namely, that men must be in a position to live in order to be able to 'make history'. But life involves before everything else eating and drinking, a habitation, clothing, and many other things. The first historical act, is, therefore, the production of material life itself. This is indeed a historical act, a fundamental condition of all history, which today, as thousands of years ago, must be accomplished every day and every hour merely in order to sustain human life.

Karl Marx and Friedrich Engels, *The German Ideology* (1846)

Until the 1960s, no section of the scientific community was devoting itself in any consistent way to unravelling the mysteries of human social origins. Like Freud before him, Lévi-Strauss with his peculiarly sex-oriented theory was an isolated figure; he was interested in neither archaeology nor evolutionary biology, and despite his immense influence worked very much on his own. His social anthropological colleagues had eschewed 'origins' for fifty years, for reasons which were discussed in Chapter 1. Meanwhile, although scientific books and papers on human origins were still being published, they did not even claim to deal with the social aspects but examined bones and stones with the aim of arranging them within chronologies and typologies.

All this began to change in the 1960s and early 1970s. The popular books of writers such as Konrad Lorenz, Robert Ardrey and Desmond Morris were arousing public controversy with their emphasis on the positive aspects of aggression, territoriality, uninhibited sexuality and other 'natural' tendencies in us all (Chapter 1). More important, however, were other developments. Extremely exciting new discoveries of fossil hominids were being made at Olduvai Gorge and at other sites in East Africa. Field studies of primates in the wild had begun revolutionising our understanding of the biological background to human physiological and social evolution. Fuelled by revolutionary new dating techniques, archaeology was in a ferment of revolt against what were claimed to be tenacious traditions of gentlemanly insularity and amateurishness governing site excavations and their interpretation. Finally, the rise of anti-racism, feminism and vigorous 'new left' Marxist political currents meant that the focus of social anthropological interest was dramatically changing. A new generation of anthropologists was anxious to make a clean break with the discipline's colonial traditions and isolation and make links with anti-imperialist struggles, with the rest of the scientific community and with the concerns of the wider world.

Social accountability and cross-disciplinary fertilisation were the catchwords of the time, and the study of human origins was the topic which, more than any other, seemed to provide the focus for such a coming together. Soon, young anthropologists, archaeologists, primatologists and others were committing themselves on a new and higher level to a project which had been left unattended for over half a century: an onslaught on the still unresolved challenge of explaining human physical and social origins. Seminars, conferences and papers began linking social anthropology with archaeology, primatology and other disciplines in ways which would have seemed unthinkable or even outrageous a few years previously.

1966 saw the most ambitious and significant event in this connection – the 'Man the Hunter' conference (Lee and DeVore 1968). This was devoted to the study of the hunting-and-gathering way of life which – the participants broadly agreed – had dominated human life for about 99 per cent of our period of existence on this planet. One of the main organisers – Richard Lee – was a Marxist who, with Eleanor Leacock and a small number of others, had kept alive the spirit of Lewis Henry Morgan within social anthropology in the United States. Lee had worked among the !Kung; in his view these gentle people practised a version of that 'primitive communism' which for millennia had been inseparable from humanity's once universal huntergatherer lifestyle (Lee 1988).

Another main organiser and coeditor (with Lee) of the symposium, Irven DeVore, was also a social anthropologist, but an unusual one. Sherwood Washburn, doyen of modern primatological field studies, had encouraged him to study the social behaviour of baboons explicitly as a model for the behaviour of protohominids. By the time of the 'Man the Hunter' conference, DeVore was already one of the main authorities on primate social life, and was in a unique position to compare and contrast this with information on human hunter-gatherers.

The 'Man the Hunter' conference was a turning point. Lévi-Strauss was present, and archaeologists mingled with social anthropologists, palaeontologists, primatologists and many others in an attempt to place the hunter-gatherer way of life in perspective as an evolutionary adaptation of immense antiquity and significance in determining the whole nature of human existence. The conference marked a radical shift in American social anthropological theorising – a virtual abandonment of Boasian cultural particularism (see Chapter 1) in favour of various forms of ecological functionalism. It also became impossible any longer for anyone to treat human evolution as the study of just 'bones and stones'. The conference made it not only legitimate but mandatory to examine early hominid fossils and artefacts in the light of ethnographic knowledge and to try to construct appropriate models of early human behaviour and social organisation.

The new school of archaeology led by Lewis Binford helped to validate this approach: Binford insisted that forms of social patterning were encoded in the material remains which archaeologists could excavate and analyse. In his view, there was no hope of deciphering these remains, however, without conducting ethnographic fieldwork among contemporary hunter-gatherers specifically to answer questions posed by the digging, without much other comparative information beyond the traditional confines of archaeology, and without sufficiently careful, controlled and thorough techniques of excavation and analysis (Binford 1983).

It was in this period, and in part through the 'Man the Hunter' conference itself, that palaeoanthropology in its modern sense was born.

However, the outcome of the conference was not all positive. Firstly, very little consciousness of gender was displayed. The title 'Man the Hunter' to many participants meant just that − the topic was not humans of both sexes, but quite literally 'man'. It would be a few years before the impact of feminism made itself felt (Fedigan 1986).

Secondly, the new realisation of the significance of hunter-gatherer lifestyles led to a rather oversimplified view of human evolution and origins. It was assumed that the evolution of humans *was* the evolution of the hunter-gatherer adaptation. Perhaps the most often-cited passage from the conference was this:

> in contrast to carnivores, human hunting . . . is based on a division of labour and is a social and technical adaptation quite different from that of other mammals. Human hunting is made possible by tools, but it is far more than a technique or even a variety of techniques. It is a way of life, and the success of this adaptation (in its total social, technical, and psychological dimensions) has dominated the course of human evolution for hundreds of thousands of years. In a very real sense our intellect, interests, emotions, and basic social life − all are evolutionary products of the success of the hunting adaptation. (Washburn and Lancaster 1968: 293)

In the following years, consequently, wherever ancient 'human' fossils were found, it was inferred that the hominids concerned must have been 'hunters' or 'hunter-gatherers' in roughly the sense in which the !Kung, the Hadza or the Australian Aborigines are. Since the latest, very exciting hominid fossil finds at Olduvai Gorge and elsewhere were being dated by the revolutionary new potassium-argon technique to two or more million years ago, the results were peculiar.

'One of the practical consequences for palaeoanthropology', as Robert Foley (1988: 207) comments, 'has been a model of human evolution that is essentially gradualistic and unilinear'. The important elements of a hunter-gatherer way of life – food sharing, hunting, a division of labour, a home base and so on – were thought to be identifiable very early in the fossil and archaeological record. In this period, it was almost as if specialists were in a race to see who could find evidence for human life, in a social as well as a physical sense, earlier than anyone else.

One result was that the differences between various hominid taxa took on the appearance of minor anatomical variations, rather than functionally and adaptively significant features. Hunting and gathering was hunting and gathering; this basic mode of production had remained in all essentials the same for countless millennia. Since all the various hominids were supposedly doing the same thing, it was not at all clear why *Homo habilis* differed from *Homo erectus*, nor why the Neanderthals and modern humans differed from one another at all. This problem will be seen to afflict most of the theories of social origins which have been put forward over the past ten to twenty years.

What is the current state of thinking on human social origins? To help put into perspective the synthesis which this book will propose, this chapter provides a representative set of position statements. Many date from around 1981, a year of intense debate on the topic of origins in academic journals. Although all of these theories are now past history, many of their insights remain valid, and any new theory will have to build on the advances they have made.

Most of the theories featured here focus on one problem – that of *getting males to provide food for females and offspring*.

To appreciate the significance of this, it is necessary to recall our earlier discussion of totemism and the hunter's own-kill taboo – and then note that in no primate species can a pregnant or nursing female in any way depend for her food supplies on a male. Although highly co-operative hunting (Boesch and Boesch 1989; Boesch 1990) and meat-eating may occur, nothing resembling 'totemic' food avoidances can be found. Primate meat-eaters, in fact, differ from culturally organised human hunters in the following respects:

1.   When a baboon or chimpanzee kills an animal for food, the killer typically eats – or attempts to eat – the meat.

2.   Sometimes one animal does the killing whilst another does the eating. But such an event is *never* a deliberate act of exchange. Chimpanzee

males who have collaborated in a hunt, and are very probably siblings or close kin, certainly *do* often share their spoils. But for a whole carcass to pass from one hunter to another would be unusual *unless* the first animal had seized more than it could possibly monopolise and was mobbed and robbed despite its efforts. Only the crudest behaviourist could claim that since the meat in fact changes hands, all this 'amounts to the same thing' as hunter/gatherer-type sharing or exchange. The most that we can speak of, probably, is 'tolerated scrounging' (Isaac 1978) or 'tolerated theft' (Blurton Jones 1984).

3.   When baboons or chimpanzees make a kill, there is no delay in starting to eat. Consumption begins on the spot – indeed, it may even precede the kill. Strum (1981: 263) observes that when baboons (at Gilgil, Kenya) start eating, the victim is typically still alive. There are no signs of even the most rudimentary or prefigurative inhibitions or taboos delaying consumption until a predetermined destination or 'home base' has been reached.

4.   If, following a kill, portions of the victim are carried away, the reason is (typically) the reverse of that motivating such transport among human hunter-gatherers. Far from carrying away the meat for others to consume, the animal will typically be scampering off with a portion up into a tree (Suzuki 1975: 262–6) or into the distance to escape from others' demands.

5.   Although it has been claimed that chimpanzees have a 'rudimentary' sexual division of labour – with females specialising in termite-fishing, for example, while males hunt (McGrew 1979, 1981: 58) – the fact is that the two sexes do not exchange with one another their respective products. Since the members of each gender group are on a nutritional level entirely self-sufficient, it is unclear in what sense even a 'rudimentary' sex division of labour may be said to exist.

In this light, it seems extraordinary that proponents of gradual evolution in palaeoanthropology should have succeeded in drawing simplistic parallels between *primate* meat-sharing and the patterns of meat distribution characteristic of modern *human* hunters and gatherers.

Following the discovery of meat-eating by primates in the wild (Goodall 1986; Strum 1987), it was argued almost throughout the 1970s and 1980s that primate hunting – which can produce very impressive levels of synchrony and co-operation in the actual *hunt itself* (Boesch and Boesch 1990; Boesch 1990) – 'naturally' leads to orderly and co-operative food sharing, and that primate field studies illustrate how easy it was for human hunter-gatherer norms of distribution to evolve.

The feminist writer Frances Dahlberg (1981: 7–8), for example, asserted that hunter-gatherer type food-sharing is nothing extraordinary: it evolved 'among chimpanzees, contemporary human foragers, and certainly ancient hominids as well'. In her view, 'the sociobiological concept of kin selection' explains this. Individuals who share food within groups which include close kin are 'rewarded by gene representation in following generations'. Dahlberg claimed that the results were particularly evident among chimpanzees:

> Adult food sharing among chimpanzees does not involve aggression; adults beg for meat, they don't grab it. The successful chimpanzee hunter shares with other males and occasionally with an adult female, especially one who is in estrus.

In similar vein, the primatologist Hladik (1975: 26) claimed that chimpanzee 'hunting and meat-eating behaviour could be compared with what is known about primitive human tribes of hunter-gatherers', whilst a colleague insisted that chimpanzee hunting 'blurs the line dividing human and non-human behaviour' (Harding 1975: 256).

Statements of this kind went almost unquestioned until late in the 1980s. They were, in effect, assertions that our ancestors had to cross no rubicon – accomplish no revolution – to establish the human hunter-gatherer configuration. It was claimed that we can see its rudiments already among meat-eating baboons and chimpanzees. To put such statements into perspective, and before turning to our survey of recent origins theories, we may usefully review some of the most celebrated case studies of primate meat-eating in the wild.

The Problem of the Hunting Ape

Jane Goodall (1986: 299) describes how Gombe chimpanzees rush up to a successful hunter and furiously struggle to seize a share of his kill. In the chaotic scramble which follows, the forest becomes filled with screams, barks, waa-barks and pant-hoots. Almost always, it is eventually a tough male who emerges victorious in any such fight; he runs off, attempting to monopolise 'his' meat.

'Meat is a highly coveted food', Goodall comments on her chimpanzee subjects, 'and often there is intense aggressive competition around a kill.' Those without meat attack those in possession, possessors counter-attack, and dominant but meatless animals attack empty-handed companions if these are of lower rank or are seen as competitors in the general conflict. 'Begging' does occur and is sometimes successful, but in any large group, there is no doubt that sheer physical struggle is a more important factor in determining how much – if anything – each animal receives.

One writer (Suzuki 1975: 262–6) describes some Budongo Forest chimpanzees who had just killed a subadult blue duiker. Ten minutes after the victim was first heard screaming,

I found the four big males in a tree crying and struggling with one another for the spoils of the duiker. . . . Several furious struggles . . . took place between the four animals; these were followed by silent periods of eating the meat.

The victim was killed through being bitten, mauled and eventually torn limb from limb in the struggles of each chimpanzee to obtain a share; the primatologist could 'hear at thirty metres the sound of tearing meat and bone'.

As an evolutionary gradualist, anxious to find parallels with the sharing-behaviour of human hunter-gatherers, the reporter who observed all this (Suzuki 1975) confidently interpreted it 'as a case of cooperative working for the division of the spoils'.

The pattern is still more competitive among baboons. 'The young antelopes that baboons sometimes kill', writes Kummer,

are almost exclusively eaten by the adult males, and fighting over such prey is frequent. The inability of baboons to share food is a behavioural characteristic that probably prevents them from shifting to hunting as a way of life. (1971: 59)

The whole situation places females at a severe disadvantage. 'In baboons and chimpanzees', notes Harding (1975: 253), 'the killing of small animals appears to be an activity carried on only by adults and almost exclusively by males.' Much the same applies to bonobos (Susman 1987: 82). Since the killers are also likely to be among the main eaters, and since the eating begins on the spot, the result is a foregone conclusion. Even should a female manage to make a kill, she will typically be robbed of it by some aggressive male very soon.

This last point needs to be emphasised. Whatever the force of 'the sociobiological concept of kin-selection' (Dahlberg 1981: 7–8), it does not mean that male chimpanzees in a typical group spontaneously give each other meat or provide meat for females. *Far from bringing meat for females to eat, the usual pattern is for males to rob females of whatever meat they may have been lucky enough to obtain.*

Among Gombe chimpanzees, even the toughest female cannot count on holding a piece of meat for long. 'Gigi' was one whose ability to defend herself against males was quite remarkable:

On a number of occasions she maintained possession of her meat despite determined assaults by adult males. Once, for example, she caught a large juvenile colobus [monkey] when it fell or jumped to the ground during a mixed-party hunt. Satan instantly leaped down, chased after Gigi, and attacked her vigorously as she crouched over the prey. She managed to escape and rushed up a tree with her prey. (Goodall 1986: 307)

Satan – a particularly strong male – followed her up the tree and attacked her. Both chimpanzees fell ten metres to the ground. Gigi ran off, chased by Satan, who was then momentarily distracted – some other chimpanzees had made a second kill nearby. However, he was still empty-handed eight minutes later; again, he chased Gigi up a tree; again, both fell heavily to the ground. A third chimpanzee, 'Goblin', then attacked Satan, allowing Gigi to escape back up into some branches. Another male, 'Sherry', charged up and grabbed the prey. Gigi did not let go; 'both pulled, screaming loudly'. Satan charged back, attacked Sherry and inadvertently allowed Gigi once more to escape up a tree with her piece of meat. Satan raced after her; Gigi crashed to the ground, and Sherry – waiting below – managed to grab the prey and tear off a large part. Finally, Satan robbed Sherry, allowing Gigi, 'for a while at any rate', to eat a little of her hard-won spoils.

Given this kind of 'sharing', in which physical struggle far outweighs the importance of communicative subtleties such as 'begging', it is no surprise to find that among common chimpanzees (Hladik 1975: 26; Goodall 1986: 301–12), bonobos (Susman 1987: 81–2) and baboons (Harding 1975: 249; Strum 1981: 276), meat-eating is largely monopolized by the more powerful males.

It is true that females can gain meat by sexual means. A common female chimpanzee tactic is to present her rump to a meat-possessing male; the more alluring this sexual offering, the better her chances of gaining something. As Jane Goodall (1986: 484) observes, the bodily contortions involved in this kind of 'sharing' can be remarkable:

> When a female in estrus is begging meat from a male at Gombe, it is not at all unusual to see the male, carcass clutched in one hand, pause in his feeding to mate her – after which she is usually allowed to share his prey. I have even seen females, during copulation, reach back and take food from the mouth of the male.

Note that the female 'may' be allowed a share in the meat – but only *after* she has paid in the currency of her own flesh. Note also that because offerings of meat and other privileges are bestowed on females who display oestrus swellings, 'the swollen state has been prolonged well beyond the biological need for female receptivity and attractiveness to the males around the time of ovulation' (Goodall 1986:484). As Goodall puts it, the female chimpanzee's swelling 'in a way, serves as a sexual bargaining point. . . '. There are some costs – for example, being fought over by rival males and perhaps severely wounded – but the benefits evidently outweigh these.

Much baboon evidence illustrates a similar logic, but here in particular we see how it is not only females, but males who are faced with certain difficulties as well:

> Sumner in consort with Peggy was a classic case. Peggy stared fixedly at a nearby carcass as Sumner copulated with her. When he was done, she

determinedly circled back to the carcass – which was surrounded by males – while again and again Sumner tried to chase her in the opposite direction. (Strum 1987: 131).

Sumner's problem in this case was that 'his' female would gladly trade sex with any male who could tempt her with meat. His only hope of stopping such liaisons was to physically drive her the other way.

As Shirley Strum (1981: 269) strikingly points out, the whole situation can subject a successful male to stressfully conflicting pressures and temptations:

> For example, when a male was in sexual consort with a receptive female and then conflict occurred between maintaining proximity to the female and eating meat, the male chose to continue consortship. At times the male appeared to be deliberating, looking back and forth between the meat and the female, but finally chose to follow the female.

Thirty-five times in one year, Strum observed dominant males apparently torn between meat and sex, reluctant to decide between the two but eventually abandoning the meat. Resolution of such conflicts ranged from males 'entirely ignoring meat-eating opportunities' to their simply allowing associated females to keep and eat the carcass. 'Even males with very high predatory scores chose estrous females over meat.'

In the context of hominid evolution, any such logic would have played havoc with males' freedom to hunt. It is simply not possible to guard or chase a female and chase a prey animal at the same time; a dominant male is in a strong position provided he does not have to be in two places at once. 'The trouble with that system', as Lovejoy (cited in Johanson and Edey 1981: 338) puts it,

> is that the alpha male's authority is enforced only by his presence. If he goes down to the river for a drink, he loses it. Some other watchful fellow is always hanging around. By the time the alpha male gets back, his chance for having any offspring may be gone.

If a similar system existed among early hominids', Strum (1981: 299) comments, 'a major change in reproductive strategies would have been necessary before males could give predation the priority it needed as a prelude to further division of labour between the sexes.'

All the evidence indicates that such a change would have been immensely difficult to achieve.

Origins theories of the 1980s

With this primatological background in mind, we are now in a position to look at our sample of origins models, almost all of which focus on the issues we have just discussed.

1. Glynn Isaac

Glynn L1. Isaac (1971) 'The diet of early man: aspects of archaeological evidence from lower and middle Pleistocene sites in Africa'

Glynn L1. Isaac and Diana Crader (1981) 'To what extent were early hominids carnivorous? An archaeological perspective'

Glynn L1. Isaac (1983), 'Aspects of human evolution'

Isaac was a brilliant palaeoarchaeologist who worked under Louis Leakey in 1961, and became responsible, before his premature death in 1985, for interpreting several of the most crucial East African sites linking hominid activities with animal remains. His 1971 paper was one of the opening contributions in what has become an on-going multidisciplinary attempt to relate specific hominid-related archaeological sites with models of foraging strategy.

Of the East African sites which provide our entire fund of information on early hominid life, Olduvai Gorge contains by far the largest body of evidence. The various excavations at Olduvai are in geological deposits spanning an extremely long period – from about 1.8 million years ago to 600,000 years ago. The older deposits, known as 'Bed I', are among the best preserved, providing evidence of activities beside a lake whose margins were gradually receding.

In his 1971 paper, Isaac argued that the Bed I deposits indicate that humanity's distinctive hunter-gatherer lifestyle – featuring a sexual division of labour and reliance on a home base – stretches back some 2 million years to the early Pleistocene or late Pliocene (p. 281). He describes 'concentrated patches of bone' and comments:

> It seems certain that hominids were the prime agency creating these concentrations. The sites document a behaviour complex that is fundamentally human: tool manufacture, a partly carnivorous diet achieved by hunting and/or scavenging, and the practice of bringing meat back to a home base for sharing amongst the members of a social group.

In common with most other participants in the 'Man the Hunter' symposium, Isaac linked the origins of bipedalism with the first appearance of the 'home base'. The assumption was that walking upright evolved because it freed the hands for carrying things to and from the base.

Isaac in particular argued that (1) food-carrying using baskets or other containers and (2) the occupation of home bases as places where food was shared and consumed are the two distinctive practices by which we can distinguish humans from other primates. Chimpanzees simply eat as they go, consuming what they find on the spot. When they have eaten enough for their own private needs, they stop collecting. Hence they have no need for bags or other carrying aids. By contrast, human hunter-gatherers find food and instead of immediately eating it, carry it (or some of it) to another place for others to eat. This 'other place' is the home base, which may be quite some distance from the foraging-area. Repeated carrying of food to such specific locations results in the localised accumulation of food refuse, and it is this 'which has made archaeological study of prehistoric life possible' (Isaac 1971: 279).

One of the Bed I Oldowan sites, known as FLK 'Zinj', has for long been a focus of particular interest because several hominid bone fragments were found in its various levels, including the remains of a robust early hominid known initially as 'Zinjanthropus'. This 'Zinj' level, dated to about 1.8 million years ago, has preserved by far the densest concentration of archaeological materials from any Bed I level, including many pebble tools and tens of thousands of tiny splinters of bone (Potts 1988: 18, 29). An even earlier lakeside site, known as DK-3, has been dated to about 1.9 million years, and included a 4-metre in diameter roughly circular jumble of rocks frequently interpreted as the earliest known evidence of a man-made structure (but see Potts 1988: 257–8).

In his earlier papers, Isaac (1969, 1971) argued that the presumed hominids responsible for such debris patterns were hunters whose prey included large game animals. Later (Isaac and Crader 1981: 103n), he pleaded guilty to having overstressed this model, admitting that there was little real evidence for it. His more cautious formulation was that the hominids at this early stage 'were opportunistic scavenger/hunters and that, given the simplicity of the technology of the time, the flesh of medium and large prey was probably obtained more by scavenging than by hunting' (Isaac and Crader 1981: 86).

However, Isaac continued to insist that even at this very early stage, hominids were engaging in 'active food-sharing'. He envisaged small social groups occupying temporary base camps from which individuals or subgroups travelled over a home range each day foraging. Food surplus to the gatherers' needs was brought back and shared. This was quite different from so-called 'sharing' as practised by chimpanzees:

> We distinguish *active food sharing* from the kind of behavior reported for chimpanzees. . . . 'Sharing' is in part a misleading label for what has been filmed and reported among chimpanzees; that would be better designated as 'tolerated scrounging'. (Isaac and Crader 1981: 103n)

In Isaac's view, real food-*sharing* is a deliberate bringing of food for others to enjoy, and is a form of economic life characteristically and uniquely human. It is this which was occurring almost 2 million years ago by the lakeside at Olduvai.

Discussion

Isaac's interpretations quickly met with many detailed objections. One of the first into the fray was Lewis Binford, who poured scorn on the notion that Plio-Pleistocene hominids were departing daily from a home base, using food-carrying bags or baskets, the males conscientiously foraging or hunting in order to provide meat for the females and young waiting back at home. He pointed out that the actual evidence for any of this was non-existent. His view was that while a few of the bones showed signs of hominid activity, the hominids (rather diminutive ape-like creatures) must have been cautious and opportunistic foragers and scavengers, not hunters, and there is no proof at all that the concentrations of bone represent living floors or 'home bases'. Binford (1983: 59) in fact argued that the Bed I Oldowan hominids did not hunt and had only very small components of meat in their diet. 'The signs', as he put it, 'are clear. Earliest man, far from appearing as a mighty hunter of beasts, seems to have been the most marginal of scavengers.'

It soon became agreed that Isaac's interpretations had underestimated the dangers which would have been presented by ferocious competing carnivores around this East African lakeside. Noting that 'an odorous collection of food remains would rapidly attract other carnivores', two specialists with much experience of predator and other mammalian behaviour in Africa (Schaller and Lowther 1969: 335) had earlier pointed out that not until defensive arrangements had been made secure would it have made sense for hominids to bring carcasses to the places where infants and young were being cared for. Binford (1983), Potts (1984a: 136; 1988: 259–60) and Shipman (1983, 1986) endorsed this view, and it is now widely agreed that since Oldowans were small and vulnerable creatures, apparently lacking fire, they could not have afforded to sleep or rear young anywhere near large, fly infested carcasses smelling of blood – and least of all risk sleeping by a lakeside teeming with prey where lions and other nocturnal predators habitually made their kills.

Binford (1983: 68) wrote that the lakeside Oldowan so-called 'working areas' were probably places where non-hominid predators habitually attacked drinking prey; hominids may occasionally have gone to such places to scavenge animal remains which had been left behind, using stones to smash the bones.

Early in the 1980s, Richard Potts re-evaluated the Olduvai evidence and concluded that none of the so-called 'living floors' represented a home base. The famous stone circle at the DK site, he argued, was probably produced by the roots of a large tree, and was certainly not a shelter or 'home' (Potts 1988: 257–8). He argued that the 'working areas' were points where stone tools were cached – tools which hominid hunter/scavengers left at lakeside sites and at other points about the landscape. Whenever an animal of convenient size was killed or a dead one found, it would have been dragged to the nearest cache of ready-made tools so that it could be cut up. Something approaching caching of stone tools – for example, stone hammers used to open palm-oil nuts – has been observed among West African chimpanzees. Despite the absence of real logistic planning, they may at least remember where they dropped a particularly useful stone the last time they used it (Boesch and Boesch 1983). If caching were what the Oldowan hominids were doing, it was really only a modest advance on what chimpanzees can do, and certainly implies neither home bases nor a hunter-gatherer-like sexual division of labour (Potts 1984a, 1984b, 1986, 1987, 1988; Potts and Shipman 1981; Potts and Walker 1981).

On the question of meat-eating, Binford (1981, 1983, 1984) carried out a statistical analysis of the patterns of animal bone damage and loss at the FLK 'Zinj' and other Olduvai sites, concluding that the patterns were more often consistent with animal predators' gnawing and crunching than with human butchering. In fact, the animal bones have been minutely investigated for signs of possible hominid hunting or meat-eating, using a scanning electron microscope. One research team (Bunn 1981; 1983; Bunn and Kroll 1986) described a series of very fine linear grooves on bone surfaces, which most specialists now agree represent cut-marks made with knife-like stone flakes when hominids detached meat from the bones. Another find was of a bone on which a cut mark made with a stone edge can be seen to cross an underlying carnivore tooth mark. It has been inferred that the carnivore had the bone before the presumed hominid did, the implication being that the hominids scavenged meat remains that other predators had already discarded (Shipman 1983, 1984; Binford et al. 1988). More recently, percussion marks on bones have been added to the list of scratches, cut-marks and other possible diagnostics of early hominid behaviour at Olduvai Gorge (Blumenschine and Selvaggio 1988).

In his earlier writings Binford probably overstated his case, but although his was perhaps an 'extreme' position, denying that the Oldowan hominids were hunting even small game or doing anything impressive at all, virtually all archaeologists now agree with most of his critique. The consensus is that a sexual division of labour associated with even a temporary home-base arrangement did not emerge until considerably later than the Pliocene or early Pleistocene (see Brain 1981; Gowlett 1984; Shipman 1983, 1984, 1986; Potts 1984a, 1984b, 1988).

2.   Tanner

Nancy Makepiece Tanner (1981), *On Becoming Human*.

Nancy Makepiece Tanner (1987), 'Gathering by females: the chimpanzee model revisited and the gathering hypothesis'.

Nancy Tanner, of the University of California at Santa Cruz, put forward a more feminist perspective on human origins. Her book (Tanner 1981) was in two parts. Firstly, she reviewed the chimpanzee studies to date, and outlined her reasons for taking chimpanzee patterns of social behaviour as a reasonably accurate model for early human life. The second part of her book attempted to relate this 'chimpanzee' model to the palaeontological and archaeological evidence for human evolution.

Tanner argued that as our early ancestors – australopithecines – moved out from the forest into more open savanna environments, it was the females who were most under pressure to innovate in the food quest, since these had responsibility to feed their offspring. Their response was to develop the digging stick, along with other tools used for plant foraging, while males continued to forage for themselves in more traditional ways.

Tanner envisaged a matrifocal group of a few females with offspring, including older juvenile males, as the central social unit. Adult males were at first peripherally involved, but became gradually 'incorporated' during the Pliocene as hominisation proceeded. Tanner did not see males as particularly necessary for protection against predators, since female chimpanzees seem to be as good at driving threats away as males are. Big game hunting did not enter into this picture at all, although the author accepted that small animals would have been part of the diet, and there may have been some scavenging.

This situation, according to Tanner, would have selected for intelligence and resourcefulness on the part of females, and also for stamina and carrying ability.

Changes in sexual behaviour would have occurred. Whereas chimpanzee females, like many other primates who have evolved in 'multi-male' settings, advertise the fertile period with large sexual swellings around their rumps, in hominids these would have disappeared. Tanner saw this as a simple and mechanical consequence of bipedalism: as the female stood upright, her vaginal area would no longer have been visible from behind, and so ape-like 'oestrous swellings' would no longer have served any signalling function (1981: 209). We will discuss oestrus loss in greater detail in Chapter 6.

Still writing of the time when bipedalism was evolving, Tanner stressed: 'It was the mothers who had reason to collect, carry, and share plant food; at this time males were likely still foragers, eating available food as they went' (p. 141). However, over time, males would have found that they were more likely to be granted sexual favours if they learned to travel with females and share food with them.

The females would have tended to select as their sexual partners not aggressive, dominant males but the more friendly, co-operative types, who would have been relatively lightly built and with progressively smaller canines. As Tanner puts it: 'Perhaps early hominid females preferred males who used their mouths to kiss, rather than the ones who bared sharp teeth' (p. 210).

'Females and males', in this picture, 'might become sexual friends who sometimes travelled together, and finding a temporary sex partner could easily occur in the larger groups that camped near water, along river beds and lakes' (p. 209). In these larger groups, just as in the smaller ones, there were few sexual conflicts, jealousies, fights or problems.

In his review of origins theories, Graham Richards (1987: 166) paraphrases Tanner's argument succinctly:

> for Tanner males are helpful occasional visitors to the matrifocal group; on entering this busy domestic world they had better make themselves useful and behave, for the females exercise a high ethical standard in evaluating them and choose to mate accordingly.

Only on the eve of the emergence of *Homo*, in Tanner's view, did hunting appear, playing a minor but increasing role in hominid food-acquisition. Tanner says very little about the later stages of evolution, her argument being that the basically human configuration was already in place from earliest times (Tanner 1981, 1987).

Discussion

Tanner's book was a healthy corrective to the male-centred bias of most previous palaeoanthropologists. With all the emphasis on 'Man the Tool-Maker', 'Man the Hunter' and so on, the female of the species had barely been noticed before. As Tanner (1981: xiii) put it:

> In exploring the roles of members of my own sex along with the roles of males in early human social life, this model seeks to correct what has been both a ludicrous and a tragic omission in evolutionary reconstructions.

But although she played down early hominid hunting whereas Isaac over-estimated its role, her thesis suffered from many of the defects of Isaac's. Tanner's was a *gradualist* picture, based, apparently, on the assumption that evolving society presented its members with few difficulties. Hominids from very earliest times were essentially decent and even 'human' in their basic lifestyle. Males were mostly 'helpful'. Not a lot had to happen to make these distant ancestors (australopithecines) fully human in the sense in which modern hunter-gatherers are.

Too often, Tanner used a verbal formulation to hide a difficult problem. Take a passage such as the following:

> Overall, females apparently were choosing males who were sociable, cooperative, willing to share, and protective. In general, then, sexual intercourse would not be disruptive of either ongoing group interaction or organizational flexibility. (1981: 210)

But *why* was sexual intercourse suddenly 'not . . . disruptive'? Can it really have been because the males chosen by females were genetically more 'sociable'? And if that were the case, why were hominid females so discriminating whereas baboon and other primate females continued 'choosing' males of a different kind? Tanner offers no plausible explanation. Gathering as such cannot have been the cause. Not just humans but all primate females, after all, practice 'the gathering adaptation' in one form or another, even if most do not use digging-sticks.

Tanner's theory is essentially about the supposedly more co-operative genetic constitution of protohumans, particularly in relation to their sex lives. Yet it is hard to believe that through female selection – operative to this effect in the case of the early hominids but no other species – men became *genetically* 'sociable . . . protective' and so on. If what is at issue is male genetic 'nature', many feminists would surely ask whether there is any evidence that human males ever *did* become as nice as this! The fact is that sex can be immensely disruptive of social harmony, not only for all known primates, but for humans in most cultural contexts, too – including, of course, our own. Evolutionary selection pressures as such seem to have done little to render sex non-disruptive or males sexually tolerant in a genetic sense, and we would therefore seem to require a totally different kind of explanation in order to understand how the problem of sexual conflict was dealt with in the course of human evolution.

In short, while Tanner's book helped to change the whole tone of discussions on human origins, focusing attention on females as no previous contribution had ever done, its underlying theory was simply not adequate. Most of the book was about gentle and co-operative chimpanzees, and the basic argument was that only the most minor of changes from a chimpanzee lifestyle were required in order to set the hominids along the road towards cultural humanity.

This will not do, for two reasons. Firstly, chimpanzees are not intrinsically gentle and co-operative, as used to be imagined twenty years ago, but often murderously aggressive, infanticidal and cannibalistic (Bygott 1972; Teleki 1975: 169–72; Goodall 1986: 488–534). It all depends on circumstances, not genes, just as it does with us.

Secondly, a theory which says that the problems were in essence solved already, before culture, by primates such as chimpanzees, is really not a theory. It does not explain why culture as such – with its taboos, its rituals, its symbolic systems, complex kinship systems, grammatical systems and so on – ever became needed at all.

3.   Lovejoy

Owen Lovejoy (1981), 'The origin of man'

Lovejoy, Professor of Anthropology at Kent State University, Ohio, centred not on ecological or technological changes, and not on the development of hunting, but on reproductive factors. His view was that human evolution required above all intensive parenting, and that the most essential prerequisite of this was male involvement in getting food for females and young.

Lovejoy was primarily concerned to find the ultimate factor at the very start of hominid evolution which began requiring that most distinctive of hominid anatomical traits – our adaptation to upright gait. In this context, he dismissed various previous theories. Hominids, he wrote, did not begin walking on two legs to hold or use tools, to hunt game or to escape from predators once the protection of the forest had been abandoned – all such factors postdate the earliest evidence for bipedalism in the fossil record. Walking upright, Lovejoy emphasised, arose extremely early in the course of hominid evolution – millions of years before the emergence of stone tools or hunting. The earliest evidence for it is a series of footprints in the mud found at Laetoli in Tanzania, dating to about 4 million years ago (Johanson and White 1980). What was it which, from such very early stages of hominid evolution, necessitated this peculiar and (for mammals) unprecedented primary mode of locomotion?

Lovejoy argued that far back in the Miocene, before our ancestors had even begun leaving their (presumed) original forest environment, the basic social, sexual and reproductive patterns which were to determine the course of all subsequent evolution had already been laid down. Man's 'unique sexual and reproductive behaviour' had already been established. Sexual competition between males was minimised or even eliminated at a very early stage through an arrangement which made it possible for every male to have exactly one sexual partner – no more, no less. According to this scenario, conflict was minimised and our species made human by monogamy and the nuclear family. Lovejoy argued that it was in the course of adapting so as to be able to bring provisions exclusively to his mate and offspring that the monogamous hominid male began walking on two legs.

In presenting his model, Lovejoy sought to explain (a) why males began systematically provisioning females and (b) why this necessitated monogamous pair-bonding and a strictly 'nuclear' form of family.

In approaching the first question, Lovejoy spotlit a problem which he thought would have been faced by the ape-like Miocene ancestors of the hominids. This was an extraordinarily slow rate of reproduction.

The evolution of the primate order as a whole – from lower to increasingly 'higher' forms, with larger and larger brains – is achieved only at some cost. This is borne mainly by the female of the species, who must go through an increasingly prolonged pregnancy and must nurse her offspring for longer and longer periods of time. As primates become more intelligent, so they require more nurturing and learning before they are capable of surviving on their own at all. To obtain this nurturing, they slow down their biological clocks, as if to give themselves more time. In other words, there is a progressive prolongation of gestation, infancy and all other life phases.

Lemurs are at the lower end of the scale, with a fast clock. Following conception, they are quickly born, quickly mature and usually die before they are 20 years of age. With macaques, the whole process is slowed down; birth, maturity and death are all delayed. Gibbons delay everything further,

and chimpanzees delay each life stage further still, often remaining reproductively active until about 40 years of age. Humans have delayed the
attainment of each stage furthest of all. Gestation lasts 38 weeks (compared
with 34 for chimpanzees, 18 for lemurs), childhood dependency continues
for a decade and more, female reproductive life lasts until around fifty, and
female life expectancy extends (uniquely for any primate) many years even
beyond child-bearing age.

The extreme and prolonged dependency of their offspring poses a particular problem for female chimpanzees. Even at the age of five or six years, a
young chimpanzee may still be getting rides on his mother's back while she
is foraging for food. Admittedly, the burden borne by female chimpanzees is
less than that of human mothers, but it has to be remembered that the chimp
mother has to do all her foraging for herself, with no economic support from
others. No woman in a human hunter-gatherer context is forced to be so self-
reliant.

The combination of intense mothering and foraging burdens makes it
impossible for a chimpanzee to give birth to several infants in quick
succession. Any chimp mother who did this would have to neglect many of
her offspring. Field studies at Gombe in Tanzania in fact show the average
period between successive births to be 5.6 years. A chimpanzee female does
not reach sexual maturity until she is about 10 years old; if she is to
reproduce herself and her mate – that is, if a stable population level is to be
maintained – she must therefore survive to an age of 21 years. Within any
given population, various factors – accidents, predation, infection and so on
– tend to lower the average life expectancy of all individuals, and in the case
of chimpanzees, there is very little tolerance in the system. If chimpanzees
were to enter a new, more dangerous, environment, how could they avoid
increased infant mortality or avoid average female life expectancy from being
pushed below the critical figure of 21 years?

Lovejoy envisaged that the ape-like ancestors of the hominids faced some
such problem. Conditions in East Africa in the period when bipedalism was
evolving, he wrote, involved increased seasonality and the development of
diversified mosaics – that is, a variegated landscape of patches of woodland,
grassland, rivers, riverbanks and so on. Hominids in this context would need
to be omnivorous and capable of exploiting a range of different types of
environment; they would also need to boost their rate of reproduction to cope
with occasional harsh conditions or severe seasons.

Crucial factors contributing to infant mortality in chimpanzees include
inadequate mothering and (even in the case of 'good' mothers) injuries caused
by falling off the mother's back. Many of these problems stem from the fact
that the mother has to keep moving from place to place as she looks for food;
Lovejoy (p. 344) saw this as a significant cause of infant mortality and 'the
most important restriction on primate birth spacing'.

Hominids during the late Miocene (according to Lovejoy) may have had at least as slow a rate of gestation and maturation as chimpanzees. Unless they were to regress to smaller brains and faster clocks, there would have been only two theoretically possible ways of producing more surviving offspring. One would have been to reduce the interval between one birth and the next; the other would have been to reduce infant mortality in some way. Yet both would have posed immense problems – demanding more intense and vigilant mothering, distributed among yet more offspring, on the part of females who were already heavily burdened.

There was only one radical solution: a completely new distribution of parenting responsibilities between the sexes, involving an end to the primate male's ancient freedom from the responsibilities of parenthood. The hominid female had to be released from the need to be perpetually on the move in search of food. She had to be allowed to rest, to choose a safe sleeping and living area in which to care for her offspring, to stop having to carry infants around over long distances – and devote the energy thereby saved to intensified mothering. This meant that the male had to enter the picture and actually start providing food. His privileged status as a member of the leisured sex would have to be brought to an end.

Lovejoy argued that this was the breakthrough on the basis of which hominid evolution set off on its distinctive course. Quite unlike other primates, the earliest hominid females stayed at or near a 'home base' while males ranged further afield. As each female with her offspring remained near a fixed base, her male consort would go out periodically in order to bring back food. The reduction in female mobility was an immense gain, reducing the accident rate during travel, maximising female familiarity with the core area, reducing exposure to predators, and allowing intensification of parenting behaviour (p. 345).

But why monogamy? Lovejoy saw this as the only solution to the chaotic problems of sexual conflict which any other system would have involved. For example, how else could a male depart periodically from his sexual partner, free of the anxiety that some rival male might take advantage of his absence? According to Lovejoy (p. 345), only monogamy and a one-to-one sex ratio could provide a solution: each male would then be sexually satisfied, competition for mates would no longer disrupt everything, and the male who went away to forage would not risk losing his mate.

Other considerations (according to Lovejoy) point in the same direction. In a polygamous harem system, the female population is attached to only a small proportion of the males potentially available. Within each harem unit, in other words, the sex ratio is two or more females to every male. Any such system would have obvious drawbacks for females in need of male-derived food. On the one hand, much of the energy of the dominant males would be wasted on the constant fights needed to keep control over each harem. On the other hand, the remaining males – the losers in the competition for mates – would be excluded from the breeding system, unattached and therefore not used by the females as a source of food. These groups of 'bachelor' males would roam about, unmated and in a sense 'wasted' as potential food-getters ('an untapped-pool' of reproductive energy: p. 346). Emerging protohuman females, in Lovejoy's argument, needed the services not just of a fraction of the adult male population, but the totality. Each female needed a whole male all to herself. Monogamy satisfies this condition, and also guarantees paternity to males.

Because of this, Lovejoy saw the matrifocal basic unit of non-human primates as of little relevance to human origins. In his view, it gave way at an early stage to pair-bonding. As he wrote: 'there would be a gradual replacement of the matrifocal group by a "bifocal" one – the primitive nuclear family' (pp. 347–8). The nuclear family was described as a 'prodigious adaptation' central to the success of early hominids, and firmly established in the Miocene (that is, 5 million and more years ago).

The new system would have made it possible and adaptive for each male to provide food strictly for his monogamous partner and his own genetic offspring, and no others. Whereas chimpanzees, when they find food, utter a 'food-call', inviting others to come and share the find, human males would not have done this. 'In the proposed system', in Lovejoy's words,

> selection would not favor this behavior: instead, selection would favor a behavior that would benefit only the male's own reproductive unit. The simple alternative to the food call would involve collecting the available food item or items and returning them to the mate and offspring. (p. 345)

Human males would have been careful to keep the food to themselves and to their own nuclear family.

The better each male was at provisioning his mate and her offspring, the more likely were his genes to be immortalised. Since monogamy meant that each male was assured that all his food-getting efforts enhanced the survival prospects of his own offspring and no one else's, such behaviour was powerfully selected for. Lovejoy (p. 345) was at pains to point out that this would have nothing to do with 'reciprocal altruism', since 'it would only benefit the biological offspring of the male carrying out the provisioning and thus would be under powerful, direct selection'. Lovejoy explained bipedalism as arising from males' need to carry food to their mates and offspring.

Meanwhile, the females who were in sexual terms most willing and desirable would have been those best able to motivate their mates to provide for them. This led to attractive breasts, buttocks, skin and so on – females being quite markedly differentiated from males in such terms – and also to 'continual sexual receptivity'. Evolving hominid females, well cared for and not obliged to travel and forage so much, could now give birth to increasing numbers of increasingly dependent, slow-maturing offspring. The effect of intensified parenting, protracted learning within the nuclear family, and enhanced sibling relationships (resulting from more offspring of a similar age being brought up within each family) enhanced each child's chances of survival in the world.

Discussion

'The Origin of Man' was in its time an authoritative article which quickly became a favourite following its publication in the prestigious journal, *Science*, in 1981.

It focused immediately on what is still recognised as the basic problem: the primate male's traditional unwillingness or inability to provide food for his mate and offspring. Lovejoy's theory highlighted the immense burdens of motherhood imposed on the evolving primate female, and saw human evolution in terms of this figure's emancipation from some of the difficulties involved in combining foraging with child care. Institutionalising the 'home base' was seen as the key condition of this emancipation.

Moreover, Lovejoy showed awareness of the problems which would have been posed by inter-male sexual competition in any 'harem' type of mating system. He pointed out that if females were to take maximum advantage of the provisioning services of males, and if inter-male sex fights were to be minimised, then the male population as a whole must have been brought into the mating system and a one-to-one sex ratio established.

But while Lovejoy's selection of problem areas was perceptive and often convincing, his scenario has in the end fared no better than its rivals. The most devastating fault was one which also demolished the other theories, and has been touched on briefly already in our discussion of Isaac. Lovejoy's dates were seriously wrong. Studies of tooth-eruption schedules in immature fossil australopithecines have shown that their maturation rates were not significantly different from those of living chimpanzees (Bromage and Dean 1985). Whatever it was, therefore, which lead to the emergence of bipedalism, it certainly had nothing to do with the reproductive factors Lovejoy envisaged. Linked with this, there is no archaeological evidence for the emergence of a home base arrangement even in the Pliocene, let alone the Miocene. Even in the Middle Pleistocene, there is little firm evidence, and there is now a virtual consensus that a clearly demarcated home base and sexual division of labour did not appear until very late – possibly as late as the arrival of anatomically modern humans. This is much too late for it to have anything to do with bipedalism, large brains or any other specifically hominid as opposed to pongid anatomical traits.

Beyond this, however, Lovejoy's argument was quickly criticised on various grounds.

Females and bipedalism

Lovejoy's theory is a good example of what the feminist writer Fedigan (1986: 29) describes as the 'coat-tails' theory of human evolution: traits are selected for in males, and then females evolve by clinging to the males' coat-tails. Lovejoy attributes the evolution of upright gait entirely to the food-carrying activities of males. Females in this model are given little to do except feed, reward their partners sexually, give birth and nurture their young. The fact that they, too, walk upright is not accounted for, except to the extent that their shared genetic inheritance makes the females of any species tend to 'keep up' with males as a matter of course.

A more serious problem concerns the very antiquity of bipedalism. In the 1960s, writers on evolution almost invariably saw human origins as a single complex process involving such elements as hunting, tool use, food sharing, the emergence of a sexual division of labour – and bipedalism. All these developments were supposed to have been directly and simultaneously interrelated, in the sense that no single element could fully evolve without the others. In particular, bipedalism could not have evolved prior to the making and carrying of tools, because until tools began to be made, there was no need to free the hands 'in order' to hold and use them. All this seemed plausible enough in those years, when it was thought that fully evolved bipedalism was a late development, emerging at about the same time as stone tool-making. However, now that the Laetoli and other finds push back the origins of upright walking to 4 or perhaps even 5 million years ago, we have two choices. Either we conclude that upright walking evolved independently, long before systematic stone tool use, hunting or other characteristically 'human' activities. Or we are forced to say that the basically 'human' way of life began immensely far back in the past – long before anyone had previously thought.

Unfortunately, Lovejoy took the second course. He acknowledged that hunting and tool use could have had nothing to do with the origins of bipedalism. But he still tried to save the old paradigm by arguing that the 'essentially human' lifestyle – involving intense parenting at a home base, made possible by a sexual division of labour within a primordial 'nuclear family' – indeed stretches back 4 or 5 million years, far enough into the past to qualify as an explanation for bipedalism. More obviously even than Isaac, Tanner or Hill (see next section), Lovejoy fell into the trap of telescoping the various quite distinct, widely separated phases of human evolution into one decisive 'moment' which – because bipedalism had to be included – was necessarily thrust back into the Miocene.

In reality, as Richards (1987: 193–204) points out in his survey of origins theories, it is seeming increasingly likely that we need a non-social, non-'human' and extremely simple *physical* explanation for bipedalism (see Chapter 7). We need an explanation rooted in an understanding that what we are trying to explain, at this stage, is not 'human life' in a social or political sense at all, but the initial evolutionary divergence of one particular zoological species – the hominids – from the ancestral pongid (ape-like) stock. All attempts to explain this divergence by reference to a 'uniquely human way of life' are a retrospective imposition of our own preoccupations on to the lives of creatures whose priorities were rooted in their own times, not ours. Such arguments are part of an old paradigm which must be abandoned in its entirety.

Lovejoy and monogamy

The old idea that early humans were monogamous continues to have its proponents. 'However,' as the feminist sociobiologist Sarah Blaffer Hrdy (1981: 175) put it when Lovejoy was writing, 'taking this position now necessitates a certain anthropocentrism and special pleading'.

Among non-human primates, monogamy produces not advanced forms of sociability but a very elementary, simple and sparse social life, with little variety or political complexity to select for novel forms of self-awareness or intelligence. Compared with other primates, those which are monogamous appear to eat lower-quality diets, have an inferior ability to perceive social relationships and have minimal levels of role differentiation (Kinzey 1987: 109). Moreover, monogamous primates are known to be 'behaviorally more conservative, and ecologically more restricted' than their non-monogamous counterparts (Kinzey 1987: 105). The behaviour of gibbons, for example, is stereotyped, with little regional variation.

Among non-human primates, in fact, a monogamous mating system appears to have the least long-term adaptive value, and it has been argued that this may apply to humans, too. In a powerful contribution on the whole subject, Kinzey (1987: 106) writes:

> The lack of social networks is the major disadvantage of monogamy per se. Promiscuity does not normally occur in *any* human society, but polygyny and polyandry taken together are much more frequent than monogamy. They encompass a greater extension of social networks than monogamy; they have greater long term adaptability, and consequently they are more common. Probably the majority of cultures in the world practice some form of extended family in which the living group contains more than a single pair and their children.

The palaeontological evidence, such as it is, does not seem to fit the monogamy theory either. It seems that there may have been pronounced sexual dimorphism among early hominids (Johanson and White 1979), and it was not all of the 'epigamic' kind which Lovejoy described in his article — the female having large breasts and buttocks, the male a prominent penis, and so on. These 'soft-tissue' characteristics which Lovejoy envisaged do not fossilise and so we lack evidence either way; what does fossilise is bone, and where male skeletons are to a marked extent larger and heavier than females, as seems to be the case with the australopithecines, then some kind of polygamous mating system with inter-male competition seems likely (Foley 1987: 171).

We can agree with Lovejoy that if the birth interval were to be reduced whilst the period of childhood dependency were lengthened, then mothers would need additional social support. But why assume a totally isolated Miocene or Pliocene female, utterly dependent on support from 'her' male, when all the indications are that these evolving ape-like hominids would have been highly sociable animals, living in groups? Might there not have been close female-to-female kinship bonds within such groups – bonds which could have been drawn upon by intelligent mothers in times of need? Hrdy (1981: 98, 217) documents multi-parenting ('allo-parenting', as it is termed) among non-human primates, showing that a variety of related females may assist the mother in caring for her infant, sometimes freeing her for unencumbered foraging. Could not evolving hominid females have formed quite extensive coalitions, and might they not also have tempted various males to give them support, perhaps even deliberately confusing issues of paternity in order to get as many males as possible to offer protection to their offspring?

In discussing such features as the physiology of the human clitoris, Hrdy (p. 176) argues that human females have been 'biologically endowed with a lusty primate sexuality', their ancestors displaying 'an aggressive readiness to engage in both reproductive and nonreproductive liaisons with multiple, but selected, males.' Her belief (Hrdy 1981: 153–8) is that many unexplained features of female sexual physiology and anatomy may have evolved in the service of a deliberate female strategy of confusing paternity! The idea is that females manipulate their sexual relations with a succession of different males, sometimes several simultaneously, so as to make a large number respond positively on the basis that her offspring just *might* be their own! This certainly seems to be common among numerous primates, and it is an idea supported by others besides Hrdy – for example, Hill and Kaplan (1988: 280), who rely in part on their social anthropological fieldwork among the Ache. In all this, Lovejoy's line of reasoning is precisely reversed.

We know (see previous chapter) that neither monogamy nor polygamy is rooted in any simple way in a species' genes. All primate males – including humans – are or would be mainly polygamous in some situations, primarily monogamous in others. Human males today are not particularly monogamous, and it is far from certain that females are very different, although mothers with heavy child-care responsibilities may have fewer opportunities or inclinations to prioritise their sex lives in the way some males in many cultures can afford to do.

In any event, as Hrdy (1981: 179) points out, men in patriarchal cultures have never had much confidence in women's instinctive monogamy, and have invented chastity belts, clitoridectomy and draconian penalties in their attempts to impose 'fidelity' on their wives, meanwhile practising rather different standards themselves. 'Whole chapters of human history', Hrdy (p. 179) writes, 'could be read as an effort to contain the promiscuity of

women'. In no human culture does monogamy appear to be sustainable
without powerful cultural, religious, legal and other sanctions.

Meanwhile, hunter-gatherers such as the Aborigines of Western Arnhem
Land, Australia, openly celebrate sexual freedom, each woman on ceremonial
occasions taking advantage of her traditional right to enjoy extra-marital
sex – including, sometimes, relations with a string of different lovers in a
night (Berndt and Berndt 1951). Similarly, Eskimos during their prolonged
winter ceremonies traditionally engaged in sacred orgies which approached
very close to complete 'sexual communism' (Mauss 1979: 60, 68). !Kung
San women in the Kalahari desert increase their sexual activity, with lovers
as well as husbands, particularly at mid-cycle, around the period of ovulation
(Worthman 1978, cited by Hrdy 1981: 139). According to Malinowski
(1932: 221), marital and extra-marital love-making games and celebrations
among the Trobriand Islanders reached their climax each month at around
full moon.

Erotic festivals involving sexual 'licence' form a recurrent pattern in
hunter-gatherer and other ethnographies from all parts of the world. Even
groups stereotypically conceived as rather sexually restrained or even prudish
– such as the Hopi Indians of New Mexico – are known to have had the
wildest 'secret dances' dubbed 'vulgar and wicked' by the Spanish authorities
as well as by later government and religious officials (Eggan et al. 1979).
Beyond this, moreover, it is simply the case that the nuclear family is not
even recognised as a unit, terminologically or conceptually, in many non-
western cultures; so-called 'extended' forms of kinship with 'classificatory'
terminologies are almost universal, with sibling bonds usually accorded
greater symbolic or ritual value than the (usually) all too fragile bonds
uniting husband with wife.

Despite its different assumptions, Lovejoy's theory suffers from many of
the defects of Tanner's. We know that in the long run human males were, as
Lovejoy says, drawn into a form of behaviour unknown among other higher
primates – systematic provisioning of their offspring and sexual partners.
This human pattern, then, is one which certainly has to be explained. But it
is not at all clear why we should introduce the male as a 'naturally' co-
operative parent and food exchanger at the very beginning of the hominid
line, unless it is to salvage the now discredited idea that bipedalism emerged
contemporaneously with the evolution of 'culture'. Few specialists nowadays
still argue this case, but if this idea is abandoned, then Lovejoy's theory
implies that symbolic language and culture were simply not necessary in
order to draw the male into performing his provisioning role. The implication is that it was all a matter of natural selection operating upon male
genetic characteristics. This continued until there had evolved a male who
was 'naturally' monogamous, and who 'naturally' devoted his time to finding
food for his offspring and mate. The argument that such a monogamous male
exists – even in the present, let alone 4–5 million years ago – is surely not
conclusively proven.

Lovejoy placed 'human social and reproductive life' far back into the dawn of hominid existence, and elevates it to the status of prime mover. In his model, social life does not evolve out of its own material conditions. It does not evolve out of the transition to bipedalism, the emergence of tool use, changing ecological circumstances, movement into new environments, increasing reliance on meat etc. etc. Rather, it is established at the very outset, in the form of 'the nuclear family', at a time when the earliest hominids occupy an ecological niche similar to that of modern forest-dwelling chimpanzees. Lovejoy wrote in the concluding lines of his paper that his model 'implies that the nuclear family and human sexual behavior may have their ultimate origin long before the dawn of the Pleistocene' (p. 348).

In fact, he was referring to the Miocene. In this view, a sexual division of labour operating within the boundaries of the nuclear family is the one constant feature of the whole of human evolution, a 'prodigious achievement' central to the success of the very earliest hominids and the context within which all subsequent advances have been achieved. Given all that we know about monogamy in both primates and contemporary hunter-gatherers, given the time scales, and given the complete absence of any archaeological evidence for a home base until at least the Middle Pleistocene – it seems unlikely.

4. Hill

Kim Hill (1982), 'Hunting and human evolution'

Kim Hill (1982), a sociobiologist at Emory University, Atlanta, set out to reaffirm the hunting hypothesis in opposition to Tanner and other supporters of Woman the Gatherer. Hill's model assumed an early male monopoly of hunting, but was designed to explain how, nonetheless, females could have gained access to at least some of the meat.

Hill (1982: 533) envisaged a very early population in a game-rich environment where returns from predation were particularly high. Carnivorous males, it was argued, would then be able to satisfy their hunger in a few hours, whereas females – denied access to meat – would still need to forage all day. Males would then have much free time, and new strategies might evolve in an attempt to use this to increase fitness:

> One strategy that might be very successful for males would be to continue hunting during the day, and provide females with food resources in an attempt to increase the possibility of copulation with receptive females. The pattern of males hunting while females continued to forage primarily for plant items, would be the beginnings of sexual division of labour.

In Hill's model, promiscuous mating was assumed. On the one hand, males competed against one another on a direct behavioural level for meat and sex. On the other, females competed against one another sexually, the most desirable and constantly available attracting the best hunters. Noting that among both chimpanzees and baboons, females displaying oestrus signals receive more meat than non-oestrus females, Hill argued that an accentuation of this kind of selection pressure would have led to the continuous 'shamming' of oestrus among constantly receptive human females. In short, it was argued that the primate pattern of oestrus soliciting (see Chapter 6) would only have needed accentuating and systematising for something like the human hunter-gatherer pattern to have evolved.

Males, according to this model, did not at first fully provision females but consumed most of the meat they obtained themselves (Hill 1982: 537). As pregnancy and child care limited female mobility, an increasing reliance on meat food ensured that the males as a whole were in a stronger bargaining position than the females. An implication was that the females, badly needing meat which only males could provide, were prepared to do almost anything to get it. Females who offered copulations to males could induce them to fetch meat for them. The more continuously females could copulate and display oestrus signals, the more meat they got. They therefore eventually adapted so as to be able to display oestrus signals – both real and 'sham' – all the time. Meanwhile, bipedalism evolved as males ran to and fro using tools and fetching meat, those males best at running or walking upright being able to carry most in their hands and therefore enjoying most reproductive success.

At the end of this paper, Hill (1982: 540) summarised the theory under eight points:

1. A sub-population of Miocene apes found itself in a region where easy prey made it logical to specialise in hunting.

2. Unencumbered by offspring, males were better at this than females. With time on their hands, males hunted beyond their own needs, bringing meat to oestrus females so as to 'trade' it with them for sex.

3. As the males used artificial weapons in the hunt, the size of their canines decreased, since these were no longer needed and hampered the chewing of meat.

4. Because sexiness was useful for getting meat, females developed longer and longer periods of sham 'oestrus', obscuring the real moment of ovulation and evolving towards the human condition of continuous sexual receptivity.

5. Sexual competition between males was high, with some males very poor at hunting or gaining mates while others were extremely successful. Those males who could best carry meat to females reproduced best. Since meat-carrying and tool-use required hands which were freed from locomotory functions, bipedalism in males evolved.

6.   Once tools could be carried, it made sense to rely on them more. Tool-making led to changes in the shape of the hand.

7.   Tool-use and predation – especially upon other primates – developed intelligence.

8.   Thanks to male provisioning, there was a decline in infant mortality, leading to increased mean longevity, increased juvenile dependency and therefore an increased need for grandmothers to assist with child-care. For this reason, females started living on beyond their reproductive years.

Richards (1987: 166–7) aptly and inevitably dubbed all this the 'prostitution' theory of human origins. He summarised the differences between the Tanner and Hill models as follows:

> While both see food-acquisition as central in selecting for bipedalism, for Hill it operates on the male, for Tanner on the female. For Hill the sexual deal is sex-for-meat, for Tanner it is sex-perhaps-for-good-behaviour (bringing meat being good behaviour of course).

Discussion

Hill's article cannot easily be dismissed. Indeed, this book will outline a theory closely related to Hill's, with a similar emphasis on the 'sex for meat' principle of exchange.

However, like Isaac's and Tanner's models, Hill's telescoped bipedalism and the basic social changes involved in becoming human into a single complex occurring in the late Miocene or early Pliocene. Hill saw the 'sex for meat' scenario as nothing radically novel, but as the extension of a tendency characteristic of baboons and chimpanzees – the tendency of oestrous or sham-oestrous females to invite copulations in exchange for male-procured provisions.

The article provided an intriguing explanation for male bipedalism and for the male contributions to food-carrying, tool-making and the sexual division of labour. It did not seem quite so convincing in explaining the role of females in all of this. The main qualities apparently required of females were that they should reproduce, prove good mothers and be continuously receptive to the most successful hunter-males.

Hill's theory suffers from a number of problems. We will not dwell on 'oestrus shamming' here, since oestrus loss and the evolution of the human female reproductive cycle will form the subject matter of Chapter 6. Suffice it to note that human females do *not* accentuate, extend or 'sham' oestrus at all but, on the contrary, have dampened down primate oestrus signals to the point at which they have completely disappeared. If there is one thing about human females which needs to be explained, it is not that they act as if they were in oestrus all the time – which would mean that they were forever unable to say 'no' – but that quite unlike any other primate, women can say 'no' at any time whatsoever, even when ovulating. Competitive prostitution would not seem to be a very good explanation for this.

Beyond this, however, there are other problems. Lovejoy's theory posited monogamy as an answer to the problems presented by inter-male sexual conflict and the consequent 'wasting' of males who, potentially, might have been used by females to provision them. Hill assumed promiscuity and polygamy, but unfortunately simply failed to address the associated problems that Lovejoy had drawn to our attention.

Although Hill spoke of a sexual division of labour, it is far from clear how competitive sexual soliciting could have produced any such result. A sexual division of labour implies that males bring food to females and offspring. But given Hill's premises, a male hunter in possession of meat would have had very little incentive to carry or drag his catch to a pregnant or nursing female waiting for him at some distant point. In the absence of either monogamy or generalised inter-female solidarity, there would always have been a certain number of 'free' females chasing after the best hunters so as to be first on the spot when a kill was made or when meat was being butchered at a tool cache or processing site. It seems strange that Hill overlooked this logical consequence of this 'free competition' model, because it would have had severe reproductive consequences of precisely the kind Lovejoy had envisaged. Young and/or non-pregnant females would have had a competitive advantage, whereas females burdened with offspring would have been the least mobile, the least readily available and the last to get meat, even though their needs would have been greatest.

A further problem is that public oestrus shamming implies continuous public sexual interest and the incitement of competition between males. The picture conjured up is not one in which co-operatively organised males are left free of sexual cares and worries — left free to make planning decisions on where to find distant game, how to track it, or how to invest in building up a detailed shared knowledge of the surrounding area. Rather, with competition making every male afraid to leave 'his' females unguarded, the picture is one of insecure and anxiously competitive males trying to snatch game as quickly and continuously as possible from the immediate surroundings. In this situation, an array of conflicts and contradictions can be envisaged. The moment one male had left 'his' female to go hunting, would not some rival have taken advantage of his absence? When a male had killed an animal, would not fights have broken out over the spoils? And if females were only interested in meat, without caring who hunted it or where it came from, would not males who robbed their companions often do as well as or even better than genuine hunters?

It is not that there would have been no answers to such problems. It is simply that any long-term stable answers — evolutionary solutions involving the establishment of a home base and genuine sexual division of labour — would have necessitated extensive coalition forming and gender solidarity, taking us beyond Hill's scenario into a very different one not based on 'prostitution'. We will return to these issues in a moment. In the meantime, let us examine a more recent variation on the 'prostitution' theme.

5   Parker

Sue Taylor Parker (1987) 'A sexual selection model for hominid evolution'

Parker's model is very like Hill's, showing little if any feminist influence. Parker's is a sophisticated, well-documented Plio-Pleistocene sex-for-meat scenario, explaining bipedalism as 'a male adaptation for nuptial feeding of females' (p. 235). The origin of 'higher intelligence' and 'language' in *Homo sapiens* is attributed to 'male competition through technology and rule production to control resources and females' (p. 235). Parker places greater emphasis than Hill on gathering and scavenging as opposed to hunting, at least in the early stages of evolution. Moreover, she differs from Hill in recognising that early hominid females could not have motivated males to bring food to them while they waited behind at a fixed home base. In Parker's scenario, the picture conjured up is that of females having to chase after males in order to be the first present when kills were made or meat butchered at a processing site. But if anything, this is an even more explicit and uncompromising 'prostitution' model than Hill's.

Parker unfolds her scenario as follows. Plio-Pleistocene hominid males, she writes (p. 243), would go out foraging at a distance and use the food – for example, roots extracted with digging-tools – for sexual purposes: 'Through courtship or nuptial feeding of estrus females, males could entice females to go away with them on "safaris" or honeymoons where competing males were not a threat.'

Later, Parker (p. 244) continues, the coveted foods would have included increasing amounts of meat. Brains taken from hunted animals are particularly valued by chimpanzees, but are difficult to extract through hard skulls which first have to be smashed (Teleki 1973: 144). Hominid males who used rocks or hammers for the purpose may have helped solve this problem, discovering a particularly useful enticement for attracting females.

Still later, according to Parker (1987: 245–6), males would have dragged whole carcasses of animals, not to a 'home base', but to special sites dotted about the landscape:

A male subsistence strategy of bringing carcasses of scavenged prey to special sites where processing tools were stored (Potts, 1984b) would have paid off reproductively by attracting females to locations where they could be guarded at least temporarily.

By adapting to walk on two legs instead of four, writes Parker (p. 243), males would have been able to get, transport, defend and display such coveted foods:

This pattern could have arisen naturally through female choice of males who responded to their begging for favored food; presumably males who were able to get more preferred foods unavailable to females, e.g., meat, would have been preferred by females.

Like Hill, Parker assumes promiscuity; 'nuptial feeding' implies not long-term parental investment but each male's short-term provisioning of numerous females in exchange for casual sex (p. 244). Like Hill, Parker also sees male dominance as having intensified owing to the male monopoly on meat (pp. 243, 246).

What counter-strategies would females have evolved? Parker accepts that females of all species generally 'prefer not to be controlled', and would have attempted to maintain their own freedom, particularly where choice of sexual partner was concerned. In her view, increasingly sexy and intelligent protohuman females would have played off males against one another in order to pursue their own ends. They would have incited inter-male fighting 'by using one male as a foil to get the attention of another', males battling with one another with increasing intensity for 'control of females through provision of meat' (1987: 246–7).

Discussion

Parker's article was informative and well researched, and at the time of publication was a state of the art expression of sociobiological and neo-Darwinian thought on human origins. Nonetheless, her scenario conjures up a picture of sexual chaos on precisely the scale necessary to prevent human culture from emerging. We are told, for example, that at food distribution points there would have been intense 'aggressive competition among males', adding to 'the value of using aimed missiles in combat'. Put bluntly, this 'nuptial' picture is one of males hurling stones or spears at one another in fights for temporary control over females at butchering sites, with females actively inciting males to intensify the violence! Parker seems not to have considered whether it would have been in the genetic interests of females with increasingly vulnerable offspring to collude in such fights.

We may leave aside the many problematical aspects of all this and concentrate on one issue. Regardless of how much or how little inter-male violence we assume, the system Parker envisages is one of ruthless competitive sexual selection, placing a very high premium on the ability of females to become fully mobile as they chase after meat-possessing, highly mobile males. Now, it seems undeniable that such a system would favour sexually available, non-pregnant females at the expense of burdened mothers. But this means that females with large-brained, slow-maturing offspring would be discriminated against. The best-provisioned female meat-eaters would be those fastest at presenting themselves sexually at kill sites or butchering sites. Females would have to compete with one another in racing to such sites as kills were made; they would also have to compete in appearing sexually tempting to the males.

The problems with all this are considerable. Pregnancy, breast-feeding and other reproductive responsibilities would all interfere with both sexual availability and mobility. The 'losers' in such a competition would probably include the best mothers, the 'winners' the worst. Certainly, Parker explains no better than Hill how any such system could generate mechanisms to ensure that females with increasingly dependent offspring had priority of access to meat. And as females who prioritised meat-eating had to scamper about chasing males and therefore had fewer or smaller-brained surviving offspring, we might imagine that in each generation, the females most abundant in the population would be those whose genetic constitution best enabled them to *avoid* becoming too reliant on meat.

Yet the core objection to both Hill's and Parker's scenarios is a still more fundamental one. It concerns the manner in which both models conceptualise 'sex-for-meat' exchange. As noted earlier, in the form in which it is presented, this kind of 'trading' does seem to resemble 'prostitution'.

Now, the anthropomorphic description of primate oestrus-soliciting as 'prostitution' is not new. Solly Zuckerman popularised the usage in his pioneering book, *The Social Life of Monkeys and Apes*, published in the 1930s (Zuckermann 1932: 233). After a discussion of primate sex-for-food and sex-for-status exchanges, the author commented that if a particular response of a sexual nature 'is always followed by the acquisition of some social or material advantage', then 'it is legitimate, for purposes of description, to refer to the response as a form of sexual prostitution'.

The question we must now ask, however, is whether 'prostitution' – as Zuckerman's words might imply – is something intrinsic to all forms of sexual bargaining for economic gain. Is it an inevitable consequence of the fact that nursing females needing male support may have nothing to 'sell' but their bodies – or are totally different forms of sex-economic exchange actually possible?

Zuckerman wrote many years ago, and there is nowadays no need to give any particular weight to his formulations. However, the difficulty is that few contemporary palaeoanthropologists apparently feel any need to draw a distinction between primate sex-for-meat exchanges and human hunter-gatherer practices such as 'bride-service'. Indeed, as in Sue Parker's case, the two may be explicitly linked. Parker (1987: 244) writes of her 'nuptial feeding' model: 'This scenario has the virtue of connecting chimpanzee behavior with modern ethnographic behavior [e.g., meat for sex as described by Siskind (1973a)]. . . . '

By 'chimpanzee behavior', Parker means the oestrus-displaying and 'presenting' behaviour of female chimpanzees as they beg for meat from males.

Hill (1982: 533) notes a similar pattern among both chimpanzees and baboons, and continues:

> The widespread reports in ethnographic literature [e.g., ... Siskind 1973a] that human males frequently trade meat for sexual access or that good hunters obtain more wives suggest that this is the optimal solution for 'hunting apes' to increase their fitness.

Again, a direct primate–human parallel is drawn. In each case, in other words, the writer draws a parallel between primate females who competitively present their rumps to meat-possessing males, and hunter-gatherer women who make marital relations dependent on their menfolk's hunting success.

The 'sex-for-meat' concept will by now be familiar to the reader; it is central to the theoretical construct of a sex strike and therefore to the whole argument of this book. More specifically, we encountered sex-for-meat exchange in our discussion of bride-service in hunter-gatherer societies, and concluded that it lay at the root of men's 'avoidance' of their own kills (Chapters 3 and 4). Hunters normatively avoid eating their kills precisely because the whole point of hunting is to surrender the meat so as to earn goodwill from their spouses and/or in-laws and thereby qualify for marital relations.

In responding to Hill and Parker, we need to think very carefully about all this. It seems important to determine precisely what is the relationship between hunter-gatherer bride-service and what Zuckerman long ago termed primate 'prostitution'.

Although the topic has not been exhaustively debated, it seems that the majority of social anthropologists would deny any simple parallel between these two. Certainly, application of the term 'prostitution' seems problematical in the human case. 'The exchange of something for sexual favors is not considered prostitution', writes one cultural anthropologist (Witherspoon 1975: 25), referring to the viewpoint of the Navaho Indians. 'On the contrary, sexual relations without exchange are considered immoral.'

This last point seems vital: amongst almost all hunters and gatherers, as well as in more developed tribal cultures, it is actually considered wrong for a woman to have sex *without* extracting some material gift from her spouse or lover. To this we can add that wives with their kin rather than husbands or lovers are in the forefront in enforcing this rule, and that there is a sound economic basis for it. For a woman to offer sex 'free' would be for her to let down her sisters and her kin. It would undercut their sexual bargaining power, and consequently they would collectively react.

Regarding the situation among the Trobriand Islanders – among whom, as usual, men have to 'pay' for sex – Malinowski comments:

> This rule is by no means logical or self-evident. Considering the great freedom of women and their equality with men in all matters, especially

that of sex, considering also that the natives fully realise that women are as inclined to intercourse as men, one would expect the sexual relation to be regarded as an exchange of services in itself reciprocal. But custom, arbitrary and inconsequent here as elsewhere, decrees that it is a service from women to men, and men have to pay. (1932: 269)

Malinowski does not link this obligation to pay with 'prostitution', but neither does he repudiate such a parallel. Witherspoon (1975: 25), in his discussion of a similar situation among the Navaho, does tackle the issue and explicitly warns that we must be careful not to impose western concepts of morality which might lead us to see 'prostitution' wherever we find apparent 'payment' for sex. It is tempting to agree. But assuming that the 'prostitution' label is rejected on more than purely moral or political grounds, what exactly is the scientific basis for distinguishing between 'prostitution' and so-called 'moral' patterns, when in both cases females grant sexual favours in exchange for material benefits?

Different observers may arrive at different conclusions, but if we use solidarity as a touchstone, some new and perhaps more satisfactory insights can be obtained. Instead of concerning ourselves in the abstract with whether women engage in sex with an eye on economics, we can look at the concrete social effects and ask: do women's demands for 'payment', under the specific concrete circumstances, enhance social solidarity – or undermine it? No one has ever argued that the 'prostitute', in the contemporary European sense of this term, is an active agent of social solidarity. By allowing men to 'buy' sexual access to her body with money, prostitution in fact allows men to play off one category of women against another; in the eyes of the female community as such, it is this which undercuts all women's bargaining power in relation to 'their' men.

At the end of Chapter 4, we concluded that an element of female gender solidarity, implying a measure of collective sexual self-control, was an important mechanism through which women in many traditional cultures help sustain the own-kill rule. By this means, in other words, women ensure that they receive gifts of meat from men. An alternative strategy which may be combined with gender-solidarity is for women to maintain strong links with brothers or other kin. In either case, by not being too 'loose' sexually – in other words, by maintaining solidarity and the right to say 'no' – women help ensure that hunters do not take them for granted but instead have to work for their marital rights, surrendering their game and (usually) carrying the meat all the way to a home base where women can process it without having to travel far.

Although women must be attractive and capable of enjoying sex for this logic to work, it is equally true that an essential ingredient is an element of sexual negativity – sexual resistance. It is this second element which no sociobiological model of human evolution has as yet properly taken into account. Almost all contributions from sociobiology in the 1980s stressed 'continuous receptivity' and the evolution of female 'sexiness', yet seemingly forgot that none of this would be tolerable to any female unless her increasing ability to signal 'yes' became matched by an equal and opposite capacity to signal 'no'. Having lost her hormonal cyclical period of anoestrus or incapacity for sex, she urgently needed to be able to signal 'no' with at least equal effectiveness in other ways. In the typical hunter-gatherer bride-service configuration, as we saw in Chapter 4, this second capacity is evidently central. Solidarity enters in at this point because if women are to be effective in signalling 'no', they cannot afford too much inter-female rivalry and competition. If one woman were to signal 'no' only to find another beside her signalling 'yes' to the same man, her bargaining position would be completely undermined. Put crudely, women need each other's support in controlling the supply of sex.

A central argument of this book is that far from constituting 'prostitution', such collective control over sex lies at the root of all sexual 'morality'. Janet Siskind (1973b: 235) shows an understanding of this when she perceptively points out: 'If women are to be the incentive for male hunting efforts, they must be scarce. . .'. One way for women to become scarce, as Siskind continues, is 'to limit sexual access by social rules of sexual morality. . .'

Now, in conceptualising the evolutionary origins of this, we do not need to envisage anything symbolically sophisticated: all that would be required, as an absolute minimum, would be the capacity of female coalitions or groups of kin to inhibit unwanted male sexual advances. The mere fact that such resistance were collective – supported in principle by women in general, without breaches – would give it the embryonic status of a 'rule'.

At this point it seems appropriate to bring the Sharanahua directly into our discussion, partly because the reader will be familiar with them from Chapter 4, partly because both Hill and Parker explicitly appeal to them in support of their scenarios.

Two points stand out. Firstly, gender solidarity among the Sharanahua is pronounced. What Siskind (1973a: 109) terms the 'combination of same-sex solidarity and antagonism to the other sex' permeates the social structure.

Secondly, by any conventional definition, a 'prostitute' among the Sharanahua would be a woman for whom solidarity was not a priority. If the 'price' offered to her were high enough, she would break ranks with the other women of her community, offering her body for personal gain regardless of the collective female consensus. If the Sharanahua women as a whole decided on a sex strike, motivated by collective dissatisfaction with the hunting performance of their menfolk, the prostitute would be a strike-breaker. She would be the one to offer her favours on an individual basis to whichever male(s) could provide her with enough meat. For example, she might be prepared to meet one or a few men privately outside the village – perhaps far out in the bush – to exchange sex for economic benefits, cheating the sex-striking women back 'at home'. Moreover, if solidarity between the men and hence their capacity for co-operation in the hunt were in part founded on their respect for the women's sex strike, the prostitute would be a threat in another respect, too. She would tend to undermine this male collective resolve, appealing against solidarity to the private sexual self-interest of males. In all these respects, the 'prostitute' would stand in opposition to the bulk of her gender group.

To equate the normal Sharanahua 'sex-for-meat' logic either with primate oestrous soliciting or with human prostitution seems in this light an extraordinary confusion of opposites. One strategy involves prioritising gender solidarity under all circumstances; the other involves dispensing with solidarity in pursuit of competitive personal gain. In this context – and bearing in mind the previous arguments of this book – we can adapt the words of Durkheim (1961[1925]: 59) in linking 'morality' quite simply with solidarity: 'Moral goals, then, are those the object of which is *society*. To act morally is to act in terms of the collective interest.'

No matter how much this classic formulation can be queried or refined (see, for example, Ingold 1986: 222–92), at the simplest, most elementary level, human sexual 'morality' can have no other basis. Durkheim himself may not have been thinking particularly of gender solidarity, but his principle is all we need. The 'moral' hunter-gatherer woman is the one who keeps in step with her sisters, her kin and/or her gender group, on occasion refusing sex unless or until the male(s) in her life can be induced to behave acceptably, for example by providing meat. The 'immoral' woman, by contrast, is the selfish one, who exploits her body's attractions in competition with other women, using sex for her own personal gain at the expense of her sisters, undermining gender solidarity and thereby weakening the position of her gender group as a whole.

On this basis and no other can we decide upon the morality of a sexual act, or decide upon whether or not to call it 'prostitution'. Whether material benefits are involved is entirely secondary: what matters is whether, in pursuit of any benefits, solidarity is enhanced or undermined. Admittedly, no social system is ever a manifestation of either pure solidarity or pure competition – both tendencies will always be present to some degree. But in any stable system, one logic or the other will prevail. It is the basic argument of this book that only one logical thread, carried through to its conclusion, leads us towards central-place foraging, a home base, sexual morality and a genuinely human lifestyle. The other thread is a competitive, primate-style 'prostitution' pathway, leading social life in wholly non-cultural directions. Hill's and Parker's models of human origins pursue only this second pathway, and provide us with an interesting object lesson for that very reason.

Zuckerman (1932: 233) described primate 'prostitution' as 'mainly an effect of the system of dominance upon which sub-human primate societies are based'. This is an important insight. As Pateman (1988:189–218) has eloquently re-emphasised, females can systematically prostitute themselves to males only if the overall social structure is one of male dominance, resting as this does upon divisions and rivalries between females who then have to compete to gain privileges from members of the dominant sex.

We saw in Chapter 4 that the only effective answer to male dominance is female solidarity. Neither Hill nor Parker says anything about female gender solidarity or collective *resistance* to male dominance or exploitation. Their two related models in fact imply a massive shift or even 'counter-revolution' away from some of the basic primate patterns discussed in Chapter 4. It was noted there that female primates tend to determine social structure by arranging themselves spatially in accordance with their own foraging requirements, leaving the males to map themselves secondarily on to the female-defined distribution pattern. In the origins scenarios of Hill and Parker, however, protohuman females can no longer obtain their own food. The space over which females forage no longer has the same value, and female decision-making no longer has the same power in determining overall social structure. Males now monopolise access to the basic economic resources. It is they whose foraging strategy becomes primary, and the females have to 'map' themselves on to this pattern, adjusting their sexual behaviour to match the new male-defined economic realities. Female 'prostitution' – in this case as, perhaps, in all cases – is an expression of female economic dependency and weakness.

One thing is certain. If this really were the prevailing logic within a population of evolving hominids, the 'home base' institution with its accompanying female-defined parenting priorities would not evolve. The centre of gravity would be male-defined hunting space or processing space, and females would have to revolve around this, offspring or no offspring. Whenever game was caught, females would be in a race with one another to get to the kill site or butchering site, since those first to arrive would have the best prospects of obtaining a share. This is the exact inverse of the human hunter-gatherer pattern, in which *despite* the importance of hunting, women can and do centre their lives around a home base to which males laden with game are forced to return, and in which despite physical and reproductive distinctions between women, solidarity ensures that all share in the provisions which the opposite sex brings home.

Mobility, Group Size and Home Bases

It will have become apparent by now that the core concept central to all the models which we have surveyed is that of the 'home base'. Before we can finally put these theories into perspective, we need a better understanding of what this really entails.

Although in technological terms it rests on many factors including the domestication of fire (Oakley 1958; Wymer 1982; James 1989), what has all too often been overlooked is that the home base as an institution is equally rooted in a fact of sexual politics – the fact that human females do not 'chase after' males out hunting in the bush. In effect, hunter-gatherer women stand their own ground. Even if they gather over a wide area, they do so usually quite separately from men, typically in all-female groups. Their activities and solidarity may give them considerable autonomy and power. Female status among hunters and gatherers varies widely according to conditions (Hayden *et al.* 1986), but whatever the precise mode of foraging, women almost invariably organise their lives around 'their own' space, whose focal point is the hearth and campsite.

For all models of human origins, the concept of the 'home base' has always been and still remains central. As DeVore (1965: 33) put it several decades ago, no monkey or ape has such a base; when a baboon troop leaves its sleeping place in the morning, all the troop members must move together. There is no assurance that the troop will return to the same sleeping place in the evening, and every individual, even though sick or injured, must keep up with the others or risk permanent separation from the troop. Moreover, because the whole troop moves together, DeVore continued, it is not possible for baboons to hunt other animals effectively:

> Even more important, the absence of a home base makes it impossible for males to go in one direction in search of game while females and juveniles disperse to gather vegetable foods – a system of food-getting which seems universal among hunter-gatherers.

Although hardly anyone now talks about home bases in the Pliocene or Early Pleistocene, its significance for modern hunter-gatherers and for our understanding of the transition to symbolic culture remains undiminished. Its particular importance in the present context is that it tells us something about the role of early women.

For all hunters and gatherers, the home base is the central focus of activity. Its precise location usually selected mainly by the women, it is a known, predetermined point on the landscape to which all the members of a given group, however widely scattered, can consistently return and meet. It is the place to which provisions are brought, and at which food is prepared and consumed. 'The home base', as Potts (1988: 249) puts it in his book devoted largely to this topic,

> is also the place where group members sleep, make tools, and perform other maintenance activities. It is the primary spatial arena of social activity: the exchange of stories and information, the redistribution of

food, the rearing and protection of young, and the reciprocal exchange of resources or services.

A division of labour along gender lines is integral to the home base concept. It is at the base that marital sex normally occurs and that two categories of resources, 'meat' and 'gathered foods', can be systematically exchanged between two well-defined and usually rather rigidly demarcated groups – men on the one hand, women on the other.

Some feminists, for example Fedigan (1986), have rejected on ideological grounds the linkage of women in so many origins models with 'home'. This reaction is understandable in view of the manner in which anthropologists have tended to allow nuclear-family, western images of passive domesticity to pervade the concept. But perhaps this whole topic can be evaluated in a different way once it is realised that the 'home base' for hunter-gatherers has little to do with 'home' in its western cultural sense as a privatised space peripheral to the centres of social and political power. In terms of the evolution of human culture, to be centrally involved in establishing the base camp was to be in a pivotal position, in effect carving out and defending a collective space which was to become the controlling centre of all politics, all social solidarity and all economic exchange.

If we take into account the transient camps of tropical hunter-gatherers, it becomes clear that a home base is not necessarily a single permanent location. It may be occupied for only a few days. In most cases, the degree of permanence of the camp varies according to the season. But regardless of whether a camp is occupied for months, weeks or only days, the basic point is that the camp exists as a space which has been marked out as a distinct sphere and set apart from the foraging trail as such. A chimpanzee sleeping site is just one point in a chain of points along a foraging trail. A home base, for the duration of its occupation, is the beginning and end of all such trails.

Almost universally, this distinct social sphere is particularly associated with femininity. Once established, its value is that it exempts many members of the group – such as the young, the sick and the elderly – from having to move on each time an expedition to explore distant foraging grounds is mounted. Women in particular can base themselves in the same defended, watered, sheltered and pivotal spot for days or even weeks before moving on, specialist hunting parties or other foraging groups continually being sent out and welcomed back with supplies. This is the essence of what Lewis Binford (1980) terms 'logistic mobility', which he contrasts with the 'residential mobility' (that is, the constant shifting of sleeping sites) of primates and pre-cultural hominids.

Why can humans occupy the same camp for days or even weeks continuously, whereas primate groups, such as chimpanzees, have to keep moving their sleeping sites on a day-to-day basis? The reasons are complex, but an important dimension is the fact that the hunter-gatherer group does not simply forage in the area immediately adjacent to its sleeping site. There is therefore no need to move on once immediately local resources have been used up. Instead – as Lewis Binford (1983) has vividly described in the case of the caribou-hunting Nunamiut Eskimo – a constellation of far-flung localities can be combed for food whilst retaining the same base camp. Certain members of the group can forage at great distances, leaving other members, particularly immature offspring and their mothers, behind. When necessary, the distant foragers – typically hunters – may even stay out over-night, after which time, if successful, they return to the base-camp laden with food (Binford 1983: 130). Because an extremely wide area may be combed for food, there is no need for the base camp as such to be constantly moved.

All primate foragers, by contrast, experience a conflict between being residentially stable on the one hand, and being sociable on the other. The two are simply not compatible. As group size increases, so the foraging group as a whole – males and females – has to become more continuously mobile. This is because primates have to eat as they go, each individual relying essentially on whatever food it can find for itself in the space adjacent to its own body. The more individuals there are in each foraging group, the smaller is the available body space, the greater the internal competition for food, and the sooner the temporarily occupied area is 'eaten out'. The larger the group, in other words, the briefer must be its stay at any one place (Dunbar 1988: 305–22).

A consequence is that in proportion as primates are sociable, so they are compelled to devote more energy to moving around, the females having to bring their immature offspring with them (for a full discussion see Dunbar 1988: 292–322).

In any discussion of the evolution of hominid patterns of foraging and group living, this logic must be taken into account. The connection between large brains, slow maturation rates and added burdens of motherhood has been discussed already in this chapter. As brain size and childhood dependency increased, evolving protohuman mothers would have been confronted with increasingly severe infant-transport problems. But the difficulty is that on this logic, the evolving protohuman female whose intensifying burdens tempted her to cut down on travel would have had to forage in a relatively isolated way, keeping other females at a distance from each feeding spot as it was discovered. Depending on the local availability of food, this would have made it difficult for groups of females to do something which is common-place in modern human camps of hunters and gatherers – support one another in child care and other domestic tasks. It would certainly have placed strains on close links with all relatives, including grandparents; the more relatives present in each foraging group, the less easily could it afford to stay

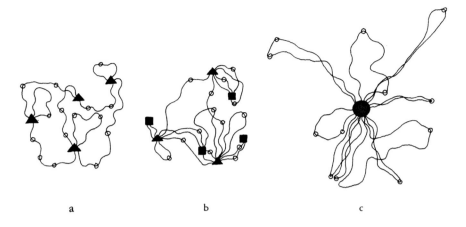

a   b   c

Figure 3 Foraging and spatial patterning. ▲ = sleeping sites. ■ = areas for resource-processing, typically centred on tool caches. ○ = points along the trail at which food is obtained.

a A common primate pattern: sleeping sites are distributed at intervals along the foraging trail.
b Hypothesised early *Homo* pattern. Focal points now include stone tool caches as well as sleeping sites.
c Modern hunter-gatherer 'logistic' pattern. Sleeping, tool storage, food processing, child care, information exchange and all activities except actual food procurement can be focused on a single semi-permanent base camp.

for a period in any one place.

By the standards of these primate-derived considerations, human hunter-gatherer females have achieved something quite remarkable – combining intensified group life (and almost always some significant sharing of child care and/or other household burdens) with facilities for resting and nursing offspring at a home base. Despite living in large social groups, human females do not have to travel across the landscape from dawn to dusk in search of food, carrying their offspring with them and ending each day at a new location. They have in this sense broken through the whole system of constraints governing primate social evolution. Group-living human females can afford to centre their lives at and around a home base area largely because, as we saw in Chapter 4, they have adopted a strategy of 'standing their ground' and making the opposite sex do some or much of the necessary foraging for them. The problem, of course, is to explain how this breakthrough could have been achieved (figure 3).

The 1980s in Retrospect

Isaac, Tanner, Lovejoy, Hill and Parker share one assumption in common. This is that our task is to explain the origin of the hunter-gatherer way of life by means of a single all-embracing theory which covers a vast timespan since it must also explain bipedalism and the slow, supposedly culturally inspired divergence of the hominids from the pongids. It is this simplifying gradualist assumption underlying all the theories which the latest fossil and genetic evidence has undermined, leaving the field in a state of some confusion and uncertainty.

The key issue is the approximate date of emergence of a recognisable 'hunter-gatherer' social configuration centred on the institution of a 'home base'. No one now disputes that the early hominid tool-makers ate meat. What matters is how significant this component of their diet really was, and at what stage there emerged anything resembling the contemporary hunter-gatherer pattern in which females control the domestic area and gather while males go out hunting at a distance and bring food 'home'.

The truth must reside somewhere between two 'extreme' possibilities. The first of these extremes is Isaac's view, supported with varying emphases and varying views on the relevance of hunting by Tanner, Lovejoy, Hill and (in part) Parker. This is an 'early' scenario. Human evolution was always gradualistic and unilinear. The sexual division of labour stretches back into the distant Plio-Pleistocene (or even the Miocene) because it was something which hominids as a species just 'did', perhaps in connection with their evolving bipedalism and relatively large brains. If there was any 'human revolution', within the paradigm of these writers, the expression refers not to an unprecedented and momentous Late Pleistocene political transformation, but to an essentially zoological process of accelerated genetic evolution which got under way two or more million years ago, when hominids were emphatically no more than one animal species among others. Such a way of looking at matters would imply that the characteristically 'human' system, however novel, was not dependent on fully symbolic culture for its success; it would be something which chimpanzees, for example, might have managed if only they had been subject to slightly different selection pressures – if only they could have walked upright more easily or displayed a little more intelligence, generosity and/or dexterity.

The contrasting possibility is a 'late' scenario. It would seem to imply a process of conflict, struggle, set-backs, local extinctions – and occasional bursts of explosive evolution once radical solutions to pressing problems had been found. This would be in keeping with Lewis Binford's recurrent theme that for change to occur, 'the system . . . must be under stress in some way, must face some problem' (1983: 222). In this context, we would need to know: What was the zoologically 'insoluble' problem whose ultimate solution was language, the incest taboo, the 'home base' arrangement, a sexual division of labour, ritual, art and, in short, symbolic culture?

Acceptance of the late scenario would imply that establishing a home base arrangement with concomitant sexual division of labour was delayed – seemingly endlessly – because it was something profoundly difficult to achieve and sustain. It did not simply 'evolve', immediately, whenever environmental pressures made it in our eyes theoretically 'optimal'. Instead, because of the difficulties inherited from the past, evolution was held back. For a million or more years, hominids – including even the large-brained and skilled tool-maker, *Homo erectus* – remained unable to make what with hindsight we see as the 'necessary' breakthrough. As a consequence, population levels remained fairly low, technological development reached a plateau and then stopped, and the various hominid species or subspecies stayed locked within a relatively narrow band of habitable ecozones within Africa, Europe and Asia.

In this book, it will be shown that something approaching the second scenario now looks more likely. Even so intelligent a creature as *Homo erectus* seems to have got stuck in a rut for about a million years, the process of advance being 'quite clearly constrained', as Clive Gamble (1986b: 6) puts it, 'by factors other than simply technological competence'. This 'late' scenario would envisage certain ancient and deeply rooted socio-sexual and political constraints restricting what even the most competent, intelligent, 'sociable' hominids could achieve. The theoretically or retrospectively 'optimal' system of establishing a sexual division of labour/home base was not attained. Although to us it seems logical, for evolving hominids themselves it was not optimal for the simple reason that it was not even possible – its material preconditions had not evolved. It required not just bipedalism, tool-making, basket-making technology, larger brains or good-naturedness, but a massive social and sexual revolution culminating in the firm establishment of collectively agreed moral regulations and symbolic culture in something like the form in which it governs the lives of hunter-gatherers to this day. The neural, anatomical, physiological, technological, ecological and other preconditions which had to be met before all this could work were numerous, and it took two million or more years from the first manufacture of stone tools before they were all in place simultaneously in the case of any one population.

An effort of the imagination is needed if we are to comprehend what was at stake. The fact that contemporary hunter-gatherers manage the sexual division of labour easily should not blind us to the difficulties – contemporary humans, after all, are the beneficiaries of millennia-old established rule systems and traditions which are the products of the human revolution and did not exist prior to it. Demarcating the 'home base' area from a much wider foraging range was not just a conceptual or technical challenge. It presupposed on the part of females a powerful capacity for solidarity and a resistance to any attempts to make them move from their chosen 'home' whilst hunting was in progress. It presupposed on the part of males a respect for this resistance, and sufficient self-control to avoid either rape or temptations to eat their own kills on the spot. It meant being able to separate the act of *production* systematically and regularly from a postponed act of *consumption*. Above all, it presupposed that males could travel long distances away from their female sexual partners for periods of time, *realistically able to dismiss the worry that rival males might take sexual advantage of their absence.* To the extent that any primate legacy of male behaviourally competitive sexuality still prevailed, all this would have presented a vast set of challenges.

If such considerations were valid, we might expect evidence for a firm sexual division of labour – that is, a clearly demarcated home base area implying the complete liberation of hunters to forage at great distances – only late in the archaeological record. Evidence for it would be bound up with the first firm evidence for other dimensions of mental and social collectivity such as ritual, religion and conventionalised symbolic art. That would mean that even archaic *Homo sapiens* – accomplished tool-maker, fire-user, hunter and possessor of a massive brain – never quite found a stable and effective solution to the sexual and political problems involved, leaving the final perfection of this arrangement to await anatomically modern humans possessing fully symbolic culture. If there was a 'human revolution', its final successful consummation came remarkably late.

Conclusion: Economics, Meat and 'Higher Purposes'

Before we leave the origins theories of the 1980s, it seems worth tying up some threads with a final thought. It is often pointed out that a sizeable contribution to the diets of many modern hunter-gatherers is food obtained while actually foraging. This is the so-called 'snack factor'. Foods are often eaten immediately upon obtaining them, instead of being shared at campsites (Hayden 1981: 419).

It is a fact, however, that such foods tend to be of vegetable products rather than meat, and of smaller categories of game rather than large ones. In general, the larger the category of prey animal, the more powerful are the inhibitions against eating one's own kill (Chapter 3). Moreover, it is certainly not the non-tabooed types of food – berries, nuts and so on – which occupy a central place in traditional symbolic or ideological systems. Vital as gathered foods may be – just as air is vital, or water – they are likely to be 'free'. All members of the social group tend to have equal access to them, and taboos and avoidances are less imperiously required. It seems reasonable to suppose that dependence on such necessities has always been a feature of human and pre-human life, yet for that very reason – *because* gathering was so vital whether before, during or after the transition to culture – it cannot qualify as the new factor precipitating the establishment of culture in its modern sense. This new factor must have been women's success in harnessing the hunting capabilities of men.

The baboon and chimpanzee evidence surveyed earlier in this chapter indicates that initially, meat would have been 'free' like other foods, except for the fact that its distribution would have been particularly 'unfair'. Young offspring and their mothers would have been in effect penalised, but to begin with, no one would have been in a position to impose collective norms of 'avoidance' or 'respect' ensuring meat's equitable circulation and exchange.

But if this were so, then hominid life would still have been in a pre-economic phase. Until collectively imposed norms of sharing and exchange began to make their presence felt, the realm of 'economic' life in the human sense would still have been non-existent. As the early economic anthropologist Thurnwald (1932: xi) put it:

> The devouring of newly killed beasts. . . . certainly cannot be called economics. More than this is implied in the term. If there ever was a time when man, or his ancestor, lived from moment to moment on what he killed or caught, it was a time without economics.

Or as the archaeologist Robert Braidwood (1957: 122) observed, a man who followed animals 'just to kill them to eat' would be 'living just like an animal himself'.

An implication is that whatever the importance of 'foraging', to be human is to go beyond this – it is to engage in relations of 'production', a position linked historically with the names of Marx and Engels:

> Men can be distinguished from animals by consciousness, by religion, or by anything else one likes. They themselves begin to distinguish themselves from animals as soon as they begin to *produce* their means of subsistence. . . . (1947[1846]: 7)

In Marx's terms, it is the dimension of systematic social *exchange* which defines food procurement as 'production'. Marx writes: 'although isolated labour (its material conditions presupposed) can also create use-values, it can create neither wealth nor culture' (1951[1875]: 2,18) The isolated individual, outside society, feeds himself on what he finds. 'In society, however', Marx continues,

> the relation of the producer to his product, as soon as it is completed, is an outward one, and the return of the product to the individual depends on his relations to other individuals. Nor does the direct appropriation of the product constitute his purpose, when he produces in society. Between the producer and the product distribution steps in, determining by social laws his share in the world of products; that is to say, distribution steps in between production and consumption. (1971b[1859]: 27–8)

Returning, now, to our discussion in Chapters 3 and 4, we may say that if hunters in fully human cultures 'produce', there is a direct connection with the existence of the own-kill rule. Adapting Marx's words, we may say that to the extent that the hunter avoids eating his own kill, 'the relation of the producer to his product, as soon as it is completed, is an outward one. . . ', so that 'the direct appropriation of the product' is not production's purpose.

We have seen that in human hunter-gatherer cultures, hunters do not kill game in order to eat the meat. In fact, they often consume very little of it.

Where psychological motivations are concerned, men hunt less to eat than to win self-esteem and to be perceived as generous and skilled hunters, particularly in female eyes. That is, they hunt for complex reasons connected with their self-esteem, their sexuality and their general social status and prestige. These 'higher' purposes can be pursued successfully only to the extent that each hunter can avoid being so greedy and short-sighted as to consume his own kills – a fault which would be seen as something akin to incest (Chapter 3). Only to the extent that individuals 'respect' their own produce (procreative and economic) can the realm of human life, with its cycles of circulation and exchange, come into being. Because primates, by contrast, start to eat food immediately as it is found or as soon as it is physically possible to do so, circulation cannot develop and economic life cannot even begin to arise.

Were it not for the own-kill norm, then, it might seem legitimate to equate human hunting activities with primate predatory behaviour. Once the explanatory value of the 'own-kill' concept is recognised, we can no longer afford to blur conceptual boundaries in this way. We have seen in earlier chapters that human hunters typically 'respect' or 'avoid' their own kills, at least on some symbolic level even if not always in more literal ways. Even relatively 'selfish' hunters in most cultures offer up animal 'sacrifices' to the spirits, or they take care to avoid 'totemic' flesh, or they 'respectfully' hunt creatures puzzlingly defined as 'kin'. As Leslie White (1949) put it long ago, humans can even distinguish 'Holy Water' from 'water' – a litmus test of symbolic capacities if ever there was one. All this is a basic condition of true economics; and it indicates something which is by primate standards extraordinary. Since non-human primates show no signs of the necessary self-restraint, civic consciousness or ability to observe ritual avoidances, we must conclude that before the hominisation process was completed – bringing with it the establishment of 'economics' for the first time – a truly revolutionary restructuring of primate behavioural norms had to be achieved.

Chapter 6
Solidarity and Cycles

> Revolution is necessary not only because the *ruling* class cannot be overthrown in any other way, but also because only in a revolution can *the class which overthrows it* rid itself of the accumulated rubbish of the past and become capable of reconstructing society.
>
> Karl Marx and Friedrich Engels, *The German Ideology* (1846)

It has been a consistent implication of my argument that for this restructuring to be accomplished, women had to take the power. As members of the oppressed sex, they had to develop their coalitions, curb internal rivalries, stand by one another regardless of reproductive condition or personal circumstance – and compel males to bring meat on pain of exclusion from sex.

There was no way that males could adequately transform their behaviour whilst females were still colluding in their own oppression. As we will now begin to see, the evolving human female therefore had to define her own space, enforce respect for this, inhibit male exploitation and rape, signal her inviolability in her own blood and – in effect – seize power in the emerging institution of the 'home'. In this chapter, I will focus on a preliminary condition of this process – ovarian synchrony and the evolution on that basis of a specific and very unusual kind of reproductive physiology and anatomy.

Biologists have long been puzzled by the evolution of the human female menstrual cycle. E. O. Wilson (1975: 547–8) saw it as an example of 'extraordinary evolution'; menstruation, he wrote, has been intensified whilst the 'estrus, or period of female "heat", has been replaced by virtually continuous sexual activity. . .'. Primatologists Washburn and Hamburg (1972: 277) voiced what was until recently a consensus in noting that oestrus loss rendered human females 'quite different' from any other primate.

Strictly speaking, lack of oestrus is now seen as a feature shared by all the higher primates, in that sexual intercourse among them is not rigidly confined to the female's fertile moments. Nonetheless, the earlier writers were not entirely mistaken. In all primates, sexual motivation fluctuates cyclically, reaching a peak during ovulation, which may be announced with a public signal. With the exception of women, all primates also exhibit cyclical vulvular swellings of some kind (Dixson 1983). While in some species these are hardly noticeable, in others they are pronounced and/or accompanied by striking changes in sexual skin colouring, special scent emissions and so on (Zuckerman 1932; Rowell 1972; Dixson 1983). Such displays – which are related in an obvious way to the oestrus signals of other mammals – may be regarded as uncontrollable, involuntary 'yes' signals sent out by primate females at around the time when they are most likely to conceive. No mature male in the vicinity can resist the temptations of a female in such a state. In what follows, the term 'oestrus' will be used in a loose way to refer to this female condition which characterises many primates but which humans have completely lost.

Mating Systems and Ovarian Cyclicity in Primates

Chimpanzees ovulate for one day out of the thirty-six of their cycle, but prominently inflate the area around their genitals for about ten days beforehand. The female's sexual fervour intensifies as her swellings rise. As she approaches peak oestrus, she becomes, typically, surrounded by numerous males. In the early stages of full swelling, these take turns to copulate, one after the other, showing little aggression or competitiveness. Towards the moment of actual egg release, however, she becomes increasingly monopolised by a single dominant male who is likely to succeed in fertilising her (Goodall 1986: 450–1).

Throughout the remainder of her cycle, such a female does not arouse males or show much interest in sex (Graham 1981; Tutin and McGrew 1973; Tutin and McGinnis 1981; Goodall 1986: 443–87). Whereas oestrous females typically follow around after highly mobile males, anoestrous ones tend to stay behind in the company of other females, although they are often rather solitary (Wrangham 1979).

Among baboons, cycle lengths and other details differ, but there is the same tendency to reach a peak of excitability – 'gadfly madness', as Hrdy (1981: 156) puts it – as sexual swellings rise.

In any species, the female's sexual physiology is shaped by selection pressures specific to her usual mating system. This means that the modern reproductive physiology of womankind – which cannot have changed much over the past few tens of millennia – should tell us something about the mating system on the basis of which she evolved.

Female primates monopolised in stable one-male harems, such as gelada baboons, tend to evolve shorter periods of receptivity and less striking swellings than do chimpanzees and others adapted to multi-male systems (Dunbar 1988: 153; Dixson 1983). To understand why, primatologists have attempted to work out the costs and benefits of extended receptivity and/or pronounced swelling under different social conditions.

Flaunting one's attractions during oestrus may prompt males to grant special favours, but it also invites harassment from resentful same-sex companions, as happens among geladas (Dunbar 1980a). The risk can be minimised by trying to signal to the alpha male only on those days when other females are hormonally least interested in sex. We might say that if there is a shortage of males and nothing radical can be done about this, the females might as well ration themselves to avoid too much harassment from one another. Asynchrony, relatively modest signalling and receptive periods of only a few days – the gelada pattern – will tend to result.

On the other hand, it may not be that the shortage of males is an immutable fact of life. It may be possible to break out from the 'harem', or invite other males to come in. One-male monopolies over large harems tend to be enforceable only with difficulty. 'Illicit' matings with outsiders occur, and in the case of some species in some ecological contexts, these become the norm.

To the extent that a one-male monopoly proves untenable, the mating system which replaces it can in theory evolve towards (a) monogamous pairing, (b) polyandry or (c) a promiscuous 'multi-male' system. Monogamy is not found among terrestrial, savanna-dwelling primates (Hrdy 1981: 36), whilst polyandry is found only among tree-dwelling marmosets and tamarins (Goldizen 1987). For ground-living primates, the basic alternative to a 'one-male' harem system is a system of promiscuous 'multi-male' units.

Instead of competing to obtain once-for-all control over a whole group of females, males in multi-male contexts are faced with the fact that they can never permanently 'win' their females. There are various alternatives, including the formation of special long-term friendships with particular females, but in general fidelity is not to be expected and males have to compete more or less continuously for each copulation as and when a female comes into oestrus (Dunbar 1988: 176).

In this situation, since there is no shortage of males, females come under less mutual pressure to avoid reproductively unnecessary sex, so that there is less need for females to display their receptivity only briefly and in sequence. If sexual relations with multiple male partners enable females to gain added male support, receptivity will extend markedly beyond each female's fertile days.

In itself, this would not explain prominent oestrus displays. Indeed, it might be thought that where males were easy to get, there should be no need for females to enter into fiercely competitive sexual self-advertising. In primate multi-male contexts, however, while the greater availability of males initially reduces inter-female competition for them, the evolution of extended receptivity by the same token builds up the competitive pressure once more, even though this pressure now acts in a different way. When a number of females are receptive simultaneously in a multi-male context, they compete not for males as such – after all, any receptive female can get those – but for the most desirable males at the most crucial moments. In fact, as they approach ovulation, females in such situations compete vigorously for access to the most dominant males. Faced simultaneously with a number of 'yes'-signalling females, each such targeted male makes his choice on the basis of the surrounding females' explicit sexual 'advertising'. Females adapted to such pressures display, as Alexander and Noonan (1979: 446) put it, 'the most dramatic advertisements of sexual receptivity, the most obvious and intense sexual competitiveness, and . . . the most striking cases of receptivity outside the ovulation period'. It then becomes rather difficult for a male to distinguish true ovulation from what might be termed 'sham oestrus', but selection pressures naturally favour those males who are best at doing this.

The Puzzle of the Human Female

We have seen that non-arboreal, non-forest-dwelling primate mating systems are stretched out between two opposite conceptual poles – so-called 'one-male' harem systems on the one hand, 'multi-male' systems on the other. Concrete mating arrangements approximate towards one pole or the other, with females evolving the forms of their cycles and reproductive physiologies accordingly.

Now, the problem is that the human female seems to belong to neither pole; nor does she fit in at any point in between. She could not have evolved in a harem system – for that would have endowed her with strictly limited, cyclical, hormonally governed periods of receptivity. But neither could she have evolved in a 'multi-male' system based on promiscuity and female competition for insemination by dominant males. We can infer this because, lacking either oestrus or sham oestrus, the human female appears ill equipped to compete with her sisters in the requisite way.

The human female is in principle sexually receptive, regardless of fertility, throughout the whole of her cycle. Her interest in sex, despite possible slight peaks at ovulation and/or menstruation (Udry and Morris 1977; Adams et al. 1978), never becomes as overwhelming as it is for primates in peak receptivity and remains essentially unchanged. Conversely, she is equally able to refuse sex at any time: at no point during her cycle is she the slave of her hormonal state.

In fact, the human female does not signal 'yes' with her genitals at all.

Instead of being externally marked as a public display, ovulation has evolved in the reverse direction, to the point at which the moment of maximum fertility has become effectively concealed. In neither appearance nor behaviour is it possible to determine a human female's fertile period. Far from males in her presence being made publicly aware of her ovulation, the human female's special condition is kept so close a secret that unless she is unusually aware of her own physiology she will not even know the moment herself.

Theories of Oestrus Loss

In the human case, direct, blatant sexual competitiveness within a promiscuous mating arena has evidently been subject to strong negative selection. This is supported by two primatological observations. Firstly, monogamous primates, most notably gibbons, show extended receptivity and concealed ovulation, although not in so extreme a form as in the human case. Secondly, concealment combined with very extended receptivity characterises tamarins and marmosets, whose mating systems are versions of 'cooperative polyandry', each female consorting with more than one male partner (Goldizen 1987: 39–40). Neither monogamy nor polyandry necessarily implies interfemale solidarity; both, however, minimise situations in which females are in direct sexual competition for successive copulations with the same male. In searching for the type of mating system responsible for the human female condition, we can therefore rule out polygamy. We are drawn instead towards monogamy, polyandry – or some unsuspected pattern resting on inter-female solidarity on a level unknown among non-human primates.

The theme of a 'sex strike' was broached in Chapter 4; it is now time to consider its possible relevance. If female gender solidarity were increasingly being prioritised as a means of upholding collective sexual bargaining power, what kind of mating system and associated physiology would females evolve? Can we imagine an oestrus-governed female easily observing the discipline of a sex strike under pressure from her companions? Or would selection pressures in this context favour those females more liberated from their cycles – those better able to signal 'yes' or 'no' at any time, dependent not on hormones but on the requirements of inter-female political calculation and solidarity?

Although answers at this stage must remain tentative, merely to ask this question is to begin to glimpse the possibilities in a new way. As will be shown more fully towards the end of this chapter, the concept of gender solidarity allows us to begin to unravel some of the more difficult theoretical problems. Perhaps surprisingly, however, this solution has only recently been suspected. Meanwhile, numerous very different theories to explain the human female condition have been at the centre of scholarly debate.

Alexander and Noonan: the 'female deception' theory

Probably the most popular has been the 'female deception and self-deception' theory, which in its best-known form was put forward by the American sociobiologists Richard Alexander and Katherine Noonan (1979).

These authors set out from the crucial fact – as central to sociobiology as the class struggle is to Marxism – that females and males may have radically different reproductive interests. Typically, the female needs to get 'her' male to stay with her once she is pregnant; the male needs, on the contrary, to inseminate as many females as he can. In the course of hominid evolution, the argument runs, it was the female of the species who eventually won this battle:

> We suggest that concealment of ovulation evolved in humans because it enabled females to force desirable males into consort relationships long enough to reduce their likelihood of success in seeking other matings, and simultaneously raised the male's confidence of paternity by failing to inform other, potentially competing males of the timing of ovulation. (Alexander and Noonan 1979: 443)

The crucial idea here is that by losing their public signals, females succeeded in 'tricking' males, denying them any means of knowing when to impregnate them. For males, the only sure answer was to have sex with one and the same female throughout her cycle, whilst keeping all rivals away; nothing else could provide confidence in paternity.

The authors stress that had females betrayed the slightest sign of the moment of ovulation, their whole strategy would have collapsed – males would have abandoned their mates the moment they felt sure they had fertilised them. But it is difficult, they continue, to keep something from your partner if you are conscious of it yourself. The best deceivers are the self-deceived. Consequently, the evolving human female had to suppress even her own awareness of the vital moment. 'Concealed ovulation', the authors conclude, 'we view as a particularly powerful and instructive case of deception of others, linked with self-deception and made more effective by it.'

This theory is an ingenious one and, as will be seen, needs only to be enhanced in the context of a rather different model of early human mating-systems (Turke 1984) to appear very convincing. Before noting some criticisms, we may go on to consider another version of the same theory.

Stoddart: odours and the sexual division of labour

D. Michael Stoddart (1986) of the University of Tasmania links vaginal odours and their reduction with the evolution of hunting. He suggests that extended hunting trips combined with 'gregariousness' brought problems for the originally monogamous protohuman couple – particularly since, in the early stages, the would-be faithful female was unwittingly giving off sexually irresistible odours to all about her each time she ovulated. The problem was

> that if some males left the home camp on hunting trips which might last for several days at a stretch . . . bonded females remaining at the home camp would not infrequently produce odorous ovulation advertising signals while their mates were absent and while other males were present as guards.

As the nearby stay-at-home males ('guards') were aroused by such odours, sex would unavoidably have occurred whilst the dutiful but unsuspecting hunters were absent. This (according to Stoddart) would eventually have undermined the hunter males' confidence in paternity, discouraging them from investing care in their partners' offspring. To avoid this outcome, females had to stop involuntarily soliciting sex at the wrong times. Olfactory sexual signals consequently had to be suppressed.

It will be noted that Stoddart's model assumes a kind of 'sex strike' hypothesis, to use the terminology of Chapter 4. Females have to build up the sexual confidence of hunters by, in effect, 'promising' not to have sex with anyone else while they are away. The assumption is that ovulatory odours were inhibited to enable females to do this.

Benshoof and Thornhill: the 'cuckoldry' theory

But there have been criticisms of the notion that oestrus loss evolved to confer certainty of paternity. Responding not to Stoddart but to earlier versions of the oestrus-loss-sustains-monogamy theory, Benshoof and Thornhill (1979) contest the notion that concealed ovulation could have helped at all in increasing a male's confidence in his paternity. On the contrary, they say, the early human male's ignorance of his mate's condition would have caused intense problems. Each male would have needed to guard his female against covetous neighbours, never knowing whether he should join the hunting party and risk being cuckolded or stay at home on the off-chance that this would be her fertile week.

No system, these authors argue, could be more poorly designed to guarantee paternity than the system of concealed ovulation. The system means that no male has any idea when his partner might conceive. Taken in isolation, this actually *decreases* any male's ability to link his intercourse with the pregnancy of his partner. Indeed, the whole point of Alexander and Noonan's argument is that this is so: it is said that *because* of the newly accentuated male paternity uncertainty, counter-measures – in particular, the maintenance of round-the-clock vigilance over the female sexual partner – were required. But if paternity assurance were the deciding factor and monogamy the consequent mating system, humans would surely not have created such problems in the first place. They would have evolved the pattern common to other monogamous primates: a short, well-defined oestrus with very little advertisement of the fact. Under this system, the female's monogamous partner knows perfectly well when she is in heat, whereas rival males are kept ignorant because they are kept at a distance and the signals are not sufficiently public. Then the female's mate need only guard her for the few vital days; after that, he can go hunting secure in the knowledge that however unfaithful she might be, he will be the father of any baby she has (Shaw and Darling 1985: 82–3, citing Benshoof and Thornhill 1979). Again, it will be noted that this is a kind of 'sex strike' hypothesis, at least in the sense that the female does not engage in relevant or genetically threatening sex whilst her hunting partner is away.

Benshoof and Thornhill argue that this initially happened: protowomen were in a limited sense 'monogamous' in that, despite their many possible 'affairs', they had *fertile* sex only when their chosen partner was at home. Reducing their public sexual signalling to ward off unwanted males, they signalled just sufficiently to let the favoured partner know the correct moment to inseminate.

The authors acknowledge that this would still not explain the actual human condition which we find – complete oestrus loss, in which even the favoured partner has little if any idea when his partner is ovulating. To explain this 'later' development, the two researchers follow a complex course, arguing that when couples began living in large social groups (it is assumed that they did not do this before), the females found themselves surrounded by a wide choice of males. It then became in their interests to deceive their partners, getting impregnated by males who were in genetic terms the 'best', regardless of whether these gave help in provisioning or child-care. So human females had sex with their 'faithful' partners for most of the cycle, but during ovulation sneaked off to get pregnant by the best obtainable mate. Concealed ovulation made this possible, since the 'faithful' partner had no way of knowing that his sexual intercourse was not fertile; assuming the offspring to be his, he provided the support and child-care that the mother required. This has been termed the 'cuckoldry' theory of oestrus loss (Shaw and Darling 1985: 84).

The fatal flaw in all this, however, is that women would not have known of the correct moment to 'sneak off' and get themselves pregnant by an illicit lover. Despite all their good intentions, they would have kept getting pregnant accidentally by their faithful partner, with whom they spent so much time. 'Although some women think they can tell when they are ovulating', as Shaw and Darling (1985: 84) put it, 'the vast majority most decidedly cannot, and even with our current technological ability to measure basal body temperature and to sample and categorise cervical mucus, the time of ovulation is notoriously difficult to pinpoint'. Benshoof and Thornhill try to fall back on the 'self-deception' argument, but it is difficult to understand

how women could have cuckolded their partners at ovulation without knowing it – impelled by some inner hormonal force of which they were unaware.
'Surely', as Shaw and Darling (1985: 84) have written, Benshoof and
Thornhill's proposed system 'would function infinitely better if the female
herself knew when an egg was ready and confined her *affaires de coeur* only to
that time'.

Nancy Burley: the anti-birth-control theory

Starting out from the fact that the moment of egg release is concealed from
women themselves, yet another frequently cited hypothesis holds that such
concealment was necessary – to stop culturally motivated women avoiding
motherhood completely. Given half a chance, argues Nancy Burley (1979),
women, who for cultural reasons are in a unique position to understand in
advance the pain and dangers of childbirth and the burdens of child-care,
would simply never get pregnant. If they knew when they ovulated, they
would simply avoid sex at that time. Concealed ovulation has evolved to
prevent women from practising such a disastrous form of birth control.

Burley cites much evidence that abortion/infanticide in traditional cultures must be practised by women secretly, husbands being overwhelmingly
unsympathetic. But – even assuming earliest cultures knew of the connection
between sex and pregnancy, which is to say the least uncertain (Montagu
1974) – is it true that, left to themselves, culturally aware women would
avoid motherhood completely? Surely not. Birth control as a positive
measure to improve parenting quality would come far closer to most
women's genetic interests *and* cultural ideals than the desire to escape
motherhood altogether – certainly in pre-industrial cultural contexts, and
surely in our own as well. And if this is taken to be the case, ovulation
concealment becomes a mystery once more. For women's self-knowledge of
the moment of ovulation would be an immense benefit in terms of conscious
fertility control. As Burley (1979: 841) herself acknowledges, the woman
who was aware of her cycle would seem to possess all kinds of advantages in
comparison with her more ignorant sister. She would be more free to have
sexual affairs with multiple lovers, without having to worry about pregnancy
at an inopportune time. But on the other hand, she could also get pregnant
more quickly when it suited her. In other words, she could consciously
organise optimal spacing between births, without having to resort to the
extraordinarily wasteful and emotionally harrowing techniques of abortion
and infanticide.

In this light, it remains difficult to understand why ovulation should have
become concealed in the human case to so remarkably complete an extent.
Concealment is a form of ignorance. From whichever standpoint it is
examined, this particular form of ignorance would seem at first sight to be a
handicap imposed upon both sexes rather than an asset.

Menstruation

Despite oestrus loss, hormonally controlled sexual signals are *not* entirely missing from the human female menstrual cycle. On the contrary, menstruation in the human case has been *accentuated* as an external display. It is at menstruation rather than ovulation that the human female experiences her behaviour as hormonally influenced to a certain degree. Although this is not unique among primates – rhesus monkeys display behavioural changes mainly around menstruation (Rowell 1963) – it remains an unusual phenomenon, which any full theory must explain.

A woman loses considerably more blood during menstruation than does any other primate. This shedding of blood, although small, represents a significant loss – a loss which has to be made good by additional food intake, particularly of iron. The adaptive advantage of this has not yet been explained.

Although there is no biological imperative to avoid sex during this period, in traditional human cultural contexts, menstruation in fact signals 'no' (Chapter 11). It would seem that in proportion as she *lost* her long periods of hormonally determined *non*-receptivity, the evolving human female was obliged to compensate with some other powerful means of signalling 'no'. Among contemporary hunter-gathers, menstrual taboos are particularly intense in northerly latitudes, where meat dependence tends to be heaviest (Kitahara 1982). In this context, Stoddart's (1986) theory that a loss of ovulation odours underpinned the sexual division of labour finds it complement in the mirror-image theory that an *accentuation* of negatively interpreted *menstrual* odours can achieve the same result, keeping the sexes apart during those periods when men need to concentrate on the hunt (Dobkin de Rios 1976; Dobkin de Rios and Hayden 1985; Testart 1985, 1986). In other words, the elimination of oestrus odours and accentuation of menstrual odours may be head and tail of the same coin. The bearing of all this on the concept of a culture-generating monthly periodic 'sex strike' will be explored in Chapters 9 to 11.

In western contexts, of course, menstrual taboos have to an extent been relaxed, but compensatory constructs such as 'premenstrual syndrome' (Dalton 1977, 1979; Lever 1981) may lead to not substantially different results. At least one feminist strand of thought (Martin 1988) insists that the 'once-a-month-witches' (Donelson and Gullahorn 1977) who strain their marriages under the banner of this syndrome are not sick – merely intolerant of marital or other stress which may seem more acceptable at other times. In the premenstrual period, in other words, women are less able to tolerate society's and their partners' pressures and demands. There is an enhanced bodily self-awareness, a lower tolerance threshold – and so a stronger tendency to rebel. Western culture-specific constructs such as 'PMS' may on this analysis represent attempts to come to terms with such realities, given that traditional menstrual taboos no longer perform that protective, gender-segregating function.

There are doubtless some counterparts to all this among primates. But with the exception of rhesus monkeys (Manson 1986: 26), primate females give an impression of being behaviourally governed by hormones not so much at menstruation as at the opposite point – during and around ovulation. As Shaw and Darling (1985: 58) put it:

> although monkeys menstruate, it is an insignificant event, overshadowed by a more important event taking place at a different time during the cycle – the periodic sexual heat, which happens at the time of ovulation.

When she is not due to ovulate, the primate female may simply withdraw from sex or from consortship with males, without having to struggle against expectations to the contrary. We might say that she does not have to struggle to assert her periodic 'right to strike' – because her physiological periodic anoestrus does it for her.

For reasons which have yet to be explained, in any event, the evolving human female concealed ovulation and its associated odours almost completely, extended her receptivity as never before, and accentuated both the odours and visible manifestations of the menstrual flow. Taking these features together, the human configuration appears not just different from the usual primate pattern, but its inverse. *Whereas the basic primate pattern is to deliver a periodic 'yes' signal against a background of continuous sexual 'no', humans emit a periodic 'no' signal against a background of continuous 'yes'.* This reversal indicates something of the nature and scale of the sexual revolution central to the process of becoming human.

Synchrony: Seasonal and Menstrual

Among mammals generally, breeding seasonality is a form of reproductive synchrony which has long been recognised. In this case, it is the sun which is the ultimate determinant, producing the seasonal cycle and with it a definite schedule of resource availability. By contrast, menstrual synchrony implies, etymologically at least, a link with the moon.

Primates do not show the strict breeding seasonality of most other mammals. Nonetheless, all primate reproductive cycles vary seasonally because they are sensitive to light and other environmental cues. Among macaques, geladas and patas monkeys, for example, the onset of reproductive activity is triggered by a seasonal flush of vegetation produced by rain (Dunbar 1988: 65, citing Fa 1986; Dunbar 1980b; Rowell and Richards 1979). The reproductive cycles of gibbons are phase-locked with seasonal variations in available fruits (Dunbar 1988: 281, citing Chivers and Raemakers 1980).

When births all occur at a definite time of year, it is because giving birth at this time is optimal for the mothers concerned. Birthing at the commencement of the lean season – when the offspring would certainly die – would be a waste of time and energy. The restricted time window for giving birth then presupposes an earlier restricted season for fertile matings – and hence for roughly synchronised ovulations at that time.

In many cases, however, reproductive synchrony can be an effect less of environmental than of social factors. In such cases, births may show an even annual distribution for the population as a whole, yet marked synchrony within particular local groups (Dunbar 1988: 65). Among patas monkeys (Rowell 1978) and geladas (Dunbar 1980b), the cause is often the sudden appearance of a new male who takes over a harem, prompting the females to come quickly into oestrus together. Another factor may involve lactation. If a group of breast-feeding langurs (Hrdy 1977) or yellow baboons (Altmann *et al.* 1978) all wean their infants at the same time, then they will soon resume cycling together. Wallis (1985, citing Goodall 1983) notes that wild female chimpanzees at Gombe resume postpartum cycles near the end of the dry season – which corresponds to the period during which the peak number of oestrous swellings is detected. She suggests that after weaning their infants, females schedule their first oestrous swellings using cues from other females, who may not have been mothers in the recent period. This is interesting because it shows how cycling and non-cycling, pregnant and non-pregnant females can in the long run become synchronised to the same rhythm.

Macaques are seasonal breeders regardless of the habitat occupied, whilst monkeys such as langurs and howlers emphasise or minimise seasonality according to local conditions (Rudran 1973, Jones 1985). The seasonal transition from a non-reproductive to a reproductive condition can result in synchronised matings followed by a batch of synchronised births. Even in non-seasonal breeders, synchronised cycles can often be inferred by keeping a tally of births from year to year. If females tend to give birth once every two years, any synchrony between their cycles will lead to one year with very few births, one year with numerous births, the next with few again, and so on. Evidence for such year-to-year birth oscillations suggests that females in many non-seasonal species locally synchronise for social or other reasons (Dunbar 1988: 65).

Humans are even less seasonal than other primates. Yet we are certainly not immune to traces of reproductive seasonality. Finnish birth records show a peak of conceptions and of twins, triplets etc. in summer and a trough in winter (Daly and Wilson 1983: 339, citing Timonen and Carpen 1968). The higher the latitude – and hence the greater the contrast between summer and winter day lengths – the greater the effect. 'The obvious conclusion', Daly and Wilson (1983: 339) comment, 'is that light exposure has at least some influence on reproductive function in our own species'.

We may now turn from primate breeding seasonality – whose condition is only that births are restricted to within a few weeks of any year – to the stricter phase-locking effect of menstrual synchrony, which implies the synchronisation of menstrual onsets accurately to within days.

Little is known of menstrual synchrony in primates, but it seems to be rare – partly because many primates in the wild cycle only for a brief period every few years before getting pregnant again, and so fail to experience the necessary series of successive menstrual onsets. Among chimpanzees, the potential for synchrony is evidently present: an experimental study found significantly synchronised oestrus onsets among female chimpanzees caged together and spending social time with one another (Wallis 1985). But in the wild, adult female chimpanzees tend to forage in isolation, and so synchrony stemming from close association would not be expected to occur even among unmated females.

Within any group of primate females, the way their reproductive and/or menstrual cycles relate to one another may be a sensitive barometer of power relations between the animals. If one female is dominant over another and in conflict with her, a phenomenon known as 'suppression' tends to occur. Among captive marmosets, for example, when a dominant female ovulates, this itself seems to inhibit the ovulation of her female subordinates (Hrdy 1981: 44, citing Hearne). Far from the ovulation of one female attracting or helping to trigger that of companions, in other words, one female's ovulation occurs at her rival's expense.

It is not known what would happen if a subordinate female in such a relationship did begin to breed. Hrdy asks:

> Would the dominant female drive her away? Or perhaps murder the subordinate's offspring, as wild dog and chimpanzee females are known to do? In either of these events, it would behove the subordinate to defer reproduction – which, after all, is a costly and risky enterprise – until she has a territory of her own. (1981: 44)

Among savanna baboons, geladas and many other monkeys, the presence of a dominant female may induce delays in maturation, inhibition of ovulation or even spontaneous abortion by subordinates (Hrdy 1981: 99, 106). Dunbar (1988: 69) comments that even very low rates of physical aggression can induce reproductive suppression; the subordinate's *perceived* self-status within the group may be enough to produce the effect, providing it is reinforced by attacks at least occasionally. There is probably no better example of just how subtle and complex competition between females can be, Hrdy notes, than the effects of one animal upon the ovulatory cycle of another.

Menstrual Synchrony in Humans

Since the 1970s, medical science has begun to acknowledge what countless women must already have known for generations – that when women who are friends associate closely with one another, their cycles begin to synchronise. Remarkably, in contemporary western cultures, most of the male sex even today remains unaware of this potentiality, despite its being 'common knowledge' (Kiltie 1982, citing McClintock 1971, Weideger 1976) among women themselves.

The effect was first scientifically documented in 1971, in a paper in *Nature* by Martha McClintock (1971). Having noted that social grouping can influence the balance of the endocrine system, she went on:

> Menstrual synchrony is often reported by all-female living groups and by mothers, daughters and sisters who are living together. For example, the distribution of onsets of seven female lifeguards was scattered at the beginning of the summer, but after 3 months spent together the onset of all seven cycles fell within a 4 day period.

McClintock herself worked with 135 young residents of an American women's college. Each was asked to record the onset of her periods. At the start of term, new entrants were cycling on different schedules, whereas by the end of the year, friends' and roommates' onsets were occurring within a few days of one another, friendship rather than proximity being apparently the most important factor.

Comparable findings were soon confirmed (Quadagno *et al*. 1981; Skandhan *et al*. 1979; Graham and McGrew 1980). Admittedly, a study by Laura Jarett (1984) of 144 mainly Catholic subjects at two all-women colleges produced less clear-cut results: 86 women did not significantly synchronise with their roommates. But here the mean cycle length of the total sample was 35 days, probably because of the women's Catholic-regulated, relatively sex-negative, all-female environment. Studies have shown that networks of female friends who also enjoy regular intercourse with men have shorter, more regular cycles and consequently synchronise more easily than women who have female friends but are celibate (McClintock 1971; Cutler *et al*. 1979a).

In seeking to isolate the olfactory or other communicative mechanisms responsible for menstrual synchrony, one research team (Russell *et al*. 1980) took sweat from the armpits of a volunteer who had discovered that she could 'drive' a friend's cycle into correspondence with her own. Eight women were exposed nasally over four months to a solution containing this volunteer's sweat, while a control group were given a neutral solution. Those in the control showed no change, whereas four of the five women in the experimental group were soon beginning their periods within a day of the donor's.

Unfortunately, the sample used here was small. Moreover, the technician applying the sweat solutions was herself the volunteer who had produced the sweat, opening up the possibility that something else about her presence was influencing the subjects (Doty 1981). Others attempted to repeat the experiment under more rigorous conditions. Conclusive positive results were at first claimed (Preti *et al.* 1986), but the statistical treatment of the subjects' menstrual calendars was in turn devastatingly criticised (Wilson 1987), leaving our understanding in a state of some confusion. We know that menstrual synchrony occurs. The mechanisms causing it and its possible functions are not clear.

We have seen that amongst competing female primates in dominance/subordinance relationships, cycles may clash with and suppress one another rather than synchronise. This has general theoretical implications.

In discussing menstrual synchrony amongst humans, Richard Kiltie (1982), a zoologist from the University of Florida, asks us to consider the case of a group of co-wives in a polygamous household unit. Even if several of these females were close friends and synchronised, he writes, they would always be at the mercy of any female prepared to 'cheat' by ovulating and soliciting sex during her companions' non-fertile period. The 'cheat', on this analysis, would have a clear field; whenever her companions were sexually unavailable, she would be signalling her receptivity. At such times – as the only female available out of the whole harem – her chances of extended relations with the polygamous male would be unfairly high. Given the usual Darwinian genetic assumptions, it is difficult to see how evolution could avoid selecting for 'cheating' in this context. Synchrony could never establish itself.

Kiltie's (1982) view is therefore that human menstrual synchrony may be 'an evolutionary vestige' of something which had significance at some earlier stage in evolution – perhaps when hominid females bred more seasonally. Alternatively, he suggests, synchrony could be a trait that never had an adaptive effect in its own right, being merely a side-effect of some other adaptation. Certain physiological cycles of men – for example, cycles in basal body temperature and hormone levels – tend to become synchronised with the menstrual cycles of their wives (Kiltie 1982: 417, citing Doehring *et al.* 1975; Persky *et al.* 1977; Henderson 1976; Vollman 1977). When two men cohabit, their cycles also tend to synchronise (Henderson 1976).

Kiltie (1982) suggests that like such phenomena, the potentiality for menstrual synchrony is probably 'epiphenomenal', being of little adaptive significance. In support of this, he observes that hunter-gatherer women may only rarely experience a sufficient number of successive menstrual onsets for synchrony to become established, since like other mammals including non-human primates, they tend to spend most of their reproductive lives either pregnant or breast-feeding (Short 1976). Kiltie acknowledges, however, that synchrony ought to be strong within groups of closely associated adolescent females, who experience frequent anovulatory cycles and hence continuous menstrual cycles for several years following first menstruation (Nag 1962; Short 1976).

In any group of humans, normal cycle length can vary quite widely, ranging from about 21 to 40 days. This variation is confined to the preovulatory (follicular) phase; some women take scarcely a week to build up a uterine lining, while others may take up to three weeks. It is this part of the cycle which is sensitive to outside influences. Stresses and emotional disturbances can bring forward or delay ovulation to a marked degree; extreme and sustained anxiety can delay or suppress ovulation indefinitely. In contrast, the postovulatory (luteal) phase takes two weeks in almost all women. Once ovulation has occurred, in other words, menstruation is likely to occur two weeks later, whatever the emotional situation (Bailey and Marshall 1970; Presser 1974; Vollman 1977). It seems, then, that synchrony is at the most basic level not menstrual but ovulatory synchrony (McClintock 1978). This means (to anticipate) that if emotion-structuring cultural rituals were to have an effect in inducing continuous menstrual synchrony, they would have to act first and foremost upon the preovulatory phase.

Despite individual variation, repeated statistical studies consistently show that the average human female menstrual cycle length is 29.5 days (Gunn et al. 1937; McClintock 1971; Vollman 1977; Cutler et al. 1980). The average duration of pregnancy is 265.78 or 265.79 days, counting from conception to birth (Menaker and Menaker 1959). As Menaker and Menaker (1959) point out, this is nine times the menstrual cycle length (9 multiplied by 29.5 gives 265.5).

The fact that women have a 29.5-day average menstrual cycle length and a precisely ninefold gestation length suggests that generalised reproductive synchrony — a single rhythm involving all women equally, regardless of whether they are pregnant, lactating or cycling — may have been adaptive at some evolutionary stage. Not only arithmetic but astronomy seems supportive in this connection: there are unmistakable suggestions of a correspondence between human reproductive periodicity in general and the 29.5-day cycle length of the moon (see Chapters 7 and 10). No other primate shows so close a correlation between menstrual cycle length and the lunar month, nor between any whole-number multiple of the menstrual rhythm and the length of gestation.

What is certain is that human females, no less than other primates, are sensitive to time and possess within their bodies the means to schedule ovulation, conception, birth and other reproductive events quite accurately. Where it pays her to do so, the human female can to a significant degree shape the profile of her reproductive life to a pattern communicated through a variety of external cues, including those provided by neighbouring females of her own species.

Human Origins, Concealment and Synchrony

With all this in mind, we are now in a position to examine a final theory of human origins which was put forward in the 1980s. It has been left to the present chapter because it converges closely with the solution which this book will propose.

Paul Turke (1984) 'Effects of ovulatory concealment and synchrony on protohominid mating systems and parental roles.'

Turke is a sociobiologist at the University of Michigan, and has collaborated with Kim Hill and others in extending sociobiological methodologies into the traditional terrain of social anthropology (Betzig *et al.* 1988).

In working towards a new synthesis, Turke draws on the findings of Hrdy, Lovejoy, Hill and others (Chapter 5). His starting point is the observation that human males provide far greater provisioning services for their mates than do other primate males. He assumes that early females must have played a role in establishing this situation, and sets out to investigate how they did it. By what means, in other words, did evolving human females succeed in making males 'earn their keep'?

In proposing an answer, Turke sets out to explain the following features of human female reproductive physiology:

(a)   concealed ovulation
(b)   continuous but discriminating sexual receptivity
(c)   the potentiality for menstrual synchrony.

The author takes it that 'the earliest protohominids' (wisely, no dates are suggested) lived in chimpanzee-like multi-male troops, the females advertising ovulation and receptivity with conspicuous swellings. The females did not synchronise their cycles. Sex relations were promiscuous, with perhaps occasional temporarily exclusive consortships. General promiscuity meant that males had low confidence in paternity, and did not invest much in their offspring.

This situation began to change in a human-like direction as scrub and grasslands encroached on these creatures' former forest habitat. Increasingly, predators posed a danger, individuals sought safety in numbers, groups became large, competition between neighbouring groups intensified and foraging strategies became more complex.

It will be remembered from Chapter 4 that in this situation, Dunbar (1988) envisages the formation of female coalitions, these becoming the stable core of early hominid social groups as they moved into open terrain. This suggestion dovetails closely with Turke's model, which assumes that adult reproductively active females – those who were not already pregnant or breast-feeding – became sufficiently close to one another for their cycles to begin to synchronise.

Turke assumes increased infant dependency, slower maturation and substantially increased burdens on mothers. In this context, he asks: How did females compel males to provide more child-care help? His answer is that females began to extend their oestrus signals, so that the signals from one female would be more likely to overlap with those of her sisters. They simultaneously dampened down the gaudiness of their signals, reducing the distinction in appearance between one part of the cycle and the rest. Finally, they began to synchronise their ovulatory cycles within each local unit.

In explaining how all this would have strengthened females in their efforts to secure extra help from males, Turke asks us to imagine two young females who have just begun cycling. Slight genetic variation has rendered the oestrus signals of one more dampened and more extended than those of her companion.

During each period of receptivity, Turke points out, the more gaudily displaying female should attract the more high-ranking male (dominant males, under the old system, monopolise the females most obviously ovulating). The more modest female should obtain a more lowly male partner. However, he would be more likely than others to give his mate his continuous time. This would be partly because his lower status would restrict his mating opportunities elsewhere, partly because the longer duration of his partner's receptive period would force him to stay with her longer – and partly because she herself would be less likely to entice high-ranking males to come in and disrupt their togetherness. As a result, the lowly male would have a higher than average confidence of paternity in any resulting offspring, making it particularly worth his while, genetically, to invest his parental care in them.

Turke proceeds to ask what would happen if this modest female also began tracking her more provocative sister's hormonal status, synchronising her periods of ovulation with hers. Using modern human females as a reference, he suggests that a statistically significant degree of synchrony would exist after four cycles, the process of convergence beginning after just one cycle. Suppose that at the start of the process, one female ovulated when the other was menstruating. This would mean that the lowly male became threatened at precisely the moment his partner was ovulating, for the other female in the system would be in a relatively unattractive condition, tempting 'her' male to look elsewhere for a mating opportunity. Now suppose that the two females began to synchronise, their moments of ovulation converging more and more closely. As synchrony developed with each cycle, Turke argues, the modest female's male partner would find the sexual competition at the moment of ovulation less intense. This would be simply because at the crucial moment, each female, simultaneously with her female companion, would draw to herself a male who might otherwise be on the lookout for a mating opportunity elsewhere. Each male's prospects of mating with 'the other' female at the moment of ovulation would by the same token be reduced (Turke 1984, citing Knowlton 1979).

Turke (1984) suggests that female hamadryas baboons, who synchronise markedly within local units, exemplify this logic to a certain extent. They in effect co-operate in order to prevent harem owners from monopolising more than about two females per harem. It is as if monogamy were a desirable ideal, but that having only one other female in one's harem were the next best thing. Synchrony in this context helps keep the alpha male under some control. Predictably, Turke notes, hamadryas dominant males rarely attempt to philander with intratroop females, harems are stable and uniformly small, and the protection and care males afford to their mates and mates' offspring is substantial and well documented. In other words, Turke sees hamadryas baboons as taking some steps along the road hypothetically travelled by female protohominids in the course of becoming human.

Turke's conclusion is that it would be in the interests of any overburdened protohuman female to gain a male for herself and extract maximum help from him by synchronising as far as possible with her female companions. If females did this, then the old male strategy of competing to maximise the number of females inseminated would be thwarted, while higher than average confidence of paternity would add to the rewards of male investment in existing offspring (Turke 1984; Knowlton 1979). If the environmental/ ecological conditions envisaged — movement into open territory, greater predation danger and so on — were intensifying group life and putting a premium on parental care, then the result should be a spread of ovulatory synchrony and concealment through the population (Turke 1984: 36).

Although evolution towards one-to-one relatively stable coupling is envisaged, Turke's model differs from Lovejoy's in that females are closely associated with one another and act together in constraining their male partners to behave appropriately. Turke sees this as involving a reversal of hominid female sexual preferences: females who synchronise begin to seek out lower-ranking males. They bring previously excluded males into the system, where they become of value in assisting with child-care and provisioning. This implies a political process is which the status of dominant polygamous males is subverted in favour of previously lower-ranking males more likely to meet changing female requirements.

We can now fit the jigsaw-piece supplied by Turke alongside a complementary item encountered early on in this chapter. We noted then that if a large group of females are condemned to share only one male between them, then they should lessen the costs of competition by avoiding one another's sexual space. They should sharply demarcate their time into clearly segmented portions, using unmistakable but brief oestrus signals for this purpose. Then each female could carefully avoid impinging on the sexual time of her sisters, each one's ovulation perhaps suppressing that of her sisters. Maximised asynchrony would of course be the result. Turke's argument represents the opposite side of the coin: if the females in a harem can break out and gain access to a male each, then they should logically lessen internal competition and tie their mates more continuously to themselves precisely by blurring all cyclical distinctions to the maximum possible extent, whilst simultaneously synchronising with one another. Such female oneness across time and space would confront philandering males with an all-or-nothing choice, preventing them from picking and choosing between different females or between the fertile and infertile moments of any one female.

It is worth adding that human females' permanently enlarged breasts – unlike the small, wrinkled ones of chimpanzees which enlarge only specifically for lactation – can perhaps be regarded as adaptive in the same context. Human breasts develop at an early stage in a young woman's life, often long before she actually begins lactating. Thereafter they remain full-looking at all times – giving little clue as to real reproductive status. They are therefore in a sense 'egalitarian'. They help to make pregnant, lactating and cycling females all seem equally maternal, or alternatively, equally sexually inviting. They would therefore have helped females to maintain synchrony in the emission of sexual signals.

In fact, enlarged breasts can be regarded as sending out a 'no' signal, at least on one level. Enlarged breasts mimic lactation. To that extent, the signal emitted is that the female concerned is anovulatory. Yet in humans – and humans alone – this signal (like ovulation concealment) has become confusing and deceptive. With her large breasts, a female who is really fertile in effect signals *as if she were breast-feeding and therefore unlikely to conceive*. A primate or protohuman male interested only in achieving immediate fertilisation ought to be discouraged by this (although, of course, a male with a longer-term parental interest in supporting this particular female and her offspring need not be). The ability to emit precisely such a highly selective 'no' signal would be very much in the interests of females who needed to persuade certain types of males to leave them sexually alone (Ffitch 1987). And the pattern would fit in neatly with Turke's ovarian synchrony model. Like ovulation concealment and ovarian synchrony, in other words, lactation-mimicking breast enlargement can be understood as an adaptation through which females prevent males from picking and choosing between them on a short-term basis in accordance with varying prospects for fertile intercourse. Although there are probably additional reasons for breast enlargement in non-lactating human females, possibly involving the storage of body fat, this extension of Turke's model may help us to understand what has long been regarded as an extremely puzzling problem (Caro 1987).

Turke's theory rests on no palaeontological or other direct evidence for reproductive synchrony in hominid evolution. The hypothesis is not buttressed with findings from archaeology or from the study of contemporary hunter-gatherers. The various archaeologically testable staples of other theories of human origins – hunting, tool use, the home base, a sexual division of labour – are not mentioned. Synchrony is inferred, rather, on purely theoretical grounds, drawing on studies of (a) shrimps (Knowlton

1979), (b) non-human primates and (c) women in contemporary western college dormitories.

The value of Turke's model is, however, that it introduces a new concept. Alone among the models discussed so far, it implies a form of inter-female solidarity ('reciprocal altruism' to use the sociobiological term) as a factor contributing to evolution in a human-like direction. We can now see that females who blur/extend their signals competitively (the chimp pattern), or who sharpen signal definition and restrict receptivity to avoid harassment (geladas), are evolving in wholly non-human directions. To this we might add that those whose monogamy is premised on the complete spatial isolation of females from one another – the gibbon pattern – are if anything still further removed from the evolving human norm. The human revolution was pioneered by females who combined pair-bonding with intensified gender solidarity, so that sexual attachments were not at the expense of wider forms of connectedness. The influx of males, extended receptivity, the added time available for love-making and the consequent reduced competition meant that associated females could develop relations of sisterly trust, achieving harmony not through sexual self-restriction or mutual avoidance but through reciprocally upholding one another's sexual success.

In Turke's model, females do not exactly go on 'sex strike' together. But ovulation concealment implies the same logic at a deeper level. What is collectively withdrawn from males is not sex as such, but knowledge of which female is ovulating when. Females use synchrony to provide leverage against dominant polygamous males, involving all available males in providing parental care. By not competing against one another in emitting sexual 'yes' signals, females in each group are in effect refraining from undercutting one another in sexual competition for each other's males. We might at this point adapt Marxist terminology and view the females as expressing a form of 'class solidarity' (although of course 'gender solidarity' is the correct term). Each female is asserting her own reproductive interests, but she is doing so in ways which simultaneously serve the interests of her sisters.

Conclusion: Synchrony and Revolution

If evolving human females at a crucial stage synchronised their cycles in the manner Turke supposes, this must have been within the context of powerful inter-female coalitions, the conditions of which were touched on in Chapter 4.

Robin Dunbar's (1988: 319–20) view is that as the ancestral hominids emerged from their former forest environment into more open territory, the females would have tended to cluster together in larger groups, seeking safety in numbers. Within the female groups, coalitions would have been formed, as subordinate females suffering from harassment attempted to find allies. At first glance, as Dunbar points out, it might seem that all this could have enabled dominant males to monopolise quite large groups of females.

But for all species in which harems occur, there is a limit to the harem size a male can manage. In large harems, rebellions tend to break out, the most subordinate females becoming dissatisfied first. 'As harem size increases', in Dunbar's words, 'more and more of the females begin to suffer from reproductive suppression and are consequently more willing to desert their harem male' (1988: 167).

It is not just the number of females in any harem that matters, Dunbar notes, but their cyclical state. A male might be able to manage, say, five females – provided never more than two came into oestrus at any one time. Should all five start displaying their receptivity together, their demands would swamp him and he would risk losing them to rival males. In this context there is always a threshold number of *receptive* harem females beyond which an alpha male will be unable to cope. As Dunbar puts it: 'Once the probability of co-cycling females rises above this critical threshold, the harem-holder will be unable to prevent other males entering his group and mating with his females' (1988: 141). So by synchronising, the females in a harem could theoretically organise a 'revolution', enticing in new males and thereby propelling themselves into a different social order – a different mating system – for a while.

Among various primates, such revolutions have actually been observed. In the case of two well-studied groups of redtail monkeys and blue monkeys, for example, 'there were rare occasions when up to six females were cycling together. During these periods, the harem-holder was unable to prevent other males from joining the group and mating with the females.' Once the females had ceased cycling, however, the extra males left the group, which reverted once more to being a conventional one-male harem (Dunbar 1988: 141, citing Cords 1984, Tsingalia and Rowell 1984). It is therefore no surprise to find that among primates generally, multi-male groups tend to be found where reproductive synchrony is high – for example, where there is a short breeding season each year – whereas one-male units tend to occur in year-round intermittent breeders (Ridley 1986).

In this light, we can discern two strategic options open to females in a harem system which they experience as restrictive. One is to accept the system. This may be the best course if ecological constraints make attachment to a single polygamous male an optimal solution to problems of foraging, communal defence and so on within the environment. If there is no long-term viable way of breaking out or of bringing other males in, then the dominant male's position is secure, in which case inter-female competition for his favours or services is imposed on all inescapably. In that event, Kiltie's (1982) arguments against the possibility of establishing synchrony would apply. To synchronise would be misguided, since even if a few co-operative females managed to entrain their cycles, any female wishing to get ahead in life would simply cheat, ovulating out of step so an to gain as unfair advantage over her companions.

The alternative, which certain ecological conditions might favour, would be to resist the whole system and change it – either by setting a lower limit on harem size, or by making even the smallest kind of harem ungovernable. The latter solution, of course, is the more radical. If the harem-holder is frail or vulnerable, and if previously excluded males can be reached at his expense, then dissatisfied females might synchronise as part of a break-out plan, the aim being to link up with previously marginalised males. In that event, the 'cheat' could be simply outflanked – left to get on with seeking favours from the once-dominant male whilst everyone else ignored him and broke away to liaise with other males at the peak moment of synchronised ovulation. Dunbar (1988: 148) points out that it would probably be the more sub-ordinate females – those suffering most from reproductive suppression – who would have the greatest interest in subverting any system based on single-male monopolies. It is they who would be most inclined to incite outsider males to come in and form liaisons with them, synchronising with coalition allies in order to do so. 'Even if only some females synchronise their cycles', Dunbar comments, 'they may be able to attract enough males into the group to meet their needs'.

Where homind evolution is concerned, we have no direct evidence that a link-up between oppressed females and previously excluded males along the lines suggested by Paul Turke occurred, nor that female ovarian synchrony played a part in achieving this. Nonetheless, on purely theoretical grounds, we may begin to detect quite a revolutionary potential in such synchrony – this biological capacity which human females nowadays possess, and which they have doubtless possessed throughout the span of hominid evolution.

At the very least, taking synchrony into account extends our under-standing by widening our view of the possibilities available to evolving female hominids. Whether synchrony occurred in the period referred to by Turke, we do not know. What we do know is that to the extent that it did occur within any population at any time, it would have tended to subvert male attempts to monopolise large harems of females. Dominant males, on this analysis, would have maintained their power only where they could operate a policy of 'divide and rule'. Where their cycles were randomised, females could be dealt with one by one and thereby managed and controlled. Synchrony, by contrast, would have been a manifestation of inter-female solidarity; its achievement would have granted females a special kind of power, enabling them to escape being privatised by dominant males either monogamously or in harems.

Chapter 7
The Shores of Eden

The jealousy of the male, representing both tie and limits of the family, brings the animal family into conflict with the horde. The horde, the higher social form, is rendered impossible here, loosened there, or dissolved altogether during the mating season; at best, its continued development is hindered by the jealousy of the male. . . . Mutual toleration among the adult males, freedom from jealousy, was, however, the first condition for the building of those large and enduring groups in the midst of which alone the transition from animal to man could be achieved.

Friedrich Engels, *The Origin of the Family,*
Private Property and the State (1884)

Paul Turke's ovarian synchrony model not only helps explain the human menstrual cycle. It also sheds unexpected light on some central problems of human biosocial and cultural origins. It enables us to appreciate that the final, culture-inaugurating phase of the human revolution – the phase during which the male sex was at last forced to abandoned its former sexual competitiveness and assist females in accordance with new, solidarity-based rules – was in a profound sense 'nothing new'. Underlying it was a logic of intensifying sexual synchrony and control which had roots deep in the past, when the basic features of modern human anatomy and physiology were being determined.

Synchrony and the Fossil Record

Early hominid fossils are found from end to end of the East African Rift Valley – an immense geological system of volcanic mountain ranges, valleys and interconnected estuaries, rivers and lakes stretching from the Gulf of Aden almost to the southern Cape. Such fossils are found in no other part of the world. A possible implication of Turke's model would be that conditions unique to the Rift Valley enabled females to synchronise on a scale not possible in other locations. This in turn would lead us to ask what these special conditions may have been.

We can at once eliminate Paul Turke's own suggestion – that ovulatory synchrony became established when a forest-dwelling ape for the first time began moving out into open savanna territory. This scenario is now as outdated as others which locate the decisive events leading to a modern lifestyle as far back as in the Pliocene or early Pleistocene (Chapter 5). Even if survival in the savanna were possible at such early times, dense aggregations (such as those of baboons) would not have been. Whilst many savanna-dwelling primates can eat virtually anything, human digestive systems are highly selective (Milton 1984; Stahl 1984). To a chimpanzee-brained, ape-like creature whose hunting capabilities were relatively undeveloped or associated basically with males, movement into semi-arid savanna would have meant entering a vegetationally impoverished habitat, incapable of facilitating synchrony through sustaining large groups of females all foraging in the same vicinity. Even the idea that more meat would have been available in the savanna is mistaken. The most recent primate evidence totally undermines the assumption of any necessary connection between movement into open savanna and the beginnings of co-operative hunting. Contrary to the preconceptions of the savanna theorists, it has been demonstrated that dense rain-forest-dwelling chimpanzees (such as those in the Taï National Park in the Ivory Coast) eat much more meat and hunt much more co-operatively than do their savanna-woodland or savanna-dwelling counterparts. It is the rain-forest chimps who are most likely to plan their hunts in advance and set out seeking for prey, organising an elaborate ambush, instead of just chasing an animal when one happens to be encountered (Boesch and Boesch 1989; Boesch 1990).

Robert Blumenschine (1987) has become known for his careful observations on predation and the fate of carcasses in the present-day Serengeti. His conclusion is that if early hominids were in part scavengers – as most analysts now assume – they could not have been savanna-dwellers. The open savanna would have been well populated with hyenas. These superbly equipped animals would easily have out-competed hominids within any scavenging niche. On the other hand, hyenas tend to avoid the dense woodlands which surround rivers and freshwater lakes, despite the fact that carcasses may be abundant in such places. Feline predators make overnight kills of zebras and adult wildebeest close to the waterfronts, leaving plenty of marrow-rich bones and other high-quality foods along the wooded shores. Leopards have a habit of storing their partially eaten kills – usually gazelles and other small ungulates – high in trees, and hominids would have climbed up to steal these (Cavallo and Blumenschine 1989). For Blumenschine, in short, 'riparian woodlands' – a habitat of trees bordering lakes, rivers and estuaries – are the most likely dry-season setting in which scavenging early hominids could have survived.

In the case of all evolving hominids, ovarian synchrony, where it existed at all, must have depended on the ability to maintain area-intensive foraging patterns. Females could only associate closely with one another where there was enough food to sustain their togetherness within each small patch of temporarily occupied territory. The moment the climate cooled, turned dry or for some other reason reduced the primary productivity of the local terrain, more space would have been required per foraging individual. Under these conditions, group life of any kind – and with it, synchrony – would have become more difficult to sustain. If we concur with Turke that the precursors of the hominids must have been forest-dwellers, and that their divergence from the apes was based on a move into some other habitat, then the synchrony scenario means that an alternative to open or semi-arid savanna must be found.

Turke's model would lead us to link variation in consistency of ovulatory synchrony with key aspects of hominid evolutionary diversity. We cannot know whether any single population of fossil hominids was synchronising in accordance with Turke's model. But given the lack of evidence for sub-stantially delayed maturation, neoteny or encephalisation in the Pliocene, it seems unlikely that his model can be applied to the early stages of evolution which he himself envisages.

Over the period of hominid evolution as a whole, the presence or absence of synchrony between co-resident females would doubtless have been uneven. Females in some localities would have synchronised weakly or not at all, while in other areas they phase-locked more consistently. Opportunities for female gender solidarity and synchrony would have been influenced by local resources and associated patterns of foraging – in other words, by ecologically determined patterns of female aggregation or dispersal. If synchrony were a condition of long-term genetic approximation towards anatomical moder-nity, this variable pattern would in turn have meant that while certain hominids were evolving in 'modern' directions, others were adapting in divergent ways. In any event, we can reject the notion that Plio-Pleistocene hominids were under any obligation to advance unilineally towards moder-nity. Each of the various different species and sub-species was following its own trajectory, most of which led in directions rather different from the road which we can retrospectively trace as leading to ourselves (Foley 1987, 1988).

Turke's model would imply, then, not that all females behaved in the same way; only that those which synchronised best were the ones to evolve in the most anatomically modern directions. The most consistent synchronisers would have secured the most male support, and in this context would have been the most effective mothers. The added support would have enabled mothers to become more slow-moving, more attached to sheltered, well-watered spots or to camp-fires affording warmth – and consequently more able to prioritise child care. Relatively premature babies would have survived better, leading to increased neoteny and hence the possibility of larger brains (Turke 1984).

At the opposite extreme, on Turke's logic, failure to synchronise would have been associated with higher levels of sexual conflict, philandering, monopolisation by alpha males – and the exclusion of subordinate males from the breeding system. The adaptive pressures of mating systems of this kind tend to select for physical fighting capacities in males – 'brawn' rather than 'brain'. One result is high levels of sexual dimorphism. Another is minimised male involvement in parenting. In this light, the model might attribute some of the less gracile or less human-like products of evolution (for example, the robust australopithecines, or some of the more robust and/or dimorphic species of *Homo*) with the probability that as radiating hominids colonised what were by previous standards impoverished or arid areas, female ovarian synchrony became difficult to maintain. Groups of foraging, largely self-sufficient females would have had to space themselves out in the search for food – perhaps in small 'family'-type groups which aggregated only infrequently if at all. The possibilities for widespread female gender solidarity would therefore have been weak or non-existent, and in most situations this may have allowed males to monopolise individuals or small groups, setting up boundaries dividing one breeding unit from another. It is tempting to speculate that in the more barren or more marginal environments occupied by *Homo erectus* or archaic *Homo sapiens*, patterns of this kind became established. Such developments would in turn have set up locally specific selection pressures driving hominid evolution in non-modern directions.

According to Richard Wrangham (1987: 68), the common ancestor of apes and hominids had hostile, male-dominated intergroup relations, polygamy, and a social system which allowed for few alliance bonds between females. In the view of Robert Foley (1987: 171), this situation did not change fundamentally even when the hominid/ape evolutionary divergence occurred. Foley argues that 'the early hominids possessed a social organisation not dissimilar to that of other terrestrial primates – large group size and competition between males for access to females'. He suggests (p. 172) that like geladas and other baboons, 'early hominids may have had a single-male, polygynous reproductive system'. *Australopithecus afarensis* does seem to have been heavily sexually dimorphic, the males having rather large canines (Johanson and White 1979), and it is generally true that a high level of dimorphism tends to correlate with a harem system, or at least with strong sexual competition between males. More controversially, however, Foley (1988: 219) extends his model into the Late Pleistocene, arguing that humans during the last ice age practised 'a harem system of polygynous mating' or, in any event, 'a system of patrilineal control and organisation of females'. It is, of course, a view diametrically at variance with that advocated here.

It is true that a move into open territory – at least among many primates – can lead to the setting up of one-male dominated 'harems'. However, we have also noted an apparent incompatibility between such mating systems and the evolution of large brains. This would make a harem model perhaps consistent with the cranial anatomy of *Australopithecus afarensis*, but certainly quite inconsistent with that of evolving *Homo*. It would seem that any kind of harem monopolisation would have been particularly incompatible with the evolution of large brains under seasonal or other conditions of climatic stress. Any fall in the primary productivity of the local terrain would have added to child-burdened females' need for foraging assistance from mobile males – at the very moment when these same factors were excluding many of these males from the breeding system. As a result, selection pressures would have acted against mothers who produced slow-maturing, ultra-dependent, large-brained offspring. Endlessly moving, autonomously foraging, hard-pressed mothers would have been under pressure to produce smaller-brained babies – precocious survivors with plenty of stamina and brawn. If with the hominid digestive system it was impossible to survive in the harsher areas without immense intelligence and hence large brains, the result would have been extinction or retreat into richer habitats.

In fact, we know that in all periods prior to the Middle and Later Pleistocene, hominids were restricted to relatively resource-rich and predictable ecosystems. *Homo erectus* tested and in places extended the limits of such constraints, but did not transcend them. The ecosystems exploited by the hand-axe makers of Africa and Eurasia were quite diverse – grassland or woodland savanna, the steppe, montane grasslands and the sea coast, among others. But they avoided cold regions with seasonally sparse vegetational cover or resources. Even the Neanderthals were forced to retreat from severe cold, remaining restricted within ecological zones able to sustain their relatively area-intensive foraging patterns. It was only symbolic culture-bearing, anatomically modern humans who eventually broke through all such constraints (Gamble 1986a; Shea 1989; Whallon 1989).

We have noted Foley's one-male harem model of early hominid sociality. Foley himself would concede, however, that his attempts to reconstruct early mating systems are speculative. In particular, he makes no attempt to reconcile his theory with the seemingly incompatible findings of Alexander and Noonan (1979), Paul Turke (1984) and others who have taken into account the unique features of the human female reproductive cycle. Perhaps the most we can be certain of is that like contemporary primates if not more so (Dunbar 1988), *Australopithecus* and *Homo* would have been quite flexible, setting up one kind of mating system under some conditions, other kinds under others. Paul Turke's model does not help us here – it is not concerned with the fossil evidence – but his argument would lead us to suppose that

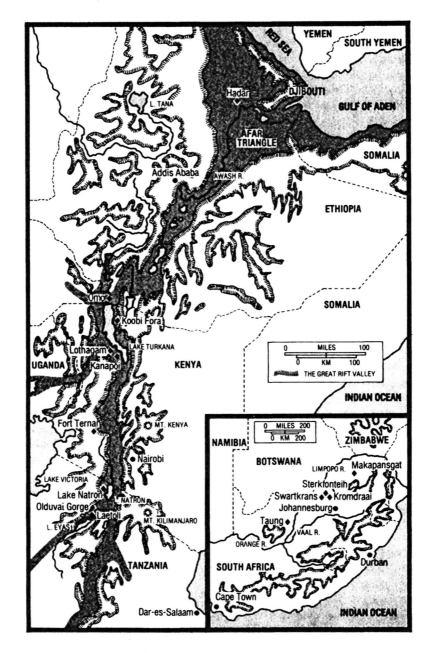

Figure 4 The East African Rift Valley. Today, its floor – shaded in this map – has for the most part dried out, leaving a landscape of bush and dry grassland, although a string of lakes remains. Between 3.5 and 2.5 million years ago, the shaded areas were wetter and in many places flooded, with swamps and dense woodlands bordering the numerous lakes and rivers (map after Johanson and Edey 1981: 13).

where ecological conditions enabled females to synchronise as a means of compelling males to intensify provisioning, larger brains, reduced sexual dimorphism and a more human-like reproductive physiology would have evolved. The interesting question is to ask what these synchrony-favouring ecological conditions might have been.

Synchrony and Subsistence

We may suspect that there must have been something rather special about the East African Rift Valley 'savanna-mosaic' ecosystem of woodlands, grasslands, lakes, estuaries, sea-inlets, islands and rivers in which the earliest hominid fossils have been found (figure 4). Whilst it is possible that this is only an impression created by depositional bias – rivers and lake-shore settings are far better than others in helping to ensure that organic remains fossilise and are preserved – it now seems likely that early hominids really were restricted to roughly this region. Above all, early stone tools, which need no such special conditions in order to be conserved, seem on present evidence to replicate much the same distribution pattern as the fossilised bones. It has been pointed out (Blumenschine 1987: 393) that all known East African Plio/Pleistocene hominid *activity* sites are located in or along ephemeral or perennial watercourses and/or lake shores. These sites would have been in riparian woodlands denser than the tree/bush cover which is found further away from water sources.

Throughout their evolution, hominids seem to have been exceptionally water-dependent primates. The early Oldowan hominids have been labelled 'The People of the Lake' (Leakey and Lewin 1979). What little we know of the function of the battered 'hammers' found from the early levels of Olduvai Gorge seems to indicate that they were used for pounding up *aquatic tuberous plants*; phytoliths (the silicified remains of such tubers) have actually been found on the hammers (Binford 1989: 27, citing Isaac pers. comm. 1985). In reporting this finding, Binford adds that the frequencies of these tools 'seem to vary with the presence in the environment of this type of plant, and they are found in the spots where the plants occurred'.

Wymer (1982: 125) comments that throughout human evolution in the Pleistocene, including in Europe and Asia, 'there was a definite preference for rivers and lakes'. Evolving *Homo*'s association with water seems to have lasted right up until the appearance of anatomically modern forms. Among the earliest-known fossils of anatomically modern humans from anywhere in the world are those from Klasies River Mouth Cave on the southern coast of South Africa. These large-brained hominids, who were on the very threshold of establishing culture in its modern, symbolic form, were feeding on a rich diet which included an abundance of sea foods (Wymer 1982: 157; Binford 1984: 19–20). This would have meant high productivity as well as an easy accessibility of foods, potentially leading to that 'mobile sedentism' discussed earlier as a precondition of synchrony. Seals, it should be pointed out, would have provided a wonderful source of very rich, portable food including valuable fats. Clumsy and defenceless on land, they can be picked up and killed with tools as crude as stones or sticks when colonies are assembled on small islands, rocks or reefs along the coast (Lanata 1990).

The most primitive known hominid fossils are those of *Australopithecus afarensis* – 'Lucy' as her most famous representative is known (Johanson and Edey 1981). These fossils come from the East African Rift Valley's northerly end – in particular from the floodplain of an immense, now largely desiccated estuarine region known as the Afar Triangle, stretching between the Gulf of Aden and the lower end of the Red Sea.

The lower-lying areas of this geologically unstable region were partly flooded during the early Pliocene, although rising out of the sea in the Afar Triangle at the northern end would have been a large island – now the Danakil Alps (LaLumiere 1982 [1981]). Adjacent to this island at its northeast end, the Danakil Depression – which was first invaded by marine waters about 6.7 million years ago – only became finally desiccated about 30,000 years ago (LaLumiere 1982 [1981]: 128–32).

If any apes had lived in this initially forested but periodically flooded riverine and estuarine region between the Miocene and Early Pleistocene, we would expect selection pressures to have favoured a creature who could not only climb trees, but also on occasion walk bipedally, swim when it occasionally fell into the water and, when necessary, wade waist-high in search of food, holding the head above water. In other words, whilst there may be little or no real evidence to support the more exuberant, early versions of the 'aquatic hypothesis', according to which unknown Miocene hominids were living an almost dolphin-like or seal-like existence in the sea (Hardy 1960; Morgan 1972), it seems reasonable to suppose that the earliest hominids actually known from the fossil record were well adapted to the wetland, riverine and shoreline environments in which their remains have in fact been found. If despite the attractions lakes, rivers and marine shores evidently held for these hominids, they could not swim – then we would want to know why! It is surely the savanna theorists' idea that our ancestors *could not swim* which is the intrinsically improbable hypothesis that needs to be questioned and tested most sceptically, not the more likely view that, as in our own case, swimming was one of the things that these creatures could do.

In this respect, *Australopithecus afarensis* causes no apparent problems. Lucy – being a female in this sexually dimorphic species – was rather diminutive, with a small, chimpanzee-like brain, straight spine, relatively long arms, a mobile ankle, curved toes and ape-like toe joints. Her feet were broader and larger than those of modern humans – 35 per cent of leg length instead of 26 per cent – giving her a gait described by Roger Lewin (quoted in Morgan 1990: 34) as 'not quite as bad as trying to walk on dry land wearing swimming flippers, but in the same direction'. These features argue against a savanna-dwelling habitual biped, suggesting instead something of an all-round gymnast – a walker who still spent much of her time climbing in trees (Stern and Susman 1983; Susman *et al.* 1984; Susman 1987). Assuming that she could also swim (Morgan 1986, 1990; Verhaegen 1985), her repertoire would be a suite of activities requiring retention of many of the characteristics of brachiators, including the position of the *foramen magnum* (indicating the angle of the head) and a pelvic connection allowing the legs and trunk to form a straight line.

Fossil remains of early hominids along the Rift Valley are found in water-deposited sediments associated with the valley's many ancient lakes, rivers and swamps. The bones and stone tools occur in association with bovids (frequent visitors to waterholes and lake shores), pigs (which root for their food in swamps) and also aquatic species such as fish, turtles, snakes and crocodiles (Potts 1988 and references). When pieced together, the evidence as a whole suggests adaptation to a mixed waterside ecology of foraging and scavenging (Blumenschine 1987) quite different from the 'burning savanna' scenarios of popular writers such as Robert Ardrey in the 1960s.

Despite this, authoritative textbooks still repeatedly use such phrases as 'the hot and arid low-lying floor of the Rift Valley' (Wymer 1982: 63) when discussing the background to hominid evolution. Even so well-informed an evolutionary ecologist as Robert Foley (1987: 189) uses the term 'semi-arid savanna' to describe what he terms 'the particular environment in which the fossil hominids seem to have lived'. Such formulations appear to owe more to the weight of disciplinary tradition than to the data as such.

Palaeoenvironmental reconstructions are notoriously controversial and subject to change almost from year to year. But in terms merely of the sources and conclusions drawn on by Foley himself, the evidence does little to support his model. The site of Tabarin, according to Foley (1987: 195, table 8.1), was a lake margin. The Middle Awash provided 'fluvial condi-tions'. The site of Hadar, home of 'Lucy', was a lake and associated floodplain, with 'braided streams and rivers'. Omo was a region of dry-thorn savanna 'flanking river banks with gallery forest and swamps'. Koobi Fora was a freshwater lake with floodplains, gallery forest and dry-thorn savanna. Peninj consisted of open grassland surrounding a salt lake, fed by fresh rivers.

Admittedly, in all these localities the climate was subject to pronounced seasonal variation, with many rivers and waterholes becoming desiccated during the driest months – but this only adds to our understanding of the factors compelling early hominids to keep close to the more permanently watered lakes, estuaries and tree-shaded shorelines. In fact, of ten early hominid-occupied Rift Valley habitats listed by Foley (1987: table 8.1), only the reconstruction for Laetoli would seem dry enough to qualify straight-

forwardly as 'grassland savanna'. Although the evidence is as yet uncertain, it
may turn out that this and similar dry and/or elevated areas were occupied by
hominids only during the rainier parts of each year. Should this possibility be
established, it would confirm our picture of an extremely water-dependent
animal.

Olduvai Gorge, in the middle of the Serengeti Plain, is the best-known
site. At its centre, about 1.9 million years ago, was a perennial, saline lake
about 22 km across. All around were the lake's floodplains, traversed by
freshwater seasonal streams and rivers. Fossil pollen, microfauna, geochem-
istry and bovids from the oldest horizons in Bed I indicate a moist lakeside
environment with about 1,000 mm of rainfall per year, closed-canopy
vegetation, and isolated patches of grassland and marsh (Potts 1988: 193).
Papyrus and other shore grasses were plentiful, and the remains of birds
include abundant grebes, cormorants, pelicans, ducks, gulls, terns and
wading birds such as flamingos, herons and stalks (Potts 1988: 22). This was
a semi-aquatic, mixed-waterside environment if ever there was one. We
might indeed suspect it of having been so boggy and prone to flooding as to
be best avoided during the rainy months.

It is true that on rare occasions, Developed Oldowan tools have been
found on high plateaus above the Rift Valley proper, a good example being a
string of sites along the Plain of Gadeb, Ethiopia, where an immense lake
existed in Late Tertiary times (Wymer 1982: 63). But again, the lake-shore
setting is significant – the tools were found in its sediments – and there is no
evidence that this habitat was in any sense arid. In fact, over East Africa as a
whole, it seems certain that where dry-savanna regions, high plateaus or
mountain slopes were occupied at all, this testifies not to a preference for
semi-aridity but to the mobility and adaptability of early hominids – their
ability to move from excessively flooded regions during the rainier months
when water was everywhere, returning to lower-lying regions as desiccation
increased. Even an ape who could wade and swim could be drowned in a
sudden flood – and in any event would not want to be wet all the time!

In the Transvaal region, which is also outside the Rift Valley proper, it
may be more appropriate to speak of 'savanna environments', but here, too,
the term 'mosaic' must qualify this (Foley 1987: 196). The valley of the Vaal
River is wide and gently sloping. Gravels in the riverbanks are remnants of
former, higher courses, and it is in the oldest of these that early chopper-core
tools have been found (Wymer 1982: 72–3). If any these sites was really in
open savanna territory, it was certainly not 'semi-arid'. 'Most of the South
African sites', as Foley (1987: 196) himself comments having examined the
details, 'seem to be at the wetter end of the environmental spectrum'.

Such associations are neither fortuitous, nor a product only of depositional
bias. Not a single excavated Plio-Pleistocene site anywhere in Africa supports
the view that semi-arid savanna was remotely favoured by the earlier
hominids. We have noted that Oldowan stone tools have been found to be

distributed in essentially the same ecozonal patterns as fossilised bones — a fact which helps rule out the possible objection that we are mistakenly inferring waterside environments only because fossilisation is favoured by such conditions. In short, it is clear that early hominid subsistence activities were in some necessary way linked to well-watered, well-wooded, highly variegated habitats such as the Rift Valley to an unusual extent provided.

Extremely fertile, volcanically enriched soil and hence abundant vegetation was no doubt one factor which made the Rift Valley such a uniquely favourable spot in which hominids could evolve. The availability of rivers, streams, springs and hence perennially available water was another. 'Man is the most dependent on thermal sweating among the mammals thus far investigated', it has been observed (Newman 1970: 379), 'and may well be the most dependent on a continuing source of water. . . '. Whilst culturally organised modern hunter-gatherers can often survive for many months in seemingly waterless regions such as the Kalahari Desert, obtaining their water supplies from melons, the insides of game animals and similar sources, for pre-cultural hominids such capacities would have been inconceivable.

In the hot, seasonally rainless region which was Plio-Pleistocene East Africa, uninterrupted proximity to water was for evolving hominids an absolute necessity (Foley 1987: 106–7). Humans shed mineral-rich body salts in addition to precious water through their profuse sweating, and must drink copiously for this reason as well as because human urine is dilute and little water can be stored in the body (Verhaegen 1985). None of these features suggests a savanna adaptation. In fact, the precise salt/water composition of human urine (a quite different mix from that of dry savanna- or desert-dwellers, whose water-conserving urine is sticky and concentrated) leads Verhaegen to conclude that our ancestors 'probably lived once near salt or brackish waters or at simultaneously or successively different aquatic habitats, e.g. first in a freshwater and afterwards in a salt water environment . . . but certainly not in a very dry habitat (savanna)' (1985: 25).

To the extent that hominids were situated along the shores of saline lakes (such as many of those in the Rift Valley) or the sea, they would have needed to focus around estuarine regions which provided drinkable water. The evidence is that they did.

Drinking water would have been only one utility associated with such sites. Water has other uses, too, and it must be significant that early hominids situated themselves not just along riverbanks or springs but more specifically at the points at which these entered large, often saline, lakes. What could have been the special value of such sites?

Some modern human analogies are pertinent here. Unless cultural norms, freshwater crocodiles or other factors intervene, humans from childhood onwards find bathing an enjoyable way of keeping cool, of cleaning the body and of playing. Diving can be pleasurable once learned. The traditional coastal peoples such as the diving women of Korea and Japan (Hong and Rahn 1967) go as deep as 75 feet to gather shellfish and seaweed, while Polynesians can dive into deep water, hide behind plants – and catch passing fish with one hand. Given that humans are clearly genetically equipped to cope extremely well with swimming, diving and even underwater childbirth (Morgan 1982), we have every reason to suppose that such facilities have been at least intermittently adaptive for millions of years.

Subsistence considerations point in the same direction. Human brains are large and brain tissue is 60 per cent polyunsaturated fat. Such brains are in energetic terms exceedingly expensive and need constant replenishing. The savanna grasslands of early and middle Pleistocene Africa would have held only a miserable supply of the fats essential to nourish such organs. Some nutritional chemists (Crawford and Marsh 1989) have pointed out that this effectively rules out a savanna adaptation for hominids who were as yet unable to practise efficient hunting. Hominids whose brains were expanding, these authors find, must have been collecting marine foods and gathering seeds and fruits along rivers, lakes, seashores and estuaries which contained not only foods rich in polyunsaturates but also a wealth of essential trace elements and minerals washed off the land. We could perhaps link such considerations with the fact that whereas the small-brained robust australopithecines apparently evolved their huge grinding teeth and other special adaptations in the drier regions of East Africa, the gracile forms and *Homo* evolved in the wetter parts, close to rivers and lakes (Foley 1987: 210–14).

In fact lakes, marshes and shorelines can provide abundant foods of all kinds – weeds, edible bulbs, aquatic birds and their eggs, turtles, small reptiles and much else. As Plio-Pleistocene African lakes and pools contracted or even sometimes dried out in the driest, most difficult, months of the year, they would often have been teeming with stranded fish and other creatures; collecting these in addition to birds or other small-to-medium-sized game would have been for hominids a high-yield strategy in otherwise stressful months. It is worth adding that because of the salinity, plant resources may have been sparse in many such areas, prompting an increasing need to exploit non-vegetable foods (Foley 1987: 209, 212). A very omnivorous diet would conform with what we know about the gracile hominids' teeth (Foley 1987: 211).

Little technology is needed to exploit shoreline resources. In Australia, coastal Aborigines using extremely simple tools combine the eating of molluscs with fish, turtles, birds, wallabies, snakes and lizards, and they collect yams, water chestnuts, fruits, eggs and wild honey. The economics of mollusc gathering are revealed by a study on the shores of Arnhem Land (Meehan 1977), in which women and children were each able to take 8.5 kg of shellfish per trip, of 29 sorts, but mainly of a single species,

Tapes hiantina. For the energy expended, Ebling (1985) comments, it seems unlikely that male hunters could have secured a better return. Although they may have a rather low food value for their weight (Bailey 1978: 39), shellfish contain valuable minerals as well as other nutrients, and as part of a varied shoreline diet can play an important role. Over Australia as a whole, in any event, the pre-contact population density of Aborigines is closely correlated with rainfall – except along coasts and on islands, where it is higher than would be predicted (Birdsell 1953).

It used to be thought that an absence of Plio–Pleistocene shell-middens indicated that early humans were not using aquatic foods. But this was in the 1970s, when theorists were still looking for 'home bases' as diagnostic features of early hominid activity. The collapse of this paradigm has radically changed the picture. It is now realised that if early hominids were diving or wandering along shores, sometimes catching fish in shallow waters, selecting edible weeds or seaweeds, or cracking crabs or bivalves with stones and eating the flesh as they went, locally concentrated middens would never have arisen. Indeed, since stone tools need not have been used, at most sites it would be extremely surprising to find any archaeological traces of such activities at all.

Hominids, Evolution and Water

There is nothing extraordinary about the theory that in a coastal, estuarine or riparian woodland environment, water as such would have been an important component of the total system of environmentally linked selection pressures acting on evolving hominids. Wild chimpanzees are much less water-adapted than humans, but even they have been seen wading in streams, drinking from lakes, feeding on aquatic plants – and mating ventroventrally in very shallow water (Nishida 1980). On the other hand, if chimpanzees waded any deeper or foraged and travelled through trees overhanging rivers and lakes, they would frequently fall in and drown. Chimpanzee infants as well as adults lack the fat-based buoyancy of humans, their bodies are not streamlined – and for numerous reasons connected with breathing control, the shape of limbs and so forth, no one has ever trained a chimpanzee to swim. The only primate known to be a good habitual swimmer is the proboscis monkey, which inhabits an ecological zone comparable to that which Blumenschine and others have envisaged for Lucy and other early hominids. Proboscis monkeys live in mangrove trees in the coastal swamps of Borneo. They climb trees which overhang the water and swim, but occasionally, and especially at low tide, they are seen on relatively dry land – on a mud flat or sandbank. It can hardly be a coincidence that proboscis monkeys are the only primates able to practise a form of sustained bipedalism very similar to that of humans, in one Japanese documentary film being shown 'walking calmly on the ground through the trees in single file' (Morgan

1990: 46). Periodic inundation of their habitat is, of course, the incentive for such bipedalism. As Morgan (1990: 46) points out:

> For proboscis monkeys crossing a stretch of water a couple of feet deep, walking upright offers only one single advantage, but it is an offer they cannot refuse. It enables them to breathe, whereas if they walked on four legs, their heads would be under water.

Bonobos are widely regarded as the most human-like of all the great apes. Whilst they are not known to be swimmers, their near-bipedalism has seemingly evolved under comparable selection pressures. Bonobos often feed whilst wading along streams in their periodically inundated natural habitat (de Waal 1991: 182−6).

Any hominids evolving in the northern regions of the Rift Valley would have been under selection pressures shaped in part by the waters which periodically flooded wide areas − particularly when the Danakil microplate became detached from both the African and Arabian plates at the beginning of the Pliocene, allowing waters from the Red Sea and Gulf of Aden to flood into the Afar Triangle (LaLumiere 1982 [1981]: 128). Lucy's skeleton was found among the remains of crocodile and turtle eggs and crab claws. It is perhaps also worth noting Foley's (1987: 26) support for the view that a mixed *Australopithecus afarensis* group who died in this region 3 million years ago was a whole family, whose members had all been drowned together in a flash flood (Johanson and Edey 1981; Johanson *et al.* 1982). In fact, most experts now believe that the bones are not those of a single family but were accumulated separately over many years. Nonetheless, drownings must often have occurred, and certainly the need for wading or occasional swimming would explain why the very earliest hominids failed to adopt the restrictively terrestrial but otherwise extremely efficient locomotory technique of quadrupedalism.

The need to move within three contrasting media − trees, open ground and water − would have hastened the tempo of evolutionary development, particularly if small populations became stranded for periods on islands with water all around. As less efficient swimmers occasionally drowned, the survivors would have displayed increasing hairlessness, a thick subcutaneous fat layer, chubby and buoyant babies, streamlined body contours, downwards-facing nostrils, a descended larynx, unusually good control over breathing, enhanced diving abilities − and the many other clearly water-adaptive characteristics which make humans such unusual primates (Hardy 1960; LaLumiere 1982 [1981]; Morgan 1972, 1982, 1984, 1986, 1990; Morris 1977; Verhaegen 1985). *It is simply impossible to believe that hominids who selected the Afar Gulf and various Rift Valley lakesides as their favoured habitats could have been unable to swim.* On the other hand, if they could swim, it is impossible to believe that selection pressures associated with this mode of locomotion could have been irrelevant to their evolution.

Admittedly, attempts have been made to explain some of the features listed above without reference to water-associated selection pressures. But in general they have not stood the test of time.

In the 1960s, the development of bare skin and profuse sweating as a thermoregulatory system was ascribed to the exigencies of survival in a hot, tropical, dry savanna environment. This was seen in terms of the needs of overheated males hunting or foraging strenuously under a hot sun (Morris 1967). The fact that leopards, lions, hunting dogs and other savanna-dwelling predators failed to lose their fur under such conditions was not seen as a problem.

In a recent variation on this theme, Wheeler (1984, 1985, 1988) argues that both bipedalism and humans' relative hairlessness evolved as a thermoregulatory system enabling foraging hominids to run out into the open savanna to obtain food under the noonday sun – when rival scavengers and predators were keeping cool in the shade. Wheeler (1988) makes the important observation that chimpanzees with their short muzzles are poorly equipped to keep their brains cool by panting, and that the ultra-large human brain is particularly heat-sensitive. He suggests that by keeping upright, retaining heat-reflective hair on the head and by sweating from the rest of the body in the absence of fur, humans have developed an efficient set of mechanisms for keeping the body and hence also the brain cool and avoiding sunstroke during activities under a blazing sun.

This hypothesis is interesting and valuable, yet taken in isolation it is inadequate. Firstly, the loss of body-warming fur would have affected hominids on a day-round basis – including in the bitter cold of night – as well as at noon. If shivering in the small hours were the price to be paid for comfort under a blazing sun, it is not at all clear that in the habitat envisaged, the benefits of the new system would have outweighed the costs (Morgan 1990: 60–1). In fact, of course, it is known that enhanced body fat has in humans compensated for fur loss, so at least the plumper furless hominids might have kept warm. But fat-insulation is not discussed by Wheeler (1985, 1988). Humans' enhanced subcutaneous fat layers – whilst useful for a swimmer – would surely be unwelcome during strenuous activities under a tropical African noonday sun. It seems mysterious how this *particular* configuration could have been the product of the selection pressures that Wheeler envisages.

A further objection is that human females have less body-hair than males. They are also on average substantially fatter (Pond 1987). Wheeler does not posit a sexual division of labour for his noonday foragers, but still his model would surely predict the opposite. Had humans lost their body hair primarily in order to monopolise a foraging niche involving running in search of highly-clumped food over partially sunlit ground (Wheeler 1988), then males – as the more mobile sex – ought surely to have evolved furthest in this direction. They ought to be less hairy than human females – the reverse of what we actually find.

In other ways, too, Wheeler's speculation fails when it comes to the fine detail. As Morgan (1990: 80–91) has intriguingly shown, human sweating is actually nothing like that of a chimpanzee which began foraging under a noonday sun. Humans have lost most of the scent-emitting *apocrine* glands which are found all over the bodies of chimpanzees, and through which they (like other large mammals) produce their temperature-regulating sweat. Extraordinarily, humans sweat using the *eccrine* glands which in other primates are relatively few in number and are found mainly on the palms of their feet and hands, where they produce tiny amounts of moisture to assist in gaining a grip and have nothing to do with thermoregulation. In contrast to other primates, humans have eccrines which vastly outnumber the apocrine glands. These eccrines (which in chimpanzees are scattered thinly over the whole body) produce a form of sweat which – bizarrely for a savanna-dweller – takes several minutes to appear in response to over-heating and is also extravagantly wasteful of both salt and water. Incomprehensible in a savanna context, this would make sense if humans were the descendants of an early hominid which – like any mammal adapting to water – lost most of its apocrines. Scent trails cannot be left in water, whilst sweating of any kind is less necessary for habitual bathers. It would seem that in proportion as our ancestors later began foraging in hot, dry conditions and needed to sweat profusely to keep cool – they had nothing but their eccrines to fall back on. Add to this the fact that humans have an astonishingly weak sense of smell (Stoddart 1986 and references), anomalous in a savanna scavenger but quite typical of swimming mammals (Morgan 1982: 97, citing Martin 1979) – and the pieces of the jigsaw nicely fit.

In short, the aquatic hypothesis (Hardy 1960; Morgan 1972, 1982, 1990) offers far simpler explanations than Wheeler's, and has the added advantage of accommodating Wheeler's own substantive findings. Wheeler (1988) himself is not averse to postulating very early selection pressures *pre-adapting* evolving hominids for the bipedalism whose thermoregulatory advantages he has documented:

> Our ancestors may well have been predisposed to walking upright by virtue of the time that their ancestors had spent hanging about in trees. Brachiating – swinging by the arms – means the animal has to hold its body in a vertical position for long periods of time; primates that brachiate often adopt a more upright posture on the ground than true quadrupeds (Wheeler 1988: 62).

Add 'moving through water' to 'brachiating' in the above passage and the problems are solved. Wading through water no less than swinging through trees would require the traveller 'to hold its body in a vertical position for long periods of time'. The upper body's buoyancy in water would help sustain such a stance. It is well-known that semi-aquatic creatures tend to adopt a more upright posture on the ground that true quadrupeds – as the examples of penguins, proboscis monkeys and beavers nicely show (Morgan 1982: 53–4). Postulating at least occasional swimming, moreover, has the added advantage that it explains the development of the characteristically human layer of subcutaneous insulating blubber about which Wheeler says nothing at all. Interestingly in this context, and puzzlingly in view of his concerns over hominid overheating, Wheeler (1985) dismisses the idea that early hominids could have been swimmers on the basis of a single unsupported supposition. A hairless primate the size of an early hominid, he writes, would have got *far too cold* in the tropical waters of East Africa!

Bipedalism doubtless helped minimise overheating, just as it is useful in food-carrying, tool-use, peering over long grasses and many other activities. But understanding the many ultimate benefits is one thing; tracing the *initial* functions and selection pressures – as Wheeler in his discussion of brachiating in effect concedes – is quite another. We can accept that an increased capacity to forage under a hot sun would have conferred selective advantages – without, however, postulating 'noonday foraging' as the novel niche responsible for the ape/hominid evolutionary divergence. It might be thought difficult under any circumstances to persuade heat-sensitive, large-brained and increasingly fat-insulated hominids to choose noon as the time of day to maximise their foraging activities in the tropical African sun! On the other hand, apes becoming bipedal under combined arboreal/terrestrial/aquatic selection-pressures, drinking copiously, keeping cool by washing, by finding a shady tree or by taking a splash – such apes would have been under strong pressures to evolve precisely the out-of-water thermoregulatory system which Wheeler has so usefully described. In the water, our ancestors would have had few problems in keeping cool. Each time individuals emerged, evaporation would have extended the cooling effects. Enhancement of the technique of drinking copiously and intermittently so as to be able to 'bathe' when necessary through sweat-evaporation can in this light be seen as an extension of the bathing adaptation. The blubber which would gradually have evolved would have served as an aid to buoyancy (particularly necessary for young babies, which are surprisingly fat in the human case) and also as an out-of-water insulation functional in cool periods and at night. To this it should be added that whilst a marked absence of subcutaneous scalp fat combined with abundant heat-reflecting scalp hair fit Wheeler's scenario nicely – such features would equally be predicted of an ape whose postcranial body-hair initially diminished to reduce water-drag. The head is the one part of a swimmer's body which remains above the water-line, and which would therefore need cooling (or alternatively, keeping warm) in a completely different way from the rest of the body. In short, whilst the thermoregulatory hypothesis has some strong points, it is not a complete solution to the problems which need to be addressed; in this context, there seem to be no good reasons why Wheeler's and Morgan's complementary insights should not be combined.

The advantage of taking aquatic selection-pressures into account is that it allows us to view early hominids not as specialists adapted to just one narrow niche – but as flexible creatures capable of climbing trees, foraging on open ground and food-gathering in water as well. It is perhaps possible to envisage sex-linked differences in this context, with males at one evolutionary stage or another more likely to forage inland on dry savanna because of their greater mobility, while females with their offspring stayed closer to protective trees overhanging water and/or resource-rich shores. The sex-linked pattern found in modern humans – with women on average both fatter and less hairy than males – would be consistent with the possibility that evolving hominid females were marginally more dependent on swimming and/or shoreline foraging, although a more probable explanation for women's extra body fat is simply that it provides an energetic fallback needed particularly for mothers who must carry babies in the womb and provide milk at the breast in bad seasons as in good. That might mean that the subcutaneous fat which evolved in the first instance under semi-aquatic selection pressures at a later stage turned out to enable human females more reliably to feed their young.

The restriction of early hominid sites to just one riverine, lake-ribboned and estuarine geological zone confirms the scenario. In Plio-Pleistocene Africa, there were plenty of savanna environments outside this restricted region, particularly in the colder periods (Foley 1987: figure 5.10, citing Bonnefille 1984; Roberts 1984). Tropical rain forests were much less widespread than was previously thought, disappearing almost completely during each ice age although from time to time covering a large swathe of central and south-western Africa (see figure 5). Most of Africa has for a very long time been savanna, and the proportion has been increasing over the past 10 million or so years (see references in Foley 1987: 110–17). If the survival of evolving humans presupposed no more than good hunting or scavenging conditions in this kind of environment, then the geographical distribution of early hominid sites ought at various times to have extended widely across almost the whole of the African continent.

The actual, highly restricted distribution pattern suggests that open savanna-foraging played little role. We have seen that humans' poor sense of smell, reduced apocrines, salt-and-water wasting eccrine sweat glands, constant thirstiness and generally extreme water dependence in tropical climates would have been maladaptive and indeed inexplicable in the context of a simple savanna adaptation. On the other hand, an ordinary, non-aquatic forest or woodland adaptation would leave us wondering why our ancestors ever stopped being apes. We can conclude that evolving early hominids – unlike culture-bearing anatomically modern humans – were extremely discriminating as to where they could live. The quite peculiar mosaic of conditions prevailing in the Rift Valley between the Miocene and Late

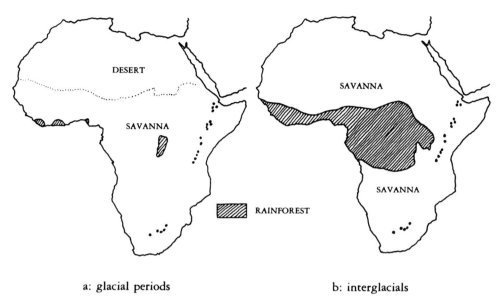

a: glacial periods   b: interglacials

Figure 5   Approximate ratio of rain forest to savanna in Africa during the Pleistocene. In earlier
periods the rain forest shown in the second map extended still further. Mountain forests and additional
woodlands bordering lakes and rivers are not shown. Superimposed on both maps, the dots indicate the
points along the Rift Valley where early hominid stone tools and/or fossil remains have been found
(modified after Foley 1987: 112–13).

Pleistocene uniquely met their requirements. It was these specific conditions
which were responsible for the initial divergence and unique characteristics
of the hominids – characteristics increasingly differentiating them from their
ape-like cousins.

The Shores of Eden

Some of the best-known early hominid fossils date back to as much as 3.8
million years ago, and were found in the Afar Triangle (Johanson and White
1979). No South African fossils as old as this have been found. Within the
Afar, 'Lucy' and her associates settled some 3 million years ago along the
Awash River, which flows down the Rift Valley at its northern end.
Although fully bipedal (even if not quite in a 'modern' sense), they had no
more than chimpanzee-sized brains, and were not yet making stone tools.
With neither fire for cooking nor a stone technology for bone-breaking, they
could hardly have been proficient open-country scavengers. A diet radically

different from that of chimpanzees, however, is indicated already by their rather different teeth. There has been little agreement among palaeontologists on what these teeth were for. Electron scanning microscope use-wear studies indicate micro-flaking, pitting and scratching. It is as if Lucy were a chimpanzee-like fruit-eater – except that she also ate many other kinds of food, including coarse, gritty items which have not so far been identified (Johanson and Edey 1981: 363–4). An unconfirmed possibility is that these were often sand-contaminated lake shore foods including bulbs, aquatic tubers (Binford 1989: 27), and perhaps shellfish.

Others of Lucy's kind must have followed the Awash up to its source and beyond. As they did so, such hominids would eventually have discovered other inland shores, leaving their remains at such present-day sites as the Omo River, Koobi Fora, Lake Turkana, Olduvai Gorge, Laetoli, Makapansgat, Sterkfontein, and Taung (LaLumiere 1982 [1981]; Leakey and Lewin 1979). Those who remained behind, on the other hand, appear to have continued evolving under probably more strongly aquatic selection pressures along the banks of the Awash or in the partly flooded Afar Triangle itself, with offshoot groups periodically moving up the valley and sometimes finding ways of surviving in drier regions as the earlier robust australopithecines seem to have done.

The process of evolution and migration along the valley continued through the Pliocene and into the Pleistocene. Some of Lucy's ape-like but relatively intelligent tool-making migratory descendants – earliest *Homo* – stopped about two million years ago beside lakes at Koobi Fora and Olduvai Gorge (Leakey and Lewin 1977, 1979). Later still, hominids with even larger brains began moving along the valley; around a million years ago, some were able to migrate right out of Africa altogether (figure 6a), eventually reaching China and Java, where they acquired more and more of the derived features of *Homo erectus* (Wood 1984; Groves 1989).

Even later, anatomically modern humans had begun evolving within the Afar/northern Rift Valley area. Among currently favoured candidates for the earliest anatomically modern humans are some fragmentary fossils from Omo Kibish, Laetoli and Lake Turkana, some of which may be up to 130,000 years old. The precise age and status of these fossils may need corroboration (Rightmire 1989), but it is at least possible that anatomically modern humans came to exist in the middle-to-northern part of the Rift Valley some tens of thousands of years before they appeared anywhere else. They would then have moved northwards and southwards, gradually replacing or perhaps sometimes interbreeding with the native populations in each newly entered area (figure 6b).

Much of this is speculative. New evidence is likely to change our picture substantially. Nonetheless, what seems stably established is that from the Miocene onwards until the Last Interglacial, the Rift Valley retained its unique position as the evolutionary cradle of large-brained, gracile hominids.

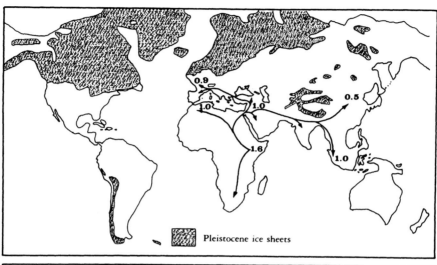

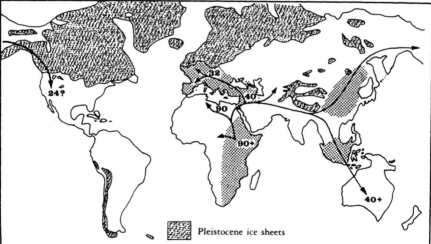

Figure 6 'Out of Africa'. *Top*: dispersal of pre-sapient humans. The lines suggest routes and local dates of arrival (in millions of years before the present). Hatched areas indicate ice-cover at glacial maxima. *Bottom*: dispersal of anatomically modern humans (dates in thousands of years). Also indicated (dot-patterned areas) are resident archaic populations encountered by the moderns: archaic *Homo sapiens* in Africa; Neanderthals in Europe and the Near East; East Asian archaic populations in China and Java. Note that in all periods the ultimate source of dispersal is seemingly from the northern end of the Rift Valley (modified after Foley 1987: 264–5).

In this region and nowhere else in the world, selection pressures – which I am here linking with Turke's ovarian synchrony scenario – promoted intensified parenting (including a growing *paternal* input) and hence gave rise to a succession of bipeds with more and more neotenous features, and larger and larger brains. Each time a new type was produced, certain descendants of these evolved hominids may have been forced by population pressure to migrate southwards and sometimes northwards in successive waves, replacing their less neotenous, usually smaller-brained local antecedents – hominid cousins who in their local (drier) habitat had not evolved in similar directions or at the same rate. Acceptance of Turke's model would imply that the northern half of the Rift Valley had something about it which enabled pre-cultural or proto-cultural hominid females to sustain ovarian synchrony more consistently than was possible elsewhere.

Synchrony, Tides and the Moon

It was noted earlier that women's higher levels of body fat and decreased body hair are both water-adaptive features, suggesting that evolving females may have had some special need to maintain proximity with expanses of water. In the light of Turke's model, we may speculate that this was connected not only with the requirements of an area-intensive mode of foraging – but also with females' need for environmental cues unique to shoreline habitats, and of direct relevance to the maintenance of ovarian synchrony over wide areas.

In recent decades, researches have substantially increased our understanding and awareness of biological clocks (Cloudsley-Thompson 1980). Almost every living organism can become entrained by – locked in step with – oscillations in its natural environment, provided these have set up selection pressures which have endured for long enough for the capacity to evolve, and provided social factors such as the prevailing mating system do not produce counteracting pressures to avoid synchrony.

Tidal movements provide an extremely reliable, predictable environmental rhythm (or *Zeitgeber*, to use the technical term) for all organisms which live close to large expanses of water (Cloudsley-Thompson 1980: 74, 75, 91–5).

Tides are of course a lunar effect, spring tides occurring twice a month – at full and again at new moon, when the gravitational pulls of both moon and sun combine. Contrary to some classical writers including Darwin (1871: 1, 212n), most terrestrial mammals have physiological cycles showing no link at all with such rhythms. Primates, however, have menstrual cycles. Whilst with few exceptions these are not in fact genuinely lunar, there is at least the basis for tidal phase-locking here – should selection pressures act in that direction powerfully enough and for sufficiently long. For what it is worth, a minor medical study of human births at St Thomas'

Hospital, London – chosen for the analysis because of its situation beside the tidal Thames – showed significantly more deliveries at the flood tide than at the ebb (Rajasingham et al. 1989). Confirming that the tides may have been directly involved, a similar study at a hospital 3 km from the river showed no such effects (Chamberlain and Azam 1988). Such isolated findings of 'lunar effects' using small samples are notoriously variegated and unreliable, however (Rotton and Kelly 1985; Culver et al. 1988). In the absence of improved statistics, any grounds for suspecting tidal selection pressures operative in the evolution of the human menstrual cycle must come from logical considerations based on rather different kinds of data.

The most important logical consideration is simply that any form of sustained and generalised reproductive or menstrual synchrony would require a reliable external cue. Many environments – such as the floor of a tropical forest – would not provide environmental cues of the kind necessary for consistent menstrual synchrony to work. The open and often moonlit shores of lakes and seas would provide such cues. In this context it seems worth recalling that the theoretical underpinnings of Turke's theory rest essentially on Nancy Knowlton's (1979) studies of shrimps, her findings constituting perhaps the only conclusive demonstration yet made that females can impose monogamy on males by totally synchronising their reproductive cycles . In the case of shrimps, at least – as of prawns, sea-horses and many other sea creatures (Cloudsley-Thompson 1980: 91–8) – it is definitely tidal and/or directly lunar influences which provide the proximate cues necessary for females to synchronise with impressive precision.

In the case of evolving human females, we can construct a narrative along similar lines. *Females who synchronised to escape monopolisation by alpha males found themselves drawing on tidal cues.* The earliest hominids, we have seen, arose and for several million years evolved in the Rift Valley and along the shores of the Afar Gulf. Assuming that females were already tending to synchronise for sexual-political reasons (Turke 1984), the ovarian cycles of closely associated females in this setting could hardly have escaped selection pressures to mesh in with the movements of the moon and any tidal rhythms, however slight. *Indeed, we might even turn matters the other way around, and suppose that it was some kind of tidal effect which provided the necessary cue for ovarian synchrony on Paul Turke's model to become set up in the first place.*

Direct lunar/tidal influences on the human body (for a survey of the medical and psychological literature see Rotton and Kelly 1985; Culver et al. 1988; Kollerstrom 1990) are at best weak (see the following section). Even on clear nights or at the sea's edge, they would be easily overridden by other factors such as those of sexual politics. Regardless of the moon or the tides, synchrony would *not* occur if the prevailing mating system rendered it maladaptive.

But conversely, if coastal females were beginning to synchronise with each other for their own sexual-political reasons, then any external cues with an appropriate periodicity would automatically have acquired special significance. If it was important not only that local groups synchronised on a local basis, but also that neighbouring groups synchronised to a single schedule over a wide area, then it would have become vital for all to converge around a shared external rhythm capable of acting as a 'clock'. It would hardly have mattered how weak were the signals – if females needed to receive them, then selection pressures would have acted powerfully to develop the necessary senses. Oysters, shrimps, prawns and other natural organisms which synchronise through internal body-clocks must continuously reset these using environmental cues – which may be vanishingly weak to human senses. Deprived of such cues, the organisms tend to drift out of phase over time (Cloudsley-Thompson 1980: 6–21), although sea-horses rather amazingly continue to lay their eggs at full moon even when in laboratory tanks, deprived of any evident source of information on the lunar cycle. (For a discussion of this and other examples see Kollerstrom 1990: 157.) When the early human populations of this book's narrative migrated along or up the sides of the Rift Valley, eventually ending up far from coastal shores, faint tidal effects in lakes or even direct cues from the moon itself would almost certainly have proved sufficient to preserve the synchrony essential to their mating system – although direct lunar cues would have been weaker and less reliable than tidal ones, the moon's light being blocked out during periods of thick cloud.

In this context, the ovarian synchrony model is strengthened by the fact that the human female menstrual cycle – virtually alone among primate cycles – is a body-clock with precisely the correct average phase-length to enable lunar/tidal synchrony to be maintained.

Lunar Cycles

If the human menstrual cycle were genuinely linked with the moon it would be rather surprising, for such a correspondence is not normal, either for primates or for mammals in general. Although many invertebrate marine animals, certain fish and some frogs and toads concentrate their reproductive activities at specific lunar phases (Bunning 1964; Cloudsley-Thompson 1980: 90–100), few terrestrial mammals appear to be in any way synchronised with the moon.

We saw in Chapter 6 that hamadryas baboons synchronise not only within harem units but also more widely, a degree of synchrony characterising whole bands and even troops (Kummer 1968: 176–9). However, there is no generalised synchrony: troops in different localities are cycling on different schedules from one another. Hamadryas baboon menstrual cycles are longer than those of humans – on average between 31 and 35 days (Hrdy and Whitten 1987: 372–8) – which suggests that neither lunar changes nor the tides have entrained baboon cycles to a locality-independent fixed rhythm, at least not in evolutionarily recent times.

Mating at full moon has, however, been reported of certain diurnal prosimians, such as *Lemur macaco*. In one often-quoted study (Cowgill *et al.* 1962), researchers reported that of 15 matings observed in their laboratory, 13 fell within 5 days before or after a full moon. Their lemurs' first three oestrous periods, after they were moved from Madagascar to the northern hemisphere, were out of phase, perhaps because of disorientation caused by travel, but after this, six of seven oestrous periods overlapped a day of full moon.

Alison Jolly (1967: 3–14) subsequently studied wild lemurs of a different species, *Lemur catta*, and concluded that evidence from the wild 'agrees with the moon hypothesis, but hardly proves it'. In each troop, the females came into oestrus annually, mating for a few days, all at the same time, the period roughly overlapping with full moon. But this may have been coincidental, and Jolly (1967: 13) simply concludes that 'there is a challenge to elucidate the mechanism of synchronous breeding, whether social, by day length, or by the moon, as well as the evolutionary function of synchronous breeding.'

Isolated reports aside, consistent lunar synchrony appears to be rare among primates and perhaps non-existent. Neither do many primate cycle lengths match the 29.5 day duration of the synodic lunar month (see Table 7.1).

It could be argued that the figures for primate cycle lengths indicate a roughly lunar/tidal pattern, but if so there are numerous divergences. Any hypothetical lunar baseline would have to be seen as a trait which has been largely overridden in the course of primate evolutionary speciation. From the table it would appear to be principally the smaller primates which have departed most radically from what one might suppose to be a rough 28-day to 30-day norm.

In humans the situation is intriguing. Although few contemporary western women cycle in a way which has anything to do with the moon (see next section), woman's reproduction physiology differs from that of most other primates in being theoretically consistent with tidal synchrony. The key biological condition for synchrony of successive cycles is of course that the cycle length should match the moon's. In women, this condition is met with precision.

Among the most careful investigations of human menstrual cycle length ever conducted was that of Gunn and associates (1937); their data, when properly arranged, gave a mean of 29.5 days (see Arey 1954; Menaker and Menaker 1959; Menaker 1967; Criss and Marcum 1981; Dewan *et al.* 1978). This is exactly the length of time it takes for the moon to pass through its phases as seen from the earth. The figure has been confirmed by Treloar (1981; Treloar *et al.* 1967), who compiled well over 270,000 cycle lengths of

Table 7.1 Cycle lengths in non-human primates

Species	Cycle length (days)
Ring-tailed lemur	39
Tarsier	24
Common marmoset	15–17
Lion tamarin	14–21
Goeldi's marmoset	21–24
Red howler	16–27
Squirrel monkey	7–25
Gray langur	27
Barbary macaque	31
Rhesus macaque	29
Japanese macaque	28
Vervet monkey	33
Talapoin	33
Patas monkey	32
Yellow baboon	32
Olive baboon	31–35
Chacma baboon	31–35
Hamadryas baboon	31–35
Gelada baboon	35
Lar gibbon	30
Orangutan	31
Common chimpanzee	37
Pygmy chimpanzee	28–37
Mountain gorilla	28
Lowland gorilla	31

Source: Hrdy and Whitten (1987: 372–8).

women throughout all ages of reproductive life. In a more recent study, Cutler et al. (1980) again confirmed the 29.5 day average.

In western contexts, human menstrual cycle lengths vary widely. Only about 28 per cent of reproductively active women show a 29.5 ± 1 day cycle length. On the other hand, cycles of this length tend to be the most fertile ones (Vollman 1968, 1970, 1977; Treloar et al. 1967, Treloar 1981). The finding that there is a positive correlation between fertility and precision of lunar phase length has been described as an 'intriguing biological coincidence' (Cutler et al. 1987).

A related finding is that heterosexual women who have regular weekly sex tend to have significantly more 29.5 ± 3 day cycles than women who have either sporadic or celibate sexual patterns (Cutler et al. 1979a, 1979b). According to Cutler and her colleagues (1987), weekly sex is usually sufficient to set up 29.5 ± 3 day cycles. Male pheromones may be involved (Cutler et al. 1986; Preti et al. 1986).

Lunar Phase-locking: Negative Evidence

Much evidence suggests that if women needed to phase-lock themselves to a lunar schedule and could set up the appropriate conditions for this, physiology would do the rest. In other words, there is nothing in women's genetic constitution to prevent the moon from acting as a *Zeitgeber* (exogenous synchroniser) of their cycles. Whether or not the moon in practice acts in this way depends on many factors – above all, it would seem, on the prevailing system of kinship and marriage, which may either sustain or preclude the possibility of women's remaining in close contact with one another after marriage.

The fact that women *in contemporary cultures* fail to synchronise is well established. In an analysis of 11,807 menstrual onsets at the turn of the century, the Swedish researcher Arrhenius (1898) concluded that these were more frequent while the moon was waxing than when it was waning. But nearly forty years later, when Gunn and associates (1937) analysed 10,416 menstrual events, they expressed their disappointment in having to conclude that there was no justification for asserting any connection with the moon. A more recent investigation by Pochobradsky (1974) analysed over 6,000 menstrual onsets, mostly of women living in Czechoslovakia, and concluded likewise that 'women in the study menstruated and ovulated independently of the phases of the moon'.

There is of course the theoretical possibility that non-western statistics would produce different results. In a study conducted in 1982 (Law 1986), 826 young female volunteers with normal menstrual cycles living in Beijing and Guangchow in China were asked to record their cycle lengths and dates of menstrual onset over a period of four months. It was found that 'most menstruations occurred during 4 days around the new moon'. This was quite a strong statistical effect. When the lunar month was divided into equal periods averaging four days each, the results broke down as shown in Table 7.2.

In other words, over twice as many menstruations occurred during the new moon four-day period as during the four-day full moon period. But until comparable studies have confirmed such results, few conclusions can safely be drawn.

One female researcher in the United States has regularly found the opposite effect to that claimed by Law (1986), women in her sample showing a tendency to menstruate at full moon whilst ovulating at new (Cutler 1980a; Cutler et al. 1987). A possibility is that these women were more subject to artificial lighting than the Chinese subjects studied by Law, but even then, the results would seem puzzling. In any event, there is a clear need for large-sample statistical studies which control for variables such as

Table 7.2 Correlation of menstrual onsets with lunar phase

Four-day period	No. of menstruations	%
New moon	234	28.3
New moon: first quarter	104	12.6
First quarter	87	10.5
First quarter: full moon	77	9.3
Full moon	95	11.5
Full moon: last quarter	83	10.0
Last quarter	77	9.3
Last quarter: new moon	69	8.5

Source: Law (1986).

exposure to artificial light. None has so far been conducted. Ethnographic data of possible relevance to this issue will be surveyed in later chapters of this book.

Birth Records and the Moon

If women tended to menstruate at around new moon, they should give birth at full moon, the mean length of pregnancy measured from the last menstrual onset being nine synodic months plus a half. Again, there is no evidence that this happens.

The best-known studies to test this in a western context were carried out in the 1950s and 1960s (Menaker and Menaker 1959; Menaker 1967). Records of half a million live births in New York City between 1948 and 1957 showed more births occurring in the half-cycle centring on full moon, although there was only a 1.35 per cent difference between the figures for the two half-cycles. Taking half a million births between 1961 and 1963 in the same city, it was again found that more births occurred in the half-cycle centred on full moon. In this case, however, the two half-cycles differed by only 1.01 per cent, falling only just within the standard (1 per cent) margin of statistical significance.

Others (Osley et al. 1973) later reported similar results. But daily birth data for the years 1972–3 compiled from the records of the Vancouver General Hospital gave no indication of a birth peak related to full moon (Schwab 1975). Still more recently, a French team (Guillon et al. 1986) looked at hospital records of almost 6 million births in France between 1968 and 1974. They found a slight tendency for more births to occur during the dark moon and fewer to occur during the moon's first quarter – a finding in conflict with those of the Menakers.

Possible Photic Entrainment of the Menstrual Cycle

We have examined statistical studies of women in modern industrialised cultures, and have found no evidence of a significant correspondence between lunar phase and events in the menstrual cycle. However, a circalunadian version of Paul Turke's synchrony model would not predict this. Modern cultural conditions are unlikely to resemble even remotely the conditions of shore-dwelling evolving protowomen in the East African Pleistocene. The model would predict merely that modern women should be found to possess the physiological capacity to synchronise with one another through the moon – given ideal conditions of exposure to moonlight, to the tides or to an appropriate artificial cue. Falsification of the hypothesis would require medical evidence that women lacked such physiological potentialities. It is to this question that we now turn.

In a pilot experiment to test for the effects of nocturnal light on a human female, Dewan and Rock (1969) subjected a 26-year-old woman to overnight lamplight from days 14 to 17 of her cycle (day 1 being that of menstrual onset). She had to keep her room quite dark during sleep for the rest of the month. Under this treatment her cycle, which had been varying between 33 and 48 days, regularised to between 29 and 31 days. To check that this was not coincidental, several women were then subjected for a few months to a similar regimen of nocturnal light while also supplying control data (the subjects receiving no nocturnal illumination). As before, a 100W lamp-bulb was kept on once per month overnight, from nights 14 to 17 of the women's cycles, this being 'an artificial simulation of the effects of full moon . . .' (Dewan et al. 1978: 582). Again, the treatment worked: eight of eleven subjects showed a narrower range of cycle lengths than when not manipulated, a quarter of the experimental cycles achieving a lunar cycle length.

The theory that light triggers ovulation seems well-founded, and would accord with the Chinese findings noted earlier (Law 1986). This would mean that under ideal conditions, ovulation should occur at full moon, menstruation at new.

The moon's light is some 300,000 times weaker than the sun's, and also many times weaker than the 100W bulb used in Dewan's experiments. Theoretically, however, this need pose no problem. Studies of humans living artificially in near-total darkness have shown that quite miniscule amounts of light are sufficient to entrain the body-clock which regulates the daily alternation between sleep and wakefulness (Moore-Ede 1981).

Humans are of course primates, whose ultimate ancestors were nocturnal, arboreal insectivores resembling tree-shrews. High up in trees, their periodic exposure to moonlight may have been adaptively significant. For example, movement through branches could well have been impeded on moonless nights, so that courtship behaviour tended to intensify during the better-lit nights around full moon. All this could help explain what may turn out to be a baseline of lunar periodicity beneath the variability of primate reproductive physiology as a whole. Whilst all this is speculative, we do know that in Malayan forest rats there is a strong tendency for conceptions to be most frequent in the period before full moon. This is true for the nocturnal forest species and, to a less marked degree, for house rats and the rats on an oil-palm estate, but not for day-active forest squirrels (Cloudsley-Thompson 1980: 100, citing Harrison 1954).

The hormone melatonin has been shown to inhibit ovulation in rats as well as in some monkeys. The synthesis of this hormone is inhibited by light (references in Dewan et al. 1978). Consequently, it has been argued that a possible mechanism for ovulation-synchronisation by means of exposure to nocturnal light exists (Dewan et al. 1978). If true, this would mean that early hominids in the Rift Valley could have standardised their synchrony even hundreds of miles from tidal shores, merely by sleeping out under the moon. Once again, however, it must be stressed that we have no independent evidence for this. The nearest we have to evidence is the fact that the menstrual cycles of modern females are clearly light-sensitive and have the same average phase-length as the moon.

The Moon and Culture: Some Hypotheses

J. L. Cloudsley-Thompson (1980: 100) is a leading authority on biological clocks. He keeps an open mind on the evolutionary origins of the human menstrual body-clock, declining to rule out the possibility that it may be the manifestation of what was once a true circalunadian rhythm. He suggests that a civilised, indoor life with artificial lighting may now be the factor which prevents most women from synchronising. This would make contemporary women's typical failure to keep in step with the moon 'unnatural' – a product of civilised artificial lighting and culture.

Unfortunately, this view is contradicted by persuasive evidence that a randomisation of menstrual cycles with respect to the moon has long been typical in most known human cultures, whether 'civilised' or not. Such evidence suggests that it is mating systems – what social anthropologists term 'systems of kinship and marriage' – which are the primary determinants, not light availability considered in isolation.

The social anthropologist Tim Buckley's (1982) work on the Yurok Indians of California will be examined later in this book, since it indicates the possibility of a Yurok tradition of widespread lunar phase-locking which broke down at some point in the fairly recent past. It may well be that similar patterns of synchrony were widely prevalent among Amerindians and others until quite recently, and indeed some evidence of this will be surveyed in Chapters 9–14.

Nonetheless, such patterns were not in recent times universal and probably would have been unusual even among those hunters and gatherers least influenced by western culture over the past few centuries.

Given Aboriginal Australians' long resistance to farming and horticultural influences, their continent might have seemed a good place to look for synchrony, yet it is certainly not the case that all Aboriginal women everywhere synchronised their periods with one another or with the moon in the recent pre-contact period. There is in fact little evidence for synchrony except in coastal Arnhem Land, where traditions of synchrony linked with 'the rainbow snake' have lived on until recent times, in Western Australia in the form of certain suggestive rock-paintings, and in Central Australia where myths depict synchrony as a basic feature of the ancestral Dreamtime (see Chapters 12–14). Such evidence is of course significant. But if a pattern of maintaining synchrony were once widespread, it must have started breaking down in Australia as in most other parts of the world millennia before the emergence of modern civilisation or the sustained use of artificial lighting.

One conclusion which adherents of the lunar hypothesis might draw is that gender politics and mating systems have in most regions changed dramatically since the Late Pleistocene, and that the pressures these exert have always overridden all other factors in determining whether synchrony will occur.

A slightly different view has been put forward by Cambridge experimental psychologist Nick Humphrey, a figure well known for his pioneering work on the social functions of primate intelligence (Humphrey 1976; see Byrne and Whiten 1988). Humphrey's hypothesis was put forward to explain the results of a survey which he had helped to conduct.

Together with a third-year undergraduate assistant, Humphrey (1982) asked 500 students, 150 of them women, to indicate the phase which they believed the moon to be in on that particular day. The women among them were also asked to say when their last menstrual period had occurred. The results were surprising.

The answers concerning the moon were quite wrong. The students had no real idea which phase the moon was in. Two-thirds said it was waning, when in fact it was waxing. Men had a particular tendency to view the moon as waning. But strangely, women's answers bore a systematic relationship to the positions they were in within their menstrual cycles. In the words of Humphrey (1982):

> Around the middle of the cycle, around the time we would guess they were ovulating, they showed a strong shift over to seeing the moon as waxing – a very significant effect. And during the menstrual period they showed an even more significant tendency than men, who were the control group, to seeing it as waning.

Interestingly, this was only true of women who were having normal cycles; those who were on the contraceptive pill – who were menstruating every month but not producing an egg – did not show the effect at the middle of the cycle, although they did show it at menstruation. As Humphrey himself stresses, it would seem difficult to explain these findings except on the assumption that women entrained their cycles to the moon's phases at some time in their evolutionary past.

From all these studies, the conclusion which emerges is that women are probably capable of entraining their cycles to the moon's phases, but conditions have to be ideal. If the moon's weak light were to be found entraining women's cycles unconsciously and automatically under artificially lit modern conditions, it would be surprising indeed. The evidence is that it does not happen, or happens so rarely and unpredictably as to amount to near-suppression of any 'lunar effect'.

Early humans sleeping in trees overhanging expanses of water in tropical Africa would doubtless have been more easily influenced – if, that is, light from the moon or tides can affect the human metabolism at all. But even in their case, sexual politics acting in a negative direction would have over-ridden any synchronising effects. If Foley (1987) is correct and early hominids were unavoidably organised in one-male harem units, then wide-spread synchrony would have been maladaptive, since it would have inten-sified harassment by setting female harem members in severe sexual conflict with one another for the few available males (Chapter 6). Females aiming to minimise such harassment within the constraints set by the system would have done best to ignore any lunar or tidal environmental cues.

On the other hand, in those 'multi-male' cases where such constraints had been overridden and synchrony was occurring, evolving humans are unlikely to have been passively reliant on the tides, the moon or any other cues. Some female populations would have been synchronising widely, others would have been synchronising less consistently. The physical impact of moonlight or of tidal cues would have been quite secondary in deciding such matters. If certain populations of protowomen were synchronising consistently not only with one another but also with the moon and tides, it would not have been because in the localities concerned such environmental rhythms were so powerful as to entrain or enslave women. It would have been because detecting the appropriate cues in order actively to synchronise was in these particular females' sexual-political interests.

We know from Chapter 6 that had evolving human females needed synchrony sufficiently, they would have maintained it at least on a local level even far from the coasts or under cloud-covered skies. On the other hand, where females had access to the appropriate cues and were required to synchronise, but lacked the resources to sustain their spatial proximity, problems would have arisen. Evidence from contemporary hunter-gatherers suggests, as we will see, that as anatomically modern women left their former coastal environments for the continental hinterlands in the course of the Upper Palaeolithic revolution, they did encounter severe problems. Their vegetationally sparse new habitat was not capable of sustaining large groups of females all foraging together within a restricted area. On the other hand, they needed a solution which enabled them to survive in this habitat without leaving their ancient traditions of tidal synchrony behind. Since synchrony's old conditions were vanishing, anatomically modern protowomen had to seek ways of preserving their menstrual and reproductive harmony – their 'witchcraft' or 'magic', as it would become conceptualised – in novel ways. In the end, they broke their umbilical cords, abandoned their ancient shoreline habitats – and in the new situation used massage, sweating, ritual bathing, dance, night-long firelight and moon-scheduled celebratory sexual intercourse to augment any effects that nature's weakened clocks on their own might have had. Using such extraordinary new 'artistic' devices as body-paint, sound-making instruments and elaborate choreography, they sustained and intensified their synchrony to the point where the harnessing of male provisioning energies could match the challenges of the new environment in which they lived, releasing child-burdened females from the need to find their own food for themselves. It was in the course of this woman-inspired process that symbolic culture – forged centrally in what social anthropologists term 'the ritual domain' – was at last born.

Chapter 8
Between Water, Stone and Fire

No social order ever disappears before all the productive forces for which there is room in it have been developed; and new, higher relations of production never appear before the material conditions of their existence have matured in the womb of the old society. Therefore, mankind always sets itself only such problems as it can solve; since, on closer examination, it will always be found that the problem itself arises only when the material conditions necessary for its solution already exist or are at least in the process of formation.
Karl Marx, Preface to *A Contribution to the Critique of Political Economy* (1859)

The emergence of human culture was a revolutionary event. To say this is not new: a succession of authoritative writers have spoken of 'the human revolution' in this context (Hockett and Ascher 1964; Montagu 1965; Holloway 1969; Collins 1976; Mellars and Stringer 1989). Until very recently, however, the idea has seemed less than convincing. The concept of revolution has seemed to be belied by the extreme gradualism of the prevailing palaeontological and archaeological scenarios (Chapter 5). If a human way of life began to be established in the Plio-Pleistocene, yet was still being established two million years later towards the end of the Pleistocene, how can this lengthy and very gradual process be termed a 'revolution'? Can a revolution last two million years?

As we have seen, however, the dates no longer pose such a problem. The scenarios of the 1970s and early 1980s are now largely discredited. Few believe any longer in the gradualist theory of a two-million-year long epoch of 'steady progress' towards a human lifestyle. It is now widely agreed that in the million and more years prior to the Upper Palaeolithic, any discernible cultural advance or 'progress' was in most areas exceedingly and indeed quite astonishingly slow (Binford 1984). Since late in the 1980s, on the other hand, molecular biologists have been producing exciting new evidence that all anatomically modern, symbolic-culture-bearing humans are the genetic descendants of a single fast-developing sub-Saharan African population which first appeared only some 200,000 years ago (see pp. 269–72). This new information makes postulated events in the distant Plio-Pleistocene now seem rather less relevant.

A Recent Perspective

In this and the following chapters, it is not intended to dwell further on the early biological preconditions of the human revolution. Although key elements of Turke's sociobiological model will be drawn on, it is intended to focus on the social processes underpinning the later, cultural, stages – the development of variegated tool-kits, of logistic big game hunting, cooking, systems of notation, art, dance, music, ritual and, in short, the final, stable establishment of a cultural way of life in its fully modern, symbolic, form some 45,000 or so years ago.

Compared with Plio-Pleistocene frameworks, this recent perspective imposes fairly rigid constraints upon the weaving of 'just-so' stories. Speculative narratives whose only requirement is to conclude with a picture of the known end-result can be quickly dismissed; we have far more solid information on the various stages in the transition to modern humans than for any of the earlier major transitions in the hominisation process (Pilbeam 1986; Mellars 1988). We can test our models because, firstly, modern humans are still living today so that our biological make-up can be directly studied, physiologically, psychologically, sociobiologically and in other ways. Secondly, the fossil record for the Late Pleistocene is quite good. Thirdly, archaeological finds – including evidence for the appearance of self-adornment, burial practices, ritual and art – constitute potentially decodable messages yielding information on at least some aspects of the symbolic and social structures of the prehistoric communities we are interested in.

Fourthly, a focus on modern humans renders hunter-gatherer studies fully relevant for the first time, so that social anthropologists' cross-cultural findings can act as a further check on our model-building. Whilst no surviving human culture can constitute a model of earliest *sapient* life, it is not unreasonable to suppose that certain recurrent patterns – for example the striking near-universality of 'classificatory' modes of reckoning kinship, or the prevalence of mythological patterns of something like the kind isolated by Lévi-Strauss in his *Mythologiques* – convey information on traditions stretching back to the last ice age. Actual human social formations have certainly changed and diversified virtually limitlessly since that time, but it is also true that cultures can resist change to an astonishing extent, particularly where religious ideology is concerned. An extreme example is the Northern Australian Aboriginal cult of the rainbow snake, chronicled in rock art as extending in an unbroken tradition for up to 9,000 years (Flood 1983). In the concluding chapters of this book, we will draw heavily on evidence of this kind.

Tool-making: The First Two Million Years

Stone tool-making, fire-tending and an increasing dependence on meat food were central to the human revolution. However, in their earliest manifestations these potentially momentous developments apparently did little to revolutionise social and political life. Rather, it seems that for millennia, our ancestors maintained sociopolitical continuity with their primate past – at the cost of missing out on the full potential of the technological advances they were experimenting with. It was to be two million years after the first stone tools and perhaps a million or more from the harnessing of fire before the evolution of technology, physiology and brains would eventually create the material conditions for a breakthrough to symbolic culture.

The tool-making traditions of the Lower Palaeolithic are known as Pre-Oldowan, Oldowan, Developed Oldowan, or (more generally) 'chopper-core' industries. Modified beach pebbles, such tools were of all shapes and sizes: there was no symmetry and no repertoire of standardised patterns. These first tools, according to one psychologist's report (Wynn 1988: 277), 'do not argue for an intelligence greater than that known for apes'. About a million and a half years separates the first of these industries in East Africa from Oldowan industries of Middle Pleistocene date. Crudely flaked pebble implements characterised the beginning of this immensely long period, beginning anything up to about 3.0 million years ago; tool-kits of essentially the same type were still dominant at the end of it. In the words of one specialist 'It is difficult to comprehend such slow development. Man had certainly evolved physically: he was now bigger both in stature and in brain capacity' (Wymer 1982: 98) The puzzle is to explain why, despite substantial biological evolution, very little technological advance appears to have taken place in all this time.

About 1.4 million years ago however, an industry appears with implements known as 'hand-axes'. These tend to be well-made, symmetrical, bifacial tools of pointed or oval shape, all made to a standardised pattern. Unlike the pebble tools, their manufacture has been estimated to have required levels of intelligence far beyond that of any ape (Wynn 1988).

The hand-axe traditions are known as 'Acheulean', and are the characteristic products of *Homo erectus* (who first appears in the fossil record of East Africa about 1.7 million years ago), although it is again significant that technological evolution clearly lagged behind biology, the earliest hand-axes dating back to 1.4 million years at most. Hand-axe-using groups seem to have begun moving out from Africa into southern Eurasia about a million years ago – about 500,000 years after the first appearance of hand-axes in the archaeological record.

The most extraordinary feature of the Acheulean hand-axe tradition is its monotonous uniformity. It might have been expected that local conditions – the availability of different plant resources or species of game, for example –

would have given rise to specific, localised methods of foraging, in turn reflected in locally distinctive specialised tool-kits. But instead, the same basic design for a 'hand-axe' is replicated unimaginatively all over the world – from southern Africa to northern England, from Spain to India.

Most specialists admit to having little idea of the function of these tools. The puzzle has indeed been described as 'the greatest enigma of Lower Palaeolithic archaeology' (Wymer 1982: 102). The problem would lessen if it could be demonstrated that these implements facilitated greater hunting success. But no such evidence exists.

Hand-axes were not good hunting weapons. Too heavy to be hafted to spear-shafts or thrown, they do not even look like particularly good cutting tools, although at least occasional involvement with the butchery of elephants and other large *scavenged* animals has been documented (Binford 1987; Villa 1990: 302n). Some of the large, pointed hand-axes could also have been used for digging – but as Wymer (1982: 103) points out, 'experiments show that they are not much use in this respect, and far less efficient than a suitably shaped stick'.

The commonest form of hand-axe is a very small, poorly made tool that 'does not look useful for anything' (Wymer 1982: 103). Yet in certain levels at some sites – for example Olorgesaile in Kenya, and Swanscombe in England – such axes are extremely numerous, almost to the exclusion of any other implements (Wymer 1982: 103, 106). One theory is that the 'axes' were not primarily tools at all – their basic function was to act as a source of flint from which to chip off usable, sharp-edged flakes from time to time (Hayden 1979).

It used to be argued that because they are so stereotyped, hand-axes provide evidence for true cultural life. Their standardised symmetrical shapes, according to a well-known formulation of this idea (Holloway 1969, 1981), represent the human collectivity's imposition of 'arbitrary form' upon the environment, indicating the presence of hominids capable of constructing and enforcing grammatical, social, moral and technological 'rules'. Other authors – such as Jolly and Plog (1986: 289) in their popular textbook on archaeology and evolution – envisage *Homo erectus* possessing not only hearths and home bases but also 'language, ritual, complex social relationships, and refined tool-making techniques'. They base such inferences in part on the uniformity of hand-axe designs; this is stated to be a sign of cultural-level learning, transmission and diffusion of techniques and traditions.

Such interpretations are almost certainly wrong. If the hominids of this period were cultural, we would expect uniformity on some levels – but also much greater diversity on others.

Had the hand-axe makers been involved in a truly collectivist, cultural framework of action, this would have released individuals from the need to replicate one another's activities: numerous different roles could have complemented one another in the joint pursuit of common goals. Moreover, with sufficient co-operation and trust, there is no fear that particularly valuable tools will be appropriated by some competitor or rival. There is no need to carry tools on one's person at all times – even precious implements can be left at caches or with trusted allies or kin until they are needed. Again, this allows for a much more variegated community-wide tool-kit than when each individual must guard against theft and carry everywhere a full personal survival kit. Collectivity, in other words, means less need for 'all-purpose' tools. There is no need for each individual to limit the tool-kit to the personally required bare essentials – to one or a few multi-purpose tools portable enough to be kept close to the body and guarded at all times.

Finally, although a cultural framework implies standardisation of tool-kits within local communities, it also produces wide diversity between distant communities as these adapt in different ways to contrasting local conditions. The same factors also lead to relatively rapid stylistic and other changes over time. We do not expect to find tools of essentially identical design being replicated over an area stretching from Britain to India for over a million years. The homogeneity and conservatism of the hand-axe tradition suggests 'that it as yet retained the character of a general species-specific behaviour, not subject to cultural level processes of stylistic differentiation, formal classification and fairly rapid change' (Richards 1987: 281; see also Binford 1989: 28–9).

Despite important advances (for example Villa 1990), the problem of explaining the hand-axe traditions has still not been solved. What we do know is that with the arrival of the Neanderthals, a wide variety of standardised tool shapes for the first time began to evolve, and that with the emergence of modern humans, this variety increased radically whilst hand-axes totally disappeared. The efficient and co-operative hunters and gatherers of the Upper Palaeolithic had no use for such implements at all.

To survive for a million years with basically the same technology can be seen in its own terms as no small achievement. Cranial capacity increased by about 20 per cent over those years, so presumably social complexity was also increasing. But by cultural-historical standards, the hand-axe people appear locked in a kind of 'time-warp', incapable of more than a snail's pace of technological advance. It is impossible to avoid the question: Why?

In the light of the primate evidence surveyed in Chapters 4 and 5, we can glimpse the outlines of an answer. If Lower and Middle Pleistocene hand-axe makers were socially and sexually organised in *anything like* the manner of baboons or chimpanzees, the problems posed by a weapons-technology would have been daunting. We have only to imagine Goodall's 'Satan' equipped with a hand-axe to appreciate this. The danger would have been that hand-axes or other weapons would have been used not as 'collective hunting implements', and not only as all-purpose tools for cutting and pounding, but from time to time also as instruments for settling scores, as males battled with one another for meat and for access to females along the lines which Parker (1987) indeed suggests. Our ancestors' evolving weapons technology would then have been turned dangerously inwards, instead of being directed outwards towards external nature as it is (at least for the most part) among modern human hunters and gatherers. Wymer (1982: 106) may be hinting at this sombre possibility in writing in this context that 'tradition may have outweighed rational behaviour'. He continues:

> There are so many puzzling factors about hand-axes that the answers may well be outside a straightforward, rational explanation and lie in the realms of human behaviour rather than function.

When hand-axes were first discovered in European gravel pits, they were popularly described as 'fighting stones'. Wymer comments that the implements 'would have been useless as hand weapons, unless hunters were fighting each other, which may have occasionally happened' (Wymer 1982: 103). Whatever its scientific merits, the idea that hand-axes were used in fights has always had a certain popularity (see, for example, Lorenz 1966: 208).

Archaeologists are not usually trained to think in sociobiological or primatological terms. But perhaps they have been mistaken to assume that every 'human' artefact-type must have had a positively useful 'function' in relation to 'the species' or 'the group'. Group functionality may be relevant once the cultural-symbolic stage has been reached, but there is little to suggest that tool-makers during the Middle Pleistocene were 'cultural' in anything like a modern sense (Binford 1989). Consequently, a wholly different conceptual framework seems to be required.

If we are dealing with a non-cultural evolutionary process, then it seems appropriate to use a sociobiological approach. We should set out from the individual as the unit of selection, not 'the species' or 'the group'. In this context, we should ask how possession of a hand-axe might have contributed to an individual's genetic fitness.

Homo erectus was a heavy-faced, large-jawed creature with enormous brow ridges (Collins 1986: 149–50). Compared with both *Australopithecus* and modern humans, his skull was extraordinarily thick: 12.5 mm in the case of the Swanscombe occipital, 11 mm for the parietal. Values for Zhoukoudian exceed 18 mm on occasion, whereas the figures for most modern humans are little over a third of this (Collins 1986: 148–9, and references).

No doubt the need for heavy chewing and use of the teeth as tools was partly responsible for the large teeth and jaws, but why was 'Beijing Man's' skull in places three times as thick as ours? Like the massive brow ridges, this feature suggests at least some function in terms of self-protection, possibly in the context of occasional fights. Some fighting does not seem intrinsically improbable: sexual dimorphism was by modern standards pronounced, a fact which has led many writers to infer that *Homo erectus*, like other early hominids, had some kind of polygamous mating system in which the more dominant males gained access to the most females (Foley 1987: 171 and references; Parker 1987). Could it be that the million-year-long Acheulean tradition represented a period in which, in many localities, every male simply 'had to' be the owner of a hand-axe or other weapon, as much for reasons of personal and sexual security as to facilitate hunting or foraging?

We do not have to envisage constant *Homo erectus* violence for an interpretation along the lines suggested here to seem persuasive. Although there has been a long-standing controversy over 'Beijing Man's' alleged 'cannibalism' (Poirier 1973: 140; Binford 1981), hand-axes are not found at Zhoukoudian, nor at other far eastern *Homo erectus* sites. Yet it is these specimens of *Homo* which have the thickest skulls of all. Perhaps the Eastern groups used weapons made of materials which have not survived. Where these *or* stone hand-axes were used, they may well have been all-purpose tools, used for opportunistic hunting, butchering and various other activities, but capable of being used in self-defence when necessary.

All this would fit well with Parker's (1987) 'sexual selection' model of hominid evolution (Chapter 5). In the light of all that we know of the size, shape and distribution of hand-axes, and in the light of what seems to be a picture of social and economic near-stasis throughout this immensely long period, it is a tempting (even if only partial) explanation. It links a plausible set of productive and other functions for these strange tools with male behaviour of a kind which does not seem too difficult to envisage, which is familiar from an indefinite number of primatological accounts, and which – in the period preceding the 'human revolution' – might well have constituted a sexual-political brake upon social and economic development.

Fire

The development of pyrotechnology presents a similar set of puzzles. Eventually, as we will see, fire proved an important factor assisting proto-women in defining and defending their own domestic space, this achievement in turn underpinning the immense sexual-political and symbolic changes associated with the Upper Palaeolithic revolution. But it is surprising how long it was before females apparently succeeded in making full use of cooking fire as an economic and political resource.

Except in northerly regions and tropical rain forests, fire is one of the natural hazards which most animal life must periodically face. Bush-fires are particularly common in the drier savanna regions of tropical East Africa (Foley 1987, citing Harris 1980). For most animals, such fires are extremely frightening, the only appropriate response being flight. But this is not always so. Even when flames are raging through the bush, falcons and kites may hover over them to hunt fleeing birds and insects. Later, quadruped predators visit the smouldering remains in search of prey; and later still, ungulates venture near to lick at the salted ashes. 'Most animals', comments Goudsblom (1986: 518–19), 'enjoy the warmth radiated at night by the site of an extinguished fire'. For early hominids, the task would have been gradually to build on such familiarity, extending or preserving local fires by feeding them, slowly gaining an increasing measure of control.

Without fire, meat reserves cannot be kept overnight at a campsite. Apart from other problems, it has been pointed out that bears and wolves are attracted by the smells, posing a danger to sleeping offspring (Schaller and Lowther 1969: 335; Potts 1984b, 1988). For millennia, one of the few things capable of *reliably* keeping carnivores from non-arboreal sleeping-sites may have been the visible blaze of a fire.

In addition to providing warmth, protection and nocturnal light, fire can in principle be used to dry out materials, to harden wood, or to preserve food by drying or smoking. Among fire's other uses, well-timed grass-burning may amount to something close to farming, in the sense that the new shoots may tempt game within range of hunters – a technique skilfully developed by Australian Aborigines with their firesticks (Hallam 1975). Alternatively, grassland can be fired over a wide area so as to encircle herds of game.

Finally, fire can of course be used for cooking, a process which removes toxins from plant foods (Leopold and Ardrey 1972; Stahl 1984) and makes meat and bone marrow easier to consume. In enabling each group to extract more from its surroundings, increased cooking efficiency would have allowed bands – perhaps most significantly their female members with dependent offspring – to remain longer in each occupied locality before having to move on.

Because humans are the only animals to control fire, we are handicapped in constructing models of its early use: materials for cross-species comparisons are not available. It has been suggested that several different Plio-Pleistocene hominid species may originally have been involved with fire, each using it in its own, species-specific way (Barbetti 1986; Gowlett et al. 1981; Brain and Sillen 1988; Goudsblom 1986). Chimpanzees being rehabilitated into the wild in Senegal have been observed to manage camp-fires in a rudimentary manner, and to collect and eat roasted seeds after a bush-fire (McGrew 1989: 16, citing Brewer 1978), so the idea that early *Homo* or even *Australopithecus* may have achieved this level is perhaps not far-fetched.

A recurrent mistake has been to project modern concepts of fire use back on to the distant past. Whenever early fire traces have been found in association with hominid remains, writers have imagined a dutiful husband bringing meat for his wife to cook in the glowing embers of their camp-fire.

The tendency has been to associate fire almost automatically with a home base, with food-sharing – and with a sexual division of labour on the model of modern hunters and gatherers.

In fact, there is no evidence for domestic fire until about 250,000 years ago, whilst *structured* hearths – for example, deep pits lined or banked around with heat-conserving stones – do not make their appearance until considerably later (James 1989: 9). All the evidence indicates that despite the presence of occasional shallow fires, the camps of early hominids were radically different from those of modern hunter-gatherers, being rather more akin to the temporarily occupied, ever-shifting sleeping sites of chimpanzees.

During excavations at the Swartkrans cave in South Africa late in the 1980s, burnt bones were found and dated to about 1.0 to 1.5 million years ago – an astonishingly early date if the burning indicates the artificial control of fire. The bones were found in association with tools of the Developed Oldowan tradition. The archaeologists responsible for this excavation (Brain and Sillen 1988) stress that fire in this cave was 'a regular event' in the period before *Australopithecus robustus* had become extinct; since robust australopithecine remains are also found in the same levels, it has even been suggested that *robustus* was the fire user.

Another site giving an early claimed date for fire use is Chesowanja, near Lake Baringo, in Kenya. Here, in sediments dated to over 1.4 million years, a 'hearth-like' concentration of stones is said to have been found, associated with lumps of burnt clay. However, no burnt bones were found at this site, and it may be that a smouldering tree trunk set alight in a bush-fire was responsible for the burnt clay (Gowlett *et al.* 1981, 1982; Gowlett 1984; Isaac 1982).

Other claimed early fire sites have been Yuanmou in China (Jia 1985), FxJj20 at Karari at East Turkana (Isaac and Harris 1978), and Gadeb in Ethiopia (Barbetti *et al.* 1980). Some of these sites may be more than a million years old (Gowlett 1984: 182), but even where this has been confirmed, Binford and his students dispute whether fires at such early dates were produced by hominids. It seems significant that there is a complete absence of evidence for fire use at Olduvai Gorge in Tanzania. On the basis of this and other negative evidence, James (1989: 4) has in fact argued that the baked clays, charred organic remains and other finds at sites such as Chesowanja must have been produced by natural fires or volcanic activity.

Numerous claims for European Acheulean and pre-Mousterian hearths – such as Lazaret (Alpes-Maritimes), Pech de l'Azé (Dordogne), Orgnac III (Ardèche) and Grotte de Rigabe (Var) – have been made, the sites being dated to the Riss glaciation, about 360,000 to 330,000 years ago. The site of St. Esteve (dated to about 500,000 years) in Provence has fire traces. Vértesszöllös in Hungary had charred bone in the occupation deposits of perhaps 400,000 years (Kretzoi and Vértes 1965), while scattered traces of charcoal were found at Torralba and Ambrona in Spain, dating to perhaps 360,000 years (Freeman 1975; Collins 1986: 253). Outside Europe, the deposits at Zhoukoudian probably date to about 480,000 years ago, and reveal apparent sporadic traces of fire throughout, possibly produced by *Homo erectus* (but see Binford and Ho 1985). However, a reanalysis of the literature by James (1989) suggests that many of these claims are questionable: there is no firm evidence for *domestic* fire, he concludes, prior to 250,000 years ago. Such a date would at least enable us to include one of the most celebrated (if still not fully authenticated) of all early 'campsites' – Terra Amata in southern France, which has produced the earliest claimed indication of an artificially constructed shelter of some kind associated with the use of fire. On a beach near Nice about 230,000 years ago (Wintle and Aitken 1977), several huts are said to have been built by shoreline foragers over a period of about a century, one floor above the remnants of another, often enclosing a charred area (De Lumley 1969; Villa 1983). Several burned mussel shell fragments have been found in the deposits (Villa 1983: 80–1). The claimed 'hearths', however, are usually described as 'unprepared'. It is not until much later – generally as part of the Middle-to-Upper Palaeolithic transition – that hearths shifted from being thermally inefficient shallow depressions or flat surfaces that would radiate little heat to effective structures (including stone-lined pits) which would have cooked food effectively and conserved heat for extended periods of time.

Until fire could be kindled at will, there would have been strong incentives within each local group to ensure that at least one accessible fire, somewhere, was kept constantly burning. In seeking an ethnographic analogy, Oakley (1958) notes one modern Northampton family who claim to have kept their cottage peat fire burning without a break for 200 years! To keep an Early or Middle Pleistocene fire burning for months on end would have been an immense challenge; in meeting it, a section of society – presumably mainly older individuals and females – would increasingly have had to be entrusted to remain behind during extended foraging expeditions to protect and feed the fire. Unfortunately the *political* preconditions of such a division of responsibilities have rarely been properly examined.

Wherever fire-using hominids were governed by a primate-style social and sexual logic, fire as such may only have added to the problems touched on in Chapter 5. It is even possible to envisage a scenario in which early hominids treated the resource as a scarce value to be competed for and from which to exclude rivals. Selection pressures may in this context have favoured males who strove to keep close at all times to 'their' females and, by implication, to 'their' fires. This would not have enhanced hunting efficiency. In an atmosphere of sexual mistrust, how many males would have been prepared to go away from their females and associated camp-fires, staying out in the cold overnight on an extended hunting trip? In male eyes, would the possible benefits have outweighed the risks?

Much evidence suggests that problems of some such kind may not have been fully solved until the final establishment of symbolic culture by anatomically modern humans. It seems that although they had loosely prepared, temporary hearths and camps, neither *Homo erectus* nor the Neanderthals were capable of the kind of organisation in which the group can periodically split into distinct parties each with its own logistic task (Binford 1980, 1981, 1983, 1984, 1989; Binford and Ho 1985; Binford and Stone 1986; James 1989). The probability is that females in early populations were simply not permitted to stay in charge of a constantly burning fire while males went off to hunt. At its worst, we may suspect, the picture was just the opposite. Males were tempted to keep close to the fire at all times, and because of their insecurities, kept taking 'their' females and fire with them whenever they moved. Not only would this have been bad for mothers with young babies. Constant movement dictated by foraging concerns would have done little to ensure that precarious fires stayed alight.

In other words, fire's potentialities may at first have been constrained by the limitations of a basically primate-like social system. And if all this was the case, then we can say that inseparable from all the other problems was the probability that to begin with, fire was – like much of the rest of life – basically under male political control. Females might have seemed ideally placed to take power in this domain, assuming the responsibilities of 'guardians of the hearth'. But prior to the Upper Palaeolithic revolution, the female sex had not yet wrested fire away, established its semi-permanence at a given site, and made it the focal point of a specifically female domain.

The Neanderthal Problem

The final, culturally-expansionist phase of the human revolution seems to have been entered about 45,000 years ago (Binford 1989). In the Near East and in North Africa, anatomically modern humans make their appearance in the archaeological record from about 100,000 years ago. At the time of writing, the evidence suggests that from this time onwards, they lived in the Near East *without* fully developed symbolic culture for something like 60,000 years – a period during which the long-standing Neanderthal occupation of Europe was not affected. Why the thriving Near Eastern modern humans did not break out into Europe during this lengthy period is something of a mystery (Stringer 1988). We know that towards the end of this period they spread across Asia quite rapidly – fully cultural modern humans were already in Australia as early as 40,000 years ago and perhaps even before that. One conclusion which seems reasonably safe is that events in Europe were peripheral to the processes in which culture as such was born.

The European Neanderthals only became extinct about 30,000 years ago, presumably as a consequence of changes in their environment brought about by the eventual arrival in Europe of modern humans – with whom there seems to have been little or no interbreeding (Stringer 1988). Populations of modern humans came up from the Levant and seem to have begun percolating into Central Europe from about 38,000 to 42,000 years ago, establishing a new tradition of tool-making known as the Aurignacian, which was characterised by heavy retouching and a proliferation in the production of intricate tools made from antler and bone. After some delay, these peoples then began to spread into Western Europe, completely displacing the Neanderthal former inhabitants over a period of perhaps 3,000 years (Dibble 1983; Leroyer and Leroi-Gourhan 1983; Stringer *et al.* 1984; Harrold 1988). Although this meant a relatively sharp break in continuity, the new arrivals in Central Europe at first lived sparsely and with a material culture containing significant elements taken from the Mousterian traditions of their Neanderthal predecessors (Hoffecker 1988; Straus and Heller 1988).

In the 1960s and early 1970s (Breuil and Lantier 1959; Maringer 1960; Solecki 1975), it was widely agreed that the Neanderthals offered grave goods to their buried dead, believed in an afterlife, cared for the sick, engaged in bear cults and other totemic rites, spoke complex languages, hunted big game, cooked and shared their meat – and were the forerunners of modern humans both genetically and in terms of cultural tradition. In short, there were no radical differences to be discerned between Neanderthal lifestyles and those of their 'modern' descendants, so that the notion of a sudden 'human revolution' establishing symbolic culture made very little sense.

In the 1970s and more particularly the 1980s, this view came under sustained attack. One contribution came from two researchers (Lieberman and Crelin 1971) who examined Neanderthal skulls and concluded (mistakenly, it now seems: Arensburg *et al.* 1989) that their supralaryngeal vocal tracts would not have enabled them to produce the full range of sounds necessary for human speech. Other investigations led to the claim that female Neanderthals must have had a radically different reproductive physiology from modern humans, with a gestation period of perhaps thirteen months instead of the modern human nine (Trinkaus 1984). More recently, even the long-accepted idea that the Neanderthals buried their dead has been challenged (Gargett 1989), whilst others have shown that we have little more than isolated, fragmentary and disputable suggestions of Neanderthal necklaces or other items of personal ornamentation (Chase and Dibble 1987).

Findings of this kind converged with others touched on earlier in this book. As mentioned already, from the late 1960s onwards, Lewis Binford began arguing forcefully that 'culture' in its modern sense could not have arisen until the Upper Palaeolithic revolution, and that the Neanderthals had settlement systems and subsistence strategies quite different from those of contemporary hunter-gatherers and other modern humans. Although Binford probably overstated his case, archaeologists recently have been much less ready to see evidence for hunter-gatherer-like behaviour in the Middle Palaeolithic archaeological record.

Despite these findings, until late in the 1980s it was still widely assumed that there was a direct ancestor-descendant relationship between the Neanderthals and modern humans, at least in the Near East, where the two populations had long been known to have lived close to one another in space and in time. It was therefore a shock to discover that even this idea would probably have to be abandoned.

Perhaps the most decisive event in this connection was the publication of a brief report in the journal *Nature*, in 1988. It described the use of the new thermoluminescence technique to determine the age of burnt flints in Mousterian levels in Qafzeh Cave in Israel — levels which had earlier yielded some anatomically modern ('Proto-Cro-Magnon') fossils (Valladas *et al.* 1988). It turned out that the levels and hence the fossils were 92,000 years old — twice as old as had previously been guessed. Such 'modern' people could not possibly have evolved from the local Neanderthals — because they were not younger, but about 30,000 years older than the earliest known Neanderthals in the region (Stringer 1988)! On the basis of this and other evidence, it is now known that anatomically modern humans were living in the Levant as far back as 90,000 to 100,000 years ago, whereas Neanderthals arrived in the region — perhaps retreating from the intense cold in Europe — only about 60,000 years ago. In at least one cave, there is evidence that modern humans eventually moved out, to be replaced by Neanderthals, who were in turn replaced much later by a new population of culture-bearing moderns. The Neanderthals then appear to have become extinct.

All of this information — and particularly the age of the Qafzeh fossils — gave the severest of jolts to Regional Continuity as a model of human evolution in this part of the world. As the London Natural History Museum's Chris Stringer (1988) was quick to point out:

> The palaeoanthropological implications of such an age are enormous. . . . Evolutionary models centred on a direct ancestor-descendant relationship between Neanderthals and modern *H. sapiens* must surely now be discarded, along with associated schemes designed to explain such a transition.

The finding that resident modern humans and intruding Neanderthals coexisted in the Near East side by side for about 60,000 years, apparently with little if any interbreeding, has led some writers (Stringer 1988; Foley 1989) to suggest that the two groups must have been entirely distinct species, not sub-species of *Homo sapiens* at all.

The Qafzeh dates delivered the heaviest blow to an orthodoxy which had retained at least some of its credibility until late in the 1980s. Under these circumstances, 'Regional Continuity' could not even be resuscitated by the astonishing discovery in France of fossil Neanderthals who had evidently been making and using Upper Palaeolithic stone tools. In an earlier period, this would undoubtedly have been taken as ruling out any real gulf separating Neanderthal from modern cultural traditions. But it is now widely suspected that the Upper Palaeolithic (Chatelperronian) technology of the Neanderthals at Saint-Césaire testifies not to an autonomous local attainment of full cultural modernity – but to the impact of newly arrived modern humans upon an ancient Neanderthal lifestyle. It seems as if the retreating Neanderthals at first began to learn advanced tool-making patterns from the new arrivals, although this did not prevent them from becoming extinct a few thousand years later (Harrold 1989).

Despite superficial appearances to the contrary, all of this can probably be reconciled with Marshack's (1989) eloquently argued view that the Neanderthals had for millennia been wholly in possession of the *capacity* for symbolic culture, even though this capacity in their case never became fully *realised*. We can rephrase this distinction in the light of Richard Dawkins' (1976) comparison between 'genes' and 'memes' (see Introduction). The breakthrough to cultural evolution required not just the localised replication of sophisticated symbolic memes. Memes had to be able to circulate freely over vast areas. Only this could guarantee that they did not die out with the extinction of particular local populations. And only this could guarantee the necessary element of 'immortality' – that is, guarantee that memes did not die almost as fast as they were born, but instead became widely exchanged, pooled and subject ultimately to global evolution. The late Neanderthals in each inhabited European district seem to have been in principle capable of almost any symbolic invention. But each of their most unexpectedly 'modern'-seeming artistic or other advances – many of which Marshack (1989) has beautifully documented for us – seems to have occurred only in a localised way, usually disappearing in the place of its origin *before* it could become part of the cultural heritage of all Neanderthals as such. This was the Neanderthals' handicap. The capacity for a universalistic *collective pooling* and hence *indefinite cumulative evolution* of cultural knowledge was displayed only by those anatomically modern humans who evolved in Africa and the Near East, eventually displacing the Neanderthals in the earliest stages of the Upper Palaeolithic.

African Eve

No less decisive in revolutionising our recent origins models has been the rise of palaeogenetics – the use of molecular biology to work out past genetic relationships. Although fierce controversies remain, there is now strong support for the belief that contemporary racial diversity is superficial, all anatomically modern humans being not only one species but a very homogenous and recently evolved one. Modern Chinese people – according to this view – are not the direct genetic descendants of Peking Man, any more than modern Europeans are highly evolved Neanderthals. Instead, all contemporary humans, from Hudson's Bay to Ayers Rock, are the descendants of a small population of fully modern humans from Africa who broke out and fanned across the world only a few tens of thousands of years ago.

The most influential studies in this connection were conducted in the late 1980s, most spectacularly in the form of an analysis of sequence variation in modern women's mitochondrial DNA. The mitochondria are tiny energy-generating organs found outside the nucleus of every cell, their location determining that their DNA can be transmitted only matrilineally. Whenever a female has no daughters, therefore, her mitochondrial genetic inheritance is lost – her line simply comes to an end. Rebecca Cann and her colleagues (Cann et al. 1987) deduced on logical grounds that if all of us, throughout the world, were to trace our lines back far enough, the ancestral tree would keep converging until it reached a point. In other words, the mitochondrial DNA now immortalised in us all must ultimately flow from just one ancestral mother.

When measurements of mtDNA from women of different racial origins began to be taken in the mid-1980s, the amount of sequence variation seemed astonishingly small for all modern human populations. One surprise was that the average variation between any two racially distinct groups was much lower than inter-individual variation within each group. In other words, any two Eskimos, or any two Aboriginal Australians, would be likely to have mitochondrial sequences differing much more widely than the average differences separating Eskimos as a whole from Aborigines (or Europeans, or Papua/New Guineans etc.) as a whole.

Assuming mtDNA mutations to be largely neutral – that is, assuming that they make little difference to the fitness of individuals, and so escape the influence of natural selection – then their occurrence and accumulation must be mostly a function of time. The more variability a population possesses, in other words, the older it is. Modern humans show a small (0.57 per cent) variability across all populations, indicating a remarkably recent common ancestor. Since the rate of mtDNA evolution for a wide variety of vertebrates is 2–4 per cent per million years, and since there is much evidence that this also applies to humans (Stoneking and Cann 1989), the human results suggest a common ancestor living between 142,000 and 284,000 years ago.

Although the worldwide mtDNA variation is small, within this restricted range the African gene pool shows greater variation than that of any other group (Stoneking and Cann 1989: 22, table 2.1). Caucasians, for example, show an internal variation of only 0.23 per cent, compared with a 0.47 per cent variation in African populations. This indicates that the evolution of modern humans has been occurring in Africa longer than elsewhere. In fact, it seems that the descendants of 'African Eve' – postulated common ancestress of all modern humans – at an early stage split into two major lines of descendants: (a) the ancestors of several African fully modern groups and (b) a line ancestral to the remaining fully modern African groups, in addition to all the world's other racial groups.

If the transition from anatomically archaic to modern humans had occurred more or less simultaneously in different parts of the world – as the gradualist proponents of 'Regional Continuity' had always held – then the various populations of archaic *Homo* in Asia and Europe would all have made major contributions to the modern human gene pool (Wolpoff *et al.* 1984; Wolpoff 1989). Any common ancestor of all modern humans must have lived before the period when *Homo erectus* populations were first beginning to migrate beyond Africa with their hand-axes or other tools. In that event, the observed pan-human variation in mtDNA and in other genetic phenomena should be very wide, indicating that our common ancestor lived not a mere 200,000 years ago but something more like a million years ago. The fact that such wide mtDNA variation between populations is not observed has been an important factor in persuading many specialists to abandon the theory that the world's various racial groups could have descended locally from middle Pleistocene populations of *Homo erectus*, or from the Neanderthals. Instead, within each continent or region, all contemporary racial groups seem to be recent immigrants from some restricted point of origin within Africa (for both sides of the continuing controversy, see papers in Mellars and Stringer 1989b).

Current molecular research, then, is profoundly changing our understanding of evolutionary timescales and of the genetic background to human cultural origins, and the next few years are likely to see exciting further developments. 'African Eve' herself would appear to be little more than a logical construct. She may before long fade from fashion, and has in any case recently been joined by a perhaps still more ephemeral 'Adam' (Lucotte 1989). Nonetheless, the population to which either construct refers presumably existed, and we can usefully ask what it was about this population which destined the mitochondrial inheritance of one of its number to become immortalised in every single living member of the human species.

We know that Eve's genetic constitution was under selection-pressures leading to the anatomy and physiology of modern woman. We know that modern offspring mature slowly compared with Neanderthal offspring (Trinkaus 1986; Bromage and Dean 1985; Dean *et al.* 1986), and that male parental contributions must have been increasing to cope with the consequent added parenting burdens. Linking this to our previous discussion of Paul Turke's (1984) model, we might infer that if evolving protohuman females ever followed the ovarian synchrony strategy, then Eve and her kin must surely have been doing so as they diverged from related hominid forms. Although not yet fully 'cultural', such mothers would have been prioritising child care, synchronising their cycles, concealing ovulation, extending receptivity – and thereby harnessing to an ever-increasing extent the available provisioning energies of males.

A final inference can be made. Our findings in Chapters 5 to 7 would indicate that when, finally, the 'home base' institution in its modern form did appear, it was because an age-old, primate-derived sexual-political obstruction associated with male sexual dominance had at last been removed. This obstruction had never completely prevented the rise of ovarian synchrony and therefore of a kind of 'human solidarity': but it had restricted it to those populations inhabiting a small number of rather special, semi-aquatic or in any event resource-rich habitats. Overcoming this restriction involved a revolution in the most literal sense of the word – a relatively sudden change involving a redistribution of power and a radical transformation of all social, sexual and also spatial relationships.

Background to Revolution: Foraging Strategies and Shores

It is widely agreed that the emergence of symbolic culture involved 'the replacement of ape-like systems of interpersonal dominance . . . by systems of at least relatively egalitarian, stable, and reliable relations of rights and obligations' (Whallon 1989: 449). Such an overthrow certainly merits description as a revolution. Yet however decisive an event or process this may have been, it is now clear that Upper Palaeolithic humans had no need to invent either egalitarianism or solidarity. Paul Turke's model (Chapter 6) enables us to appreciate that the extraordinary scale of internal social harmony required for the final, Upper Palaeolithic consummation of the human revolution already had an ancient evolutionary pedigree. Gender solidarity of the kind expressed in ovarian synchrony had been a powerful evolutionary factor from the moment when evolving humans' anatomy and reproductive physiology had begun acquiring modern form.

What, then, was distinctive about the human revolution's final con-summation? Much could be said about this, because the transition from Middle to Upper Palaeolithic levels of technological competence brought with it what one writer has termed 'the creative explosion' (Pfeiffer 1982) – the emergence of personal ornamentation, art, ritual, dance and much else besides. Understanding such changes in symbolic behaviour, however, requires delving into their material roots in subsistence strategies and in climatic and other environmental change.

According to my own preferred narrative, the point of departure was a situation in which evolving humans were still practising area-intensive foraging strategies. While this may not necessarily imply riverside or shoreline settings, I think there is evidence that such habitats were strongly favoured.

A glimpse into an early Mediterranean setting of this kind is provided by the site of Terra Amata, near Nice in southern France, where, as mentioned earlier in my discussion of fire, what may have been a shelter was built on the Mediterranean beach about 230,000 years ago (Villa 1983: 55). The people – probably archaic *Homo sapiens* – seem to have based their subsistence largely upon the hunting of selected young or weak animals; they also ate marine resources such as fish and shellfish (de Lumley 1969: 45; Villa 1983). The presence of water-lilies, whose bulbs are edible (Dimbleby 1978: 28), may have been another attraction of the beach-site. 'If the conditions were suitable for water-lilies', comments McKay (1988: 48),

> perhaps other edible plants with similar restrictions on their habitats were also growing. We cannot be certain, but it is not unlikely that along the salt-wasted coast there were little oases where streams created small gardens of edible plants. Gardens that could, perhaps, sustain a hunter-gatherer band for a few days, and which served as ideal camp-sites, whilst the men hunted and the women harvested vegetables and shell-fish.

Analysis of hearth positions and reuse suggest eleven perhaps-seasonal visits to this site, each of two or three days duration (de Lumley 1969; Villa 1983). All this could indicate a lifestyle perhaps not radically distinguishing these hominids from their Lower Pleistocene ancestors evolving along the shores of the Afar Gulf and the wetlands and lake shores of the East African Rift Valley. It will be remembered that one of the few hints we have as to the food eaten by the Bed I hominids at Olduvai was that they used 'hammers' to pound up aquatic tuberous plants (Binford 1989: 27).

The southern coast of the Mediterranean, especially in Morocco and Algeria, was similarly occupied, the site of Sidi Abderrahman yielding contemporary remains of the hominids themselves (Wymer 1982: 124). At the Libyan coastal site of Haua Fteah, mounds of sea-shells have been found buried with Mousterian tools dating to about 80,000–70,000 BP (McBurney 1967). Whatever else it may imply, such evidence suggests that Mousterian and earlier hominids tended to favour coastal economies and did at least occasionally eat seafoods.

In most parts of the world, shorelines have changed substantially over the past 10,000 years. Rising ocean levels coinciding with the end of the last ice age have often destroyed evidence of Late Pleistocene human occupation as cliffs, perhaps honeycombed with inhabited caves, have collapsed into the sea. But along the southern coast of Africa, tough Palaeozoic rocks have withstood the batterings of both time and crashing waves, changing scarcely at all since the Middle Pleistocene. It is the evidence from Klasies River

Mouth which has given us some of the oldest known fossils of anatomically modern humans — presumed descendants of 'Eve' — in addition to outstandingly early dates for stone tools indicating a level of lithic competence approximating that of the Upper Palaeolithic. And it was this same evidence, as Binford (1984: 20) notes, which 'forced the recognition that early man was using aquatic resources for a long period of time prior to the Late Pleistocene'.

Compared with earlier Acheulean peoples in the same region, there is evidence that the Middle Stone Age peoples at Klasies River Mouth were becoming less narrowly restricted to valleys and to the coastal platform, and were beginning to collect game and gatherable resources up in the adjacent plateaux (Deacon 1989: 557). Nonetheless, the evolved, anatomically modern but pre-cultural hominids of Klasies River Mouth lit their fires and foraged along the seashore, killing penguins, scavenging seasonally washed-up seal carcasses (Marean 1986) and eating other marine creatures in addition to vegetable foods. At the Klasies main site there is no archaeological evidence for fishing. But as a supplement to the carbohydrate-rich geophytes (buried plant foods) dug up in the surrounding mountains and apparently encouraged by controlled burning, small- to medium-sized terrestrial game animals were hunted and eaten, and quantities of shellfish were consumed as a rich and necessary source of minerals and other nutrients (Deacon 1989: 558–9).

We do not know whether the females at Klasies River Mouth at various times were organised into harems monopolised by single males, chimpanzee-style multi-male systems or other arrangements. However, Binford's (1984) healthily sobering view that they were still constrained within the parameters of a basically primate-like system seems too extreme. It would seem more likely that periodically or perhaps even continuously, the females in this locality had escaped many of the severer problems associated with competitive primate sexuality, and that they had done so by synchronising along the lines suggested by Paul Turke (1984). It is difficult to think of types of evidence which could decide between these possibilities, but information concerning sex ratios and measurements of sexual dimorphism might possibly prove relevant. There is some evidence that in the warm period preceding the Last Glacial, the Klasies hominids showed pronounced sexual dimorphism, with very robust males and much more gracile females (Deacon 1989: 556). Then, as colder weather intensified with the onset of the last Glacial, there is evidence that selection pressures against dimorphism set in. This might indicate an increase in synchrony in the later period, reducing inter-male physical competition for mates, but this is of course guesswork. Perhaps the most we can say is that since the skeletal anatomy of even the earlier Middle Stone Age Klasies hominids had become basically modern, the soft-tissue sexual anatomy and physiology of the females may also have reached modern form. If Turke's (1984) model can be relied upon, this would in turn imply that some time, somewhere, ovarian synchrony had been playing an important role in these females' lives.

If females were synchronising and by that means maximising male help – and it is hard to see how these hominids could have attained anatomically modern form without this – then along the coasts they were probably supplementing their own collected resources with occasional medium-sized land mammals brought to them by males and cooked on fires. Whilst male provisioning may have been reaching a relatively high level, however, there is nothing to indicate a rigid sex division of labour at Klasies River Mouth. Females would have collected what foods they could, and males would have done likewise as they provisioned their offspring and mates. Groups of kin and offspring may have slept in caves like those which have been excavated (Singer and Wymer 1982), doubtless enfolded in skin blankets and huddling together for warmth around a fire.

In this and similar coastal areas, population densities may have been locally high – perhaps rather higher than in the more mountainous hinterland regions which were also occupied. On that analysis, Middle Stone Age anatomically modern females would have been maintaining the togetherness necessary for synchrony thanks to the rich coastal environment and an area-intensive foraging strategy. Permanent movement into the surrounding mountains would have posed challenges which led to greater dispersal.

Out of Africa

As anatomically modern humans began to spread out from Africa across the world between 90,000 and 40,000 years ago, they were almost certainly capable of living inland from lakes or coastal shorelines where necessary. According to my narrative, however, *wherever possible* they at first opted for easier ways of feeding themselves and maintaining their togetherness – ways that involved retaining area-intensive foraging strategies close to river valleys, lakesides and shores.

The Nile Valley is the corridor along which anatomically modern humans probably filed as they moved from Africa into adjacent parts of Eurasia some 70,000 or more years ago, shortly before beginning their colonisation of the world (Bräuer 1989: 148; Howells 1988: 226). The fertile banks of the Nile, comments Howells (1988: 226), would have been 'hospitable at all times regardless of continental climates . . . '. There are alternative routes – such as the short sea crossing over the Strait of Bab el Mandeb into Southern Arabia; but these would have presupposed familiarity with swimming-logs or rafts (Clark 1989: 580).

Sea crossings cannot be ruled out, for an expertise with watercraft evidently extends back to the very earliest stages of the Upper Palaeolithic. Indeed, in order to explain the surprisingly early expansion of anatomically modern humans across Asia to Australia, it is necessary to picture small groups travelling along the edges of the Indian Ocean and other coasts, periodically following and crossing rivers, inlets and estuaries. The final step to Australia involved a daunting 90 km sea crossing between Timor (on the Sunda continental shelf) and Greater Australia (Sahul). Rhys Jones writes:

> My own scenario is that in the period just prior to the colonisation of Australia – say 40 kyr ago – there were people living on the shores of Sundaland, in the mangrove swamps and using the river mouth for resources. They had an adequate technology of inshore watercraft, perhaps rafts made of bamboo palm or other suitable materials. Random events such as storms and currents sometimes swept people off into the ocean, where under suitable conditions of wind and current they made new land falls. The odds against any one such episode being successful might have been high, yet given enough time the entire archipelago could be colonised. (1989: 755)

Once in Australia, the same coastal economy was maintained. Among the favoured hypotheses for the gradual colonisation of Greater Australia is that of Bowdler (1977, 1990), according to whom the first immigrants moved south along the coasts of this vast continent, before expanding their territory by following major river and lake systems and soon colonising the interior.

The American case was probably similar. 'In both America and Australia', comments Bednarik (1989: 109–10),

> it seems entirely plausible that first entry was by small numbers of people who were adapted to coastal economies. Hominids of the Lower and Middle Palaeolithic are generally credited with a penchant for near-coastal, riverine and lacustrine environments. . . . For a people occupying a new continent there may have been little incentive to shed their coastal economy and penetrate the hinterland until such time as coasts and major river courses were settled to capacity.

Bednarik's conclusion is important: it is likely that until coasts, estuaries and major river valleys were settled to capacity, newly settled modern humans in all continents tended to retain their ancient evolutionary preference for resource-rich estuarine and/or shoreline homes.

We have seen that shoreline economies were favoured not only by evolving hominids in the East African Rift Valley during the Plio-Pleistocene, but also by much later, large-brained tool-makers as these moved out of Africa into Eurasia, Australasia and even the Americas. It would be an exaggeration to state that a restriction to such settings characterised all sapient humans prior to the Upper Palaeolithic. But although many archaic populations of

Homo successfully penetrated the higher and drier regions of the great continental hinterlands, it would seem that this was always and everywhere achieved only at a price. If our earlier arguments about the more robust, derived features of Eurasian *Homo erectus* are correct, then in the more arid or otherwise marginal habitats which they were able to colonise, archaic humans – who owed their brains ultimately not to local conditions but to the peculiar circumstances of their African origins – would have been obliged to adapt locally in ways which did not involve significant further neoteny, gracility or encephalisation. Instead, increased dispersal, a corresponding decline in social complexity and new, strenuous physical demands would have led to enhanced robustness and to a certain emphasis on physical at the expense of highly sophisticated communicative/social skills. This, in any event, is one interpretation which can be put upon some of the super-robust features of *Homo erectus* in Asia and the earlier specimens of archaic *Homo sapiens* in Europe and elsewhere – in particular the massive limb bones, enormous brow ridges and astonishingly thick skulls (Collins 1986: 148–50).

From about 200,000 years ago onwards, these problems evidently began to be overcome. No longer did dispersal out of Africa and into cooler regions entail losing touch with those conditions (conducive to ovulatory synchrony) which, within Africa itself, had led to the initial evolution of large brains. Certainly, Eve's descendants – or at least a group of them – avoided pressures to evolve in non-modern directions of the kind characteristic of *Homo erectus* in Asia or the Neanderthals in Europe. Yet it was long before a solution was arrived at which made ice age Eurasian and other continental hinterlands positively favoured as habitats by anatomically modern humans. Such humans were biologically adapted to the tropics and subtropics, and – for as long as they remained in roughly comparable climatic conditions – it would seem that there was little pressure on them to undertake a 'cultural revolution'.

In fact, wherever the origins of the Upper Palaeolithic have been adequately researched, it turns out that an episode of severe cold, desiccation or both was in some way connected with it. It was lowered primary productivity which triggered the change – a momentous cultural transition rooted, I believe, in a cold-triggered, forced abandonment of area-intensive foraging patterns and riverine/coastal ecosystems. This involved a genuinely revolutionary 'leap' to new transpatial, non-territorial forms of social organisation, in turn made possible by symbolic communication systems of an entirely new kind.

Culture and Cold

Let us examine more closely the background to this revolution – its relationship to long-term climatological change. We will see that everywhere, the decisive events were associated with periods of combined dryness and cold.

In addition to its many other riches, the Middle Stone Age site at Klasies River Mouth has yielded some astonishingly early dates for tool assemblages which, in a European context, might almost be labelled 'Upper Palaeolithic'. The sophisticated blade-making technology known as 'Howieson's Poort' – dated to about 70,000 BP (Deacon 1989: 554) – coincides with the onset of a glacial period and worldwide regression of sea levels, bringing with it substantially deteriorating environmental conditions in southern Africa (Clark 1989: 573; Deacon 1989: 560). It was evidently this deterioration which triggered the cultural advance. The Klasies deposits reveal a sudden lowered frequency of gathered shells at this time. This coincided with a smaller proportion of seals among the faunal remains and a larger proportion of bovids, equids and geophyte plant remains – all indicating a partial abandonment of marine foods and a move towards inland collecting (Marean 1986: 366). Thereafter, the climate improved, and technology reverted to simpler forms for tens of thousands of years. Then at about 40,000 BP came the next major technological advance, which this time proved permanent. Again, cold weather had something to do with it. The change from the Middle Stone Age technological stage in southern Africa to that of the Later Stone Age coincides with the onset of the Last Glacial Maximum – the most extreme environmental conditions of the late Pleistocene (Deacon 1989: 556). This eventually led modern humans such as those at Klasies River Mouth to abandon their coastal economies altogether in favour of gathering and hunting in the hinterland (Deacon 1989).

A comparable pattern can be discerned in the northern part of the continent. Severe desertification affected the Sahara about 75,000 years ago – at the start of the Last Glacial (Clark 1989: 573) – at a time when Neanderthal populations were retreating from the severe cold in Europe and expanding or shifting their range by entering the Levant (Bar-Yosef 1989: 604). Many former inhabitants of the Saharan region seem to have migrated into the Middle East at this time. In the Central Negev Desert, the Upper Palaeolithic revolution came at a time when severe desiccation associated with global cooling was setting in; eventually, this area had to be abandoned because it was so barren – but by this time people had moved on, now equipped with revolutionary new cultural forms which they took with them (Marks 1983).

In Europe, too, a deteriorating climate seems to have tipped the scales in favour of modern humans and their associated Upper Palaeolithic symbolic cultural traditions. Gamble (1986a: 367–83) has shown that considerable differences existed in the responses of European Neanderthal and anatomically modern populations to the establishment of polar desert conditions of low terrestrial productivity. Whereas the probably light-skinned, physiologically cold-adapted Neanderthals appear to have abandoned Central Europe during the glacial advances of about 70,000–50,000 BP, modern human populations, who, given their African origins were at first probably dark-skinned or even black, persisted in the face of similar severe cold conditions between 35,000 and 12,000 years ago. The final displacement of the last Neanderthals by modern humans in central and south-west France occurred in a particularly cold phase (Harrold 1989: 689).

At first sight, it might seem that given their tropical origins, probably dark skins, warmth-adapted physiologies, ultra-dependent offspring and labour-intensive child-care burdens, anatomically modern females would have been hit particularly hard by the onset of cold weather. In addition to such requirements as thick clothing, the cold, windswept plains now inhabited would have demanded higher levels of mobility and a heavier reliance on hunting. In the previous chapter we took account of environmental factors making it difficult to imagine how Paul Turke's ovarian synchrony model could have worked under such conditions at all – certainly not if females were forced to disperse widely and forage inland and in isolation from one another. Besides undermining synchrony, the cold/dry conditions would also have undermined any competitive female strategy of granting favours to males in return for favoured access to foraging space. Of what use would a few square metres of ground have been – if insufficient food for survival could be found in such patches? What use personal feeding space, if the decisive requirement had become access to roaming herds of game?

In short, it is hard to imagine how the new conditions could have been anything other than negatively experienced by females – unless, of course, they could find some way of compelling the opposite sex to do massively more of the travelling, hunting and related tasks for them. Yet the evidence is that soon after the start of the last ice age, the harsher conditions not only failed to block the expansion of modern humans into new regions – they positively facilitated such expansion. Despite their tropical origins, modern humans with their warm clothes, semi-permanent dwellings and well-controlled domestic fires embraced the snowswept plains and tundra of ice age Eurasia as if such spaces had been made for them. We must conclude that females in these regions were guaranteeing their subsistence requirements by relating to males in a wholly new way.

Paul Turke Reconsidered: Synchrony and the Ice Age

The requirement, we can now see, would not have been for culturally organised humans to invent entirely unprecedented patterns of synchrony and area-extensive gender solidarity. Instead – as our findings in the last chapter now suggest – the task would have been *to preserve synchrony under entirely new conditions*. The sociality built up over preceding millennia and responsible for the unique reproductive physiology of the human female would have had to survive the transition from the rich tropical shoreline environments of hominid ancestry – to the much less hospitable environments of the continental hinterlands of the last glacial epoch.

In the Levant at around 70,000–80,000 BP there is evidence that whilst the Neanderthals were still restricted to moving within highly productive, often-coastal ecosystems, anatomically modern humans in the same period were able to transfer to less productive mountain and desert zones (Shea 1989: 622). Previously, entering such zones might have prompted local extinction, the retreat of hominid populations to more resource-rich areas or (if survival were possible at all) much greater mobility and dispersal into small groups, with a corresponding loss in sociality. The final consummation of the human revolution, by contrast, was achieved not through retreat but through some extraordinary process of meeting the new challenge. As a result, humans became able to live almost anywhere. In the Levant (as, perhaps, in other regions where anatomically modern humans existed), an extraordinary revolution occurred when for the first time extended communities proved that they could traverse and embrace immense areas of space – *without* losing the high levels of sociality which their area-intensive former foraging traditions had sustained.

Chapter 9
The Revolution

Finally, in times when the class struggle nears the decisive hour, the process of dissolution going on within the ruling class, in fact within the whole range of old society, assumes such a violent, glaring character, that a small section of the ruling class cuts itself adrift, and joins the revolutionary class, the class that holds the future in its hands.

Karl Marx, The Communist Manifesto (1848)

Evolving ice age woman solved her problems not by setting out into uncharted territory. She had only to discover a new, intensified application of the strategies inseparable from her entire previous evolution. Her secret was to extend, intensify and add a new cutting edge to the sexual techniques discussed in Chapters 6 and 7. Raising ovarian synchrony to new and unprecedented levels, she established a movable but semi-permanent base camp which was so well-provisioned by the opposite sex that it could be situated almost anywhere, no longer depending for its existence on the localised foraging relations or produce of females and their offspring themselves.

Paul Turke's (1984) ovarian synchrony model therefore cannot be dispensed with. Retaining it as our point of departure, we can simplify it and bring it into conformity with the relevant genetic, palaeontological, archaeological and other data by making the following changes:

1   The most decisive events in the human revolution occurred not in the Plio-Pleistocene but within the last 70,000 years. The accomplishments of symbolic culture were achieved not by forest-dwelling primates emerging for the first time on to open savanna. They were achieved by large-brained hominids – descendants of 'Eve' – who had reached anatomically modern form in African shoreline settings but were now penetrating into the harsher continental hinterlands of Africa and the Near East during the last ice age.

2   Not only the distinctive features of human female reproductive physiology but other features of both sexes, such as large brain size, reduced sexual dimorphism, increased gracility etc. can be explained using the synchrony model. A mating system based on synchrony would have minimised the selective value of violence, maximised that of more co-operative social and communicative skills. This shift in selection pressures was the most important factor underlying the transition to anatomical modernity.

3   Mating systems based on area-intensive foraging patterns and shore-line synchrony involved the formation of unusually strong and enduring coalitions. Such systems were complex and intellectually demanding, particularly with regard to time awareness. Although not cultural in a modern sense, their selection pressures amply pre-adapted 'Eve' and her descendants for the complexities of symbolic culture.

4   The consummation of big game hunting scheduled through general-ised ovarian/menstrual synchrony *in ice age hinterland conditions* was achieved only during the start of the Upper Palaeolithic revolution, the new logic reaching take-off point and beginning to spread irresistibly across the globe probably around 45,000 or at most 50,000 years ago.

5   Selection pressures in favour of heavier menstrual bleeding resulted in part from women's need for visible signals to help keep track of their own and one another's cycles. The use of blood in this context also meshed in with a focus on blood spilled periodically by men in the hunt (see Chapter 11), an idea which ties in with the view of classical scholars that the first true 'contracts' had always to be 'signed' in blood (Girard 1977). The result was a blood-centred symbolic system which linked game animals and the female body into a tightly integrated web of meanings which generated the stylistic characteristics and distribution of much Early Upper Palaeolithic art. These characteristics included periodic notation systems (Marshack 1972a, 1972b), the use of ochre as a blood substitute (Wreschner 1980), the recurrent association of vulva engravings with those of animals (Delluc and Delluc 1978), figurines which emphasise the female reproductive organs (Gamble 1982) – and, more generally, what Marshack (1972b) among others has described as the art's suggestively lunar/menstrual as well as seasonal or 'time-factored' internal logic.

6   Understanding the 'leap' to symbolic culture is not possible on the basis of an analysis which restricts attention only to conventionally 'symbolic' behaviour, such as language. Retaining the concept of synchrony, we must bring domesticity, extended and formalised kinship, fire, division of labour, menstrual taboos, hunting and meat cooking into our sexual-symbolic equations (see Chapter 11).

In this new form, the ovarian synchrony model does more than account for the biological aspects of human modernity. It also provides the key to an understanding of symbolic culture – not in the abstract, but in the specific, puzzling ritual and other forms in which it first actually leaves its traces.

The task now is to understand how shoreline-dependent, tropically derived, lunar/tidal synchrony could have been preserved by females under cold-climate conditions and far from tidal shores. In the remaining chapters of this book it will be shown that Upper Palaeolithic art, dance and ritual – all manifestations of sexual/economic collectivity and synchrony – can be understood as having arisen to meet this need.

As climatic conditions deteriorated and lowland/coastal economies were of necessity abandoned, mobile bands of males would increasingly have been needed by females to chase after large game animals. In this context, Turke's idea that evolving human females used control over their sexuality to obtain male help must be reformulated: the resource increasingly required was *meat*. This meant effective hunting. Females, particularly those nursing young offspring, had no interest in participating directly in this dangerous activity if they could possibly get males to do it for them.

This prompts us to recast the rest of Turke's theory. The reader will have noted that Turke's model is focused essentially on the ovulatory or 'positive' phase of the menstrual cycle, not its menstrual or 'negative' aspects. As Chapters 6 and 7 have indicated, however, evidence for the accentuation of menstrual signals must lead us to question this omission. In the absence of an oestrus signal, synchronising females would surely have required some alternative hormonally driven signal through which to keep track of their cycles. More importantly, it seems unlikely that synchronously cycling anatomically modern females would have evolved the capacity to signal 'yes' simultaneously, without being able to signal 'no' on occasion just as emphatically and in pursuit of the same goals.

We arrive at the conclusion that menstrual bleeding in the modern human case became accentuated to meet these demands. Just as females collectively synchronised and extended their receptivity to motivate male provisioning, so – by the same token – they collectively refused sex whenever meat supplies were exhausted or men attempted to approach without meat. It would have made biological sense to signal 'no' not during ovulation but during menstruation, when fertility was lowest, even if previous evolution had rendered females on a behavioural level fully receptive at this time. The need to signal 'no' in visually and physiologically emphatic ways would explain both the biological accentuation of menstruation and its associated symbolic negativity. The value of this model in explaining ethnographic menstrual taboos will be discussed in Chapter 11.

The Revolution

Synchrony had formerly depended on a measure of togetherness in the food quest. Area-intensive foraging patterns had brought females together and – along with other co-operative activities such as food-processing and fire-tending – enabled their body-clocks to synchronise as a result. With the onset of colder weather and with an increasing reliance on hunting, this no longer worked. Females were in danger of becoming dependent on males in new ways, and increasingly isolated from one another.

Yet there was a solution to this dilemma. Given a sufficiently powerful initial 'kick', synchrony could be made self-sustaining.

Let us imagine a group of fire-possessing females in some particularly favoured location or with particularly powerful traditions of ovarian synchrony. We might visualise them as members of an expanding anatomically modern population along some restricted stretch of coastal shore, many generations after their first arrival in the area. The climate is cooling and gatherable resources are becoming scarce. Population pressures and/or resource shortages along the coast are prompting some groups to venture further inland in an effort to find food.

The most promising new edible resource is meat from large game animals which can be cooked on the controlled fires. Highly mobile males, roaming in bands, have recently become more successful in hunting these. Such males are anxious to prove their worth to the females, anticipating sexual rewards. In this context, they are beginning to use their meat gifts to subvert the dominance of any males who attempt to maintain control over females in direct physical ways. Since the more dominance-inclined males can only be poor hunters – their mobility being restricted precisely by their pre-occupations with sexual monopoly and control (Chapter 5) – females wanting meat now have very little interest in remaining under them.

Not only are would-be harem-owners themselves poor hunters; their sexual preoccupations also exclude the monopolised females from access to other males' meat. To the extent that political relations based on 'dominance' still prevail, in other words, females are increasingly finding themselves attached to males of the wrong kind. Indeed, at its worst the paradox is that males with access to meat now have no sex, while on the other hand sexually privileged males are cut off – along with the females they control – from supplies of meat.

The obvious answer is for the two oppressed/segregated gender groups to come together at the expense of any would-be harem-owners attempting to prevent such union. To achieve this result, the females take action along the lines outlined in Chapter 6. They synchronise their menstrual cycles, perhaps phase-locking with tidal cues. As the hunter-males approach with meat for the cooking fires, the females link up with them. The revolution begins here.

It must be stressed that so far, nothing that has been described is really new: it is the conditions which are new, not the 'revolutionary' sexual logic of synchrony as such (Chapter 6). However, over a period, the hunter-males now begin to find that it pays them to time their hunting expeditions so as to harmonise with the physiological rhythms of the females. This means ensuring, for example, that each time the females are due to ovulate, they (the males) are not just about to go away on an extended hunting trip. Although strict scheduling may not always be possible, in general males try to time matters the other way around. That is, it is in their genetic interests to be returning home laden with meat just when the females are most ready for them, hunting-linked absences coinciding or overlapping with menstruation.

It will be noted that the cards are now for a variety of reasons stacked against old-style 'dominance' in males, no matter how large their hand-axes (Chapter 8) or other physical capabilities for dominance. Not only are sexually competitive, female-monopolising males excluded by their own preoccupations from co-operative hunting. There is also the problem that since the two gender groups are now normatively cycling and hunting in sympathy with one another, even any sex relations forcefully or deceitfully secured during the hunters' absence will be infertile. The time-honoured primate strategies of 'Machiavellian' deception and dominance (Byrne and Whiten 1988), in other words, no longer pay. Since old-style alpha males are no longer able to meet female needs, whole groups of females begin to synchronise across wider areas than ever before, in effect 'voting against' and perhaps also physically 'disarming' individual males who may still prove obstructive (see Chapter 4).

Now, if the females in such a situation could compel the hunter-males to scour a wide enough area in search of terrestrial game – sending hunters inland for days on end – it would soon not matter whether female foraging activities *in themselves* were sufficient to sustain the social density necessary for synchrony. The burden in this respect could be transferred to the other sex. In other words, if hunting produced sufficient meat, male provisioning could begin to sustain not only the physical, bodily existence of females and their offspring. It could sustain women's togetherness – their synchrony – as such.

Male hunting could do this if meat supplies were so reliable that females had no need to disperse thinly over the landscape in search of food, but could forage or carry on child-care duties collectively, remaining in reasonably large groups, retaining this togetherness even in seasons when gathered food was scarce or non-existent. Females could then synchronise regardless of the immediately local terrain. This would be of immense significance because it would involve positive feedback. Males would hunt and provide meat for females, enabling mothers to rear their offspring together in relatively large groups, synchronising their ovarian cycles as a result – and thereby intensifying the pressures on males to step up their hunting activities still further.

If successful, this strategy would quickly enable synchronising females to abandon their former vegetationally rich habitats altogether. It might enable them to pick on a favourable, sheltered inland spot and remain there not just for a day or two, but for weeks or even months. Such a spot would have to be strategically located, with the local availability of game and drinking water among the most important considerations. But once a camp had been decided upon, this spot and its immediate surrounds could be established as a semi-permanent and essentially female-defined (although doubtless also male-defended) area. Females with their offspring would then be able to remain in it regardless of male day-to-day movements. They would not be obliged to disperse across the surrounding landscape, some staying with their offspring whilst others followed males in search of game. The status differences between child-burdened females and unburdened ones would no longer divide women spatially. Keeping in touch, they could all prioritise not only child care but, even more importantly, the togetherness necessary for the synchrony on which their meat supplies collectively depended.

In addition to maintaining synchrony, the other basic requirement would have been for females to refuse sexual access to males who brought no meat. This would have been nothing new, in the sense that Turke's model already implies a trade-off between male provisioning and sex. But the new situation would have required more definite female action in extracting the maximum possible effort from males. Continuous receptivity would not have sufficed. Most forms of hunting are best carried out in a scheduled way, with an enhanced awareness of time and much investment in 'anticipatory' actions which yield no immediate rewards. In view of this need for what Binford (1989: 19) terms 'planning depth', it would have been best for all those about to go on a hunting expedition to have had their minds concentrated on the task in hand, with all sexual distractions removed. Females could have met this requirement in an uncomplicated way – simply by declaring themselves 'on strike' whenever they felt the need for meat.

As well as delaying gratification and thereby raising hunters' horizons beyond immediate concerns, this would have had several direct advantages for the females themselves. Firstly, striking would have meant *keeping together* in dense female-centred groups rather than dispersing in pursuit of meat-possessing males. No sex strike could have been maintained if females allowed one another to disperse in ones or twos in the company of male hunters. Although prompted initially by this collectivising logic of strike action, spatial togetherness would in turn have yielded immense additional benefits in terms of the sharing of child care, gathering, fire-tending, food-processing and other burdens.

Inseparably from this, the strategy of making males do much of the running around would have enabled females to *reduce their mobility*, staying with their own and one another's offspring and moving only when necessary, at their own child-compatible pace. It would have meant a final break with the whole tradition of having to follow around after dominant males. Males would have been forced instead to circulate around the females, returning 'home' periodically with meat.

A third advantage would have been connected with the need to reassure sexually anxious hunters that prolonged absences would not be taken advantage of (Chapter 5). A firm sex strike would have enabled females in effect to *guarantee that during hunting-related absences there would be no sex – not even infertile sex – with rival, stay-at-home males.*

Some Sexual Implications of the Model

Women created culture, it has been argued, by taking domestic power into their own hands. To do this, they had to rely on their own internal gender solidarity to back up their ability to signal 'no!'. In directly sexual terms, this may seem a negative beginning. But from the start, female sexual resistance would have been only one side of the equation.

As the logic of primate dominance was transcended and males became more consistently co-operative, gender conflicts would have assumed novel forms, with less necessity for female negativity in sexual relationships. Naturally, not all contradictions would immediately have disappeared. But once the cultural configuration had been firmly established within a given small population, conflicts would increasingly have taken on a cyclical aspect, endlessly created yet endlessly transcended and resolved. Both sexes, in short, would have begun emerging from the treadmill of endless power struggles to enter a new dimension of life governed not by physical manipulations but by language, shared symbol and rite.

With power more widely shared and with conflicts of interest no longer expressing themselves as basic irreconcilabilities, the context of women's sex strike would have become transformed. The former battle between the sexes would have evolved into teasing, banter and play. We may envisage men's mock-resistance to women's 'no!' becoming expressed in subtle, ambivalent, playful ways, with women clapping, embracing or dancing on each occasion of their coming together, and with celebrations of all kinds becoming stylised, formalised – ritualised. Given a measure of stability, economic abundance and success, what was once women's angry determination to signal 'no!' – a half-articulate political battlecry against sexual oppression – would have become so confidently expressed and so unquestioningly respected as to begin to be enjoyed in large measure for its own sake, turning thereby into a new form of activity with very little of the political element still attached to it. It would have begun flowering into that joyful activity which takes up so large a portion of the lives of all hunters and gatherers – ritualised song and dance.

Hunter-gatherer traditions of dance vary widely, but in most cases the repertoire includes a strong element of gender-polarity, with men in one group, women in another, each dancing or singing alternately, group to group. It is impossible to imagine human life with neither song nor dance, and we must suppose that both were present from the beginning. The Bushman peoples of the Kalahari, it has been said,

> dance for everything; they dance to celebrate a birth, they dance at marriages, they dance for the rituals of a girl's first menstruation or a boy's first kill in the hunt. And often, when no particular reason presents itself, they dance just for the fun of it, clapping and chanting and stamping around the fire with increasing verve as the night wears on. (Taylor 1985: 52)

At first sight, my model may invoke an image not of celebratory dancing but of sex-negative women signalling 'no!'. Had this been the basis on which humanity evolved, it might be thought that women ought to have turned out to be quite unusually sex-negative primates. We know that this is not the case – human females have greater capacities for extended bouts of love-making, for orgasm and for sexual enjoyment, quite possibly, than has any other primate, male or female (Hrdy 1981). Superficially, this might seem a problem for the whole idea of a 'sex strike' – which, after all, implies banning sex, not enjoying it!

In fact, however, such difficulties turn out to be non-existent. The sex-strike strategy would have accentuated the sexualisation of all life, rather than the reverse.

Let us return to our imagined protohuman population still only tentatively pursuing the new strategy. Genetically this population would be heterogeneous, with some females more desirable in male eyes – and more interested in sex – than others. Now, it might seem at first sight that those females with the fewest drives and attractions would be those who would find it easiest to go 'on strike'. The argument would be that those least able to express or to excite sexual interest would be those faced with fewest difficulties in simply withdrawing from sex altogether. To use a contemporary political analogy, it would be like saying that those who made a point of avoiding wage slavery because they disliked work or were incapable of it – would be those most able to form powerful trade unions based on the power of the strike.

It can be seen at once that this logic is flawed. Those incapable of work would be incapable of benefiting from the strike weapon at all. If people are to gain anything by going on strike, the first condition is that their presence at work should be missed. Correspondingly, in terms of the model presented here, minimally sexually motivated or minimally wanted females would be in the worst rather than the best position effectively to pursue the sex-strike strategy which has been outlined.

In reality, the whole purpose of female strike action would have been not to avoid sex altogether, but to make males go away only temporarily – and then *come back home with meat*. Not only does this assume that males are motivated to return to the females. It also implies that the females can enjoy sex sufficiently to have something to offer when the males do return. If – to extend our analogy – sex in the pre-cultural period had been comparable to 'wage slavery' (a chore performed to gain minor concessions from the dominant power), then following the revolution it should have shaken off this aspect altogether. Women should no longer have felt that they had to loan their bodies to dominant males on a continuous basis, simply in order to secure a steady flow of food on which to survive. The revolution should have reversed all such equations, so that females faced with economic need were motivated not to solicit sex but to resist it. By the same token, sexual play should have been all the more welcomed and uninhibited once meat was plentiful and in female hands.

In proportion as modern humans moved away from African coastal shorelines and began to spread inland and across the globe, those spear-heading such developments would have tended to locate themselves in deforested, vegetationally sparse grassland or tundra environments teeming with large game. Here, a single collective fire drive, jump kill or other hunting expedition may have produced large quantities of meat sufficient to last for weeks. Given such abundance, it is important to realise that sex should no longer have felt like prostitution – an activity carried on under pressure of economic anxiety and motivated basically by desire for material gain (Chapter 5). Under the new conditions, every successful hunt should have dissolved society's temporary economic anxieties, inaugurating an extended period of celebratory feasting. A consequence of such 'original affluence' (Sahlins 1974: 1–39) would have been to release women to feast, sing, dance and enjoy sex for its own sake – as a social and natural activity pleasurable in and for itself.

As we explore the internal logic of all this further, it becomes clear that the pre-cultural equations governing inter-female sexual rivalry and jealousy would likewise have been reversed. The earlier primate-like pattern would have been for females to have felt threatened by one another's sexual attractiveness, competing with one another behaviourally on this level. Under the new circumstances, such patterns would have been profoundly changed.

We may assume that no very early female sex strike could have been absolutely total in its effects across vast stretches of the inhabited landscape. There must always have been some females, somewhere, who were beyond its reaches – some who were still innocently signalling 'yes!' even while their sisters elsewhere were saying 'no!'.

Potentially, this would have posed a problem. If the sexually willing females possessed stronger sexual drives and more powerful attractions than those on strike, their availability would have undermined the whole system. Every time the new-strategy females tried to organise a sex strike, their much-desired female rivals or counterparts would simply have undercut them, offering themselves so that males went straight to them.

Because of this, the new system could have worked only on the reverse basis, with those females *most* wanted by the males being among the *first* to get organised. Other females wishing to make use of the new strategy would have been under pressure to link up with them.

Primate females tend to experience one another's sexuality as a competitive threat. An oestrous female gelada, for example, may be favoured by the dominant male but precisely because of this, tends to suffer harassment from her non-oestrous female companions at the same time (Dunbar 1980a). The sex-strike logic would have acted to reverse all this, and the consequences may have been decisive in enabling large groups of cultured, fully human females eventually to coexist in long-houses or other quite closely packed conditions without endless destructive jealousies and conflicts. Under the new conditions, a female regarded by males as particularly desirable would not necessarily have been resented by her coalition sisters. On the contrary, she may have been highly valued by them – provided she did not flaunt herself but remained under the discipline of the group. All women would then have benefited from the increased cutting edge now given to their strike action each time it was imposed.

By the same logic, the sexually highly valued female would have benefited from her association with good organisers, good mothers or those with long memories or special knowledge. Just as an elderly female may have gained from association with a young one, so would the young have gained from association with their mothers, grandmothers or other senior allies. Indeed, this collective valuing capacity – the capacity to pool and to share the benefits of personal resources and skills – would have been for females one of the main advantages of the new sex-striking, coalition-forming strategy.

Nakedness, Clothing and Beads

Given the logic just outlined, females set on following the new strategy would clearly have done best if they could (a) arouse the sexual motivations of males prior to each hunting expedition whilst (b) making absolutely sure that no actual sex – no consummation or fulfilment – was allowed. The need, then, would have been to find a balance, sharpening the edge of the strike weapon not by disclaiming all sexual interests – but rather by dangling before the hunters' eyes the rewards in store for them once their tasks had been performed.

Bangles, beads, necklaces and other adornments, many in the form of pierced marine shells, appear suddenly in the archaeological record in great abundance during the very earliest stages of the Upper Palaeolithic (White 1989a, 1989b). Doubtless, they were accompanied by pigments, pubic coverings, shawls, tassles and other items of ornamental clothing made of materials which have unfortunately not survived. Taken together – and leaving aside possible physical functions such as protection or warmth – these items would have conveyed symbolic information on various levels.

Firstly, they would have helped combine bodily concealment with allurement. We can imagine women deliberately dressing up – and very probably also dressing one another up – in order to mark the start of each 'strike'. Writing in about 400 BC, the Greek classical playwright Aristophanes (1973: 188) comes to our assistance in humorously bringing out this logic inherent in any sex strike: the fact that all possible must be done to make it 'hurt'. The fictional strike-leader Lysistrata spells out this oath to her followers:

> I will not allow either boyfriend or husband. . . . [repeat]
>   to approach me in an erect condition. [repeat]
> And I will live at home without any sexual activity, [repeat]
>   wearing my best make-up and my most seductive dresses, [repeat]
>   to inflame my husband's ardour. [repeat]
> But I will never willingly submit to his desires. [repeat]
> And should he force me against my will, [repeat]
> I will be wholly passive and unresponsive. [repeat]
> I will not raise my legs towards the ceiling. [repeat]
> I will not take up the lion-on-a-cheese-grater position. [repeat]
> As I drink from this cup, so will I abide by this oath. [repeat].

The sisters drink the dark red wine – explicitly likened to the blood of sacrifice – as their solemn pact is sealed. Earlier, Lysistrata had answered as follows a question about how her struggle against internecine war could be won:

> How? Well, just imagine: we're at home, beautifully made up, wearing our sheerest lawn negligées and nothing underneath, and with our – our triangles carefully plucked; and the men are all like ramrods and can't wait to leap into bed, and then we absolutely refuse – that'll make them make peace soon enough, you'll see. (Aristophanes 1973: 184)

This is uncannily similar to the mixture of seductive body adornment and sexual defiance encountered in Chapter 4, when we discussed how women among the Sharanahua of Peru paint their faces and encircle their menfolk in the course of initiating a 'special hunt'.

As the Upper Palaeolithic revolution got under way, the body-paint, beads, pendants, pierced shells and other ornaments worn during dances and at other times would not only have helped motivate the men. As removable items under social control, they would also have helped older women to control the sexual availability of their sisters and daughters. The wearing of pubic coverings may have been particularly central here. The very concept of 'nakedness' – unknown among primates – would in fact have been one of the immense cultural consequences of the new logic. However variable in its cultural manifestations – one culture's dress can be another's shameless nudity – this concept as such is undoubtedly a cultural universal. Its basis is the knowledge that society's collective stake in the sexual aspects of one's body is a very real one, and that carelessness with dress or ornamentation can make one a laughing-stock in the eyes of a public which, thanks to the human revolution, now for the first time really cares.

At the most basic level, the earliest personal ornaments would have been a guarantee for the individual in this sense: they would have been the visible sign that the wearer was not 'naked' – that his or her body was under the supervision and sexual protection of the group. In other words, necklaces, pubic coverings and/or beads would have stamped each human body with its special *socialised* nature. They would have marked the fact that its availability or non-availability was no longer a private issue between the individual and his/her sexual partner but a matter for decision through negotiation on the basis of groups. The ornaments' stylistic uniformity would by the same token have signposted each individual's gender-group affiliation, women (and in this context men, too) wearing 'female' (or 'male') ornaments to express their self-identity as members of their own particular group (cf. Wobst 1977).

As social media, then, such ornaments would not have been chosen or applied exclusively on a private basis. Just as men assisted one another in hunting, there would have been every reason for women to assist in enhancing one another's appearance and charms – sharing, exchanging and mutually applying body-paint, bangles, beads and so on. The collective nature of style in women's personal ornamentation would have reflected such communality, just as stylistic uniformities in hunting outfits would have been prominent in reflecting the gender-group communality of men.

In short, the sex-strike model does not assume sex-negative females. Indeed, it allows us to agree with those earlier models of human origins (Morris 1967; Hill 1982; Parker 1987) which have insisted that evolving protohuman females must increasingly have learned to signal 'yes!'. But women could not have afforded to do this in any simple, unconditional sense. There would have had to be teasing, paradox, ambiguity. Every 'yes' must have implied the threat of an equal and opposite 'no'. Such a cultural point of departure explains why it is that where human sex is concerned, the positive must always emerge *from behind* the negative – like desirable flesh made all the more tempting by adornments which partially conceal. It helps to explain the seeming paradox that when the Sharanahua women referred to in Chapter 4 form into a man-challenging 'picket line', each is defiantly looking her very best, her body temptingly adorned with paint and beads (Siskind 1973b: 233–4). It helps us to understand why, when a Sharanahua participant teasingly says 'no!' to her preferred 'special hunt' lover (Siskind 1973a, 1973b), her whole body is simultaneously and on another level signalling a future 'yes!'. By contrast, those crude 'Naked Ape' theories (Morris 1967; Hill 1982; Parker 1987) which have assumed an endless, open-ended female 'yes!' – 'yes' in the form of 'extended oestrus' or so-called 'continuous receptivity' – are simply implausible; they explain neither the specific features of human female reproductive physiology, nor morality, nor culture.

Synchrony and the Skies

Close inter-female solidarity and resistance of the kind required by a sex strike would not only have presupposed synchrony along Paul Turke's lines. It would have presupposed an intensification of synchrony – in particular a phase-locking of cycles across much wider areas than would have been strictly necessary previously.

This would have been because of the need to curb cheating. Lysistrata made her followers swear on oath precisely because she was aware of the threat posed by the likelihood of strike-breakers (Aristophanes 1973: 185). In the early Upper Palaeolithic, our model would lead us to infer a similar logic. Few males would have felt constrained by a localised sex strike if they could simply look elsewhere for sex. To put matters another way, it would have made no sense for a female to attempt to force out 'her' male to go hunting unless she had chosen her moment well, and was sure that her sisters would be with her, sending away their men as well.

In fact, to be sure of success, the women in any one camp would have done best to pick their moment in relation to an external, transpatial standard. Even if all those in a co-residential group were synchronising, it would have been unwise to choose a moment when those in some neighbouring camp were sexually available. Much better for women to wait or to pick a time of month when it was known that those in neighbouring and even far-distant localities would be with them. Otherwise, once again, philandering would be possible – males might pretend to go hunting, but really seek sex elsewhere. Local synchrony, then, would not have sufficed. To the extent that hunters were now highly mobile and quite capable of crossing local boundaries, generalised synchrony – the Lysistratian equivalent of a 'general strike' – would have been required.

In the absence of tidal cues, this would have meant standardising by direct reference to the moon. Regardless of the strength of lunar signals or the reliability of cloudless skies, women would have had to maintain an awareness of lunar changes, using the moon to reset their body-clocks from time to time. Only in this way could women have prevented men from taking advantage of their divisions as they gradually drifted out of phase. In

Chapter 10, we will see how this helps to explain a basic feature of traditional rituals and cosmologies – their astrological insistence that good fortune on earth can be ensured only by keeping human action fundamentally in tune with observable astronomical events. 'On earth as it is in heaven'. Again and again, we find this belief that the template for the ancestral 'Way' or 'Law' lies in the skies.

From Nature to Culture

The most difficult step would have been to initiate the new logic. There is no denying that there would have been problems in sustaining gender solidarity long enough for the new selection pressures to begin operating in its favour. How such problems could have been overcome is not easy to understand. But this is a philosophical and methodological problem for all theories of cultural origins – a problem shared equally by hypotheses which attempt to explain the origins of life. The existence of culture, as of molecular self-replication through DNA, at a certain point emerges in the evolutionary record as something quite new. An immense number of preconditions appear to be required for this emergence, and the problem is that many of these preconditions seem to presuppose the new life-principles in the first place. Too many hypotheses that seem plausible consequently turn out to be circular – they assume at the outset precisely the conditions which a scientific theory would need to explain. This problem may never be entirely surmountable – any theory must rest on the introduction of some element of novelty at a certain point – but if this new element can be made to seem less complex and improbable than it did, the theory is a good one.

The present hypothesis assumes female solidarity. It does not assume language, or the incest taboo, or a sudden flash of insight, or an extraordinary mutation producing 'conscious thought'. Naturally, the hypothesis assumes that as a result of previous, non-cultural evolution, advanced, large-brained hominids exist. An advanced threshold level of manual dexterity, tool-using and tool-making skills, vocal and gesticulatory communicative abilities and cerebral agility would have been required before 'culture' in the sense used here could even have begun to take off. It is certain that very advanced fire-tending skills would also have been required, for reasons which will be more fully discussed in Chapter 11. But it is methodologically permissible for such developments and others to be assumed, since, as we saw in Chapter 8, they do not themselves presuppose symbolic culture.

In principle, it would only have needed two females – perhaps sisters, perhaps mother and daughter – to have set in train the movement towards culture as an unstoppable force. If these two always backed each other up, always acted in concert, synchronised their menstrual cycles and were able to motivate two or more males to hunt for them by making sex dependent on it, then they might have been so much more successful in securing meat than other females in the population for their strategy to act as an attractive model, and for any genetic characteristics facilitating such solidarity to spread through the population.

To begin with, the resulting group might have been a small unit. But unlike other 'family' or 'band' units in the population, this one would have been capable of recruiting new members to its ranks almost indefinitely. There are limits to the viable size or territorial range of any horde or family type grouping, but with a strike – the bigger the better. Strike action cuts across parochial boundaries spontaneously and of necessity. The striking group would have had a powerful motive to extend its influence and recruit, since with each sex strike – as with any strike, including those within contemporary culture – there could have been no tolerance of neutrality. If the surrounding females could not be brought into the strike, then they were a threat to it. Every female encountered or liable to be encountered by any male was on one side or the other. And the more females brought into the fold, the more powerful the strike on each occasion, and the greater the attractions of joining the movement next time.

A further consequence of this logic would have been decisive. The females adopting the new strategy would have been linked not to one or more dominant individual males but to an immeasurably more effective force, both for hunting and defence. In addition to whatever links they had with offspring or biological kin, they would have been attached sexually to a male group whose capacity for joint action would have far exceeded that of unorganised males still prioritising their individualistic struggles for status, sex and food. With female synchrony sustaining much-enhanced inter-male solidarity, the rapid accumulation of effective long-distance hunting techniques would then have been in a position to begin.

Although potential rapists or dominant males may in the early stages have constituted a problem, there are no grounds for doubting that the females in their strike action would have received male support. The organised hunter-males, like the females, could not have been indifferent to the behaviour of the surrounding male population. Any male who could not be brought into synchrony with his fellows would have constituted a potential danger. The dominant individual male, the loner, the rapist, would have been perceived as a sexual threat. Such a potential 'harem-holder' might easily have been treated in principle like any other animal predator – chased away, wounded or possibly killed. In any event, where conflicts occurred, no violent male would have been able to match the coercive power of the well-organised, experienced and motivated hunting band. The traditional male sexual strategy of immortalising one's genes through assertions of behavioural dominance would no longer have worked. And if this were the case, then the cultural configuration, once established, would have spread through the population rapidly, sweeping all before its path and precipitating the extinction of all competing groups unable to adopt the new way of life.

The Universe of Rules

The females in any hypothesised protohuman population would have been divided into (a) those who were more liable to 'break ranks' and mate regardless of their sisters' attempts at a sex strike and (b) those more liable to form coalitions with other females, following the sex-strike strategy, placing pressure on other females to follow suit and submitting to similar pressures themselves. Of these two female types, there seems little question which would most plausibly have led social life in the direction of culture. We need hardly ask which would most have needed new communicative and signalling skills or which would have been most receptive, potentially, to the notion of a 'rule' or 'taboo'. Assuming that long-established traditions made it possible to control fire (Chapter 8), it seems hardly necessary to ask which females would have been most likely to succeed in keeping it alight or to maximise its uses within the context of a 'home base'. And assuming that the complex of activities implied above – speaking, rule-making, fire-tending, hunting, gathering and so on – represented a viable mode of production, we need hardly speculate as to which category of females would have succeeded in producing the largest number of surviving offspring.

The sex strike would have provided the most fundamental and obvious feature of human culture, and the one which underlies all the capabilities for joint action which have been suggested here – the fact that it is based on 'rule' (Lévi-Strauss 1969a). Here, the crucial point is not whether conventionalised patterns of behaviour exist. Such patterns, which can perhaps misleadingly be called 'rules' by external scientific observers, are discernible throughout the animal world. Baboons and chimpanzees behave in predictable ways, according to conventionalised patterns determined both genetically and in complex interplay with the social and external environment. But this has nothing to do with 'rules' as defined here.

A cultural rule exists when there is genuinely *collective* agreement to secure adherence to it. Admittedly, as was seen in Chapter 3, rules are in one sense 'there to be broken', since without infringements and their publicised punishment it is difficult to define exactly where the boundaries are drawn. Nonetheless, where the rule as such is concerned, indifference, tolerance and neutrality are of necessity abandoned. Every individual who has entered the agreement must in principle submit to its terms. A violation is supposed to outrage not just the few directly affected individuals but the community at large, gossip focusing on sexual or other 'scandal' being used to keep people in line.

Such a situation does not prevail among non-human primates. To touch on a central issue – incest in sexual relations – let us imagine a dominant male gorilla with three females. Two of these are his daughters. The question is not whether or not he has sexual relations with all three females. That would be a matter of behaviour – not of rule. The question is this: *in the event* of this male's having or attempting such relations, what would be the reaction of the other gorillas in the vicinity? Would they express some gorilla version of collective moral outrage? Would they come to the defence of the daughters? Would the females as a gender group feel that an abuse of one was a threat to all? Or would they simply show indifference, leaving individuals to get on with things as best they could in their own way, each basically preoccupied with its own affairs?

As the social anthropologist Robert Lowie (1919: 113) made clear long ago, it should be immediately obvious – and all recent primate research indeed confirms this – that there would be little in the way of community outrage in the face of the incest. Primate 'public opinion' in this sense does not exist. Admittedly, individual primates in a local community may take sides, involve themselves in others' affairs, express anger and attempt to involve allies in their emotions or schemes – but despite all this there is no overarching collective body which makes it its business to interfere with its members' private affairs. Although coalitions (as among chimpanzees) may come into being, they are formed around dominant or threatened individuals seeking immediate advantage for themselves, and allegiances and coalition boundaries shift as perceptions of self-interest change. The result is that individuals are left to follow the possibilities opened up by social interaction; they do what they can get away with doing. There is certainly no collectivity which endures beyond and despite the flux of alliances and coalitions be- tween individuals. No social group can be relied upon either to arbitrate impartially or to assert the validity or otherwise of universally acknowledged categories of behaviour. There exists, consequently, no collectively imposed system of constraints, no supra-individual force to impose sanctions – no 'rule', no 'law'. We can put this another way by saying that in chimpanzee society, coalitions indeed form – but every coalition is always sectional, opportunistic and unstable, none being capable of embodying 'society' as a whole.

Human culture, in its traditional forms particularly, is above all the 'rule of law' in this sense: that the behaviour patterns culture prescribes emanate from a source beyond instinct and beyond private enforcement by sectional interest groups or by individuals. In a human cultural system with its harmonising collective rituals and its formal structures of kinship we find something which transcends the parochial, petty level of interaction to which primates are confined. Beyond all private coalitions or alliances is a wider one – a set of shared understandings uniting the community as a whole. Whilst it is true that practical experience may often fall short of ideals, and that 'developed' class-societies are indeed characteristically conflict-ridden, the fact remains that *shared* perceptions and understandings are what language, ritual and culture in its traditional forms are essentially about. No hunter- gatherer community, in any event, can be understood without reference to this level of its being, which tends to be the most meaningful for its members themselves. And the essential point being made here is that it is inconceivable that primate 'dominance' could have led to such a level. It could never have led to shared symbol and rite, because it could never have led to a wide enough or representative enough coalition. It could never have sustained the wholly necessary element of collective responsibility and collective *intolerance* which characterises human cultural rule-making at its best – intolerance of rape, of murder, of incestuous abuse, of antisocial greed.

Primate 'dominance' is from this perspective the antithesis of culture. It is the pseudo-law, the pseudo-order of alliances in the service of purely sectional interests – the patterned, structured outcome of self-seeking interaction based on inducement, threat and fear. Such a situation leads each individual to look to itself, to use its intelligence only in the most 'Machiavellian' of ways (Byrne and Whiten 1989), to attempt to bend others to its sectional interests (interpretable ultimately as those of its genes) and to display ultimate indifference to the fate of the wider community of which it is a part. There is no way that this could have led to culture – except along the road of revolutionary, point-by-point negation and overthrow of its logic.

On the other hand, if we are looking for a source of collective, impersonal intolerance leading to the 'universe of rules', we can have no better model than that of the strike. Like chimpanzee alliances, the strike is a coalition. But it is a coalition with a difference. The strike by its very nature undermines the dominance of private interest. It has its own logic, sweeping along individuals caught up in its current. It cannot be indifferent. It must impose 'the law' – its own law of solidarity – with implacable intolerance, its survival depending on it. It has to extend, intrude, embrace and include ever more widely to avoid being thrown into reverse. And yet the concept of the strike avoids the anti-Darwinian mysticism or veiled theologism which has accompanied previous attempts to assert in humanity a spiritual, moral or psychological uniqueness demarcating us from the animal realm. The concept does not lead us to assume anything genetically or socially unrealistic in terms of altruism or morality. The individual seeks her/his material interests – which may well include those of reproduction and genetic self-perpetuation – *through* those of the collectivity which is involved in the strike. At this point, kin selection indeed transcends itself, for in principle the striking individual must be motivated to defend and identify equally with all 'kin' – who must now be defined as all those involved in the strike – instead of discriminating in favour of those genetically most 'close'. The model leads us to the concept of culture because it provides a realistic framework within which biological interests can finally transcend themselves – a point of intersection at which genetic, personal and collective interests can be seen to coincide.

Morality and the Model

If the model of the strike in general provides us with an ultimate logical source of concepts such as 'law' or 'rule', a strike on the part of *females* – the reproductively most-burdened sex whose foraging strategies are basic determinants of all primate social structure (Chapter 4) – promises revolutionising society from the bottom up.

The strike model in particular provides us with an intellectually satisfying explanation of sexual morality, both in a general sense and with regard to specific anthropologically attested forms.

It was noted earlier that the test in deciding whether or not sexual morality exists has nothing to do with individual behaviour. What matters is the attitude of others towards such behaviour. The female 'no' strategy immediately gives us the essence of sexual morality in this respect.

From the moment when two or more protohuman females went 'on strike', supporting one another in the maintenance of such action, the context of their sexuality had become transformed. No longer could each such female do with her body as she liked. She had to take account of her strike 'sisters', whose own pressures were derived from the requirements of the strike. All around her, then, was a set of 'artificial' constraints. From that moment on, all sexual behaviour became at least potentially divisible into one of two basic categories – 'right' behaviour and behaviour which was in 'moral' terms 'wrong'. Even a private act of love-making, far away in some secluded spot, would now risk being seen as an outrage if it occurred during what was supposed to be a general sexual strike.

Such morality would have been all-intrusive. By going on strike, the females were extending their claims ever outwards, stretching their influence into all corners of life, exerting a collective stake in the value which their sexuality now represented for them. Such collective sexual self-control – which is the antithesis of primate oestrus behaviour – was the source of their pride, their status as women, their economic and social power. Each female could no longer do with her body as she pleased, or allow her instincts to carry her where they would. As a sexual being, she was now socialised – an asset to her gender group as a whole. Her body was no longer just that of a physical individual. It was the incarnation of something collective, something universal, or, to use the terminology of later religions, something 'divine'. It was part of the most precious, irreplaceable, inviolable treasure of all – the body of Womankind, which was to be guarded ferociously against all male attempts at seduction or privatisation.

But the model not only generates female sexual morality. It also gives us male morality as the mirror image and counterpart of all this. For once two or more males were acting as co-operative hunters, respecting the inviolability of their sexual partners' periodic strike, they too, by the internal logic of the situation, would have felt threatened sexually by any defiance of the rules. Any male displaying tendencies towards sexual strike-breaking, dominance or rape would have constituted a threat. Allowed his way, such a male – particularly if armed with hunting weapons – might have raided the community of women and seized one or more females for his own private use. If he succeeded in this, other males might have followed suit. Along this road, culture would quickly have collapsed. But we cannot expect the group of co-operative hunter males to have exercised vigilance against this possibility purely out of concern for the future of culture. They had a more direct, very tangible motive. Without vigilant self-defence against the spectre of the dominant male, they might have lost their women. Before the whole community became extinct through cultural collapse, the members of the hunting band would have become sexually expropriated – reduced, perhaps, to something like the status of baboon-like 'bachelor males' excluded from female contact by a few dominant 'overlords'. Such, in any event, might have been the fear. It was this very material factor of collective fear – of jealous collective motivation to defend their sexual interests – which gave force to the men's moral vigilance.

The hunters' new sexual security was founded on an inversion of previous patterns of female sexual preference. What females found sexually appealing in male behaviour now was neither aggressiveness nor dominance, but adherence to rule and success in co-operative hunting. If strength or muscularity remained a sexually appealing feature in males, it was now of necessity each male's power as a member of his group which was valued – not his capacities as one individual in opposition to others. This meant that even a 'weakling' could be appealing if he was valued by his hunting comrades for his eyesight, tracking ability, accuracy of aim or other group-functional talents.

This pattern, although logical in the new circumstances, was not 'natural'. It was a reversal of the more 'normal' primate pattern, and could be sustained by each individual woman only to the extent that she felt herself to be in a wider system which worked and which reciprocated her trust. To state this in sociobiological terms: females could only afford to mate with unusually 'sensitive' or muscularly 'weak' males if there was a good chance that the resultant 'weak' male offspring carrying their fathers' genes would also be reproductively successful in succeeding generations. This whole logic could easily be undermined: indeed, given a local restoration of power to a few dominant males and the breaking of women's resistance, individual females ought quickly to abandon the quest for solidarity and revert to the pattern in which they found behavioural dominance attractive once more. The male gender group, then, had as great a collective interest as the females in upholding the new order at all points – in recruiting members to its ranks, exercising vigilance, defending Womankind's periodic inviolability and placing constraints upon the sexuality of all its members. Ever since they had followed such a logic in falling in with the women's revolution, the hunters had won for themselves collective sexual security – without struggles for dominance, without 'haves' and 'have nots', without fear of complete sexual expropriation. It was a treasure they could not afford to lose.

Incest and Exogamy

The model not only gives us sexual morality in a general sense. It also accounts for the culturally enshrined incest taboo, although not in quite the 'nuclear family' forms which prevail in western societies today. More precisely, thanks to the manner in which the model links sex and hunting, it explains the 'totemic' equation of incest avoidance rules with rules governing the distribution of meat (Chapter 3).

Females, according to the model, are inhibiting the sexual advances of non-hunter males. Within any representative group of females, there will always be some immature males still attached to their mothers. The females are inhibiting the sexual advances of all males who do not separate themselves and go off to hunt. Their own male offspring come into this category. Therefore, the females are inhibiting the sexual advances of such males. In other words, women's imposition of a kind of 'incest rule' – which in this case is merely the sex strike as experienced from the standpoint of women's male kin – is the inescapable result of a refusal or inability to threaten the strike or otherwise complicate matters by making an 'exception' of stay-at-home brothers or sons.

No other hypothesis can account for the emergence of culturally enshrined, totemically conceptualised incest avoidance so simply and neatly. Within the terms of the model, we are not asked to believe that female protohumans at a certain stage began complicating life by adding an 'incest taboo' to the already-existing configuration of artificial constraints. Still less need we follow Lévi-Strauss (1969a) in postulating the sudden appearance of sexual generosity and altruism on the part of woman-exchanging groups of males. We need suppose only that females remained consistently faithful to the logic of a meat-gaining strategy which was already established in their own material and economic interests. Within the terms of the model, inhibiting the sexual advances of stay-at-home, non-hunting males – of all such males, regardless of status or affiliation – was precisely what the women's sex strike was all about. There could be no sex except with males who brought meat. By remaining faithful to this principle even with regard to their own immature male offspring, the females involved were simplifying life, not complicating it. The inhibition of young males' 'incestuous' advances was the result.

In a general and preliminary sense, then, the incest rule – central and intractable problem for twentieth-century theories of human origins from Freud (1965 [1913]) onwards – has been explained. But the model does not stop there but proceeds to define matters more closely, specifying related core components of the cultural configuration by its own internal logic. We will see in a moment that it explains, for example, why the incest rule continues from childhood into adulthood, so that even when they mature and become hunters, sons and brothers still cannot relate sexually to their mothers or sisters. More importantly, it explains exogamy, which is the specific context within which incest avoidances in traditional cultures are normatively enforced.

When the females are on sex strike, they are insisting that the adult hunter-males separate themselves off and go out to hunt. These males will for obvious reasons be reluctant to go unless they are secure in the knowledge that the ban on sex applies to all of them without favour or discrimination – and in particular that the females will remain during their absence in control of the situation back at home. They need to know that no young males left behind, for example, will be allowed to gain the upper hand in securing sexual relations with any female. As part of their sex strike, then, the females must inhibit their sons and show that yielding sexually to them would be unthinkable.

But there is more to the sex strike than this. Remember that females would not have seen their male offspring merely negatively – as potential sexual partners who were in fact prohibited. Sons, like brothers, would have been valued as allies and sources of support. Women would have actively involved them in their own solidarity, and therefore in the organisation of each sex strike. Inevitably, given joint action by women of different generations, this would have brought male kin of all ages into the same broad category – that of male allies in women's sex strike. The model would explain mother-son and brother-sister cultural kinship solidarity as starting here.

Admittedly, it might at first sight be thought that an alternative pathway could have been followed. In theory, could not the females have repudiated the logic which has just been described, deciding that at a certain age, sons and brothers underwent a role reversal, becoming suddenly available as sexual partners after all? Such a 'solution' could not have worked. Apart from the possible psychological objections to so complete a role reversal, women would have lost out because the price to be paid would have been the loss of their adult male kin as coalition allies. It is simply not possible to organise a sex strike in alliance with individuals who are in fact one's sexual partners.

The logical choice would have been to leave things as they were. No collective decision need have been made. Sexual relations defined as 'unthinkable' in terms of the requirements of strike action would simply have remained so. Young sons and brothers who in their immature years had been involved in the solidarity of their mothers and sisters would have remained so involved, no matter how much they matured, married or grew old. Once a sex-strike coalition ally of a woman, always one – for life. Since this 'inertial' pathway would have generated the unilineal clan and lineage results actually found in the ethnographic record (see below), we will assume that it was the one which women (supported by their male kin) actually followed.

Let us follow through the implications. To the extent that sexual freedom in relations with their mothers/sisters is impossible, the males in each coalition become conditioned against perceiving their female coalition allies as potential sexual partners, and must look elsewhere for partners as they mature. They cannot join the hunting band of their fathers, because this would mean sharing in their fathers' coalition solidarity and therefore thinking the unthinkable – seeing their mothers/sisters as women to whom gifts of meat are brought, the implications of this being explicitly sexual. To join their fathers would also be difficult inasmuch as it would mean joining what previously had been 'the opposition camp', and ceasing to be coalition allies of their mothers/sisters. In short, in the absence of some complicated process of social restructuring, these males must preserve their kinship relationships in the forms inherited from childhood. Unable to join the hunting band of their fathers, they must either join another hunting band or, if none exists, form one of their own. In fact, there is no need for the males to form any new set of institutions. The cleavage between 'fathers' and 'sons' exists already within the specifications of the model; it has only to be perpetuated as the sons mature and begin hunting for there to emerge a division of the male community into two counterposed camps, each with its own internal solidarity. The model would lead us to see in this the beginnings of a 'moiety system' or 'dual organisation' – a community divided into only two intermarrying clans.

The recently matured hunters seek sexual relations outside the community of their own women. But which other women exist within the system for them to turn to? The answer is simple. Their fathers must have been nurtured in a female group of mothers and sisters with whom sexual freedom was (for these 'fathers') 'unthinkable'. In seeking sexual relations, the sons must turn to this female group, since there are no other women in the system. Assuming that they seek partners of their own generation, the sons will relate to the daughters of this group – 'fathers' sisters' daughters', who would also be 'mothers' brothers' daughters'. This is an example of 'restricted exchange', a pattern which is taken to be the simplest, most elementary structure of kinship by Claude Lévi-Strauss (1969a).

Moiety systems of the kind predicted have long been known to represent a very stable and peculiarly archaic level of kinship structuring (Morgan 1881: 5; Lowie 1920; Lévi-Strauss 1969a: 69–71). For one archaeologist (Deetz 1972: 283–4), 'the closest approach to Palaeolithic social units in the ethnographic present is to be seen in the Australians, the Ge, and to a somewhat lesser extent, aboriginal Californians'. When the native cultures of these three regions were first observed by social anthropologists, they had been only minimally influenced by surrounding farmers. It was an isolation allowing them to evolve, preserve and share in common many structural features which may have been universal when the world was populated only by hunters and gatherers. 'Most striking', comments Deetz, 'is the existence and strong development of moiety organisation in all three cases'.

Those social anthropologists who prefer to eschew social-evolutionary reconstructions of this kind would still acknowledge – in the words of Robert Lowie (1920: 135) – that a dual organisation 'is certainly the simplest that can be conceived'. Malinowski put it somewhat differently:

> The dual principle is neither the result of 'fusion' nor 'splitting' nor of any other sociological cataclysm. It is the integral result of the inner symmetry of all social transactions, of the reciprocity of services, without which no primitive community could exist. (1926: 25)

'A dual organisation', continued Malinowski,

> may appear clearly in the division of a tribe into two 'moieties' or be almost completely obliterated – but I venture to foretell that wherever careful enquiry be made, symmetry of structure will be found in every savage society, as the indispensable basis of reciprocal obligations.

The notion of dual organisation as emerging out of 'the inner symmetry of all social transactions' seems consistent with the sex-strike hypothesis being outlined here.

Matriliny Versus Patriliny

The model specifies not just moieties in general, however, but specifically – at least to begin with – moieties based on matrilineal descent. Whilst this adds to the risks involved in testing the model, it is not necessarily inconsistent with the evidence. For example, although we cannot reconstruct prehistoric kinship systems with much confidence, there are independent reasons for supposing that the kinship-based extended 'chains of connection' established by the earliest, expansionist hunters of early ice age Europe had a certain matrilineal bias.

An advance in kinship theory was made over twenty years ago, when Mary Douglas (1969) linked patriliny with area-intensive foraging patterns, *matriliny with area-extensive ones*. Comparing numerous African cultures of different kinds, she found that matriliny flourishes wherever there is an expansionist economy demanding flexibility of association, but in which despite material abundance 'the value of material goods is much less than the value of persons'. Matriliny collectivises and distributes male labour widely across space. This is because (unlike patriliny) it splits the nuclear family, making a woman (for example) remain dependent upon her brothers even when she is married. A man's 'own' child is his sister's, not his wife's, and a woman is given numerous real and classificatory brothers on whom she can call for support – not just a husband.

Douglas (1969: 128) established that this is adaptive wherever collective male labour is very productive, highly valued and must be mobilised in situations requiring loyalties to be distributed widely across space:

> To sum up the argument so far: matriliny provides the framework of a corporate descent group without making exclusive demands on the loyalties of males. It even forces men, whichever pattern of residence is adopted, to move from their natal village to another. It forces the local unit to accept newcomers within its bounds. It requires all males to accept conflicting responsibilities. In short it is a more dilute form of corporate grouping, less exacting than patrilineal descent. The latter merely permits weak female links between descent groups. Where residence harmonises with descent it is at the cost of wider forms of allegiance. Matriliny is a form of kinship organisation which creates in itself cross-cutting ties of a particularly effective kind. This is not to suggest that societies with patrilineal systems do not have such ties: they can produce them by means of cult or other associations, but matrilineal descent produces them by itself. This is in its nature. If there is any advantage in a descent system which overrides exclusive, local loyalties, matriliny has it.

These space-embracing, non-territorial, gender-segregating, coalition-forming characteristics of matriliny would have emerged directly from women's sex-strike action as specified in this work. Whilst concrete manifestations would naturally have depended on local circumstances, this means that on the most formal, abstract level, matriliny's features as described by Douglas do not need to be separately explained.

A more direct source of possible evidence concerns the gender of the many ice-age 'Venus' figurines which, according to Gamble (1982), allow us to infer the existence of a vast, integrated fabric of marital alliances stretching across central and northern Europe. If the associated cross-cutting kinship ties operated through interconnected patrilineal clans, it would seem strange that red-ochred females or 'mothers' should have been used to symbolise such ties. In fact, there seems to be remarkably little evidence of phallic symbolism in the Early Upper Palaeolithic. Of course, this does not disprove patrilineal descent, but it is an argument against its symbolic primacy. Assuming unilineal descent of any kind, it does seem intrinsically more likely that the ties were conceptualised as being through 'blood' rather than 'semen', ancestral 'mothers' rather than 'fathers' – and that they were therefore thought of primarily as matrilineal. We will return to the topic of the 'Venus' figurines in Chapter 11.

The sex-strike model gives us both matriliny and a kind of embryonic

patriliny – the first pattern whenever the sex strike is actually operative, the
second when hunters return, taboos are lifted and males are allowed to regain
access to their wives and young offspring. To the extent that the model
assumes a movement to and fro between alternative kinship states, kinship
itself may be seen to alternate between these two poles. Only if the sex-strike
pattern became permanent and unremitting would all traces of patrilineal
kinship-solidarity be eliminated from life. Conversely, only if what we
might term the 'marital conjunction' (post-sex-strike) phase were permitted
to stabilise and become permanent would cognatic and/or patrilineal forms of
kinship solidarity begin to assume primacy in place of the former state of
balance or alternation.

Despite this apparent evenhandedness, however, the model stipulates that
clan coalitions emerged first and foremost to organise monthly female sex
strikes, and that these were (a) conducted by women in alliance with male
and female offspring and (b) directed 'against' in-marrying husbands/fathers.
Since such action by definition would exclude fathers from primary solidarity
with their daughters and sons, any kinship solidarity so formed would have
been exclusively matrilineal. In this sense, to accept the origins model as
presented here is to accept the existence of matriliny as central to culture's
initial situation.

Once this has been accepted, alternative forms of kinship can be ac-
commodated by treating them as transformations worked upon the model's
basically matrilineal point of departure. It would be beyond the scope of this
book to discuss ethnographic kinship systems in any detail, but since Gamble
(1982, 1986a) in his authoritative reconstruction of early ice age 'mating
networks' draws extensively on Australian analogies, it seems worth noting
that Australian Aboriginal section and subsection systems – in other words,
those components of their kinship systems which most decisively cut across
local, parochial ties – are in essence systems of matrilineal descent. As Elkin
(1938: 130) phrased matters long ago, 'the section system expresses the
native belief that social affiliation or grouping is derived from the mother,
and not from the father'. Male-dominated 'cult' groupings and associated
loyalties, by contrast, tend to be territorial, local, parochial – and
patrilineal. It is also well known that clan exogamy virtually throughout
sub-Saharan Africa was mainly matrilineal until the relatively recent
introduction of cattle ownership (Murdock 1959: 376–8).

The link between matriliny and dual systems is also well-established. In a
cross-cultural survey, Murdock (1949: 215) long ago showed that 'matri-
moieties are . . . much more common than patri-moieties despite the
considerably greater frequency of patrilineal descent'. If strictly exogamous
moieties are counted, these are almost always matrilineal, although there are
some communities with exogamous patri-moieties and double descent 'in
which the earlier matri-moieties presumably served as the model upon which
the patri-moieties were formed' (Murdock 1949: 215). The general finding

that matrilineal moiety systems must be given both logical and historical primacy has recently been demonstrated with particular force in the context of Aboriginal Australia (Testart 1978).

Intergenerational Relations

However, all this would still not explain the prohibition of father-daughter sex. Matrilineal exogamy as such does not preclude this, since it defines the father as a 'stranger', coalitionwise, in relation to his own daughter. On the basis of this criterion alone, therefore, a man could theoretically be allowed sex with his daughter. Being in the same coalition or clan as her mother, she should logically be just as available.

Real communities with strong matrilineal clan organisation do not in fact go this far, but they do distinguish between incest which violates the internal solidarity of the matrilineal clan and other prohibited forms of sex. An example are the West African Ashanti, among whom the greatest moral horror imaginable is *mogyadie* – 'the eating up of one's own blood' – which means sex with anyone of the same matrilineal clan, however remote. For this, the correct punishment is death. Father-daughter sex and other irregularities, while strongly discouraged, are not seen as *mogyadie* and are in theory not supposed to deserve quite the same retribution (Rattray 1929: 303). To Westerners, this might seem slightly shocking, but it must be remembered that in a strongly matrilineal society, the father is not a particularly powerful figure in relation to his daughter, so sexual misconduct on his part does not carry quite the same connotations of *an abuse of power* as it does in the context of the nuclear family or a society with strong patrilineal lineage-loyalties. In a matrilineal society, a girl's most authoritative male guardian is normatively her mother's brother. Among the Ashanti as in other comparable cultures, consequently, the particularly draconian sanctions deterring this uncle from sexually 'eating his own blood' seem entirely appropriate.

In all societies, however – including matrilineal ones – father-daughter sex is also outlawed. Why should this be? There may be some genetic reasons, but if so, the mechanisms through which genetic information or knowledge is acquired and translated into cultural action remain mysterious. The prohibition can be derived from the model if we remember that a coalition of related mothers would need their daughters to 'marry well' – to attach themselves to young men whose hunting skills would contribute additional meat to the extended household or lineage as a whole. These older women – mothers – would already have their own spouses of roughly the same generation as their own, and these men would have been bringing in meat for perhaps years. The objective of augmenting these supplies would be undermined completely if such existing older spouses were to be allowed 'additional' sex – sex with their own daughters – when they would remain unable to bring in any more meat than previously. The additional earning potential of the daughters would then be wasted completely. This would, indeed, amount to the beginnings of a real counter-revolution – for the older males' additional sexual privileges could only be at the expense of younger males who would be denied sexual access to women of their own age. In any context in which women's strategy was to maximise the harnessing of male labour power, such monopolisation of many females by small numbers of older males could not conceivably be permitted.

A final way to appreciate the mechanisms at work is to think in terms of a man's relation to his mother-in-law. To begin with, we cannot assume that this woman is tabooed to a man – that is something which the model must explain. Let us simply take it that men have sexual relations with women, and that these women have mothers. The question, now, is this: can a man who enjoys sex with a female also have sex with her mother as well?

No genetically based theory can have much to say on this question: there can be no possible danger of genetically defined 'inbreeding' in connection with sex with one's wife's mother. But it should be immediately obvious that our model accords with ethnography by wholly excluding this.

The sex strike implies that coalitions of women collectively control one another's sexual availability and, in particular, that they control the availability of their own daughters. A certain authority-structure is implied here. At all times, women must retain the power to exclude their sons-in-law from sexual access to their daughters. At all times, moreover, a woman in dispute with her spouse must be able to appeal to some 'higher' female authority in the form of her mother or some other more authoritative female relative. If a man were allowed marital relations either with his own daughter, or with his wife's mother, this could only undermine the possibility of such authority. In either case, the boundaries between generations would be blurred and the status of 'wife' would be rendered indistinguishable from that of 'mother-in-law'. The female figure entrusted with the authority of the sex strike in relation to a given man would herself be a sexual object in his eyes. And if a young woman could not rely even on the authority of her own mother in a sexual dispute with her husband, to whom could she turn?

Once again, we see that there is no need to seek a separate, additional explanation in order to produce the required outcome. The model as already defined suffices. It specifies that women have solidarity and power. As each new generation of young women come of age, their mothers (supported by other kin) ensure that their daughters marry males of the appropriate, subordinate, younger generation. That way, mothers can exercise the necessary authority over their young sons-in-law – authority without which no sex strike could assert its force. And as the sex-negative authority of the older generation of women asserts itself in relation to the junior generation of in-marrying males – 'sons-in-law' – so-called 'mother-in-law taboos' are among the natural results.

Classificatory Kinship

The model not only generates exogamy and the incest taboo; it specifically generates 'classificatory' kinship – the kind of kinship logic characteristic of most hunter-gatherer and other traditional cultures (Morgan 1871; Fortes 1959: 156). Classificatory kinship expresses the principle of sibling equivalence (Radcliffe-Brown 1931: 13). It is the kind of kinship we would expect to emerge if sibling solidarity were carried to its logical conclusion, overriding the primacy of pair-bonding.

Classificatory kinship is so widespread that modern social anthropologists tend not to discuss it, tending to assume that the readers of their monographs will simply understand all kinship terms in their classificatory sense. For earlier generations of anthropologists, however, the whole issue was still a novelty, and heated debates surrounded the significance of this seemingly extraordinary and cumbersome mode of conceptualising and organising kinship terms and relationships. An unfortunate consequence of the recent lack of interest in this topic has been that palaeoanthropologists and sociobiologists (with outstanding exceptions such as Hughes [1988]) are simply unaware of its existence, and construct their origins theories as if the task were to explain modern western forms of kinship. In order to correct such possible misunderstandings, it seems appropriate at this point to review some of social anthropology's basic definitions and findings concerning classificatory kinship – findings which have never been repudiated, but have in recent years become overshadowed by other concerns. Although the sources may seem unavoidably rather dated, such a review of the classical literature will help to clarify that the sex-strike model predicts this 'unfamiliar' kind of kinship, not the forms which prevail in contemporary westernised societies.

The essence of classificatory kinship is that siblings occupy similar positions in the total social structure. Their 'social personalities', as Radcliffe-Brown (1931: 97) put it, writing in this case of Aboriginal Australia, 'are almost precisely the same'. Where terminology is concerned,

> a man is always classed with his brother and a woman with her sister. If I apply a given term of relationship to a man, I apply the same term to his brother. Thus I call my father's brother by the same term that I apply to my father, and similarly, I call my mother's sister 'mother'. The consequential relationships are followed out. The children of any man I call 'father' or of any woman I call 'mother' are my 'brothers' and 'sisters'. The children of any man I call 'brother', if I am a male, call me 'father', and I call them 'son' and 'daughter'. (Radcliffe-Brown 1931: 13)

By the same token, if a woman has a relationship, any of her sisters may in theory join her in exercising the rights or fulfilling the obligations which that relationship entails. As far as this level of formal structuring is concerned (other levels being ignored for the sake of argument), she may stand in for her sister (just as any of her sisters may stand in for her) in any kinship capacity, whether it be it as mother to her (the sister's) child, as mother-in-law to her sister's daughter's husband – or even, theoretically, as wife to a sister's husband. Moreover, since sisters are each other's 'equivalents', it follows that theoretically, no mother should discriminate in favour of her own biological children as opposed to those of her sister. All of their joint children are addressed as 'daughter' or 'son' indiscriminately, and all are in theory collectively 'sisters' and 'brothers' to each other.

In societies with strong sibling solidarity, the logic of treating siblings as terminological equivalents becomes immediately apparent. If a woman has a child, her sister can 'stand in' for her as that child's mother. Indeed, the mother's sister is already the 'mother', for the expression 'my daughter' means indifferently either 'my daughter' or 'my sister's daughter' ('my sister' and 'I' being 'the same'). A good example are the Hopi Pueblo Indians:

> Sex solidarity is strong. . . . The position of the mother's sister is prac-
> tically identical with that of the mother. She normally lives in the same
> household and aids in the training of her sister's daughter for adult
> life. . . . They co-operate in all the tasks of the household, grinding corn
> together, plastering the house, cooking and the like. . . . Their children
> are reared together and cared for as their own. (Eggan 1950: 33, 36, 35)

It is as if coalitions of sisters had such solidarity that they refused to distinguish between 'mine' and 'thine' where maternal relationships were concerned, each saying, in effect, 'my sister's child is my child'. And as this logic is followed over the generations, the class of people who can be considered theoretically one's 'sisters' (or 'brothers') may expand indefinitely. It is as if society were made up entirely of immense coalitions of 'brothers' acting in solidarity with immense coalitions of 'sisters', all those in each coalition refusing internally to distinguish between 'mine' and 'thine' where kinship-defined rights and duties were concerned.

It was Lewis Morgan's (1871) discovery and cross-cultural analysis of this seemingly 'anomalous' mode of kinship reckoning and organisation which established social anthropology as a scientific discipline (Lévi-Strauss 1977: 1, 300). The basic principle of classificatory kinship – the formal equivalence of siblings – initially seemed merely 'confusing' to investigators. As a certain Reverend Bingham wrote to Morgan, describing an example from Hawaii (Morgan 1871: 461):

> The terms for father, mother, brother, and sister, and for other relation-
> ships, are used so loosely we can never know, without further inquiry,
> whether the real father, or the father's brother is meant, the real mother or
> the mother's sister. . . . A man comes to me and says *e mote tamau*, my

father is dead. Perhaps I have just seen his father alive and well, and I say, 'No, not dead?' He replies, 'I mean my father's brother'. . . .

In fact, the problems encountered by anthropologists in attempting to fathom the logic of classificatory kinship were in large part ideological. As Robin Fox (1967b: 184) has perceptively explained:

> It is because anthropologists have consistently looked at the problem from the ego-focus that they have been baffled by it. They have placed ego at the centre of his kinship network and tried to work the system out in terms of his personal relationships.

They have been puzzled because classificatory kinship simply does not work like this. The ego or 'I' is not its point of departure. Neither is the marital couple. Although such kinship does not eliminate intimacy or individuality, it operates on another level – a level on which large-scale coalition relationships have primacy over personal interests or bonds. On this level, there is a profoundly meaningful sense in which it really does not matter who the individual is. What matters is everyone's participation in the solidarity and collective identity of a class or coalition of people in similar positions, each class defining itself through its relationships with other classes. *This, it will be recognised, is the fundamental feature of our sex-strike model, in which the women of a community as a whole form into an immense coalition and say 'yes' or 'no' in relating collectively to their sexual partners taken as a whole.*

A further expression of the same basic principle is the levirate (or sororate) – inheritance by a person of his or her deceased sibling's spouse. Many Europeans are familiar with this primarily from the Bible:

> If brethren dwell together, and one of them die, and have no child, the wife of the dead [man] shall not marry without unto a stranger: her husband's brother shall go in unto her, and take her to him to wife, and perform the duty of an husband's brother unto her. (Deuteronomy 25: 5)

Both levirate and sororate seem to have been universal throughout Aboriginal Australia (Radcliffe-Brown 1931: 96). In the rest of the world the levirate is or was so common that 'it is easier to count cases where the custom is positively known to be lacking than to enumerate instances of its occurrence' (Lowie 1920: 32).

In the levirate/sororate, a person steps into the marital role of his or her deceased sibling with little or no ceremony and as a matter of course. In a sense, the living sibling was 'married' to the spouse already, since siblings are kin equivalents and marital contracts are arrangements not between two private individuals but between the kin coalitions on either side. Among the North American Navaho, for example, where the levirate and sororate once existed, the payment of bride-price 'made each partner the potential sexual property of the rest of the clan . . .' (Aberle 1962: 121, 126).

Sibling Solidarity and the Model

In concrete social situations – at least in the contemporary ethnographic record – the 'equivalence of siblings' is rarely carried through to its logical conclusion, which would be to give every woman tens or even hundreds of 'sisters' formally equivalent to herself, and a comparable number of 'potential husbands'. In practice, this equalising logic tends to be weakened or distorted in its implications by other factors, such as day-to-day foraging necessities, marital bonding, emotional compatibility, distance or closeness of relationship and residence. In practice, for example, women do tend to favour their own biological offspring over and above those of their sisters, although this may be publicly played down or denied. And in practice, in most secular contexts, individual spouses take and assert their special sexual rights in individual partners of the opposite sex.

Strictly speaking, however – that is, to the extent that 'classificatory' principles prevail – the logic implies that in each generation, the parties which enter into relationships are neither individuals nor marital couples. They are groups of sisters and of brothers: 'The unit of structure everywhere seems to be the group of full siblings – brothers and sisters' (Radcliffe-Brown 1950; quoted by Fortes 1970: 76). In quoting this statement, Fortes offered his own opinion that it constituted 'one of the few generalisations in kinship theory that . . . enshrines a discovery worthy to be placed side by side with Morgan's discovery of classificatory kinship . . .'. He added that, like Morgan's discovery, this generalisation 'has been repeatedly validated and has opened up lines of inquiry not previously foreseen.'

In further concordance with our model, Radcliffe-Brown (1952: 19–20) noted that where 'the classificatory system of kinship reaches a high degree of development', husbands and wives are always grouped apart from each other. On a formal level – that is, where terminology, jural theory and publicly professed ideals are concerned – husband and wife do not merge or combine their social identities. They do not share in using the same kinship terms towards others. They do not form a corporate unit in sharing relationships, property or even offspring (which, in some formal sense, will always 'belong' on one side of the family at the expense of the other).

To this picture of pronounced *separation* between spouses we may add that in a very large number of cultures, particularly in South America, Africa and Oceania, spouses are not even allowed to eat together – 'an arrangement', as Lowie (1919: 122) put it, 'almost inconceivable to us'. In Africa, it is a common Bantu custom that 'the husband and wife do not eat together after marriage' (Richards 1932: 191). Among the Bemba:

> The first division of the community at mealtimes is along the lines of sex. Men and women eat separately. Even husband and wife never share a meal, except at night in the privacy of their own hut. It is considered shameful for the two sexes to eat together. (Richards 1969: 122)

Very often, the rationalisation is that meal-sharing is a sign of kinship – only kin should share food, so that for husband and wife to share meals would make them kin – that is, would tinge their relationship with incest. In various parts of the world, menstrual avoidances, menstrual huts, post-partum taboos, in-law taboos and 'men's house' institutions frequently help ensure that gender distinctions are not blurred, incestuous confusion is guarded against – and spouses are effectively kept apart for much of the time. Uncomfortably for those who argue for the universal cultural primacy of the 'nuclear family', in other words, we find a widespread pattern according to which it is the disjunction of spouses, not their conjunction, which is the most strongly emphasised ritual and structural norm.

Where the formal structuring of social life is concerned, sibling solidarity, then, overrides pair-bonding. There can be no doubt that this feature is central not only to classificatory kinship but also to ritual structure in most traditional cultures. It can quickly be seen that the model of origins proposed here would produce an emphasis on group-to-group relationships and sibling solidarity of just this kind. *The periodic sex strike would put wives with their blood kin in one great camp or coalition, husbands with their matrilineal kin in an opposing coalition.* We need only assume a subsequent weakening or patrilineal overlaying of this logic – detailing the causes and consequences of this for each culture or locality – for the ethnographic record as actually found to be explained.

Sex Strikes and Settlement Patterns

The revolution outlined above seems to have occurred in a region embracing parts of Africa and the Near East between 60,000 and 40,000 years ago. This is when most archaeologists believe they can first discern unmistakable signs of true central-place foraging based on a firm sexual division of labour and the logistic hunting of big game. If the preceding arguments are accepted, such a development implies that, by this time, the two gender groups in each community were separating out and becoming differentiated, making it possible for women to perform one set of tasks in a given location whilst men performed other tasks far away.

Outside Africa and the Middle East, there are good grounds for associating this with the transition from Middle Palaeolithic to Upper Palaeolithic tool-making traditions. In Western Europe, this occurred some 30,000 to 32,000 years ago and was a sharp, sudden transition associated with the intrusion into the area of modern humans who displaced the region's former Neanderthal inhabitants (Clark 1981; Howell 1984; Stringer *et al.* 1984; Smith 1984). In this region, the 'Upper Palaeolithic revolution', as it is often called, was not a revolution in the strict sense but only a secondary ripple effect stemming from a profound set of changes which had originated elsewhere at an earlier date. In Central and south-eastern Europe, we seem closer to the ultimate source of such ripples: the lithic changes can be discerned at least 5,000 years earlier than in western France (Kozłowski 1982a, 1982b, 1988; Howell 1984; Allsworth-Jones 1986) and were not associated with so abrupt a transition from Neanderthal to modern genetic types. But it is in Africa and the Middle East that we have the best evidence for a true developmental transition. In the Middle East, the evidence is of evolving anatomically modern populations refining Middle Palaeolithic tool-making traditions some 90,000 years ago (Trinkaus 1984; Valladas *et al.* 1988; Vandermeersch 1981, 1989; Tillier 1989) and gradually beginning the transition to Upper Palaeolithic traditions, a transition consummated about 40,000 years ago.

The new female strategy would have affected settlement patterns. We saw earlier that once the exploitation of male hunting activities was taken beyond a certain threshold, it would no longer have mattered greatly what kind of terrain females occupied. Provided it was well sheltered and within reach of a water supply, the area around the home base could have been rocky or lush, sandy or clayey, rich or poor – if a significant portion of the food coming in was meat obtained from far and wide in the hunt, none of this would have mattered very much.

Nor would it have mattered whether one female was gathering or otherwise working on slightly more fertile ground than her sister a short distance away. Given a growing dependence on roaming game animals, the need for gender solidarity directed against men would have overridden such differences. Gathered food would have been shared within female-based coalitions, and internal conflicts over foraging space would have been minimised.

As noted earlier, a point would eventually have been reached at which a group of females could survive in virtually any game-rich habitat. All they had to do was to extract just that bit more energy – more 'labour', as we can now begin to phrase matters – from the active male population as a whole. Instead of having to base their synchrony and togetherness on the richness of gatherable resources in the immediate vicinity, they could then suspend their 'home' as if in mid-air, choosing a site not because of its intrinsic vege-tational richness but because of its strategic location *between* widely spaced hunting grounds, flint quarries, a nearby source of drinking water, gather-able resources and so on.

It is precisely this which characterises the transition from Middle Palaeolithic to Upper Palaeolithic settlement patterns.

When Neanderthals and moderns coexisted in the same region for millennia – as they seemingly did for 20,000–30,000 years in the Middle East – the Neanderthals apparently hugged the coastal regions and river valleys whilst the moderns could survive on higher, less fertile, ground. The Neanderthals were by primate standards excellent close-quarter hunters, but were relatively parochial in their attachments to place, moving endlessly within a restricted territory over which they may have exercised hereditary rights (McKay 1988).

One indication of the restricted nature of their networks is the fact that where grave-goods are left, they are such as could have been obtained by a single family acting alone; there is no evidence that precious raw materials, shells or other items were gathered for such purposes through extended kinship or alliance networks, or that such goods were circulated over long distances (Binford 1968: 147). The sudden appearance of abundant and often exotic shells and other ornaments in Upper Palaeolithic burials and in habitation debris, by contrast, shows that anatomically modern humans – as they moved into Europe and elsewhere in the course of their cultural revolution – became capable of forming immense chains of connection, allowing small groups to move in and out of one another's habitual foraging areas in a highly flexible way in accordance with seasonal and other environmental fluctuations. European evidence for this includes extensive raw-material movements and finds of seashells in regions far inland – shells which can only have been circulated in a system of structured gift exchange over very long distances (Bahn 1982). A leading authority on the earliest ornamentation in south-western France (White 1989b: 221 – 4) has remarked upon the sudden burst of interest in seashells in the Aurignacian compared with the preceding Châtelperronian, adding that 'linkages between south-western France and the Mediterranean were much stronger in the Aurignacian'. Such a novel pattern of *preserving coastal links* even *when hunting and gathering far inland*, and such a determined focus on marine symbolism, including an apparent fascination with certain shells' spiral designs (White 1989a, 1989b), may be significant in the light of our earlier discussion on the possibly tidal ultimate sources of the synchrony central to earliest ritual life (figure 7). This would match the Aboriginal Australian pattern in which the mythical 'rainbow snake' – in coastal regions a symbol of tidal rhythms and periodic floods – was preserved by Aborigines even far within the desert interior (Radcliffe-Brown 1926, 1930; Mountford 1978; Chaloupka 1984; Lewis 1988).

To understand the background to the Upper Palaeolithic revolution we must retrace our steps a little. In coastal parts of South Africa, North Africa and the Levant, anatomically modern humans in the later Pleistocene had long been combining scavenging with gathering and the hunting of small-to-medium-sized game. These activities had been carried on without true home bases. Instead, anatomically modern humans – just like their archaic counterparts – had apparently been shifting their base camps every few days as it became necessary to seek out shellfish, game animals, scavenged meat, tubers, flints, wood or other resources, each residential group shifting repeatedly between a set of different sites, in many cases following the same

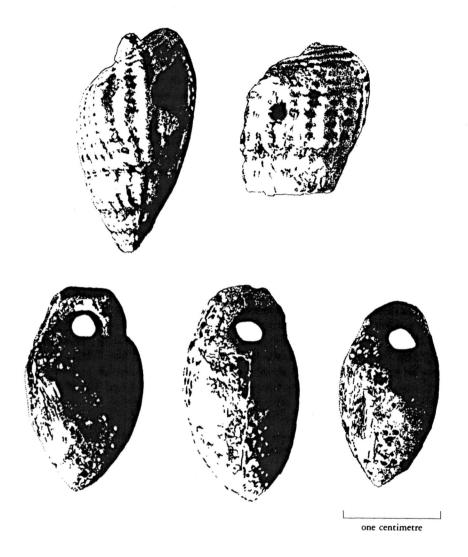

one centimetre

Figure 7   Anatomically modern humans arriving in France made ornaments from pierced sea-shells (upper); they also carved artificial 'shell' ornaments from ivory (lower), complete with spiral patterns modelled on those of the real shells. Replicas together with actual shells both recovered from the Aurignacian of La Soquette (Field Museum of Natural History, Chicago; redrawn by the author from photographs by White 1989a: 378).

local route map over countless generations (Binford 1984). Each site or temporary base corresponded to a different subsistence emphasis – perhaps hunting near one potential campsite, flint-knapping near another, tuber-digging near another and so on. No single site could be ideal for every purpose – a well-watered site, for example, might be completely lacking in flint for tool-making – and so to exploit its environment, each group had to move every few days or so from site to site within its range.

In Chapters 5 and 8 we examined reasons for supposing that patterns of some such kind remained inevitable for as long as males were tethered· by their attachments to 'their' females and offspring or, to put it another way, for as long as females with their offspring were compelled always to tag along behind 'their' males.

Between 60,000 and 70,000 years ago in the Levant, however, an important complex of cultural changes was already beginning to occur. At Mount Carmel in Israel in Late Mousterian times, two sites close to one another – a cave entrance and a rock shelter – may have been used by two collaborating groups of hunters driving medium-sized game along a narrow valley, the meat then being butchered using flake tools at the cave entrance (Ronen 1984). In the Near East we also *begin* to see evidence for personal ornamentation, as in the case of a set of drilled limestone beads found in Karain Cave in Southern Turkey and probably dating to at least 60,000 years ago (Yalcinkaya 1987: 198). There is evidence for quantitative notation, which may or may not relate to the theme of 'lunar calendars' (Marshack 1972a, 1972b; but see White 1989b: 219, who thinks such markings may have more to do with the imitation of natural seashell designs). An example is a series of regular incisions on bone at Kabar Cave in Israel (Davis 1974).

Excavations have also revealed abundant evidence for semi-permanent Middle Palaeolithic base camps of similar age. However, these were still not true home bases. Most sites consisted instead of a sprawling area of dense activity surrounded by a ring of subsidiary activity areas within a short range. Such sprawling patterns have been labelled 'radiating', to distinguish them from the 'circulating' patterns of true Upper Palaeolithic cultures (Marks 1983: 90–1). Although they were an advance on primate-style patterns in which each sleeping site along a trail is the equivalent of every other, they nonetheless indicate that spatial restrictions stemming from sexual-political constraints were still holding back foragers from going on logistic expeditions in search of game.

In the Levant, the transition to 'circulating' patterns and thus to the Upper Palaeolithic itself began happening perhaps 50,000 or more years ago. With this development, it was as if hunters had finally severed their umbilical links with the rest of the group. Instead of hovering close to home whilst making cautious 'radiating' forays away from it, individuals distri-buting their special-activities at points all around, hunters were now free to go away as far as they pleased. Once this was possible, the borders of the base camp did not have to be stretched out in all directions. Instead, 'home' could be neatly defined as a single focal point for sleeping, cooking, feeding, tool-making and many other activities – all concentrated in one spot. This point of ultra-dense activity then contrasted sharply with a surrounding 'empty' area which began immediately, and which was dotted with far-flung subsidiary sites – hunting posts, kill sites, butchering sites, quarries and so on (Marks 1983).

The transition from radiating to circulating settlement patterns marked an immense domestic and political revolution whose signature has in recent years just begun to be discerned in the archaeological record in the Levant. But it was at first hampered, according to one interpretation (Marks 1983), by an obstruction in the form of certain conservative stone tool-making techniques inherited from the past.

Lithic Implications of the Model

Pebble tools and the cruder, earlier forms of hand-axes can be made by taking a suitable lump of stone and knocking bits from it until the remainder is of the required shape. Lighter and more sophisticated artefacts are made by a reverse technique – each tool with its sharp edges is made from a flake or long blade split off from a core, rather than from the lump that remains.

Early populations of anatomically archaic *Homo sapiens* were responsible for evolving this second method into what is known as the 'Levallois' technique, whereby a lump or core is first carefully prepared, given a good striking platform and then hit upon this flat surface with a hammer to dislodge a plate-like flake. Such a flake usually has sharp edges ready made, and can be used to form the tip of a thrusting-spear or other tool. Many authorities have argued that a disadvantage is that the original lump of flint is then often useless – its size and shape frequently mean that no more tools can be made from it. This is not a problem if tools tend to be made close to a flint quarry, but the wastage may be a drawback when the knapping has to be conducted in a flint-scarce area.

One of the claimed distinguishing features of the Upper Palaeolithic is the abundance of evidence for waste-avoiding refinements of the Middle Palaeolithic Levallois technique. If the original core has been carefully selected and prepared in advance, the process of striking it with a hammer can be repeated many times, each core producing not just one leaf-shaped flake but a series of long, sharp blades. Every part of the core can then be productively used.

Although its consistent use characterises the Upper Palaeolithic, the production of blade tools from long blanks prepared in this way extends far back into the Levantine and North African Middle Palaeolithic. Over the millennia, from about 70,000 years ago, Mousterian lithic assemblages in this region show a steady change, the proportion of blade tools in each assemblage gradually increasing. Then, about 60,000 years ago in the Levant, we see cores of a certain characterisitic type. Each core has one flat platform, beneath which the flint tapers to a point. Carrying such a core from a distant flint quarry, a skilled knapper at a base camp could have transformed it into a set of good blades with virtually no wasted flint. This would have avoided the need to carry around large, burdensome lumps of flint, much of it destined to get wasted in the course of subsequent tool manufacture.

It has been argued (Marks 1983) that such concern for efficiency may tell us something about residential patterns. It may indicate that people were no longer settled in sprawling base camps with quarries or other activity areas not far away. Nor were people setting up camp near a water source one night, near a particular source of valued food a few days later, and near a flint quarry shortly afterwards when new tools had to be made. We would expect tools produced near a flint quarry to be wastefully designed. Anxiety about waste suggests the need to transport raw materials so as to manufacture tools at the knapper's leisure at a base camp which might be far from a quarry.

Piecing together the evidence as a whole, the new technique suggests that people in each locality were beginning to choose a semi-permanent site, committing themselves for a long period to this spot. A commitment to central-place foraging – involving a 'circulating' settlement pattern – would have meant selecting sites which were compromises between flint availability, water availability, the availability of food resources, shelter from the wind and so on. If a site seemed good *except* that it was nowhere near a flint quarry, it may often have had to be chosen on account of its other advantages (Marks 1983: 92). When new tools had to be made, the solution would not have been for part or all of the group to visit the nearby flint quarry. Instead, a few carefully prepared cores would have been transported over a distance to the base camp in advance. The better they had been prepared prior to transport, the more easily could they have been carried and the more blades could each have yielded.

In short, taken in conjunction with much other evidence, cores of this type seem to suggest a new type of home base consistent with the model of origins presented earlier in this chapter. Corresponding to the 'circulating' settlement pattern discussed above, its new characteristic was that it was a single permanent or semi-permanent locus for a wide variety of activities which had previously been dispersed among sites of different kinds. Instead of settling in a sprawling site adjacent to sources of flint as well as to other essential resources and moving from place to place within this small range as necessary, people embraced a far wider spatial area, settling on a single site for a lengthy period and sending out hunting parties and other detachments on far-flung expeditions from there. In terms of the argument of this book, an inference is that females had achieved sufficient solidarity and strength to pick on a good, sheltered, strategically located site for a base camp and then stay put, no longer following their menfolk around. Instead of travelling around, endlessly searching for food – they stood firm and made the food come to them!

Hunters of the Ice Age

Because of these changes, Upper Palaeolithic hunters could react to cold climate conditions in a wholly unprecedented way. Instead of responding as primates might ordinarily have been expected to do – allowing the wide open spaces to inflict a loss of social complexity and structure – and instead of falling back on the physical survival capabilities of individuals, these cultured humans were able to benefit socially as well as materially from the new, game-rich conditions. Early in the Upper Palaeolithic, the establishment of logistic hunting involved a 'shift from mixed strategies of scavenging the remains of large carcasses and hunting, to full dependence on hunting' (Bar Yosef and Belfer-Cohen 1988: 32). In other words, hunting became for the first time quite reliable, making it possible to abandon the practice of scavenging as a back-up source of food.

Jump kills, drives and similar techniques were being used in Anatolia, Jordan and coastal sites in Israel as early as 60,000 years ago, although only with medium-sized game (Bar Yosef and Belfer-Cohen 1988; Wolf 1988; Ronen 1984). In the Near East and Europe 30,000 years later, these techniques had been enormously advanced. Modern humans distinguished themselves by shifting to highly specialised forms of hunting requiring long-term advance planning, and concentrating on just a few species (Mellars 1973, 1989). No longer did people just move from place to place, occasionally killing a creature which they happened to meet: they developed specialised technologies and actively went out in search of specific prey. In Eastern Europe and central Russia, Upper Palaeolithic hunters selected in particular mammoth and wild horse; in southern Russia, bison; in Siberia, reindeer or horse. Close to the European ice-sheets, wild horse, musk-ox, steppe bison, woolly rhinoceros, ibex, mammoth and other large animals were at first abundant, and these, too, were hunted in logistic, deliberate ways.

In the new kinds of hunting, there was a much-increased reliance on the game *drive*, in which 'planning depth' (Binford 1989: 19–25) was more than ever necessary, and which demanded considerable travel on the part of highly specialised hunting teams who may often have had to stay out overnight (Binford 1983: 163). The aim of such expeditions was to ensure that whole herds of reindeer, horse or wild cattle could be stampeded over a cliff or into a bog or other trap, whereupon those that survived could easily be killed. Drawing on ethnographic analogies, such as with North American bison-hunters, most writers suppose that such mass killings would have involved elaborate ceremonial, with shamans and ritual leaders co-ordinating the efforts of large numbers of people (Fagan 1987: 199–220). Women may often have been involved in the actual driving of the game, and were certainly central in associated activities, in the ritual preparations for hunting and in the celebrations mounted as hunting parties returned.

Nearly all the known Upper Palaeolithic occupation sites in ice-age Europe were situated in the valleys of major watercourses – particularly at the shallower points which formed river crossings used by herds of migratory game. Along some of these cold rivers and streams – particularly in the vast area of tundra which then stretched from Czechoslovakia through Poland, the Ukraine and eastward to Siberia – herds of mammoth fed, migrated and roamed. Some 25,000 years ago, a group of mammoth hunters camped at Pavlov and Dolni Vestonice in what is now Czechoslovakia. Both sites were close to migration routes predictably used by slow-moving herds of mammoth; the hunters apparently lay in wait and ambushed the animals. The Dolni Vestonice people were camped at the edge of a river valley in late autumn; it is thought that they may have been laying in meat as a staple for the approaching winter months, drying out the flesh on a sunny, windswept slope. The ground was permanently frozen a few feet below the surface, which meant that meat could be stored in pits which made good natural refrigerators (Klíma 1963, 1968; Soffer 1985).

Ice, Domesticity and Fire

With the advent of the cultures of the Upper Palaeolithic, controlled domestic fire, the home base and a sexual division of labour are no longer problematic; evidence for all these dimensions is found at virtually all excavated habitation sites.

A succession of Upper Palaeolithic levels at the Abri Pataud, a rock shelter at Les Eyzies in the Dordogne, yielded particularly exciting evidence of hearths when carefully excavated in the 1960s by Hallam Movius (1966). Reanalysing Movius' data, Binford (1983: 163) notes a row of five Aurignacian hearths all neatly spaced apart with just enough room between each for one person to sleep. This floor, suggests Binford, must have been used by an all-male hunting band during overnight hunting expeditions about 32,000 years ago. Another level at the same rock-shelter belonging to the Perigordian VI phase – about 23,000 years ago – Binford also regards as representing a temporary hunting-camp. But such patterns contrast sharply with a Perigordian configuration in the same place but in a slightly different lens. Here, there are ample spaces between the rear wall and the hearths – spaces large enough to have contained multiple 'double beds' warmed by the fires and protected by a windbreak. Binford interprets this pattern as representing a mixed-sex domestic dwelling.

The Abri Pataud was one of many French excavated habitation sites which took advantage of the shelter afforded by overhanging rocks or the entrances

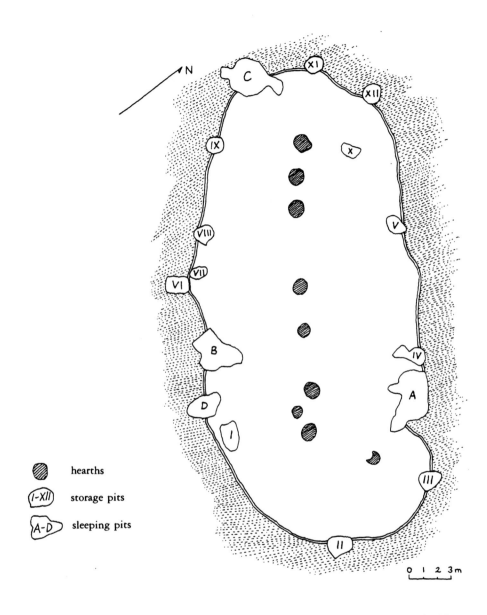

hearths

storage pits *(I–XII)*

sleeping pits *(A–D)*

Figure 8 Kostienki I-1; Ukraine. Floor-plan of an Upper Palaeolithic complex dwelling. The building materials were mostly mammoth-bones. Note the line of hearths. Venus figurines were among the objects found in the storage pits. Soviet archaeologists believe the whole immense floor area was covered by a single roof of mammoth skins. Communal living arrangements may have favoured the maintenance of menstrual synchrony between resident kin-related women tending the hearths (redrawn after Klein 1969: Fig. 33).

to caves. In most of Central and particularly Eastern Europe, however, there were few such rocks or caves, whilst in the Ukraine and Siberia, conditions were so windswept and severe that it was not until several thousand years following the Aurignacian in Europe that modern humans proved able to adapt effectively to the challenges. When they did, the hunters defended themselves against the severities of the climate by building sturdy, well-heated huts and sometimes complex dwellings.

Probably the most important of all regions for our understanding of Upper Palaeolithic domesticity is the area which includes the valleys of the Dniester, Dnieper, Desna and Don rivers in the Ukraine. Between 25,000 and 11,000 years ago, almost the entire region consisted of open periglacial grassland, not far beyond the margins of the great European ice sheets. Since there were no rock shelters, caves or other natural shelters, dwellings were constructed by digging deep pits, covering them with bones or tusks – and draping weighted hides over these supports. In the absence of wood, the builders used mammoth-bones which must have lain about in the neighbourhood for many years before being gathered for building purposes. Such bones were probably also used as fuel.

The most notable structures are of two kinds: small, round houses with single hearths, and large inferred 'longhouses' with multiple hearths. Particularly well-preserved dwellings of the second type are at Pushkari and Kostienki I and IV.

Pushkari I, on the Desna, was a shallow, oval-shaped depression, 12 metres long by 4 metres wide, with three hearths in a line along the major axis. Kostienki I-1 consists of a large and complex longhouse made of mammoth bones, with nine hearth pits strung out between 2 and 2.5 metres apart along its major axis (figure 8). The same dwelling contained numerous hollows which have been interpreted as sleeping pits, along with storage-pits dug in the floor. Some of these contained mammoth-bones – possibly the remains of meat stores – while in others were found quantities of flint tools, female figurines, animal statuettes and other objects (Klein 1969: 116–40). Charred bone has yielded a radiocarbon date of about 12,000 years (Wymer 1982: 240–2). Whether or not dwellings with very large floor spaces indicate extended matrilocally organised household units, as one archaeologist has plausibly argued (Ember 1973: 177–80), it seems that a group of about fifty people lived here through the savage ice age winter, subsisting on stored frozen meat.

Other nearby dwellings have been found, several of which could have housed a number of families living jointly. If women were not synchronising in these dwellings, it would have been surprising – unless certain of the multi-hearth camps were actually those of male hunting bands. A space of 2 metres or more separating small, neatly structured hearths, however, strongly suggests mixed-sex residential dwellings, with room between fires for couples or children to sleep together on beds warmed from each side (see

Binford 1983: 160–3). This inference is supported by the fact that many of the larger dwellings have been found to have definite 'male' and 'female' living-areas (Shimkin 1978: 278) – which incidentally is suggestive of a strongly marked system of gender segregation, implying added probabilities of gender solidarity and hence synchrony.

From about 25,000 BP onwards, rich symbolic and artistic traditions in the area from the Ukraine to Siberia are indicated by the heavy use of red ochre, by abundant female figurines associated with the more complex dwellings – and by what have been interpreted as complex lunar notation systems (Marshack 1972b). We can only guess at the traditions of shamanic dance, trance, cosmology and ritual which surely characterised cultural patterns throughout this immense region. In this context, perhaps the most extraordinary finds ever made are the apparent 'cult lodges' of Mezhirich, in the valley of the Dneipr River, about 90 miles south-east of Kiev. Dating back about 15,000 years, one of the five multi-occupied permanent buildings was evidently very special: its walls were made up almost entirely of the mandibles of mammoths (Korniets and Soffer 1984). Far to the east, an ivory plaquette from Mal'ta in Siberia has hundreds of pits engraved on it in spirals; these have long been interpreted by Soviet scholars as evidence of a system of religion or cosmology centred on the changing phases of the moon (Frolov 1977–9, 1979; cited in Bahn and Vertut 1988: 182).

Speculations about religion aside, we can be sure that women in the dwellings we have discussed had come a long, long way from the condition of their Lower and Middle Palaeolithic predecessors. Child-burdened females were no longer caught between the need to gain help from one another and the need to avoid excessive travel (Chapter 5); they had broken through the entire framework of such constraints, establishing a completely new mode of living. Groups of related women were now in a position to stay in one place for weeks or perhaps months on end, assisting one another in the tasks of household management, gathering, storing food, preparing meals, cooking, distributing provisions and caring for children – whilst drawing on the continuous economic and social support of men who could comb an immense area for game. Women could be in one place, their togetherness sustained by male activities far away. Men could be away hunting for extended periods, their logistic freedom sustained by the knowledge that their womenfolk had their own sexual defences, and were not likely to be simply 'taken over' by rival males during their absence. Each gender group was freed by the other to perform its own distinctive role, the two benefiting jointly from the human revolution's gains.

Following each hunt, the butchering, cooking and consumption of meat would have presupposed large groups and extensive systems of sharing and exchange. Roasting pits or earth ovens had to be large enough to hold sometimes considerable quantities of meat. Precisely how a mammoth would have been cooked is not known, but we can perhaps gain some idea of the associated mythology from Lévi-Strauss (1981: 623), who on the basis of American Indian materials writes of traditional cooking's

> often considerable complexity of structure, its nature as a collective undertaking, the traditional knowledge and attention needed to ensure its correct functioning and the slowness of the cooking-process, which sometimes lasted several days, and was accompanied until the final moment by uncertainty as to the outcome.

Should something have gone wrong within the great earth oven, continues Lévi-Strauss, the consequence might sometimes have been disastrous, since a whole community's provisions and prospects of avoiding starvation through the winter months might have been at stake. This is possibly overdramatised: no one would have tried to cook a whole mammoth in a single oven all at once; moreover, dried or frozen meat stores would have been carefully preserved. Nonetheless, it seems worth bearing in mind that each cooking-process would have been watched over with some anxiety. Like most other writers, Lévi-Strauss (1981: 623) concludes that it would have been women who bore the main responsibility for the momentous and seemingly magical process in which raw meat was slowly transformed into cooked. And in this connection, supernatural dangers may have been feared at least as much as others. If ethnographic menstrual taboos are any guide, there are strong grounds for supposing that all female cooks would have had to be sure that they were not menstruating at this risk-laden them – lest their blood should magically contaminate the fire and catastrophically ruin the whole process. The sexual-political logic of such taboos will be discussed in Chapter 11.

As fire became more portable with the discovery of new ignition techniques, there would have been reduced pressures on hunters to stay close to 'home'. With their own fires which could be lit anywhere, males would have been in a much better position to camp out overnight whilst hunting. As we have just seen, in the Dordogne region in France some of the excavated 'living floors' may in fact have been non-residential and occupied by all-male hunting-bands (Binford 1983: 163). It might be thought that men's independent ability to ignite fires in such dwellings may have led to some danger of them 'cheating' by roasting and eating their own kills far from camp instead of bringing it home! But as we will see in Chapter 11, this in turn would have prompted women to evolve counter-measures, including, it would seem, the imposition of menstrual avoidances restricting legitimate meat-cooking to only certain specific lunar/menstrually defined times. We will see that such female action allows us to make sense of many otherwise puzzling ethnographic linkages between menstruation, the moon and blood-linked cooking taboos.

Beyond all this, it is not difficult to appreciate the connection between the 'planning depth' essential to specialised, long-distance tracking and hunting (Binford 1989: 19–25) and the sexual logic of delayed gratification implicit in the sex-strike model. We might even say that in drastically delaying both culinary and sexual gratification, women's action made possible the 'invention' of cultural time. Banning sex would certainly have cleared aside an entirely new and dedicated sector of space/time within which human *productive* activities could occur. By decisively disjoining sex from work, consumption from production and ends from means, it must also have vastly enhanced humans' awareness of how to organise their time (cf. Wagener 1987).

A Global Species

The earliest Upper Palaeolithic peoples seem to have been quick to expand outwards, always moving so as to extend the frontiers of the then-habitable world. They had arrived in Greater Australia (then attached to New Guinea) in what by evolutionary standards seems an instant. All available evidence suggests that Australia was initially reached at least 35,000 years ago, and probably much earlier, by human migrants from south-east Asia (Jones 1989; Bunney 1990, citing Roberts, Jones and Smith). This means that fully modern humans had spread from Africa and were already arriving in Australia millennia before their slower-moving counterparts had begun entering Western Europe and displacing the Neanderthals. In Chapter 13 we will review evidence that the first Australian Aborigines who settled along the coastal regions of the new continent would have found a hunter's paradise, teeming with giant, slow moving marsupials which are long since extinct.

Why did modern humans with their Upper Palaeolithic cultures 'explode' across the world so astonishingly rapidly? The hunting way of life was part of the explanation: people were at first spread thinly over the landscape, attached not so much to particular patches of territory as to roaming herds of game – herds which human hunters were always tempted to follow. People also had powerful kinship systems which in the earliest stages stressed interdependence and space-embracing solidarity over and above local intensification or parochial territorial loyalties (Gamble 1986a). With true home bases and a sexual division of labour, each band or local group would have been able to forage over a vast area. Then only a slight increase in population would have set up pressures to embrace yet more space, both for exploration and for hunting. The post-glacial cultures associated with the origins of farming were later to prove relatively intensive in their uses of space. From then on, history was essentially made by cultures which discovered ways of fitting ever more people into ever more restricted areas. The earlier Upper Palaeolithic cultures had no need to evolve in this way: they were space hungry and resistant to any intensification of land use. Their first answer to problems of resource scarcity would have been simply to move on.

Chapter 10
The Hunter's Moon

In the final analysis, all forms of economics can be reduced to an economics of time. Likewise, society must divide up its time purposefully in order to achieve a production suited to its general needs. . . .
Karl Marx, *Grundrisse* (1857–9)

As periodic female non-availability assisted males in concentrating on hunting, menstrually scheduled sex strikes would have begun to last for three, four, six or more days. In cold, sparsely vegetated regions necessitating heavy dependence on meat, male hunting expeditions would have become more extended and well organised in proportion as female sexual pressures became intensified. Weak or short spells of celibacy would have meant ineffective, brief hunting forays; extended forays would have been undertaken in those regions where female pressures and capacities for sexual self-control developed furthest.

Extensions of female pressure would have involved longer periods of withdrawal and the steady establishment of more and more synchrony between neighbouring female groups. Short sex strikes would have been difficult to synchronise across wide areas, but longer ones would have increased the probabilities of overlap between strikes in one locality and in the next, making it harder for males to find loopholes within the system. Where females across a wide area could collectively resist sex for several days on end this in turn would have added to the pressure for increased synchronisation of activity on the part of males. Temporarily denied sex, and made aware that access to women could only be gained via success in the chase, males over a wide area would all have been motivated to go hunting at around the same time, dramatically increasing the probabilities of inter-male and inter-band collaboration in the hunt itself.

The greater the number of women who were roughly synchronising in menstrually scheduled withdrawal, the greater would have been the difficulty of compressing this collective action into a tightly delimited period. If bleeding conferred female status and power in proportion as it motivated greater male hunting efforts, there would have been selection pressures in favour of prolonged and heavy menstruation. Even before ochre or other forms of pigmentation came into use, there may have been temptations to spread the blood around – to make the most of what there was, to delay washing it off the body, or to allow women with no blood to smear themselves with blood from friends. If longer sex strikes on average produced greater quantities of meat, women would have had a strong interest in using these or other techniques to extend the duration of each strike.

Beginnings and endings may have been staggered. Even if most women had ceased to bleed after five or so days, in a large group the chances would have been high that a few were bleeding still. Far from causing a problem, however, this may have been of benefit to women in helping them to extend still further their *collective* periods of withdrawal.

Envisage, now, an early Upper Palaeolithic population in which the sex-strike strategy had been in operation for some time, and in which big game hunting had begun to become predictably successful. Larger game would have required more co-operation between hunters, and would have produced more meat as a result. It would also have meant that fewer expeditions were required within any given season, involving a slowing down of the rhythm according to which collective hunts had to be organised.

The new slow rhythm could not have been annual, for that would have been too slow: no community could have relied on just one major hunting expedition per year. But neither could it have been circadian, for a night/day rhythm would have been far too rapid. It would have been a challenge to prepare and organise a major co-operative hunting expedition even with the space of a week, let alone a day. Some intermediate standard of synchrony would have been required, its periodicity falling somewhere between a year and a day, a basic condition being that whatever the nature of the chosen 'clock', it would have needed to be capable of simultaneously regulating the cyclical on/off rhythm of the female sex.

The Moon

Now it so happens that in human cultures, menstruation – which means 'moon change' – is widely imagined to be a 'lunar' phenomenon. Robert Briffault's *The Mothers* (1927), published over sixty years ago, is the most exhaustive compilation of folk-beliefs in this connection. Although outdated in its sources and methodology, this vast cross-cultural survey still carries conviction in asserting that such beliefs are, or were until very recently, an important aspect of cosmology in just about every corner of the globe.

Briffault (1927, 2: 431) tells us of Germans in country districts who refer to menstruation simply as 'the moon', and of French peasants who term it 'le moment de la lune'. He then scours the world for comparable reports. For page after page, Briffault piles up examples – in the Congo, menstruation is spoken of as *ngonde*, that is the 'moon'; in Torres Straits, the same word means both 'moon' and 'menstrual blood' . . . etc. etc. Although many of the reports are culled not from anthropological monographs but from nineteenth-century missionaries', explorers' and traders' tales, their sheer number leaves us with little doubt as to the universality and tenacity of the cultural moon-menstruation link.

More recently, professional social anthropologists have added to our information on such beliefs, although modern writers no longer find it useful to define and isolate a 'custom' and then seek to illustrate it – independently of its context – with examples from all over the world. Since the 1920s, folkloristic findings linking the moon with menstruation have in fact rarely been accorded theoretical significance of any kind, having in the main escaped allocation within any diffusionist, functionalist, structuralist, sociobiological or other twentieth-century conceptual grid. Given the clear evidence that few anthropologists have positively wanted to discover such beliefs or known what to do with them once found, the fact that they have continued to be reported is perhaps all the more impressive as testimony to their reality.

Hunting Ritual and the Moon

The origins model developed in the previous chapter prompts us to consider the moon's possible relevance to early Upper Palaeolithic hunting schedules. In this context, two choices seem to present themselves.

It seems possible that hunting as such never had anything directly to do with moonlight, except in so far as the moon helped to make accurate timing possible and thereby assisted with the regulation of complex collective undertakings such as game drives. On this interpretation, men would have been tempted to hunt collectively whenever the need was felt or the opportunity to do so presented itself. Hunters were not astrologers. They did not check whether the moon's condition indicated a propitious moment for hunting. They just hunted whenever they saw fit. They may often have referred to the moon so as to fix in advance an agreed date (Wagener 1987), their hunting and other activities increasingly displaying what Binford (1989) has termed 'planning depth', but beyond that the moon's phases had only a random connection with the hunt. People could have decided to hunt at dark moon one month, shortly after full moon some time later, and two days following the third quarter a month after that.

On the other hand, we have already concluded that hunters would have had to fit in with what woman were doing if they wanted fertile sex. If hunters were to be away from home for long periods, it would have made biological sense for these absences to have coincided with the periods when

women were unlikely to conceive, hunters returning meat-laden and in
expectation of sexual rewards at around the time of ovulation.

This means that if women were synchronising with one another, men
would have had to synchronise with this same rhythm, phase-locking the
periodicity of hunting with the on/off rhythm of the menstrual cycle.

We saw in Chapter 7 that contemporary medical evidence linking the
menstrual cycle with the moon is inconclusive at best. On the other hand, we
noted (1) that human cycles are of the appropriate average phase length and
(2) that women can deliberately phase-lock with the moon if they expose
themselves nocturnally to correctly timed artificial light. A further finding
was that women could not have synchronised with one another over wide
areas without using some kind of clock. The moon provides the only appropriate clock which would have been available to them. If men as hunters had
to fit in with this female-defined rhythm, as outlined in Chapter 9, then the
hunt itself would have had to accommodate to this same rhythm and hence
to the moon.

That, then, is one possible way of drawing out the implications of the
model. In short: (1) women for their own reasons went 'on strike' during
their menstrual periods; (2) they used the moon to standardise their synchrony; (3) men's hunting expeditions and post-hunt celebrations had to fit
in with this rhythm; (4) hunting schedules therefore bore a certain relationship to changes in the moon. Beyond this, we need not specify how frequently men hunted, nor for how long. Provided there was no conflict with
women's rites and rhythms, men could have hunted once a month, twice a
month – or only a few times a year.

We may think of this as the moon influencing the hunt not directly – not
through the mundane, material usefulness of its light, for example – but
indirectly, through women, or through what might better be described as
the menstrual/sexual/ritual dimension of life. Before turning to the possibility of more direct influences, let us check whether there is any evidence
for this theoretically predicted indirect pathway to the lunar phase-locking of
the hunt.

Sub-Saharan Africa: Pathways to Moon-scheduled Hunting

An example suggestive of this pattern is provided by the Hadza hunters and
gatherers who occupy a particularly fertile region of East Africa in the vicinity of Lake Eyasi, within the Rift Valley (close to Olduvai Gorge).

James Woodburn (1982: 190) describes a dark moon festival (the *epeme*) as
these peoples' 'major religious celebration'. In accordance with a widespread
African pattern (Briffault 1927, 2: 422–3), all ordinary activities cease at
this time. Among the Hadza, they make way for the sacred *epeme* dance
which is held every month at night in pitch darkness. There is impressive
lunar phase-locking here, since the dance 'can only be held at the time of the

month when there is a period of total darkness without moonlight' (Woodburn 1982: 191). Leg-bells and dance-rattles are used to make noise, and after each man dances – disguised as another person – he communicates with the women, using a special whistling language. The women collectively call back using the kinship term for the relative whose role the performer is playing. This usually continues for two or three nights in succession, the basic themes being kinship, joint parentage and an attempt 'to reconcile the opposed interests of men and women which are so manifest in many other contexts'.

The dance establishes collective wellbeing and good order, and is in large part aimed at creating the conditions necessary for effective hunting. 'Failure to hold the dance is believed to be dangerous. Performing the dance is believed to maintain and promote general wellbeing, above all good health and successful hunting.'

It is important to realise that normatively – that is, in native belief – Hadza women synchronise their menstrual cycles with the moon (Woodburn, personal communication). Here, then, a logical structure begins to emerge in which synchronised menstruation occurring at dark moon puts an end to sexual conflicts and arguments, and in this context helps to establish the social and sexual-political conditions for successful hunting. Whilst it is not suggested that all this literally happens among the Hadza – menstrual synchrony on the behavioural level may be little more than a myth – it does seem as if the people are familiar with some such logic, and that they structure their rituals in awareness of it. Particularly interesting in the Hadza case is that men in these dark moon rituals are acting out alternative roles. It seems important that women should at least pretend not to recognise these men as their husbands – who, after all, if our model were to be accepted, 'ought' to be their 'blood' or kin.

Unfortunately, we have little hard evidence for either the presence or absence of real menstrual synchrony among the hunter-gatherer peoples of Africa. Woodburn has not published on this subject, and no subsequent researchers have tested to discover whether lunar phase-locking actually occurs. Woodburn's personally communicated finding is paralleled, however, by a notion reported of the !Kung. Here, people 'believe . . . that if a woman sees traces of menstrual blood on another woman's leg or even is told that another woman has started her period, *she* will begin menstruating as well' (Shostak 1983: 68). Again, it is difficult to know whether this is myth or reality. Nonetheless, the statement is interesting as an expression of what !Kung women for cultural reasons believe. When one woman menstruates, it is felt that her sisters or companions will automatically join her.

There is, then, little solid evidence for extant menstrual synchrony in eastern or southern Africa. Absence of evidence – the inadequacy of our database – is in itself not fatal for a model, however, particularly if the model poses questions which have not previously been asked. In any case, my model as such – which concerns origins – would not lead us to expect the preservation of synchrony into the twentieth century. Let us turn, now, to something which has been more solidly documented – the fact that many of the more public and observable aspects of *ritual* life in this part of the world are or were synchronised with definite phases of the moon.

The San (or 'Khoisan') peoples of southern Africa consist of a number of linguistically diverse groups whose traditions are those of hunters and gatherers, stretching from the Damara in the West to the ‖Xegwi in the East, and from the !Kung in the North to the ‖Xam in the South – a vast portion of the African continent. Uniting all these peoples is the traditional prominence, in both ritual and cosmology, of the moon (Barnard 1988).

It has often been reported that these peoples all share a particular affection for the new moon – a sentiment which in the past gave rise to somewhat misleading European reports of 'Moon Worship'. 'Their religion', as one writer put it in reference to the Namaqua (quoted in Hahn 1881: 46),

> chiefly consists in worshipping and praising the new moon. The men stand in a circle together and blow on a pipe or similar instrument, and the women clasping hands, dance around the men.

The Khoekhoe (sheep and cattle-herding San peoples) celebrated the whole night through, with 'merry-making and clasping of hands' as each new moon appeared (Hahn 1881: 38). 'At new moon', wrote another author of a related group (quoted in Hahn 1881: 39), 'they come together and make a noise the whole night, dancing in a circle, and while dancing they clasp their hands together'. Barnard (1988: 220) comments:

> There is no doubt that the Moon is important in Khoekhoe and Bushman symbolism, or that the lunar cycle marks propitious times for dancing, even today in the Kalahari, where dances are most often held at full moon; but moon-worship is largely a fantasy of European ethnographers.

The truth seems to be that since time immemorial, people throughout this region have not 'worshipped' the moon, but have felt a powerful sense of affection for and material dependency upon it, dancing in accordance with its changing phases whilst revering a spiritual entity made visibly manifest in the moon.

Among the most important San dance festivals are those triggered by the onset of a girl's first menstruation. This pattern is certainly extremely ancient. The evidence includes the remarkable painting at Fulton's Rock in the Drakensberg mountains of Natal, which David Lewis-Williams (1981) has identified as depicting a girl's first menstruation rite. A covered figure inside an incomplete circle is (according to this interpretation) a girl kept in a special hut, with three female companions clapping their hands. The

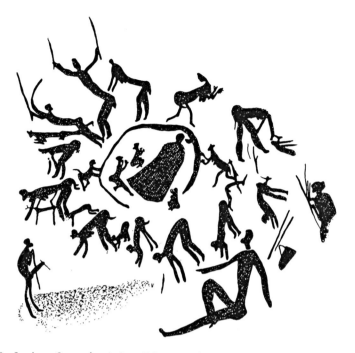

Figure 9 Southern San rock-painting. Fulton's Rock, Drackensberg Mountains, Natal (redrawn after Lewis-Williams 1981: Fig 10). According to David Lewis-Williams, the central figure is a young enrobed woman undergoing her first menstruation ceremony in a special shelter. Circling her are clapping women, female dancers and (in the outer ring) men with their hunting equipment. Two figures hold sticks; the women bend over and display 'tails' as they imitate the mating behaviour of elands. Among living San, such rituals are intimately connected with success in hunting. Note that each male figure has a bar across his penis. This is probably the artist's way of marking the marital abstinence associated with menstruation and valued as a condition of hunting luck.

figures surrounding the hut and bending forward are women performing the ritual dance, imitating the mating behaviour of antelopes. The other figures (some definitely male, others probably so) represent the few men who join in the dance, some holding sticks. It is noteworthy that the surrounding figures, are all bending over, their buttocks playfully thrust in the direction of the menstruating girl (figure 9).

All these details match those of hunt-linked menstrual rituals still practised by San and related groups in recent times (Lewis-Williams 1981). The Fulton's Rock painting comes to life in these living rituals – as described, for example, in the writings of Ten Raa (1969), who worked some decades ago among the Sandawe of central Tanzania. Although these cattle-keeping hoe-cultivators are not technically San, they have a click language, were until recently hunter-gatherers and seem to be linked culturally with San traditions in many ways.

Much of Sandawe life focuses on a series of fertility rites known as *phek'umo*. The dances of *phek'umo* are held after sunset, the only illumination allowed being the benign, 'cool' light of the moon. Linking the *phek'umo* with the eland-bull dance of girls' puberty rites among the north-western Bushmen is the native claim that such dances were organised in the past *by men who had daughters who had begun to menstruate* (Ten Raa 1969: 36). Menstruation as such is associated with *the darkness of new moon*; but the nocturnal dances get under way only as the moon approaches fullness – at around the beginning of the moon's second quarter. The dance is begun by the women, who go round in circles:

> They carry their arms high in a stance which is said to represent the horns of the moon, and at the same time also the horns of game animals and cattle. The women select their partners from among the opposing row of men by dancing in front of them with suggestive motions. The selected partners then come forward and begin to dance in the same manner as the women do, facing them all the time. (Ten Raa 1969: 38)

As the dance warms up, the movements become more and more erotic; some of the women turn round and gather up their garments to expose their buttocks to the men:

> Finally the men embrace the women while emitting hoarse grunts which sound like those of animals on heat. The men and women lift one another up in turn, embracing tightly and mimicking the act of fertilization; those who are not dancing shout encouragements at them. . . .

What the women are in fact doing, writes Ten Raa (1969: 38), is to re-enact the role of the moon in the basic creation myth, according to which the moon entices the sun into the sky for the first celestial copulation. The women are the moon; the men, the sun. The whole rite is held under the aegis of the moon, and has the explicit purpose of 'making the country fertile'.

To such descriptions, it is worth adding that among all San groups, shamanistic trance involves activating a supernatural potency which the !Kung call *n/um* (Marshall 1969: 350–3). Much rock-art from Zimbabwe shows dancers whose stomachs are distended to signify potency of a similar kind (figure 10a). Amongst the southern San, a comparable potency was made manifest as dancers began to bleed from the nose (Bleek 1935: 19, 34). Arbousset (1846: 246–7) describes Maluti San collapsing in trance 'covered in blood, which pours from the nostrils'. Numerous rock-paintings in Cape Province depict trance-induced nose-bleedings of this kind (e.g. Lewis-Williams 1981: Figs. 19, 20). If men were to express life-renewing ritual power – evidently – it was necessary either that their womenfolk should be menstruating or that blood should flow in some other way (figure 10b).

Among the extinct San groups responsible for much rock art in South

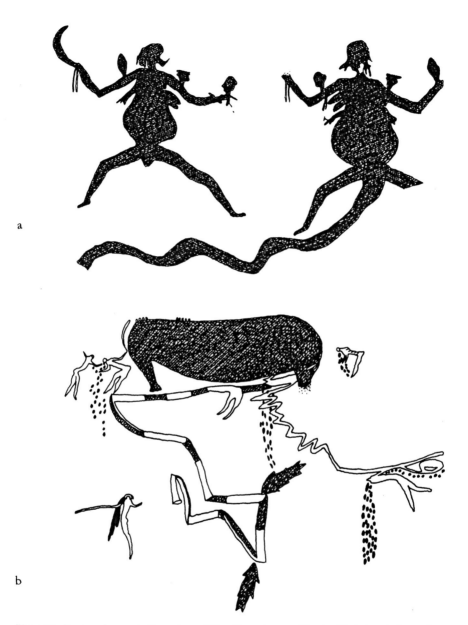

a

b

Figure 10 Dance and trance in San rock-art. *Upper*: Manemba, near Mutoko, Zimbabwe (redrawn after Garlake 1987: Fig. 78). Dance with apparently menstrual and perhaps lunar connotations. The distended stomachs indicate ritual potency, corresponding with the !Kung San notion of *n/um*. The figure releasing a flow may once have held a crescent-shaped ornament like that of her companion, but this area has now exfoliated. *Lower*: De Rust, Eastern Cape (redrawn after Lewis-Williams 1983: Fig. 18). Medicine men bleeding from the nose as they attempt to control a rain-animal. The men are in a 'wet' phase of ritual experience, as shown by the presence of two fish.

Africa, blood-linked as well as moon-linked ritual was possibly involved not
only as a subject but also in the magical process of painting. In 1930, a
woman called Marion Walsham How met an old man named Mapote who
claimed still to know the traditional painting techniques. Since his testimony is virtually the only source of information we have on this subject, it
has inevitably been widely discussed. Invited to make up the paint, he said
that the red pigment had to be Qhang Qhang – haematite, or oxidised red
ochre mixed with various other iron oxides. This, he said, had to be *prepared
at full moon outside in the open by a woman*, who had to heat it until it was red
hot and then grind it to a fine red powder. His most difficult request was for a
fixing agent consisting of *the blood of a freshly killed eland* to mix with the
ochre which had been thus prepared (Taylor 1985: 34, citing How 1965). It
appears, then – in view of the required freshness of this kill – that this eland
too, had to be killed at or around full moon.

One theoretical possibility, then, is that since culture's earliest days, the
moon's relevance was in a sense peripheral – its light did not directly influence society's basic work rhythms, but merely governed such things as the
timing of dancing, singing, shamanistic painting or other ritual. According
to this model, in a pattern still apparently perpetuated by contemporary
African hunter/gatherers, the days around full and new moon would have
been occasions for special celebrations and late-night dancing; *consequently,
productive activities such as hunting would have had to be timetabled so as to fit in
with this ritual calendar*.

At first sight – from a strictly functionalist standpoint – it might be
thought that this would have been an inconvenience. Given that preparations for a hunting trip might often have taken days, would not obligatory
all-night dancing frequently have interfered? Why would hunters have
allowed the moon to get in the way of their productive activities?

But of course our model of origins places all this in another context. We
have already seen why women would have needed to synchronise their
menstrual cycles, and why this would have meant using the moon as the only
available common clock. Moreover, we have seen that the whole concept of a
monthly sex strike implies that women would have sent their menfolk away
on a large-scale hunting expedition at least once per biological month. In
addition to all this, however, we will now see that the complex rhythmic
configuration so far arrived at would have been reinforced – in a kind of
'redundancy' characteristic of so many biological processes – by the direct,
physical action of the moon not just on women but on men as well.

The truth is that for hunters to have varied their rates of activity according
to the availability of nocturnal light would have made not just emotional/
ritual/sexual sense. It would have made sense for the most materialistic,
mundane of reasons. Far from allowing the moon to interfere with their

productive activities, hunters who clapped and sang at each dark and full moon would have been scheduling their activities so as to make maximum use of the moon's light as a resource. This would have been no more 'romantic' than the fact that agriculturalists as a matter of course use calendars to maximise their use of the sun. Let us see why this would have been so.

Hunting and Moonlight

Most lunar phases are a matter of more or less light, more or less shadow. Only at dark moon and then again at full is an extreme reached, with either all light or all shadow. At these points, moreover, there is a directional change – from waxing to waning, and then again from waning to waxing. Only at these points in its cycle, in other words, does the moon undergo a qualitative as opposed to merely quantitative change – making these two nodal points the easiest to select as cues for behavioural synchrony.

On this basis, we might predict ovulatory cycle-linked celebrations to have been timed to occur at one nodal point or the other. If we ignore the possibility of a biological photic correlation of ovulation with full moon (Chapter 7), then at first glance it might not seem to matter whether women ovulated at full moon and menstruated at dark or the other way around. Either pattern would have worked, provided one or the other direction of polarity were consistently chosen. Whether the choices were narrowed down further would depend on other factors. Here, the crucial question would be whether the moon's nocturnal light had a value independent of its value as a cue for synchrony.

As the new moon first appears, its thin wafer rises in the east early in the day but is not normally visible as it follows the sun across the sky, shining bright enough to be visible only as it sets in the west shortly after the sun. In the following days, it rises later and later during the daylight hours, becoming brighter and brighter, and lasting after sunset longer into the night. The moon's light thereby extends visibility with increasing intensity without any break, 'taking over' from the sun in illuminating the landscape from dusk onwards. At full moon itself – as eclipse-watchers will know – sun and moon are exactly opposite one another, the moon rising in the east as the sun sets in the west, and staying up all night until setting at dawn. After full moon, however, there is a break in the evening's light-supply. Following a post-full-moon sunset, there is immediate darkness before the moon eventually rises, and as the nights pass this period of darkness lengthens, the moon becoming a thinner and thinner sickle as it rises later and later after dusk.

To ice age long-distance hunters dependent on precise combinations of solar and lunar illumination, such differences between the moon's various phases would hardly have gone unnoticed. Traditional hunters frequently maintain the option of being able to extend the chase where necessary beyond nightfall – even to the point, in some cases, of going on entirely nocturnal hunts. Such hunters have sound practical reasons for valuing the moon's light. It may be relatively weak, and it may often become obscured by cloud, but except under dense cloud conditions it substantially extends the length of a working day, and helps the overnight traveller to see. Taken in conjunction with the constraints introduced by ovarian synchrony and a periodic female sex strike, the result in the case of ice age populations would have been a rigid and quite elaborate logical structure. In later chapters we will see how intriguingly this overlaps with the allegedly 'universal' structures uncovered by Lévi-Strauss in his *Mythologiques*.

For Upper Palaeolithic communal hunters, the prospect of an hour or more of near-total darkness abruptly closing off an evening's hunting would have seemed a discouraging potential handicap, particularly if the prey were active at night and in possession of good nocturnal vision. It is also worth noting that *communal* hunting, which is most effective when it involves focusing on highly clumped herds of prey, requires a considerably greater amount of *search time* than other types of hunting (Driver 1990: 25). Time would have had to be carefully portioned out. This would have been a particularly pressing consideration in northerly regions during the long winter months, when solar day-length may often have amounted to only a few hours.

In an important paper, Torrence (1983) has confirmed (without focusing on the moon) that hunter-gatherers living in high latitudes are subject to time stress. In their environment there is only a limited time or 'window' through which they have access to resources. Two concepts are critical. One is that resource availability is highly seasonal, with resources being abundant at certain times of the year but very scarce at others. The other is that because of the marked annual variation in day length, there is only a restricted quantity of *light* available for foraging and other activities during the winter.

Torrence argues that when resources are available but the time available for obtaining them is severely limited, selection will always favour strategies involving either (1) the extraction only of resources giving high returns; and/or (2) an increase in the efficiency with which resources are extracted. Torrence notes that high-latitude hunter-gatherers tend to rely on meat rather than vegetable foods, which is consistent with the view that because of time stress they are concentrating on resources giving high returns. It is also noted that such people tend to increase efficiency by developing particularly complex tool-kits and technologies. In both cases, Torrence assumes the amount of light at a given time of year to be an unchangeable factor.

In view of the model of origins favoured in this book, we can add a third suggestion to Torrence's list of possible responses to time stress. Light is provided not only by the sun but also by the moon, and thus has a periodicity which is more than simply seasonal. Hunters under time stress would surely be under pressures favouring those who could fine-tune themselves to this fact. The best survivors (who might have included anatomically modern new entrants into ice age Europe and Asia some 40,000 years ago) would be those most attuned to the fact that once a month, in the period culminating in full moon, moonlight can extend very substantially the effective length of a hunter's day. Might this explain that close interest of Upper Palaeolithic hunters in the moon which Marshack (1964, 1972b) among others has claimed to discern?

In fact this consideration, although particularly relevant in northerly regions, would have been valid regardless of season or latitude. Whatever the circumstances, time is a valuable resource. Hunters wanting an uninterrupted extended day ought logically to have maximised their activities in the period leading up to and including full moon. Likewise, they should have been aware that this period rather suddenly came to an end at full moon itself. For the reasons noted earlier, they should not have risked allowing overnight journeys or game pursuits to drag on beyond that time.

In short, wherever logistic hunting was being practised, it would make sense to ensure an overlap between the time of maximum travel and the time of maximum visibility. 'You start safaris by the new moon', notes Karen Blixen (1954: 81) in *Out of Africa*, 'to have the benefit of the whole row of moonlit nights'. Such a pattern – second nature to African and Arabian travellers, traders and hunters to this day – adds an additional constraint to our model of synchrony, over and above the need for lunar phase-locking *per se*. It selects a definite direction of polarity – a fixed set of relationships associating together ovulation, the hunt's successful conclusion and full moon.

Let us visualise the situation. The logic of a sex strike obviously dictates that sex should not be allowed until the hunt's successful conclusion. But should this be at dark moon or full?

We may take the negative case first in order to see why it must be ruled out. Suppose women were to ovulate and be sexually receptive at dark moon. In that case, men would have to reach the climax of their hunting activities when the moon was waning, and when even its diminished form did not rise until some time after nightfall. On occasions when game animals were still being tracked at dusk, there would be a much-reduced chance of catching them. Kills would tend to occur during the shortest days of each month, meaning that meat often had to be butchered and carried back over a long distance to the base camp without benefit of extended evenings. In winter, particularly in northerly latitudes, this might mean compressing numerous activities and a long journey into only a few hours.

By contrast, all such problems would be dispelled if matters were arranged the other way around – that is, with ovulatory sex at the hunt's conclusion coinciding with full moon. Such a solution would concentrate the climax of productive, distributive, celebratory, sexual and culinary activities all together – during the days when there was most time in which to complete them all.

Although it yields as intriguing and ethnographically well documented a mental logic as any of those postulated by structuralism, this set of constraints has been arrived at using a methodology which has little in common with that of Lévi-Strauss (1970, 1973, 1978, 1981). It gives us the following model:

1 Women ovulate at full moon. Hence they menstruate at dark. Menstrual bleeding signals 'no!', inaugurating a sex strike which is women's response to the absence of meat. Cooking-fire – or rather, its absence – enters into the equation at this point, since there is no point in trying to cook meat if there is none to do it with. We arrive at the conclusion that dark moon is not only a time of menstrual blood. It correlates also with 'antifire'. Cooking fires are not lit, or have been allowed to subside (cf. Levi-Strauss 1970).

2 Not all women menstruate. But the sex-strike logic requires that all act as one. In withdrawing from circulation, the cycling women in each co-residential group must therefore also withdraw their associates – women who may be pregnant, lactating, menopausal or for some reason cycling irregularly. None of this need weaken the sex strike so long as the appropriate 'no' signals can be emitted on behalf of all. We may imagine women collectively sharing in the symbolic protection afforded by the blood of those who actually menstruate. Older women, for example, might draw on the symbolic potency of younger women's first or subsequent menstrual onsets.

3 The sex strike expresses itself in the prevalence of gender solidarity, temporarily overriding pair-bonds. In fact, kinship solidarity during this phase becomes strongly 'matrilineal', in that blood alone symbolises it and men are denied access to their wives and hence to their own offspring.

4 Since the females will not lift their sex ban until the hunt's conclusion, there can be no sex for anyone on a purely personal basis. A successful hunt presupposes male collaboration. Each male therefore needs the active support of his potential sexual rivals as the condition of his own sexual success.

5 Once gender solidarity has been established and sex-based conflict has been to that extent removed (cf. the Hadza dark moon *epeme* ritual), active preparations for the hunt can begin. When these are complete, the hunt can start.

6   The hunt must be completed within a few days – before the time
when sunsets are not compensated for by moonlight. Given that women
are capable of conceiving for only a few days around full moon (see 1
above), whilst this same period is followed by a succession of totally dark
nightfalls, full moon marks the hunters' effective deadline for bringing
meat home.

7   As meat is brought back, cooking fires are prepared. The meat is
cooked. As its rawness is overcome, the ban on sex is lifted. Feasting and
lovemaking are closely associated activities, jointly expressing the lifting
of female-imposed blood taboos. Gender solidarity collapses as men and
women are allowed to pair off into couples. An embryonically 'patrilineal'
kinship dimension now appears, replacing the former matrilineal one:
semen flows, there is no blood – and men are therefore no longer 'set apart'
from their own wives and offspring.

The reader will note that this surprisingly detailed, precise monthly schedule
has been arrived at logically – through consideration of a set of constraints
derived from our abstract theoretical model of cultural origins. For all its
obvious risks, this makes for rigorous testability, and is a different methodology from the kind which works backwards from myths or from ethnographic
and other data to an assortment of conclusions, adjusting these continuously
in an effort to accommodate them to consensual findings.

The Hunter's Moon

But it must now be asked how well – if at all – this abstract, logically
derived model fits the evidence. We will begin with the question of the
moon's relationship, if any, with the periodicity of the hunt.

Although no one has attempted a systematic survey and so proper
statistics are not available, there exists scattered ethnographic evidence for
human nocturnal hunting and, in this context, for the material importance
of the moon as a source of light. In the African tropics, the full moon seems
extremely bright, and traders, hunters and others as a matter of course avoid
the midday sun, preferring to travel during the cooler hours of night,
characteristically scheduling their travels to coincide with a string of bright
moons (Blixen 1954: 81). The same pattern applies in many other parts of
the world.

'Hunting is undertaken only by men, usually at night-time when there is
a good moon', write Strathern and Strathern (1968: 196) of the Mbowamb of
Papua New Guinea. The Daribi, too, (also in Papua New Guinea) think of
the moon 'as a boon to man, for it provides clear, well-lit nights for hunting'
(Wagner 1972: 109). Although no anthropologist has thought to undertake
a survey, it would seem likely that hunters throughout Papua New Guinea
shared traditions of related kinds.

Australia is no different. 'Most hunting', writes Gould (1981: 433) of the Australian Western Desert Aborigines,

> is done by stealth, from behind simple brush blinds, rock crevices, or tree platforms close to a water source. It is frequently a night-time activity, because most of the marsupial prey is nocturnal.

When prey animals are sleeping during the day, they are usually hard to find – which is one possible reason for waiting until the moon allows hunting by night. Certainly, given the superb nocturnal vision of such animals, it would be hopeless to attempt nocturnal hunting of them in the absence of a moon. In fact, few Aborigines would dream of travelling or hunting by night without this condition (Maddock, personal communication). In Cape York in northern Australia, ghosts known as 'Quinkans' terrify members of the Gugu-Yalanji tribal grouping on moonless nights. When the full moon is shining, however, the ghosts are dispersed – so much so that it may actually become safe to talk about them, even while out in the open at night (Trezise 1969: 82, 85). A myth from the Ooldea region of South Australia makes hunting with the help of the moon sound particularly easy: it tells of an old man who simply sat down alone at night and sang. 'When he sang meat came falling from the sky, sent to him by the Moon' (Berndt and Berndt 1945: 233).

Some kinds of hunting – the net-hunting of some Central African hunter-gatherer groups, for example – need plenty of light and can only be conducted in daytime. Yet hunting techniques in most cultures vary widely according to the habits of the local prey, and it *may* make good sense in certain circumstances to hunt primarily by night. Many if not most mammalian species in all continents are basically nocturnal. Desert and savanna animals often avoid extremes of heat by restricting their activities to the night (Cloudsley-Thompson 1980: 34). Besides antelopes, many other herbivores are nocturnal, since this helps to avoid water-loss, overheating and the attentions of blood-sucking insects (Cloudsley-Thompson 1980; 72, citing Clark 1914). Some diurnal game animals, moreover, can quickly adapt to a nocturnal lifestyle when predation pressures are intense (Cloudsley-Thompson 1980: 73), although this need not necessarily save them (Kruuk 1984).

Even when the prey is diurnal, human hunting may still be a night-time activity. The Hadza of north Tanganyika (Woodburn, cited by Isaac 1968: 259–60) normally hunt singly 'but occasionally band together to surround a baboon troop at night, while the animals are asleep'. The baboons are dislodged by arrow shots and clubbed to death as they attempt to break out. In addition, Woodburn (1968: 51) writes of the Hadza: 'Occasionally animals are shot at night from hides over water and are tracked the following morning.'

Almost all man's rival predators – such as wolves, foxes and the large cats

– prefer to make their kills in the half-light or by night. Lions are active during the day, but they, too, hunt frequently by night, particulary when there is a full moon. In the case of specialised fully nocturnal carnivores with excellent night vision, however, near-total darkness may assist by adding to the prey animals' fear and inability to escape attack. In this context, what might be termed a reverse lunar effect may manifest itself, with kills becoming maximised at each dark moon. Kruuk (1984: 207–8) records a striking occasion when 82 Thomson's gazelle were massacred by a pack of 19 hyenas on the Serengeti Plain on one very dark night in stormy weather just after new moon. He relates this to a finding which he had earlier made on the Cumberland coast, when foxes regularly attacked a colony of black-headed gulls:

> It was striking that the number of birds found dead in the colony in the early morning was clearly related to the darkness of the previous night. Gulls were significantly more vulnerable around new moon than around full moon. (Kruuk 1984: 209)

This was because the gulls seemed to become paralysed and unable to flee when the night was really black.

Logically, poor nocturnal vision ought to be a disadvantage to any hunting animal. Stealth is never easiest in daylight; the techniques of deception intrinsic to many forms of hunting are most effective in darkness or in the twilight hours. A carnivore rigidly restricted to daylight hours would be unusual in nature and would not make a competitive hunter. Indeed, Lewis Binford (1983: 64, 68) sees this as a basic reason for doubting the possibility that Plio-Pleistocene hominids could have been successful hunters at all. Unlike the hyenas, lions and leopards who in the valleys of the Southern Kalahari Desert wreak their bloody carnage all through the night, humans are creatures of the daylight, our eyes being daytime organs making us ill-adapted to killing, foraging or even protecting ourselves at night.

The fears of the dark which most humans display are, however, minimised when there is a good moon. And as noted at the beginning of this discussion, modern humans would have had sound reasons to steadily intensify their hunting activities each month in the period extending from new moon to full, with the climax of night-long post-hunt rejoicing and sexual activity coinciding with full moon.

Although palaeoanthropologists have for some reason not considered the matter important, the mythology and folklore of hunting universally supports this inference. The Roman divinity Diana – 'Goddess of the Hunt' – was a moon goddess or lunar 'Mistress of the Game Animals', as was the Greek Artemis. In the basic myth of dynastic Egypt, Set fatefully discovers the sarcophagus containing his brother Osiris' body whilst boar-hunting 'on the night of the full moon' (Campbell 1969: 425–6; citing Plutarch). In North America, the Osage Indians pray to the moon 'to give them a cloudless sky, and an abundance of game' (Hunter 1957: 226). In South America, among the Makusis, as soon as the new moon is visible all the men come and stand before the doors of their huts, drawing their arms backwards and forwards in the moon's direction *so as to strengthen themselves for the chase.* Then they all run out of their huts and cry '*Look at the moon!*'.

> They take certain leaves, and after rolling them in the shape of a small funnel, they pass some drops of water through it into the eye, while looking at the moon. This is very good for the sight. (Roth 1915: 257)

Once again, good *nocturnal* vision is here implied. The G/wi Bushmen of the Kalahari (Silberbauer 1981: 108) firmly believe that good hunting depends on moonlight; they throw the bones of a game animal towards the new moon when it first appears and recite the following formula:

> 'There are bones of meat, show us tomorrow to see well that we do not wander and become lost. Let us be fat every day' (i.e., show us where there are plenty of food plants and game animals).

A similar pattern is suggested by the Southern San 'creation of the eland' myth – one version of which 'leads from the creation of the moon into a long discourse on hunting porcupines by moonlight' (Lewis-Williams 1981: 30). Writing of the Khoekhoe, Hahn (1981: 131) suggests a connection between night travel and the moon's light:

> on the dying or disappearing of the moon, especially if there be an eclipse of the moon, great anxiety prevails. . . . Those prepared for a hunting expedition, or already hunting in the field, will immediately return home, and postpone their undertakings.

No moon, in other words, means no hunt. It should be remembered that a lunar eclipse can occur only at full moon and at night, so the above words may indicate habitual hunting at this time. Comparable anxiety is reported of the Sandawe of central Tanzania, who (as mentioned earlier) are perhaps remotely related to the San peoples. The Sandawe have 'a real fear of "the powers of Darkness"' (Bagshawe 1925: 328), and for this reason joyfully welcome back the moon after her disappearance each month (Ten Raa 1969: 37). Here, the term for 'moonless night', !'ints'sa, describes pitch-dark conditions, either when the moon is in its dark phase or when clouds obscure it. On such nights, ghosts and the shadows of death are felt to reign supreme. By contrast, the Sandawe say, 'The moon shows us the path through the dark night.' The moon's benign light dispels all ogres and ghosts, just as does the mild morning sun when it dispels the night-flying bats (Ten Raa 1969: 37). Similar relief at the moon's appearance is reported of many Kalahari San; when the moon periodically 'dies', the people pray for her to return soon, 'lightening the night for our feet on which we go out and return' (Taylor 1985: 158).

Returning, now, to the Upper Palaeolithic, an implication would be that the moon became important to evolving humans not only as a clock and not only because of its connection with menstruation – but also because for several days once a month its light extended humans' options, enabling hunters to choose between or combine diurnal and nocturnal hunting according to the circumstances or the habits of the prey. This materialistic consideration would have added to the logic of synchronising hunting schedules with the moon and hence with the menstrual cycle – a worldwide pattern expressed negatively through countless seemingly 'irrational' taboos regulating the interface between the two kinds of 'bloodshed' (Chapter 11), and expressed positively in recurrent associations between young women's menstrual potencies and the 'magic' of the hunt. *There is no implication in all this that humans would normatively have preferred hunting by night. Human eyesight being what it is, the reverse seems more probable.* Taking account of the moon in this context would simply have been an aspect of humanity's basic flexibility – our capacity to avoid over-specialisation and to take advantage of whatever opportunities for hunting presented themselves. In short, although early humans would perhaps have preferred to hunt in daylight, flexibility would have paid dividends. Those hunters who could on occasion travel overnight or extend the hunt into the twilight hours would have fared better than those who could not.

Dance, Sex and the Moon

The hunt and its associated sex strike should normatively have been over by the night of the full moon. We know this, not merely because the model predicts it, but also because the suggestion illuminates data which has long been known but has never been satisfactorily explained.

All over the world, wherever the full moon is celebrated at all, the all-night dances are celebrations of life in opposition to death, and very often involve sex games and love-making. Many San groups celebrate the full moon with dancing which lasts for three whole nights. Among the !Kung, a medicine dance to ward off death or sickness 'is held usually when the moon is full, after a successful hunt or when visitors arrive or are about to depart' (Woodburn 1982: 201, citing Marshall 1969). This again indicates that hunting and travel coincide with the full moon. Among the cattle-owning Nyaturu in Tanzania, the senior woman greets the new moon by calling on all men to enter their wives' houses and all women to conceive, the climax of sexual rejoicing coinciding with the full moon (Jellicoe 1985: 42–3).

Outside Africa, the Mocová Indians of the Gran Chaco in South America call the moon cidiage: 'When the moon is full, they ask him to give them wives: and boys pulling their noses, ask him to lengthen this organ.' Mocová boys, then, seemingly feel the need for 'long' penises whenever the moon is full – the pious Jesuit chronicler (Guevara 1908–10, 5: 64, quoted in

Métraux 1946: 20) having evidently substituted 'noses' for the boys' more
relevant organs in this puzzling passage. In the case of the Rindi, on the
island of Sumba in Indonesia, 'the period of full moon is connected with the
transfer of the bride from wife-givers to wife-takers' (Lyle 1987: 14–15,
citing Forth 1981: 205–8, 376–81). Among the Nootka Indians of
Vancouver, a chief could only have intercourse with his wives by the light of
the full moon (Briffault 1927, 2: 586, citing Bancroft). In Western
Australia, in the Kimberleys, a lovesick Wagaitj woman dances secretly with
other women and signs her *Tjarada* or love charm to attract the man she
wants. This should be sung about four days before the moon is full – the
singer projecting her thoughts through the air to start an involuntary twitch
in her lover's thigh, whereupon he is supposed to look up at the moon and
see on its face his own 'shade' and hers (Elkin 1968: 148).

In European fairy-tales, likewise, the night of the full moon is the
moment when menstrual spells are finally broken, when frogs turn into
princes, and when marital relations can at last be enjoyed. In the Highlands
of Scotland, girls used to refuse to be married except when the moon was full
(Briffault 1927, 2: 587, citing Logan). Such themes echo down the ages to us
in the form of the English nursery rhyme:

> Boys and girls, come out to play,
> The Moon doth shine as bright as day. . . .

The link between marital sex and full moon is also of course lodged in our
very word 'honeymoon'.

In his book, *Before Civilization*, Colin Renfrew (1976: 264–5) quotes a vivid
passage on the Cherokee Indians of the south-eastern United States, who in
the nineteenth century built round houses like those whose remains have
been found in the stone circles of southern Britain such as Stonehenge and
Avebury. A description by a contemporary traveller of the Cherokee harvest
celebration helps to remind us, writes Renfrew, that Britain's great henges
and other ceremonial sites would have been more than just astronomical
observatories. They would also have been the scene of elaborate rituals linked
to the movements of the sun and moon.

The date of the Cherokee harvest festival was fixed as the night of the full
moon nearest to the period when the maize became ripe. 'Although it relates
to another time and another continent', Renfrew (1976: 264) comments, 'we
can almost imagine this as the description of the celebrations at a neolithic
henge':

> But the harvest moon is now near at hand, and the chiefs and medicine
> men have summoned the people of the several villages to prepare them-
> selves for the autumnal festival. Another spot of ground is selected, and

the same sanctifying ceremony is performed that was performed in the previous spring. The most expert hunter in each village has been commissioned to obtain game, and while he is engaged in the hunt the people of his village are securing the blessing of the great Spirit by drinking, with many mystic ceremonies, the liquid made from seven of the most bitter roots to be found among the mountains. Of all the game which may be obtained by the hunters, not a single animal is to be served up at the feast whose bones have been broken or mutilated, nor shall a rejected animal be brought within the magic circle, but shall be given to the tribe who, by some misdeed, have rendered themselves unworthy to partake of the feast. The hunters are always compelled to return from the chase at the sunset hour, and long before they come in sight of their villages they invariably give a shrill whistle, as a signal of good luck, whereupon the villagers make ready to receive them with a wild song of welcome and rejoicing.

The pall of night has once more settled upon the earth, the moon is in its glory, the watch-fire has been lighted within the magic circle, and the inhabitants of the valley are again assembled together in one great multitude. From all the cornfields in the valley the magicians have gathered the marked ears of corn, and deposited them in the kettles with the various kinds of game which may have been slaughtered . . . the entire night is devoted to eating, and the feast comes not to an end until all the food has been despatched, when, in answer to an appropriate signal from the medicine man, the bones which have been stripped of their flesh are collected together and pounded to a kind of powder and scattered through the air. The seven days following this feast are devoted to dancing and carousing. . . . (Lanman 1856: 424–8; quoted in Swanton 1946: 263–5)

Although it refers to a harvest festival, this passage precisely illustrates the logic discussed. Hunting directly precedes the full moon. The hunt is successfully accomplished in time for the celebrations -- the 'dancing and carousing' – which begin at full moon. A fire is lit and cooking takes place as the moon changes. After this come seven days of waning moon in which to relax, dance and feast.

A lovely account of how carnival and sex-linked festivities follow the moon's changes is provided by Malinowski (1927: 205–6) in his classic description of life in the Trobriand Islands. 'The moon', he writes, 'plays a far greater part in the life of the natives than either the sun or the stars'. Yet, he continues, unlike horticulturists elsewhere in the world, the Trobrianders have no belief that the moon magically influences vegetation. Instead, the moon's importance stems from quite prosaic factors:

In a country where artificial illumination is extremely primitive, moon-light is of the greatest importance. It changes night from a time when it is best to be at home round the fireplace, to a time when, in the tropics, it is most pleasant to walk or play, or to indulge in any outdoor exercise. This brings about a periodical heightening of social life in the village at the second quarter of the full moon. In all festivities, all enterprises, and on all ceremonial occasions, the climax is reached at the full moon.

The moon has a particularly profound influence on human sexual life. Malinowski (1932: 57) describes young boys and girls becoming aware of one another as they grow to maturity, their early friendships beginning to take fire 'under the intoxicating influence of music and moonlight'. For such lovers, the most exciting opportunities are afforded by 'that monthly increase in the people's pleasure-seeking mood which leads to many special pastimes at the full of the moon'.

'Throughout the year', explains Malinowski (1932: 201–2),

> there is a periodic increase in play and pleasure-seeking at full moon. When the two elements so desirable in the tropics, soft light and bracing freshness are combined, the natives fully respond: they stay up longer to talk, or to walk to other villages, or to undertake such enterprises as can be carried out by moonlight. Celebrations connected with travel, fishing, or harvesting, as well as all games and festivals are held at the full moon.

Each month as the moon waxes, children sit up late into the evening, amusing themselves in large groups on the village's central place. Soon older children join them, and, as the moon grows fuller, young men and women are drawn into the circle of players. Gradually the smaller children are squeezed out, and the games are continued by adults:

> On specially fine and cool nights of full moon, I have seen the whole population of a large village gathered on the central place, the active members taking part in the games, with the old people as spectators.

The main players are still the younger women and their lovers, however, and the games are associated with sex in more than one way:

> The close bodily contact, the influence of moonlight and shadow, the intoxication of rhythmic movement, the mirth and frivolity of play and ditty – all tend to relax constraint, and give opportunity for an exchange of declarations and for the arrangement of trysts.

Malinowski says nothing of menstrual synchrony, but clearly in a culture of this kind, it would not be adaptive for women to menstruate too frequently at full moon. Indeed, it might be supposed that in a culture with menstrual avoidances (see Chapter 11) of any kind, the presence of just one menstruat-ing woman in a public place at such a time would be an embarrassment. In the Trobriand Islands as elsewhere in the world, the full moon is associated not with menstrual seclusion but with travel, visiting, dancing and sexual celebration.

Returning, now, to our model, we might say that if it is indeed the case that nocturnal light helps to stimulate ovulation (Chapter 7), then all of this would make good biological sense. Celebrating out in the open late into the night would ensure maximum exposure to the moon's rays, and all-night dancing by the light of fires — as among the Cherokee — would enhance this effect. A number of different factors, then, might combine to help bring on ovulation in women, and among these — probably — would be sexual intercourse itself (Hrdy 1981: 155, 233n, citing Clark and Zarrow 1971; Sevitt 1946). In other words, the practice of timing sexual celebrations so that they coincided with full moon would probably help to ensure ovulatory (and hence menstrual) synchrony, and would also maximise the chances of fertile sex.

Possible Reproductive Functions of Dance

Contrary to some sociobiologists' assumptions, human traditional dancing is rarely reducible to courtship behaviour — at least, not in the sense that this term conventionally implies. If there is 'courtship' taking place, it is between whole groups, not private individuals. Almost always, the dancing is collective and ritualised. As noted in Chapter 9, it is in fact quite rare for marital partners to dance together as couples, or to publicise their physical bond. Rather, women dance with women and men with men. Even when the two sexes are dancing simultaneously and on the same dance-ground, and even when the dancing culminates in wild sexual abandon, the overall design of the dance is one of gender groups relating to one another as groups, not individuals. This is true of virtually all African dancing, all Australian Aboriginal dancing — and indeed, of folkoristic or traditional dancing just about everywhere. Modern western dancing which celebrates coupledom is in this context an aberration.

The usual function of dance is to harmonise bodies and emotions, to raise the spirits, to entrance and enchant, to motivate collective efforts by arousing desire — but above all to ensure that sexual enjoyment, when it is eventually allowed, takes place at the right time and in such a way as to enhance rather than undermine wider forms of solidarity and social cohesion. In this context, almost everything which was said in Chapter 9 about 'personal ornamentation' can also be said about the major context for the wearing of such ornaments — dance. We noted earlier that beads, bangles, waist-charms and so on were means by which gender coalitions helped to harness and control the value of their members' sexuality. By wearing such ornaments, each woman or man asserted an individuality whose premise was the freedom to give unique bodily expression to the collective values of her or his particular group. Dance was the basic theatre for the display of this link between sexual individuality and collective control.

Many forms of dancing among hunters and gatherers are intimately connected with hunting and hunting magic; this is particularly the case where communal hunts are frequent. Paintings in rock shelters in central India show traditions of group-dancing associated with communal hunting extending back thousands of years (Malaiya 1989).

Dancing often precedes a collective hunt (as we saw in the case of the dark-moon Hadza *epeme* ritual); it may also conclude it. Dancing to celebrate the hunt's success may immediately precede sexual rejoicing, but prolonged dancing may also be, as much as anything, an enjoyable way of delaying and offering a substitute for sexual gratification. There is an extremely close relationship, in fact, between ritual dancing and what in this book has been termed women's periodic sex strike. On the one hand, dancing punctuates time, providing any drawn-out action such as a strike with both a beginning and an end. On the other, dancing and striking may amount to the same thing, women expressing their gender solidarity and their sexual teasing of men by dancing seductively but just beyond reach, holding themselves under one another's protection. Certainly, although of course a sex strike must ultimately be 'sex-negative', there would be no reason why it should have to exclude sex of symbolic kinds. The associated dancing may even culminate in ribaldry and wild abandon, as we will soon see in the context of a West African example. But at the beginning of the proceedings, what is important is that normal *marital* relations should be prohibited and delayed; any sex which occurs to mark the onset of the strike period may arouse desire but should be wholly under female control; it should also be non-consummated, non-penetrative, infertile and/or merely acted out in play. The model would lead us to define such celebratory pre-strike intimacy as 'menstrual sex' (for an exploration of this theme in mythology and literature, see Shuttle and Redgrove 1978).

If whole-body co-ordinated activities such as dancing can influence not only emotional but also hormonal states, this may provide a clue to why dancing takes up so much of the leisure time of so many hunting and gathering peoples, and why it is so often linked symbolically with the moon. It might also throw light on the mechanisms through which women eventually succeeded in preserving their ancient traditions of synchrony far from coastal shores in the course of the Upper Palaeolithic revolution. It could be that they danced. Moreover, if dancing influenced the timing of ovulation and/or menstruation as well as of sexual intercourse itself, a further consequence may have followed. By scheduling each type of dance so as to coincide with a specific lunar phase, women could have helped ensure that their cycles were not only socially in step, but also in step with the moon. Alternatively, it may have been that by using the moon as a clock, and by dancing in time with it, women succeeded in keeping in synchrony with one another.

Before turning to some supportive evidence, our findings so far may be reviewed. It has been shown that although synchrony may always have had a certain basis in physiology and in such factors as the direct influence of moonlight, these influences acting alone would probably have been insufficient for culture's purposes. Women who for sexual-political reasons needed to synchronise would have had to keep a check on their internal body-clocks, no single one of which could have been fully reliable all the time. We may conclude that consistent synchrony would have required direct cultural intervention. The evidence is that this in turn would have presupposed (a) a major emphasis on body-harmonising and emotion-harmonising activities such as ritual and dance and (b) use of the moon as the only available clock capable of regulating the timing of these performances.

Frederick Lamp and the Temne of Sierra Leone

The Temne are the largest ethnic group in Sierra Leone. They use a lunar calendar which predates Muslim contact and is evidently ancient, the earliest document describing it being from 1506. This calendar governs all indigenous ritual, farming schedules and much of ordinary routine. 'The importance of the lunar cycle to Temne life', according to Frederick Lamp (1988: 215), 'cannot be overstated . . .'. Most rituals directly concern the moon, not the sun, whose movements seem of minor importance – 'even in the regulation of agricultural schedules' (Lamp 1988: 215). The Temne have no term for the sun as a heavenly body, although its warmth and its light are given names. By contrast, the moon has two names, one for the night-time moon, one for the daytime, and a number of metaphorical names as well. There are also eight terms for the moon's phases (Lamp 1988: 215). An eclipse of the sun is barely noted, but an eclipse of the moon occasions a furious clatter of pan-banging to chase away the cat that has caught it (Lamp 1988: 215, citing Thomas 1916: 179). In the Temne story of creation there is no mention of the sun, only of the moon (Lamp 1988: 215, citing Schlenker 1861: 12–35). The new moon is observed first with anxious anticipation and then with exhilaration at its first sighting – with hand-clapping, as at the birth of a child (Lamp 1988: 215). An early source on this topic (Barbot 1746: 125, quoted in Lamp 1988: 223) runs as follows:

> At every new moon, both in the villages and open country, they abstain from all manner of work, and do not allow any strangers to stay amongst them at the time; alledging for their reason, that if they should do otherwise, their maiz [sic.] and rice would grow red, the day of the new moon being a day of blood, as they express it; and therefore they commonly go hunting that day.

It is perhaps worth noting at this point that a total work shut-down at each new moon united the Temne with an extremely large number of other African peoples, including Zulus, Bechuanas, the Baziba, the Banyoro, the Warega and many more tribes (Briffault 1927, 2: 422–3).

The reference to hunting in the above passage seems puzzling: on the one hand, it is said that people at new moon 'abstain from all manner of work', while on the other we are told that men 'commonly go hunting on that day'. Lamp (1988: 224) suggests a plausible explanation: the reference to hunting simply means 'that the men abandoned the village women during menses'. Men who left their wives for a period beginning around the new moon were probably assumed to have gone hunting.

Aside from this, it is of course interesting that the virtual lunar-scheduled 'strike' – as we might term it – is associated by the Temne with the assumed presence everywhere of 'blood'. Women among the Temne 'abstain from work during menses, particularly avoiding cooking and working in the fields. Coitus would be unthinkable.'

Menstruation is known as 'washing the moon' or 'to be in the East' (the place of new beginnings), and is associated with wetness, darkness and with the moon's 'standing-up' phase – the Temne term for the new moon (Lamp 1988: 225). According to a mid-nineteenth-century missionary's report (Schlenker 1861: 18–19), 'all women are routinely not well at the dead moon and at the full moon'. Lamp (1988: 223) believes that Schlenker's Temne informants were referring here to ovulation – or perhaps post-ovulatory discomfort – as one period in which women were 'not well' and menstruation as the other one, menstruation occurring at dark moon and ovulation at full. In support of this, he quotes a more recent native gynaecological statement to the effect that 'the moon begins to appear on the last day blood stops' (Margai 1965: 7–8). However, Lamp (1988: 226) is not primarily concerned with biological facts but with the cultural conceptual grids through which these are socially acknowledged. Many women, he suggests, would have been at least culturally assumed to be menstruating during each dark moon period just before new moon. And he continues: 'If the Temne indeed believe that menstruation should occur at the new moon, then the implications for ritual are striking.'

Initiation ritualism was and remains very important in Temne traditional life, both for men and for women. Women are organised into an immense, community-wide association known as 'Bondo', which is under the control of a hierarchy of female officials. The details of young women's initiation ordeals are secret, but they are known to include genital operations ranging from labial scarification in some cases up to clitoridectomy in others, all the operations being performed by women. In this ultimately male-dominated culture, severe and oppressive female collective control over each individual girl's sexuality, then, seems to be the basic theme, although Lamp (1988: 213) emphasises another important aspect:

In initiation, which involves not so much practical as cultural and religious instruction through participation in ritual arts, the young learn to act cooperatively, to synchronise their behavior patterns, and to work toward a harmonious relationship with the cosmos as well as with society.

Lamp (1988: 217) soon discerned a correlation between lunar phases and the various stages of the Bondo ritual, although in defence of their secrets, the female officials themselves when questioned by him strongly denied any such connection.

An important event in the women's Bondo ritual is the 'coming out' ceremony, which lasts for two days and occurs, according to Lamp's charts, either at or just before the moon's first quarter, or at or just after the third quarter. It would seem, from this and other information, that this is in approximate terms a 'dark moon' ritual, although it falls not on but on either side of the actual days of the dark moon.

On the first day of this 'coming out' there is a ceremony 'involving transvestism in an atmosphere of wild abandon' (Lamp 1988: 221):

The dance begins in the east. The entire village takes part, including the men and children. Each person selects some article that has been destroyed or violated in some way: a rotted basket, torn rags, a bottomless bucket, a broken pestle, or dried foliage. These articles are brandished in a frenzied dance in which the crowd rushes in a counterclockwise circle around the town from east to west and back east. Honorable old women dress like lorry-boys. Young men seductively shake their padded breasts in the faces of the elders. Young girls stuff gourds into the front of men's shorts they are wearing and play the role of village stud. And everyone, from the decrepit old grandmother to the young teenage boy, engages in the most defamatory and pornographic language.

It is tempting to interpret the buckets with holes in them, the rotted baskets etc. as symbols of 'death', which – linked with the dark moon – stands in an inverse ('anticlockwise') relationship to 'life' and therefore to all 'normal' social and gender relationships.

There next comes 'the ritual sanction of the initiated person'. At this point in the dance, 'all married Bondo women are now free to have sexual intercourse with any man present without fear of reprisal from their husbands against either them or their partners' (Lamp 1988: 221). The dance goes on, but the crowd begins to thin as married women choose their male partners – who may be young, unmarried men – and go away to more private spots to exercise their rights.

Lamp suggests that this dance and other aspects of Temne ritual are not only timed by reference to the moon's phases, but may actually help to shape and regulate women's sexual cycles. It is this, he suggests, which makes such extraordinary sexual licence possible. When the married women take their special ritual lovers, the sex is most unlikely to be fertile. Lamp's materials on this topic are in fact quite complex, since he is unable to claim that women's cycles are strictly synchronised with the moon's phases. However, he succeeds in demonstrating that even if only half the women tend to ovulate in the few days leading up to full moon, while the rest do so just before dark moon – a situation of partial synchrony in which most women fall into one or other category – the observed timing of Bondo 'coming out' would make biological sense. Sexual licence would in the main coincide, in the case of both groups, with an infertile period. He also shows that on this basis the dates of final release of Bondo girls to their husbands would quite neatly harmonise with the biological facts, since there would be a strong likelihood of the girls being maximally fertile at the time of release and probable consummation of each marriage (Lamp 1988: 228).

Had Temne ideology corresponded to physiological reality, it would seem that all women would have been infertile at around the time of the dark moon. This, then – if the aim were to avoid pregnancies – would have been the best time to hold the ceremonies of gender inversion and licence. On the other hand, had synchrony begun breaking down not randomly but in such a way that some women began cycling on precisely the inverse schedule to the rest – ovulating when their sisters were menstruating – the best way to avoid pregnancies would have been to shift the timing of ceremonial licence and gender inversion so that it fell several days on either side of dark moon. This may be what the Temne have done.

Synchrony and Ethnography

Despite Lamp's Temne article and a few other published findings, we have no hard clinical evidence for dance-regulated, moon-scheduled menstrual synchrony in any traditional culture. Indeed, for reasons which obviously have as much to do with western theoretical constructs as with 'the data' as such, menstrual synchrony of any kind has remained hard to substantiate in the ethnographic record.

No one (to the author's knowledge) has as yet conducted fieldwork in a living tribal culture taking menstrual questionnaires with a view to testing whether or not synchrony actually occurs. All we have is reports on dance, ritual, ideology, mythology and belief. On one level, this absence of evidence may seem surprising; yet it has to be remembered that it was not until 1971 that menstrual synchrony of any kind was even recognised by the scientific community in *our own* culture. It then took another eleven years before the finding was taken account of in any fieldwork-based publication by a social anthropologist (Buckley 1982). We should not be surprised by this. Einstein is said to have noted: 'It is the theory that decides what we can observe'; this is certainly as true for anthropology as for physics. We 'see' what our conceptual grids enable us to see. Even assuming its contemporary or traditional existence, therefore, we cannot expect fieldwork to uncover the phenomenon of synchrony unless or until the concept enters into the body of theoretical understandings on the basis of which anthropologists become trained before entering the field.

The first anthropologist to link modern medical findings on menstrual synchrony with the analysis of a traditional culture was Tim Buckley (1982, 1988), whose account was of traditions among the Californian Yurok. It has to be conceded, however, that this case is not conclusive; although reinforced with a re-analysis of much of the classical literature on the Yurok, including some unpublished early fieldnotes, it is based largely upon the recollections of a single informant.

One evening in 1978, Buckley was invited to the house of an Indian friend for a meal. The house was a modern one within the Yurok aboriginal homelands in north-western California, close to the Klamath River. Buckley's male informant explained that he would be doing the cooking since his Yurok wife was 'on her moontime' – in her menstrual period – and they were keeping the old ways as best they could. A back room had been set apart in the modern house for his wife's monthly use; the couple neither ate nor slept together for ten days each 'moon'.

Eventually the woman emerged from her room to talk with Buckley about what she was doing and how she felt about it. She had been instructed in the menstrual laws by her maternal aunts and grandmother, who were, in their times, well-known, conservative Yurok ladies. Her understanding of menstruation came largely from these sources. She began her account by telling Buckley that as a foster-child in non-Indian homes she had been taught that menstruation is 'bad and shameful' and that through it 'women are being punished'. On her return to Yurok society, however, 'my aunts and my grandmother taught me different'.

According to the old menstrual laws, a woman should seclude herself during the flow 'because this is the time when she is at the height of her powers'. Such time should not be wasted in mundane tasks and social distractions, nor in concerns with the opposite sex. Rather, all of one's energies should be applied in concentrated meditation 'to find out the purpose of your life'. It is a time for the 'accumulation' of spiritual energy, the flowing blood serving to 'purify' the woman and prepare her for spiritual accomplishment.

In the old days, according to the same female informant, menstruating women used to communally bathe and perform rituals in a 'sacred moontime pond' up in the mountains above the old Yurok village of Meri:p. While many women performed this rite only at the time of their first menstruation, aristocratic women went to the pond every month. All of a household's fertile women who were not pregnant – according to this informant – menstruated 'at the same time, a time dictated by the moon', the women practising the bathing rituals together at this time. If a woman got out of phase with the moon and with the other women of the household, she could 'get back in by sitting in the moonlight and talking to the moon asking it to balance [her]'. Through the ritual bathing practice, and by maintaining synchrony with wider rhythms, women came to 'see that the earth has her own moontime', a recognition that made one both 'stronger' and 'proud' of one's menstrual cycle.

Just as the women collectively retreated from their husbands for ten days, so the men used ten days as the standard period for men's 'training' in the household's sweathouse. Like the women, the men bathed, gathered firewood, avoided sexual contacts, ate special foods and let flow their own blood – the men gashing their legs for this purpose with flakes of white quartz (Buckley 1982: 51). The flowing of the blood was thought to carry off psychic impurity, preparing one for spiritual attainment. Men who were in special training to become 'doctors' secluded themselves in the sweathouse and 'made medicine'; Buckley (p. 53) provides evidence that the 'medicine baskets' and dentalium shells used by men to contain their power tokens were symbolic vaginas. Moreover, elderly Yurok men told Buckley (p. 55) that 'intensive male training was always undertaken "during the dark of the moon"', while other sources indicate that this was also the time when the women may have been menstruating.

Following a re-analysis of published and unpublished material on the Yurok, Buckley concludes that there has been a consistent male bias in published interpretations of Yurok menstrual symbolism, and that his female informant's claims ought to be taken seriously. He puts forward the hypothesis, firstly, that 'the women of aboriginal Yurok households menstruated in synchrony, utilizing the light of the moon to regularise their menstrual cycles . . . ' (Buckley 1988: 207). The women's menstrual houses seem to have included large communal dome-shaped structures, heated by fires, used for sweating and capable of sheltering several women at a time. Secondly, he believes that

> both the subsistence quests and fighting patterns of all of the active men of these households, as well as their own programs of esoteric training, were keyed to the synchronous menstrual cycles of the household's women.

Buckley (1988: 204) argues that men carefully watched the skies from within sweathouses which were designed to function, at least in part, as lunar/solar observatories. There were good reasons for this. The moon had to be watched to determine the correct dates to hold the great inter-regional ritual and ceremonial events which were once held in accordance with one-, two-, and three-year cycles in more than a dozen north-western Californian centres:

> These events, customarily – if erroneously – lumped together as 'world

renewal dances', included esoteric components enacted by priests and their helpers, as well as public dances attended by very large audiences (Kroeber and Gifford 1949). Each had to be completed, in all aspects, within a single lunation and it had to end in the dark of the moon. (p. 130; Kroeber, in Elmendorf 1960: 28)

The public dances lasted approximately ten days, ending some time before the dark moon. Women were *not* supposed to be menstruating at such times. Buckley (1988: 205) comments: 'Whatever other symbolism was involved, the timing of these events makes particular sense in light of the biological model for menstruation at the new moon.'

In fact, since the public dancing followed the secret, esoteric phases, the ritual schedule appears to have mirrored the model discussed at the beginning of this chapter. In other words, 'esoteric preparations' were apparently conducted from dark moon onwards, whilst public dancing took over from full moon.

The model is also mirrored in Buckley's reconstruction of Yurok domestic practice. The inferred system, writes Buckley (1988: 205), would have meant that for ten days out of every twenty-nine,

all of the fertile women who were not pregnant were removed, as a group, from their households' mundane activities and plunged into collective contemplative and ritual exercises aimed at the acquisition of wealth objects and other spiritual boons.

Since menstruation contaminated all food, gathering as well as cooking would have had to stop. Men would not have hunted at dark moon, instead entering the sweathouse to purify and prepare themselves for later exertions. In view of such work prohibitions, Buckley writes, 'it would be logical to think that the household's subsistence quest . . . would have been brought virtually to a halt, men as well as women refraining from all but the most casual collecting of food' (1988: 205–6). In other words, the menstrual power and solidarity of Yurok women not only influenced ritual life but had 'profound, pragmatic implications as well in dictating the temporal structuring of activities for entire households on a monthly basis' (p. 207).

It was noted earlier that in Africa, reports of normative menstrual synchrony exist for both the Hadza and the !Kung. Evidence for traditions of synchrony in northern Australia is also quite strong (Chapters 12–13). In addition to such findings, Buckley's reconstruction may seem to receive some support from this description by Anne Cameron of life among the Nootka of Vancouver Island:

It was the time of Suzy's menstrual period. It felt good to be around a woman during her sacred time, good to be able to smell the special body perfume, to share in the specialness of it, expecting my own period to start any day, wondering, as it seemed I always did, how it was that the women of the village mostly all had their periods at around the same time. Finally, since I had never been able to figure it out for myself, I asked my granny. She looked at me as if she couldn't believe anybody could be so simple, and shook her head gently.

'The light, Ki-ki,' she sighed, 'it's because of the light.' Used to be, before electricity and strong light made it possible for people to stay up half the night, that we all got up with the sun and went to bed with the sun, and because we all got the same amount of light and dark, our body time was all the same, and we'd come full at the same time. (Cameron 1984: 95)

A consequence would have been that ovulations and births would have manifested lunar influence, too. There is no direct evidence to suggest that either the Yurok or the Nootka followed this pattern, but there are suggestions of this in native belief systems from other parts of the world. Two examples will serve as illustrations. Among the Desana Indians of the Vaupés, one of the major rivers of the north-west Amazon, the moon

influences beneficently the gestation of women who are pregnant. In the nights of a full moon, these women will sit talking outside of the maloca, receiving the fecund power that emanates from the lunar rays. (Reichel-Dolmatoff 1968: 72-3)

And on Melville Island in northern Australia, the belief is that births should occur at full moon. 'As soon as a woman knows she is pregnant', writes Jane Goodale (1971: 146),

she starts to 'follow moon'. 'Moon makes baby come', I was told. When the moon is full the woman knows her time is near, and she goes into the bush with a 'big mob of people, father, mother, in-laws, brother, sister'. Anyone may accompany her except her husband. . . .

In this instance, parturition is in women's eyes a collective full-moon ritual from which only the husband is excluded.

Of course, none of this has much to do with the question whether early Upper Palaeolithic big game hunters scheduled their major dances or other rituals in accordance with the moon's phases. But, as was mentioned very briefly in Chapter 9, besides additional ethnographic evidence, a certain amount of direct archaeological evidence for Upper Palaeolithic lunar time-keeping exists.

Marshack and Lunar Notation

In the 1960s, Alexander Marshack (1964) first claimed to have found evidence of lunar observation in notational sequences in Europe extending back in time from the Mesolithic Azilian in an unbroken line to the Aurignacian, a span before history of some 30,000 to 35,000 years. 'The evidence', he wrote,

> is neither sparse nor isolated; it consists of thousands of notational sequences found on the engraved 'artistic' bones and stones of the Ice Age and the period following, as well as on the engraved and painted rock shelters and caves of Upper Paleolithic and Mesolithic Europe.

His first publication presented counts of four sets of marks – two made on rock walls in Spain, one on a reindeer-bone specimen from Czechoslovakia, and one on the tip of a mammoth tusk from the Ukraine. The painted notation from Canchal de Mahoma in Spain, shows an oval shape surrounded by twenty-nine marks, many of them crescent-shaped, with a group of three rounded shapes in the middle which Marshack interprets as recording the full moon period. 'This', he comments (1964: 743), 'is a *precisely* observed lunar sequence'. Each crescent, he suggests, represents the moon, and faces 'in the precise direction it would face to a man looking south, the first crescent curving right in the western dusk sky, the last curving left in the eastern dawn' (figure 11a).

Another Azilian painted notation, this time from the Abri de las Vinas in Spain, gives a count of 30, from invisibility to invisibility (figure 11b). The month as a whole is represented in this case not by an oval but by a human-looking figure of a shape common in Magdalenian and Azilian art. 'This', comments Marshack (1964: 743), 'is the first clue towards an understanding of this "god" '.

In the same article Marshack suggests that his engraved piece of mammoth-ivory from Gontzi in the Ukraine, dating from late in the Upper Palaeolithic, likewise makes sense as a record of the moon's phases over the course of four months (figure 11c). Finally, he shows how an engraved reindeer bone from Kulna in Moravia, Czechoslovakia – displaying a row of short lines alternating with long ones – may record alternating waxing and waning phases of the moon (figure 11d). This is just one of many hundreds of comparable sequences, some dating back over 25,000 years.

Among earlier interpretations of Marshack's rows of notches was the idea that they were *marques de chasse* – 'hunting tallies' – each notch representing a hunter's 'kill' (Marshack 1972b: 35–6). An alternative interpretation is that they may have been records kept by women of their menstrual periods (Wenke 1984: 129, citing Fisher 1979). We may never know exactly who kept these tallies or precisely what they meant, but the model of cultural origins presented here would tempt us to draw on all the suggestions which have so far been made. They are not necessarily mutually incompatible. If

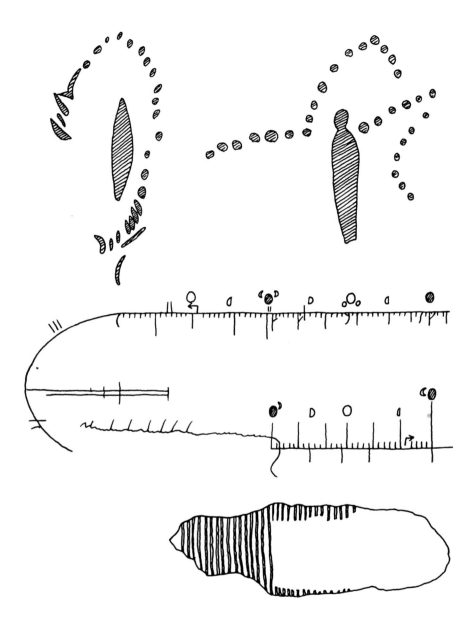

Figure 11 Some of Alexander Marshack's earliest inferred lunar calendars. *Upper left*: rock-painting from Canchal de Mahoma, Spain; Azilian. *Right*: rock-painting from Abri de las Vinas, Spain; Azilian. *Centre*: *schematised* lunar calendrical interpretation of engraved markings on a piece of mammoth ivory (original not represented here); Gontzi, Ukraine; late Palaeolithic. *Lower*: engraved reindeer bone; Kulna, Moravia, Czechoslovakia; Gravettian (redrawn after Marshack 1964).

collective dances or other rituals were connected both with female menstruation and with the sexual-political ('magical') aspects of hunting, and if these rituals were held regularly at times determined by reference to the moon, we would no longer have to choose between one interpretation and another. Ethnographic and early historical analogies suggest that ritually marked occasions frequently include moments of sacrifice or bloodshed, whether menstrual or animal (Girard 1977; Burkert *et al.* 1987). We can combine a menstrual interpretation with a hunting one by assuming a symbolic connection between menstrual blood and blood from the hunt; and we can reconcile all this with a lunar interpretation if we infer that the most propitious moments for bloodshed of any kind would have been pinpointed by reference to the positions of heavenly bodies and in particular the phases of the moon.

In his many later publications, including his beautifully illustrated book, *The Roots of Civilisation* (1972b), Marshack has developed his lunar notations theme in ways which seem consistent with all of this. He has shown above all how ice age art has left a record of Upper Palaeolithic hunters' 'time-factored' lives – lives structured powerfully by the changing seasons, the changing phases of the moon and a wealth of associated rhythmic, cyclical phenomena such as the yearly breeding of game animals, the spawning of salmon, the migration of birds and the menstrual cycles of human beings. Interestingly, he argues that what he terms the ice age artists' 'zigzag iconography' – multiple serpentine bands and meandering abstract patterns found in much of the very earliest art – are not attempts to depict real snakes, as some theorists (e.g. Mundkur 1983) have alleged. They match and often directly accompany the 'lunar notations', being expressions of the same interest in cyclicity, periodicity and, in general, the passage of cyclical, seasonal and especially lunar time. Any 'snake' in this context is cosmic and metaphorical. It is:

> The serpent of time, of process and continuity, the serpent of self-birth and origins, the serpent of death, birth, and rebirth, the cosmic serpent, the serpent of such processes as water, rain, and lightning, the *ouroboros* that bites its own tail in perpetuity, the guilloche serpent of endless continuity and turns. (Marshack 1985: 142)

Marshack (1985) argues that there are only a limited number of logically possible ways of depicting the movements of the sun and moon or the passage of cyclical time, and that among these are spirals, concentric circles, meanders and zigzags (figure 12) – motifs which may easily be though of as 'snake-like', and which in all continents are among the most recurrent prehistoric rock-art motifs.

In his most recent work, Marshack (1990) has come to see the 'female image' as the unifying symbol which integrates and harmonises all other ice-

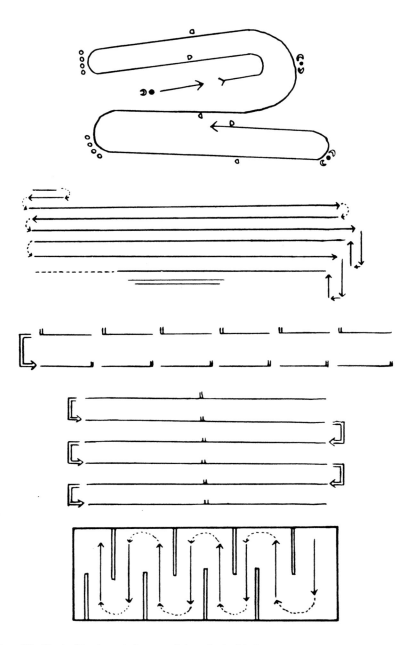

Figure 12 Marshack's schematic linear renditions of calendrical engravings (originals not shown). *From top to bottom*: Abri Blanchard, France, early Upper Palaeolithic, *c.* 28,000 BC; Grotte du Täi, France, late Upper Palaeolithic, *c.* 9,500 BC; northern Siberia, Yakut/Dolgan calendar stick, 18th–19th century; Wisconsin, Winnebago lunar calendar, early 18th century; southern Mexico, Mixtec pictographic historical record (Nuttall Codex), pre-contact period (Marshack 1985: Fig. 6; reproduced with permission).

age images of periodicity or the flow of cyclical time. He focuses on the possibility of an intrinsic semantic connection linking Upper Palaeolithic vulva-images with serpentine forms. He draws particular attention to a large limestone block from the Perigordian VI level at the Abri Pataud in which vulva and serpentine motifs are intimately combined. He also spotlights what he terms 'comet-like' angles below engraved vulvas at Kostienki II – lines which he believes may represent the menstrual flow. In general, his suggestion is that whether in association with explicit vulvas or not, the very widespread serpentine/zigzag/macaroni motif most probably represents 'the flow of water or blood'. He sees no conflict between this interpretation and the notion of a possible connection with the moon. We will return to the topic of 'wombs' linked with 'snakes' in an Australian Aboriginal context in Chapters 12 and 13.

The archaeologist Robert Wenke (1984: 129) supports Marshack in his conclusions concerning the moon, noting that without calendrical/astronomical records of some kind, winters and resource shortages would have taken people by surprise. 'The phases of the moon', confirms the cave-art specialist Paul Bahn (in Bahn and Vertut 1988: 182), 'would certainly have been the principal means available to Palaeolithic people for measuring the passage of time . . .'. Finally, Mircea Eliade (1978, 1: 23) has commented that whatever may be thought of Marshack's general theory concerning the development of civilisation,

> the fact remains that the lunar cycle was analyzed, memorized, and used for practical purposes some 15,000 years before the discovery of agriculture. This makes more comprehensible the considerable role of the moon in archaic mythologies, and especially the fact that lunar symbolism was integrated into a single system comprising such different realities as woman, the waters, vegetation, the serpent, fertility, death, 'rebirth', etc.

On the other hand, although his work has been frequently cited and is much admired, Marshack's specific claim to have discovered Upper Palaeolithic lunar 'calendars' has been treated with caution by most scholars. It is not that his arithmetical counts and calculations have been disproved (but see D'Errico 1989 on the Azilian pebbles) – rather, they fail to connect easily with the dominant paradigms of contemporary archaeologists, most of whom see culture as an 'adaptation', acknowledging seasonality but failing to appreciate why survival should have involved keeping track of the moon. With the exception of Marshack himself, archaeologists have not found any particular place for the moon in their models. Until there is independent confirmation of this aspect of Marshack's findings – confirmation arrived at on theoretical grounds, without reference to the 'notations' he has analysed – it seems unlikely that the issues will be resolved. In short, the fate of Marshack's 'lunar' interpretations will depend on the outcome of a wider debate as to how human culture emerged.

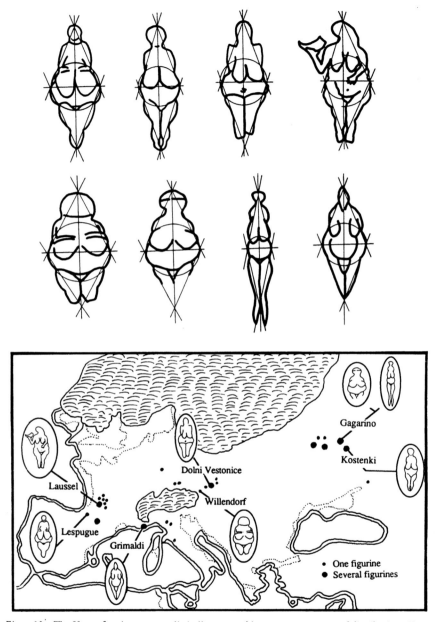

Figure 13 The Venus figurines were stylistically comparable across a vast range of distribution. *Upper*: A. Leroi-Gourhan's (1968: 92) analysis of figurines as variations on a theme. Top row: Lespugue, Kostenki, Dolni Vestonice, Laussel. Bottom row: Willendorf, Gagarino (2 examples), Grimaldi. *Lower*: Approximate locations of European Upper Palaeolithic sites yielding figurines or engravings. Coastlines (double lines) are those of the Last Glacial; shaded areas mark major Last Glacial ice sheets. Dotted lines mark present coastlines (redrawn after Champion *et al.* 1984: Fig. 3.19).

The 'Venus' Figurines

In a more theoretical approach, the study of Upper Palaeolithic art has been advanced in recent years by considering how it may have aided hunters and gatherers to adapt to their environment (e.g. Conkey 1978; Gamble 1982; Pfeiffer 1982; Jochim 1983). The emphasis here has generally been on how art constitutes a medium for the transmission of 'information'.

One topic which has been approached in this spirit concerns the hundred and more so-called 'Venus figurines' from the ice age which have been discovered in various parts of Europe and subsequently described (Abramova 1967; Delporte 1979; Graziozi 1960; Leroi-Gourhan 1968; Gomez-Tabanera 1978; Gamble 1982; Bahn and Vertut 1988). The figurines are beautifully carved, small and portable representations of women, sometimes in stone, sometimes in bone or ivory, sometimes in coal. Some are small enough to have been worn as pendants; a tiny figurine made of coal and found in Petersfels in southwest Germany has a hole drilled through the top as if for a string (Marshack 1972b: 286). Many of the figurines cannot be dated, but enough carbon 14 dates have been obtained to suggest that most were made somewhere between 25,000 and 23,000 years ago (Gamble 1982: table 1).

Perhaps the most striking characteristic of these figurines is their stylistic unity across an immense range of distribution (figure 13). They are found across a predominantly north-European zone stretching from the Pyrenees to European Russia, with specimens known from south-west France, southern Germany, northern Italy, Czechoslovakia and the Ukraine. Leroi-Gourhan (1968: 96) writes:

> No matter where found . . . they are practically interchangeable, apart from their proportions. The most complete figures have the same treatment of the head, the same small arms folded over the breast or pointing towards the belly, the same low breasts dropping like sacks to far below the waist, and the same legs ending in miniscule or non-existent feet.

Understanding how and why these objects could have remained so similar across such immense distances in space and time has constituted perhaps the major challenge of this art.

The figurines were evidently part of a wider and still older tradition. The earliest specimens of European figurative art consist mostly of 'parts of animals and vulvas engraved roughly on plaquettes or blocks of limestone . . . .' (Pfeiffer 1982: 143). Human vulva designs — sometimes oval, sometimes triangular, sometimes alone, sometimes as part of a whole-body figure — appear in France and Spain in non-decorated forms from the Aurignacian onwards, and with decorations further east. Although the depiction of female attributes climaxed with the Venus figurines of the period 25–23,000 BP, the symbolic tradition as such did not end there. It seems to have continued down through the millennia, albeit in varying forms. In the later phases of the Upper Palaeolithic, particularly during the Magdalenian, there appear numerous renditions of the female buttocks seen from the side, sometimes in long series, and often associated with other symbols or with animals (Marshack 1972b: 305). And figurines in a rather abstract style were produced over the same zone during the very last stages of the Upper Palaeolithic, between 15,000 and 10,000 years ago (Gamble 1982). Even after the ice age ended, aspects of the tradition may have lived on. A minority of contemporary archaeologists have claimed that the many clay and stone female figurines of Neolithic Old Europe – including images from Crete – are in the final analysis extensions or continuations of the same symbolic genre (Crawford 1958; Gimbutas 1982; 1989).

It has often been assumed that the figurines of ice age Europe were produced by men, perhaps for erotic reasons. But whilst that is possible, the truth is that we do not know the sex of the artists. As Paul Bahn (Bahn and Vertut 1988: 165) points out:

> The carvers of the 'vulvas' and figurines could just as easily have been female, and one can extend this argument to the whole of Palaeolithic art, invoking initiation ceremonies to explain menstruation, with lunar notation as supporting evidence.

To say that all palaeolithic art was produced by women would of course be absurd – but no more absurd than the inverse assumption which is frequently made! I will point to some evidence bearing on the gender of figurine users in a moment.

For an earlier generation of thinkers, the Venus figurines testify to the ice age existence of a matriarchal cult of 'the Goddess' or 'Great Mother': the statuettes were depictions of this mythological personage. This view is still defended by some eminent archaeologists, notably Marija Gimbutas (1982; 1989), who has traced in detail the varied forms and depictions of what she sees as an Old-European 'Moon-Goddess' who was also a 'Snake-Goddess' amongst other things. Along with Marshack (1972b) and many others, Pfeiffer (1982: 202) agrees that the figurines may relate to a myth which in its numerous local versions featured 'a widely venerated female being'.

But this entire paradigm has been heavily criticised by Peter Ucko (1962; 1968), who suggests a more prosaic interpretation: the statuettes may have been simple ornaments or even toys – rather like contemporary girls' dolls. However, Ucko goes on to suggest that even ice age or neolithic dolls (if such they were) may have functioned also as gynaecological charms of some kind, used by women to enhance fertility or – perhaps – to instruct pubescent females undergoing initiation ceremonies. Among the Igbo of eastern Nigeria, a pregnant woman until recently carried around with her a little bag containing a red-painted wooden doll:

> On her way to the market, other women seeing the bag would ask to see

her baby; she would then bring out the doll and give it to them. The women would take the doll and rub off some of the red paint on to their own bellies. . . . (Amadiume 1987: 75)

Ucko points out that small anthropomorphic figurines were used in many African societies as teaching aids in the course of initiation ceremonies (Ucko 1962; Cory 1961), whilst Zuni Indian women traditionally used magic dolls following a miscarriage or in order to get pregnant (Ucko 1968: 425, citing Parsons 1919: 279–86). All such dolls or figurines belonged – of course – emphatically within the female sphere.

Excavations of Palaeolithic settlements in France, eastern Europe and Siberia have established the characteristic position of the dolls or figurines – namely, inside the dwelling hollow, close to the hearth, and most frequently in storage pits dug into the floor. In a number of cases, the presumed guardians of the figurines had carefully covered them with bones or with stone slabs, as if to deliberately hide them from prying eyes.

Delporte (1968) comments that the specimen from the Abri Facteur was found 18 cm from the wall of a shelter, in an area where there was a marked paucity of stone tools. Was this perhaps a sanctuary of some kind? Lalanne and Bouyssonie (1946) suggest that the beautiful Venus of Laussel and other figurines at this French site formed a sanctuary some 12 m by 6 m in area. At Dolni Vestonice in Moravia (Klima 1957), the most complete Venus figurine was associated with a large hearth. The examples from Gagarino in the Soviet Union were found along the periphery of a hut (Graziosi 1960), while those from Kostienki I/1 came from a number of storage pits within a large dwelling (Abramova 1967). One figurine from Kostienki I, found in 1983 and dating to about 23,000 years ago, was upright in a small pit, leaning against the wall and facing the centre of the living area and the hearths; the pit was filled with soil mixed with red ochre and was capped by a mammoth shoulder-blade (Bahn and Vertut 1988: 140, citing Praslov 1985: 182–3). This, too, suggests a sanctuary. The excavator of two dwellings at Mal'ta in Siberia noted that the floors had 'male' (right-hand) and 'female' (left-hand) inventories. In each case, the 'female' inventories included the statuettes. Shimkin (1978: 278) comments:

The implication that the female figurines, both stylised and modeled, had some significance connected with woman's role in Upper Palaeolithic society, both in European Russia and Siberia (as well as in central and western Europe), seems obvious, but the exact nature of that significance is open to question.

The Soviet archaeologist Abramova (1967; cited by Marshack 1972b: 339) associates the figurines with the 'spirit of the hearth', suggesting a connection with traditions among the Tungus and other northern Asiatic peoples, some of whom keep in their tents a portrayal of a hearth spirit envisaged as 'a clever old, but still strong and vigorous woman'. Marshack tentatively supports Abramova here, seeing the figurines as possibly representing the 'mistress of the home and hearth, protectress of the domestic fire' and 'sovereign mistress of animals and especially game animals'. He adds that the whole ritual complex may have been rooted in ideas connecting female influences with hunting-success, commenting:

> we may suppose that the decisive role taken by the woman in the magical rituals preceding the chase had a special significance for its success in the eyes of primitive man. (Marshack 1972b: 338)

Marshack, however, sees the Upper Palaeolithic artist or record-keeper less as a goddess worshipper, shamanic specialist or astronomer, than as a story teller who needed to help regulate major activities by reference to the phases of the moon:

> Against the phases of the moon he told a story, or he told many stories. And against the phases of the moon he held at least some of his rites and ceremonies, which is another way of telling a story. And against the phases of the moon he structured his practical, social, cultural, and biological life. (Marshack 1972b: 136)

Despite Marshack's use of the male pronoun here, he is in fact conscious of the possibility that women kept records of the moon's changes in monitoring their menstrual cycles and terms of pregnancy. In this context, he refers to the Californian Yurok:

> The women apparently kept a menstrual count by dropping a stick each day into a basket and kept a pregnancy count by dropping a 'month' stick each lunar month into a second basket until they reached a count of ten. (correspondence from Arnold Pilling dated June 1968; Marshack 1972b: 337n)

Marshack (1972b: 337) also cites the Soviet archaeologist Boris Frolov (1965), who describes how contemporary Siberian peoples – traditionally reindeer-hunters – use lunar calendars in similar contexts. Among the Nganasans, for example, a mother would sew ten coloured stripes to her garment to signify the ten lunar months of her pregnancy. Referring generally to the Nganasans, Entses, Dolgans, Chukchi, Koryaks and Kets, Frolov comments that the custodians of such lunar calendars were invariably women.

It is certainly difficult to escape the suspicion that the figurines belonged to a system of which the notations were also a part, and that together they served functions within a matrifocal ritual context of some kind. The fact that many of the Upper Palaeolithic figurines were originally painted red may support the notion of an association between femininity and blood – as

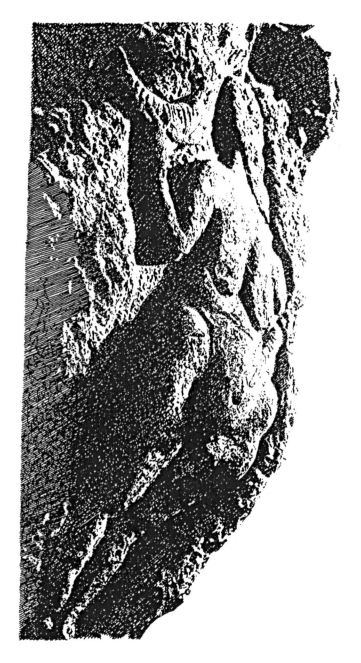

Figure 14 The Venus of Laussel, Dordogne, France. Note the typical emphasis on the mid-body and womb region. Originally red-painted with ochre (redrawn by the author from a photograph by Achille Weider).

exemplified in the custom of fertility-seeking Igbo women, who as mentioned earlier rub the redness from a pregnant woman's doll on to their own childless bellies (Amadiume 1987: 75). The topic of ochre pigmentation will be discussed in Chapter 12, but it is worth mentioning here that one well-known ochred figurine – a bas-relief from the rock shelter of Laussel in the Dordogne – is holding a bison horn marked with thirteen lines (figure 14). Marshack (1972b: 335) comments:

> The count of thirteen is the number of crescent 'horns' that may make up an observational lunar year; it is also the number of days from the birth of the first crescent to just before the days of the mature full moon.

Marshack concedes that all such interpretations are speculative, and that in the absence of informants it is impossible to say anything very definite about what ice age art may have been intended to mean. But in any event, he insists, the moon was certainly important, and 'processes, sequences, and periodicities of female, sky and season were surely recognised' (Marshack 1972b: 283).

But we must return to the topic with which we began this section – the recently popular approach which sees ice age art as adaptive in terms of the gathering and dissemination of vital 'information'.

The figurines were made during a period of extreme and increasing cold, which must have reduced population densities in many regions and placed immense strains on local populations as they attempted to maintain social, marital and ritual contacts with neighbouring groups. Taking this background into account, Clive Gamble (1982) has suggested that the stylistic uniformity testifies to the figurine-makers' astonishing success in maintaining cross-territorial chains of connection. The statuettes indicate the ice age existence of a vast mating network – an immense fabric of marital alliances and associated relations of interdependency – stretching from the Pyrenees in West Europe to the Ukraine and beyond in the east. How else could these figurines have remained so identical across such vast expanses of space, if the information encoded in them were not in some sense 'international' common currency?

Gamble (1982: 98) assumes that the figurines – some of which seem to have been worn around the neck as pendants – performed basically the same function as other items of personal ornamentation. We saw in an earlier chapter that beads, pierced shells, pendants, necklaces and similar items suddenly appear in the European archaeological record in abundant quantities at around 33,000 BP – in the earliest phases of the Aurignacian (White 1989a, 1989b). Gamble sees the figurines as portable objects which were 'components in a system of visual display involving the wearing of distinctive dress and ornament'. In contrast with later cave art, when paintings were carefully hidden, the figurines, according to Gamble, 'were made for the purpose of general display', serving as 'media through which information could be exchanged' – information allowing small bands dispersed over immense areas to remain in communication with one another despite the great distances sometimes separating them. The rationale here is that uniformity in ornamentation style enables strangers to recognise one another, even from a distance, as members of the same group. The figurines were used by people who needed to be able to recognise one another as members of the same far-flung extended mating network.

Interpretations of this kind, whilst certainly enlightening, have a characteristic drawback. As Mithen (1988: 297) has pointed out, in this as in other recent 'information'-oriented approaches to palaeolithic art, 'the term "information" is poorly defined and it is rare for any contact to be made between theoretical argument and the specific imagery of the paintings'. Granted that in this case the figurines may have conveyed information through which mating networks were cemented, we would still want to know why these particular art objects rather than others had to be produced. Why did the statuettes have to represent humans? Or, more precisely: why female humans with hidden faces, small feet and strongly emphasised reproductive parts? Or again, why were they so frequently ochred? What kind of pan-European 'information' was it which could only be communicated through details such as these?

Steven Mithen (1988) has probably done as much as anyone in recent years to redirect attention towards detail in Upper Palaeolithic art. In an impressive contribution he has shown how the manner of depiction of animals in the caves and associated mobiliary art expresses a well-informed hunter's-eye view of the world. To an experienced contemporary hunter-gatherer, the landscape is saturated with significances. Nothing is merely itself. Everything noteworthy points beyond itself to other realities – things displaced from it in space or in time. Mithen in particular notes contemporary foraging peoples' immense interest in the distinctive hoofprints of animals, their droppings, characteristic marks left on vegetation and many other details imprinted upon the landscape. He demonstrates how certain previously puzzling details of Upper Palaeolithic art make sense in this light – showing, for example, that some 'abstract motifs' long known in the art are in fact hoofprints which a tracker would instantly recognise.

Mithen is particularly convincing when he follows Marshack (1972b) in postulating a rhythmic, ever-changing yet cyclically predictable ice age world of seasonal comings and goings, each phase heralded by its distinctive signs. He points out, for example, that the birds depicted in the art are overwhelmingly waterfowl such as ducks, geese and cranes. This cannot be because aquatic birds were either the commonest species or those most frequently hunted – it is known that they were not. The more probable explanation is that such birds were migratory, their appearance each year therefore constituting an important set of cues. They were selected by the artists for their special symbolic value as indicators of seasonal time.

Mithen's claim is not that ice age hunters used such art to store information as such. Certainly, he is not suggesting that a hunter would first go to a cave or engraved rock to refresh his hunting knowledge before going out in search of game. Rather, his point is that hunters noticed certain things about animals and not others, and that the features most noticed were those which were important for survival. If tracking an animal involved noticing its distinctive faeces, for example, then such an animal might frequently be depicted in the act of defecating – as is sometimes the case in the art. Painting animals explicitly in this act may seem puzzling at first sight – but it was inevitable that the art produced by these hunters should have reflected their own particular perspectives and preoccupations.

The striking stylistic peculiarities of the Venus figurines can be understood in a similar light. Why, for example, were the 'central' portions of the human female body always emphasised at the expense of faces and feet? Mithen's approach would lead us to infer here some real preoccupations of the culture. We might suspect that faces were hidden and feet not shown because the most important, information-laden cues were in real life conveyed by other parts of the female body – the parts actually emphasised in the art. If the figurines had immense ochred bellies and thighs, along with carefully emphasised pubic triangles, it was because in life – that is, where real women were concerned – the signals of most importance to the culture were felt to emanate from such regions. If menstruating women accentuated their condition by painting themselves in red pigment – a fairly common ethnographic pattern – nature's signals could have been artificially amplified in a manner which the painting of the figurines then replicated (see Chapter 13). It is even possible that the bowed heads and hidden faces were intended to connote 'seclusion' in some sense.

Whilst all this is certainly speculative, it seems scarcely controversial to suggest that Upper Palaeolithic men as well as women needed to be aware of the times when women were in a 'special' condition, and that the figurine art reflected preoccupations of this kind. None of this would detract from the significance of Gamble's general idea – the notion that the stylistic unity expressed in the figurines reflects a vast ice age extended kinship network. In fact, this exciting finding would tie in well with the basic arguments of this book, since as we saw in Chapter 9, the model of cultural origins outlined here would lead us to expect patterns of transpatial, gender-based clan solidarity stretching across the landscape in a manner contrasting significantly with the more small-scale, localised territorial attachments of primates and (as has been inferred here) archaic humans. But it is even more satisfying when we can go beyond noting simply that the figurines are stylistically similar, to noting that the precise content of the art also supports the hypothesis. Interestingly, Gamble frequently draws parallels between ice age European mating networks and the 'chains of connection' characteristic of Aboriginal Australia. This parallel may run deeper than first appears. Figurines resembling those we have been discussing are not used, but in Australia, inter-tribal links are cemented not just through any conceivable rites and objects provided these are stylistically uniform – but quite specifically through initiation rites and associated pseudo-procreative audio-visual paraphernalia focusing heavily and insistently on the symbolic potency of 'ancestral' – very often explicitly 'menstrual' – blood (see Chapter 13).

Taking into account ethnographic parallels, archaeological associations and the model of cultural origins outlined in this book, we are led to suspect that the Upper Palaeolithic vulva engravings and Venus figurines were used on periodic special occasions. This would conform with Marshack's finding that many of the objects show signs of repeated, periodic use – under the microscope, they reveal groups and series of marks, each made by a different point (Marshack 1972b). People seem to have been meeting on successive occasions to view or to use these objects. This suggests the performance of rituals, the participants renewing their engravings or re-ochring their figurines for each re-enactment – rather as Australian Aborigines take out from their hiding places their sacred *churinga*, bullroarers or other objects, each of which needs to be re-ochred before use (see Chapter 13). Taking this idea a little further, we could link the explicit femaleness of the Upper Palaeolithic figurines with the possibly gender-specific dimensions of the rituals, taking into account also the apparent hiding of the figurines in special pits close to the hearth. We would not expect men to hide their erotic secrets from women in places such as these. A menstrual interpretation would be that the figurines were kept hidden from male eyes. They were used by women during their menstrual or gynaecological rites – their moon-scheduled periods of togetherness and segregation from male company. If the figurines were pendants, they were not simply displayed publicly, in a general, time-independent way: they were worn on special occasions. After the dance or initiation ceremony was over, they were carefully put away.

Chapter 11
The Raw and the Cooked

> Hunger is hunger, but the hunger that is satisfied with cooked meat
> eaten with fork and knife is a different kind of hunger from the one that
> devours raw meat with the aid of hands, nails and teeth.
>
> Karl Marx, *Grundrisse* (1857–9)

Culture – if the preceding arguments are accepted – originated under
pressure from what for millennia must have been the most reproductively
burdened and oppressed sex. When women as a gender group finally brought
such pressures to a head, developing sufficient internal solidarity to enable
them to assert a monthly 'strike', they thereby established the basic categories and distinctions of the cultural domain. We will see in this chapter
how such action involved, among other things, distinguishing raw meat
from cooked, imposing a taboo upon raw meat, tying feast days and therefore
cooking to specific lunar phases, and integrating the raw/cooked opposition
with that between kin and affines.

Because women signalling 'no!' had first and foremost to be inviolable, the
condition of all these achievements was the establishment of menstrual
taboos. These originated not simply as sexual avoidances, but have always
had the profoundest economic, political, ritual and other dimensions. In the
course of expressing their gender solidarity in blood, women asserted that
females were separate from males, incest different from marriage, production
distinct from consumption – and 'the raw' distinct from 'the cooked'. In fact,
we will see that women's menstrual self-identity was the generative source of
all culture's other basic categories, polarities and rules.

Menstrual Taboos

Menstrual taboos are familiar to us all. They are very much a part of our own
culture, and are in evidence as a prominent feature of most traditional ones.
Some cultures have weak menstrual taboos; the people in one agricultural
community – the Rungus of Borneo – have aroused particular curiosity

because they seem to have none at all (Appell 1988). But exceptions of this kind serve only to prove the rule. Menstrual taboos may not be universal, but they are sufficiently widespread to justify the inference that they are an extremely ancient component of the human cultural configuration.

From one point of view, menstruation may seem a relatively ordinary biological event. In modern western societies it is a bodily function not thought to require much public acknowledgement or discussion. Yet traditional cultures almost everywhere have accorded it extraordinarily elaborate symbolic attention, far in excess of that accorded to other physiological functions which might at first sight seem comparable. It is not just that menstruation is thought of as polluting. Where taboos are strong, the avoidances are enforced through spectacular institutions buttressed by often extravagant beliefs in the supernatural potencies of women's blood. It is the draconic *powers* of menstrual blood – powers which can be used for good or ill, and which may be thought to influence not only the entire earth but the cosmos, too – which stand out in traditional mythologies.

In this context, few writers on the subject have put the case more vividly than the Roman historian, Pliny (1942: 549):

> But nothing could easily be found that is more remarkable than the monthly flux of women. Contact with it turns new wine sour, crops touched by it become barren, grafts die, seeds in gardens are dried up, the fruits of trees fall off, the bright surface of mirrors in which it is merely reflected is dimmed, the edge of steel and the gleam of ivory are dulled, hives of bees die, even bronze and iron are at once seized by rust, and a horrible smell fills the air. . . .

The Gimi of the Eastern Highlands of Papua New Guinea see menstruation as a constant 'threat to male purity and superiority'; objects touched by a menstruating woman are bound to deteriorate rapidly:

> wooden bowls will crack, stone axes will misbehave in the hands of their male owners and inflict upon them otherwise inexplicable wounds, crops will wither and die, even the ground over which the menstruator steps will lose its fertility. (Gillison 1980: 149)

The Mae Enga in Papua New Guinea believe that contact with a menstruating woman will

> sicken a man and cause persistent vomiting, 'kill' his blood so that it turns black, corrupt his vital juices so that his skin darkens and hangs in folds as his flesh wastes, permanently dull his wits, and eventually lead to a slow decline and death. (Meggitt 1964; quoted in Delaney *et al.* 1977: 5)

A Mae Enga tribesman known to the anthropologist M. J. Meggitt left his wife because she had slept on his blanket while menstruating; later, still not feeling quite safe from her evil influence, he killed her with an axe (Meggitt

1964). And Maurice Godelier (1986: 58) reports that the men of the Baruya of Papua New Guinea have a similar view: 'The attitude of the men toward menstrual blood, whenever they talk or think about it, verges on hysteria, mingling with disgust, repulsion, and above all fear.'

Magico-religious beliefs only marginally less intense were active among most rural populations in Europe, at least until a few decades ago.

The belief that menstruants cause fruit trees to wither lingered on late into the nineteenth and even into the twentieth century in Italy, Spain, Germany and Holland. In the wine districts of Bordeaux and the Rhine, menstruating women were forbidden to approach the vats and cellars, lest the wine turn to vinegar. In France, women were excluded from refineries when the sugar was boiling, lest it all turn black; and no menstruating woman would attempt to make mayonnaise sauce (Briffault 1927, 2: 389). In the United States in the 1920s, women widely believed that a permanent wave would not take if they were menstruating (Delaney *et al.* 1977: 7).

In England, the *British Medical Journal* in 1878 published correspondence from doctors insisting that in curing hams, women should not rub the legs of pork with the brine-pickle during their periods (Briffault 1927, 2: 389). The contemporary anthropologist Denise Lawrence (1988: 123), reporting on fieldwork conducted in the 1970s, writes that at the annual pig-killing undertaken by families in one village in southern Portugal, 'the greatest threat to a household's economic well-being is posed by the purported destructive effects of menstruation on processing pork'. In this village to this day, almost the entire female-governed organisation of pork sausage production still revolves around such taboos.

Theories of Menstrual Symbolism

In the 1960s, William Stephens attempted an ambitious cross-cultural survey of menstrual taboos from a psychoanalytical perspective. In his view, male 'castration anxiety' lies behind the taboos. The theory was that 'the sight or thought of a person who bleeds from the genitals (a menstruating woman) is frightening to a person who has intense castration anxiety' (1962: 93). He predicted that the intensity of menstrual taboos should therefore vary cross-culturally in proportion to the intensity of male fear of castration — a prediction which he claimed was borne out.

An opposite psychological theory had earlier been put forward by the psychoanalyst Bruno Bettelheim, author of *Symbolic Wounds* (1955). Bettelheim argued that males are not so much afraid of castration as, on the contrary, envious of women's capacity to bleed from the genitals. They therefore attempt to imitate this. Bettelheim saw this as the explanation for that very important class of customs known as 'male initiation rites', many of which involve cutting the penises of boys or in other ways making them bleed. In some parts of the world male self-mutilation and bleeding is explicitly referred to in the native idiom as 'male menstruation' (see Chapter 13). While Stephens' model would lead us to see this as symbolic self-castration, Bettelheim's model interprets male initiation ritualism as an attempt by men to emulate women's peculiar blood-making/child-bearing powers.

A more recent theory with a psychological component rests on the observation that menstruation can be a rare event among hunters and gatherers. It is said that because of its rarity it would understandably have been worrying and seemingly anomalous – and therefore 'taboo'. It is said that badly nourished hunter-gatherer women reach menarche late in life, reach menopause early, and suffer frequent long spells of amenorrhoea, in addition to being pregnant or breast-feeding for much of their lives. They therefore hardly ever menstruate (Frisch 1975). The menstrual rhythm which modern Westerners think of as a frequent and regular periodic blood loss may be in other cultures, as Buckley and Gottlieb (1988: 45, citing Harrell 1981) paraphrase this hypothesis, 'a fairly rare occurrence, the rarity of which may indeed inform the great potency attributed to it and the stringency of ritual prohibitions by which it is so often surrounded'.

A different set of theories holds that psychology has little to do with the matter – people are simply being scientific in avoiding menstrual blood. The substance, according to this line of thought, really is highly toxic. This theory was first proposed in 1920 by a physician, Bela Schick, who posited the existence of what he termed 'menotoxins' in menstrual blood. Ashley Montagu (1940, 1957, cited by Buckley and Gottlieb 1988: 19) was the first to bring Schick's theory to the attention of anthropologists, asking whether menstruating women indeed wither plants, turn wine, spoil pickles, cause bread to fall and so forth – all because of the alleged chemical effects of menstrual blood.

Not one of these theories has gained more than minority support. The mutually incompatible psychoanalytical models explain neither cultural variation, nor the complexity of menstrual rituals; concentrating on the male psyche, they in fact ignore most of the social, symbolic, cosmological and other dimensions of these customs. The argument from menstruation's rarity or apparent abnormality fails to explain more than a small number of possible cases. Accepting that menstrual bleeding in some hunter-gatherer societies may be quite a rare event, we are still left with a problem. In view of the extraordinarily elaborate menstrual rituals of so many cultures, it seems all the more remarkable that what little blood is actually shed should be made to serve such vast symbolic purposes. The ideological links with the moon, with cooking, with hunting, with shamanism and so forth seem too detailed in their cross-cultural recurrences and too central to cosmology and religion to be explained as puzzled or frightened responses to an occasional perceived abnormality. Finally, the view that menstrual blood is genuinely toxic is mythical; this kind of belief is an example of menstrual superstition, not an explanation of it.

New Perspectives on Menstruation

In their attempts to find a general, cross-cultural explanation for ethno-graphic menstrual taboos, few interpreters of the 1960s and 1970s ventured far beyond the parameters of male native ideology in such matters. Much was made of the 'pollution' associated with menstrual blood, and of women's oppression through the corresponding seclusion rules and taboos. The concepts of 'taboo' and of 'oppression' were closely linked (Stephens 1962; Young 1965; Young and Bacdayan 1965). In this respect, theories intended as pioneering feminist contributions (e.g. Delaney et al. 1977) not infrequently colluded with more traditional views.

Since the early 1980s, however, in response to a fresh current of interest in the lives of women, some radically new anthropological approaches to the topic have begun to emerge. These have not yet resulted in any new general theory of menstrual symbolism, but they have added a new dimension to the debates. In some cases they have drawn on strands from an older tradition of matriarchy-theory, as exemplified for example in Robert Briffault's encyc-lopaedic, magnificent, yet almost wholly ignored cross-cultural work, *The Mothers* (1927). Other recent writers have been influenced by emergent contributions to popular culture such as Barbara Walker's impressively ambitious and scholarly compilation, *The Woman's Encyclopedia of Myths and Secrets* (1983), or Penelope Shuttle's and Peter Redgrove's imaginative psychological exploration of menstrual dreams and symbolism, *The Wise Wound* (1978).

It was above all *The Wise Wound* that presented to a new generation of emancipated women in the 1980s what seemed at first to be a daring and paradoxical message: correctly approached and understood, menstruation need not be Woman's 'curse'. It can be an empowering and indeed magical experience. Social anthropologists were slow to respond, but an edited volume published in 1988 entitled *Blood Magic; The anthropology of menstru-ation* (Buckley and Gottlieb 1988) may mark the beginning of the discipline's dawning awareness of the positive potentialities of 'menstrual power'.

Without always acknowledging matriarchalist influences, most of the anthropological contributors to *Blood Magic* seem to have drawn on the insights of Bachofen, Briffault and other early matriarchy theorists in emphasising the ambiguity of most cultural constructions of menstruation, pointing out that terms such as 'pollution', 'taboo' or 'defilement' have in the past been far too simplistically understood.

The editors of *Blood Magic* point out that the dual significance of menstrual regulations is inherent in the very term *tabu*. The Polynesian word is made up from the root *ta*, meaning 'to mark', and *pu*, which is an adverb of intensity; *tabu*, therefore, means 'marked thoroughly' (Steiner 1956: 32). In many Polynesian languages, 'holy' and 'forbidden' are inseparable concepts: a thing which is 'holy' is by the same token 'forbidden'; a thing which is 'forbidden' is also 'holy'. A Fijian woman may be termed *dra tabu* – meaning 'holy blood' (Sahlins 1977: 33).

Durkheim: the Menstrual Origin of Exogamy

The notion of 'tabu' as connoting both 'danger' and 'power' belongs in fact to a venerable tradition. One source of this is the work of Durkheim, and in particular a pioneering article on menstrual symbolism published in 1898. It is worth recalling this, since Durkheim's piece – nowadays virtually forgotten in the English-speaking world – is directly relevant to the central argument of this book.

In 'The prohibition of incest and its origins', published at the turn of the century in the first issue of *L'Anné sociologique*, Durkheim (1963[1898]) set out to explain the origins of 'the law of exogamy' – the rule stipulating that members of a clan must 'marry out'. His theory was based on a very simple idea. Social order – manifesting itself in institutions such as exogamic rules – involves the capacity to counteract the natural tendency for the sexes to conjoin. But in concrete terms, what is the force which keeps the sexes apart?

At the simplest level, there are three possibilities. Firstly, women repulse men. Secondly, men repulse women. Thirdly, the two sexes are kept apart by some overarching, external force.

Durkheim tended to favour the third option, believing that it is moral/religious ideology imposed by society as a whole which keeps the sexes apart. However, he simultaneously favoured the first option, insisting that although women in earliest times may not have possessed social or political dominance, it was nonetheless they who were the immediate agents of religious ideology's segregating action. *Earliest women established sexual morality by periodically repulsing men.* To be more precise, Durkheim argued that women established the exogamy rule by periodically *bleeding* so as to repulse the opposite sex.

The law of exogamy, writes Durkheim, is only one specific case of a much more general religious institution, known as 'taboo'. Taboo, according to Durkheim, is the ritualistic setting apart of 'the sacred'. Durkheim gives several examples – tabooed priests whom commoners may not touch, tabooed religious objects, tabooed places and so on. Just as taboo sets apart the sacred, so exogamy sets apart a woman from all men of her own clan. 'The two sexes', comments Durkheim (1963: 71) in this context, 'must avoid each other with the same care as the profane flees from the sacred and the sacred from the profane. . .'. When exogamic taboos are in force, according to Durkheim, women become like sacred beings invested 'with an isolating power of some sort, a power which holds the masculine population at a distance. . .'

In 'primitive' societies, continues Durkheim (1963: 72), it is above all with their first menstrual flows that women become 'sacred'. From this moment, and then at each recurrence of the flow, women exercise a 'type of repulsing action which keeps the other sex far from them' (1963: 75). The moral order of typically 'primitive' cultures is sustained and defined by this action. 'Each part of the population', Durkheim writes, 'lives separated from the other'. Husbands may even avoid eating with their wives. Often, husband and wife have separate kinship loyalties, and shun intimate contact of any kind in public.

All this, according to Durkheim, expresses the deepest of male fears. 'All blood is terrible and all sorts of taboos are instituted to prevent contact with it.' Since a woman bleeds periodically, a 'more or less conscious anxiety, a certain religious fear, cannot fail to be present in all the relations which her companions have with her', reducing male contacts with her to a minimum (Durkheim 1963: 85). Since sex brings a man into the closest potential contact with a woman's blood, it is not surprising that the taboos should involve sexual prohibitions above all. 'It is from this', concludes Durkheim,

> that exogamy and the serious penalties which sanction it are derived. Whoever violates this law finds himself in the same state as a murderer. He has entered into contact with blood. . . .

Durkheim saw this whole arrangement as rooted in the 'religious system' known as 'totemism' (see Chapter 3). The secret of this, in his view, was simply the belief that blood *in general* is sacred or godlike, as a consequence of which game animals, too, are felt to be the repositories of highly tabooed blood. 'Among certain North American Indians, to eat the blood of animals is an abomination; the game is passed over the flame so that the blood in it will be dried up.' Among the Jews, continues Durkheim (1963: 83–4), the same prohibition is sanctioned by the terrible penalty of excommunication. Similar beliefs were current among the Romans, the Arabs and others.

In totemism, according to Durkheim, the blood of one's mother and her matrilineal clan is identified with the blood of an animal selected as the clan's emblem. The clan members 'consider themselves as forming a single flesh, "a single meat", a single blood, and this flesh is that of the mythical being from whom they have all descended. . .' Within the shared blood resides the 'god' or 'totem' of the clan, 'from which it follows that the blood is a divine thing. When it runs out, the god is spilling over' (Durkheim 1963: 89). 'God' as an object of respect, then, is in Durkheim's model inseparable from menstrual and other blood.

It would be interesting to study the ideological and political factors which led to Durkheim's insights being virtually ignored for a hundred years. Leaving aside this issue, however, and also leaving aside for the moment the detailed validity of his particular formulations, we can agree that the potencies associated with sacrifical or other blood have for millennia meshed closely and sometimes indistinguishably with notions of 'divine power' (Girard 1977). The Siouan Dakota term for 'taboo' is *wakan*, defined in Rigg's *Dakota–English Dictionary* as meaning 'spiritual, consecrated; wonderful, incomprehensible; said also of women at the menstrual period' (quoted in Briffault 1927, 2: 412). Remaining in North America, a Muskogee informant from Oklahoma states that women naturally 'purify' themselves when they separate from men 'during their monthly time'. Men must enter monthly into a sweat-lodge to keep pure, whereas simply by menstruating, 'women are naturally purifying themselves to keep their medicine effective' (Powers 1980: 57). According to an Oglala informant, the power of woman 'grows with the moon and comes and goes with it' (Neihardt 1961: 212, quoted in Powers 1980: 62). Sacred water for ceremonial use by Oglala 'buffalo women' – sexual or pubescent women, 'those who have the power to create life' – is made by mixing water with red chokeberries. Powers (1980: 61) comments:

> Again we see the connection being made symbolically between buffalo women . . . and life. Moreover, if red is sacred and sacred water and menstrual blood are red, then symbolically sacred water *is* menstrual blood. If sacred water is life, menstrual blood also symbolises life.

A basic feature of the Sun Dance of the Arapaho and other Plains Indians was the drinking of red 'medicine water' symbolic of the menstrual flow (Dorsey 1903: 177); an informant explained that 'menses is called *ba'ataana*, which means "medicine" or "supernatural"'' (Hilger 1952: 72).

In Australia, comparable patterns are or were found. Over most of the continent, the status of women was generally rather low; however, women's 'blood-making and child-giving powers were thought both mysterious and dangerous' (Stanner 1965: 216). 'Even when ritually tabu. . .', writes Berndt (1951: 58–9) of the Yolngu of north-east Arnhem Land, 'a woman is regarded as sacred, for her blood [is] sacred. . .' The Wik-Mungkan Aborigines of Cape York describe tabooed things as *ngaintja*. Discussing the fact that women may be *ngaintja*, particularly when menstruating, McKnight (1975: 95) says: 'I think the answer to this lies in the fact that women also are associated with the Rainbow Serpent. The Rainbow Serpent is believed to be responsible for women menstruating.'

The significance of this 'Rainbow Serpent' – touched on in the Introduction – will be explored further in Chapter 13.

Frazer: Menstruating Maidens and Divine Kings

In the concluding chapter of the second edition of *The Golden Bough*, Frazer (1900, 3: 204) added his own contribution to the view of menstruants as semi-divine 'powers'. He drew attention to what he felt was an astonishing cross-cultural parallel between (a) the ritual treatment of menstruating maidens and (b) attitudes towards divine kings or priest-kings in the ancient world. It was almost as if men could be vested with cosmically potent ritual power only if they could be conceptualised as in some sense 'menstruating'. The processes of initiation through which they acquired divine power were remarkably similar to male initiation rituals in other parts of the world, whilst these in turn bore remarkable structural resemblances to the first-menstruation rituals of young women who, in being 'set apart' were thought of as secluded in 'the world beyond', often conceptualised as a place high in the night sky. For such menstruants to be in sunlight or touching 'this earth' was therefore inconceivable, and immense efforts were often made — sometimes including the elevation of young girls (like the heroine in Grimms' *Rapunzel*) into shuttered turrets or seclusion-huts on stilts — to prevent the cosmic disasters which earthly contact would invite.

The Mikado of Japan, Frazer noted, 'profaned his sanctity if he so much as touched the ground with his foot' (1900, 3: 202). Outside his palace he was carried on men's shoulders; within it he walked on exquisitely wrought mats. Neither was the Mikado allowed to expose his sacred person to the open air, 'and the sun was not thought worthy to shine on his head' (p. 203).

The same applied in Mexico to the supreme pontiff of the Zapotecs, who 'was looked upon as a god whom the earth was not worthy to hold, nor the sun to shine upon' (Bancroft 1875, 2: 142, in Frazer 1900, 3: 203). Frazer lists the king and queen of Tahiti and the kings of Dosuma, Persia, Siam and Uganda as further examples of rulers who had to be carried almost everywhere to avoid their touching the ground. His list of future leaders or heirs to the throne barred from the sun includes Indians of Guiana, heirs to the thrones of Bogota and of Sogamoso, and the future Inca of Peru.

'Now it is remarkable', continues Frazer, 'that these two rules — not to touch the ground and not to see the sun — are observed either separately or conjointly by girls at puberty in many parts of the world' (1900, 3: 204). In parts of New Guinea, for example, 'daughters of chiefs, when they are about twelve or thirteen years of age, are kept indoors for two or three years, never being allowed, under any pretence, to descend from the house, and the house is so shaded that the sun cannot shine on them' (Frazer 1900, 3: 210). Among the Ot Danoms of Borneo, a maiden was placed in a cell which 'is raised on piles above the ground, and is lit by a single small window opening on a lonely place, so that the girl is in almost total darkness'. Here she was kept secluded, sometimes for as long as seven years, without being permitted to see anyone but a single slave woman appointed to wait on her (p. 210). Amongst the Nootka Indians of Vancouver Island, girls at puberty were placed in each house in a sort of gallery, where they were prevented from touching the ground or from seeing either fire or the sun's rays. 'The general effect of these rules', notes Frazer after listing a number of similar customs, 'is to keep the girl suspended, so to say, between heaven and earth' (p. 233).

Menstruation and the Sun

Frazer's puzzling cross-cultural findings regarding menstruants and the sun have been amply confirmed. 'In Native North America', writes Powers (1980: 63),

> the two most common proscriptions regarding menstruating women are: (1) that they be secluded, metaphorically, kept out of the sun; and (2) that they not cook for their husbands, that is, that they not go near the fireplace.

These two prohibitions can be regarded as related in that the sun is experienced as fiery, menstrual blood having to be kept rigidly segregated from all 'fire'. Typically, this is less to protect the menstruant than to prevent her excessively potent blood from polluting household fires or even blotting out the sun.

Lévi-Strauss discusses a number of American Indian prohibitions segregating menstruants from sunlight in the final chapter of *The Origin of Table Manners* (1978). According to the Salish of the Cowlitz River, a menstruating girl must not look at the sky. The Tlingit of Alaska enforce the wearing of broad-rimmed hats to prevent girls who have begun to menstruate from looking up at the sky and thus polluting it (Lévi-Strauss 1978: 503). Durkheim (1963: 75) notes of these same pubescent Indians that 'in order to isolate themselves from the sun, they are obliged to blacken their faces'. Throughout the west and north-west of North America, continues Lévi-Strauss (1978: 500), 'a girl menstruating for the first time was not allowed to touch the ground with her feet, nor to look at the sun'. To keep her from the ground, the Carrier Indians conveyed her bodily from point to point. Hoods, mats, baskets, eye-shades and numerous other devices were used among various tribes to prevent such girls from looking at the sun. To Lévi-Strauss' examples we can add that among the Waiwai Indians of southern Guiana, a menstruating girl cannot look at the sky because it would cave in and crush the earth (Fock 1963: 48–53).

In the Old World, rules about keeping away from sunlight apply also in Africa among the !Xõ and other Kalahari San peoples. Taylor (1985: 62) writes of a !Xõ initiant during her first-menstruation ritual:

> During the whole time of her menstruation the girl must not touch the earth, neither must the sun fall on her. She must wear no beads or clothes. Food is brought to her inside the hut where she remains alone for most of the time. . . . No man may see her face, for if he does it is believed that ill luck will befall him.

Here in the Kalahari, such a girl 'is believed to have great supernatural power which can be harnessed for the good of the community if rightly treated' (Taylor 1985: 62). When she has just been scarified following her seclusion and is led out of her hut to become the focus of a joyful ritual dance, she keeps her eyes solemnly downcast. This is

> because in her enhanced state of potency she can affect the game that may be hunted in the coming days. If she keeps her eyes down, so too will the animals when they are hunted; they will not look up and see the hunter as he creeps up on them. (Taylor 1985: 63, citing Lewis-Williams 1981: 51)

Clearly, then, through menstruation a girl in some symbolic sense 'becomes' the hunted game which men hope to be able to kill. There is no doubt that *it is because she is bleeding* that she is identified with *game which should also bleed when successfully hunted*. We are here, of course, approaching from a new angle the 'totemism' discussed in Chapter 3.

Menstruation as Power

The contribution of Durkheim and Frazer was to have developed the concept of menstrual repulsion as a form of power – 'sacred' power in Durkheim's case, and something akin to 'royal' or 'priestly' power in Frazer's.

Neither version would deny that through menstrual taboos, women may be oppressed. In many cultures, menstruating women are subject to forms of exclusion and isolation amounting to severe and sometimes (to Westerners) horrific oppression. But, building on the insights of writers such as Durkheim and Frazer, we can begin to appreciate the extent to which men have sought to isolate and oppress women *because* of their intrinsic and much-feared menstrual powers. 'The monthly seclusion of women', as Robert Lowie (1920: 203) wrote long ago,

> has been accepted as a proof of their degradation in primitive communities, but it is far more likely that the causal sequence is to be reversed and that their exclusion from certain spheres of activity and consequently lesser freedom is the consequence of the awe inspired by the phenomena of periodicity.

Likewise the psychoanalytical interpretation of George Devereux (1950) takes as its themes 'The Menstruating Woman as Witch' and 'The Menstruating Woman as Power', drawing on the arguments of both Freud and Durkheim in insisting that 'the sacred' is also 'dangerous' and vice versa. The oppression of the menstruating woman and her power, writes Devereux (1950: 252), are by no means incompatible; indeed 'the menstruating woman can be defined as both sacred and dangerous, and in a good many ways, as "sacred *because* dangerous", and "dangerous *because* sacred"'. Devereux (1950: 252n) cites a colleague's report of an Italian peasant folk-legend according to which, although the menstruating woman has 'nefarious powers', nevertheless:

at the time of her monthly period, each woman rises a notch in the social hierarchy. The peasant woman becomes a lady, the latter a noblewoman, the noblewoman becomes a queen, while the queen becomes identified with the Madonna. In fact, menstruation specifically proclaims woman's kinship with the Madonna.

Menstruating women, Devereux concludes, 'are set apart from, and, in many ways, set above the rest of mankind'.

There is no need to multiply examples of menstrual taboos or of their recurrent magical and cosmological dimensions. It is clear that a menstruating woman may be forbidden – but she is forbidden not because of her powerlessness or degradation but, on the contrary, precisely because of the peculiar intensity of her assumed magical powers at this time.

Menstruation as Sex Strike

Throughout the traditional world, menstruation – real or pretended – has been used by women as a means of avoiding the obligation to provide sexual services in marriage. This has been the case whether or not the women have chosen to enjoy in the meantime intimacies of a different, infertile, illicit or 'incestuous' kind.

Many early accounts of menstrual taboos depict them as a woman's way of saying 'no!' Women of the Tully River district in Queensland told one ethnographer they were anxious to menstruate regularly, for otherwise 'the men would be enabled to continually pay them sexual attentions, a course to which the women assured me they objected' (Roth, quoted in Briffault 1927, 2: 406). Folk-tales of the Kiwai Papuans (Briffault 1927, 2: 406) represent men as 'enraged owing to their being repulsed by their menstruating wives'. Briffault (1927, 2) gives numerous other examples in his immense compilation, *The Mothers*, remarking that 'there is little indication that any compulsion is needed to force the women to segregate themselves at such times'. And Delaney, Lupton and Toth in *The Curse* (1977: 19) cite further cases, commenting that even today:

> If a woman does not wish to engage in sexual intercourse, her period is her one legitimate way out. . . . Using 'the curse' as an excuse, many a woman has enjoyed a dinner date free from the bothersome knowledge that she herself might be the dessert.

Katharina Dalton (1971: 26) notes in this regard that some women actually develop prolonged menstruation as a way to avoid sex.

Among the Beaver Indians, according to an early report, a menstruating woman 'pretends to be ten days in this state and suffers not her husband except upon particularly good terms. Her paramours, however, are permitted to approach her sooner' (Keith, quoted in Briffault 1927, 2: 404). For a woman to repulse her husband, only to take advantage of his absence by engaging in extra-marital love affairs (Buckley and Gottlieb 1988: 13) does not seem unusual. Citing Radin (1920: 393), Lévi-Strauss (1969a: 21) draws on evidence of this kind to argue that, contrary to Durkheim's claims, 'the horror of blood, especially menstrual blood, is not universal': 'Young Winnebago Indians visit their mistresses and take advantage of the privacy of the prescribed isolation of these women during their menstrual period.'

Similar customs are reported of the Djuka of Dutch Guiana (Kahn 1931: 130), the Warao of Venezuela (Suárez 1968: 2–6), the Kaska of western Canada (Honigmann 1954: 124), the Yolngu of north-east Arnhem Land, Australia (Berndt 1976) and many other peoples.

Many taboos shield menstruating women not only from marital obligations but also from household chores. In association with avoidances of the sun's 'fire', a ban on contact with cooking-fire is often imposed. An African example will illustrate this.

In Central Africa among the Bemba (Richards 1956: 32): 'The most constant danger to the family fire is in fact the touch of the housewife herself, when she is passing through her periods.' It is firmly believed that anyone who ate food cooked on a contaminated fire would become ill. 'It is difficult', writes Richards (1956: 33),

> to exaggerate the strength of these beliefs, or the extent to which they affect daily life. In a village at cooking-time young children are sent here and there to fetch 'new fire' from neighbours who are ritually pure. Women in their periods call their sisters to cook for them.

When a woman's menstrual period is over, the old fire has to be extinguished, whereupon a ritual act of sexual intercourse takes place and a new, ritually clean fire is lit (Richards 1956: 32). It is worth noting that marital intercourse is associated with the renewal of fire, just as – by contrast – menstruation is associated with its negation or pollution.

Anthropologists have usually seen all such mythico-ritual patterns and constraints as additional proof of the extremity of female oppression wherever menstruation is feared. The assumption is that women want marital sex, want to be able to cook for their families, and want to gather or labour in the fields – even during their periods. Given such assumptions, the taboos certainly appear to constitute irksome restrictions. But as Buckley and Gottlieb (1988: 13) point out, all this is a strange way of looking at matters. Taboos prohibiting women from working, cooking, engaging in marital relations and so on 'can as easily be interpreted as boons to women as means of suppressing them'. Often, the taboos may protect women from male attempts to pressurise them into cooking or working in the fields when in fact they have no inclination for this at such a time.

An example of how women can use and enjoy their periods of release from labour comes from the Beng of the Ivory Coast, West Africa, as described by

Alma Gottlieb in *Blood Magic* (Gottlieb 1988: 71–2). In this culture, older men – or, more specifically, men who have eaten meat from animals sacrificed to the Earth – are strictly prohibited from eating food cooked by a menstruating woman. The irony is that such men are known by women to be missing something:

> Women themselves are said to enjoy food cooked during their menstrual periods immensely and for a specific reason: women cook best when they are menstruating. In particular, there is one dish, a sauce made from palm nuts . . . , that is supposed to be most delicious when prepared by a menstruating woman. This is because the sauce gets better and better (i.e., thicker and thicker) as it cooks longer and longer – up to four or five hours for optimum flavor.

Usually a woman does not have the time to cook a sauce for so many hours because she is busy working in the fields:

> While she is menstruating and confined to the village, however, she has the leisure to cook the sauce properly – virtually all day – and she and her friends and close female kin with whom she exchanges food have the exquisite pleasure usually denied to men of eating palm-nut sauce as it was meant to be eaten.

As it cooks for hours, adds Gottlieb, the sauce's colour 'develops into a rich, deep red, not unlike the colour of menstrual blood'. Gottlieb concludes by noting that if Beng culture has *haute cuisine*, 'it is this rich, red, thick palm-nut sauce – a cuisine of menstruation'.

Menstruation as Solidarity

To go 'on strike' implies female power and – if analogies with Marxist concepts of class struggle are to have any force – collectivity at the point of production/reproduction. Nothing could seem further from this than our received image of the menstruating woman isolated in her hut. What possible connection could there be between menstrual taboos and the great collective sex strike which, according to the central hypothesis of this book, inaugurated the human cultural domain?

But the possibility of synchrony places the question of menstrual taboos in a new light. Seclusion need not necessarily mean isolation from other women. We have just seen how Beng women share out their menstrual cuisine among 'friends and close female kin'. Other ethnographic reports show how menstrual blood and its symbolism, far from isolating women, may in fact express their solidarity and kin-based sisterhood. On Mogmog Island in the Pacific atoll of Ulithi, menstrual seclusion is welcomed by women – who 'enjoy this break from their normal labors and spend the time happily talking or weaving' (Patterson 1986: 490). On this island, women's large *ipul* — the 'women's house' — is equipped with looms and serves as a community centre for women with their children (Buckley and Gottlieb 1988: 12, citing photograph by David Hiser in Patterson 1986: 490–1). Much other evidence supports the view that similar patterns may once have been widespread.

The Mbuti *Elima* Ceremony

The Mbuti people of the Ituri Forest, Zaire, are basically hunter-gatherers, though they live in a symbiotic relationship with neighbouring cultivators. Whereas their village-dwelling neighbours see menstruation as a defiling calamity, the Mbuti celebrate it positively. The onset of a girl's first flow is marked by a joyful ritual known as the *elima*, this word denoting in the first instance a large hut in which one or more pubescent girls are joined by female relatives for a period of singing and celebration. During this, the girls are taught to be proud of their bodies both sexually and in terms of reproductive potential (Turnbull 1976: 167–81).

The *elima* forges strong bonds of solidarity between girls who together 'have seen the blood'; it simultaneously achieves 'at least a temporary obliteration of the bonds of the nuclear family' (Turnbull 1966: 136).

A girl who has begun to menstruate for the first time is said to be 'blessed by the moon' and becomes the focus of rejoicing as everyone is told the good news: 'The girl enters seclusion, but not the seclusion of the village girl. She takes with her all her young friends, those who have not yet reached maturity, and some older ones.' They enter a single communal 'women's house' (the *elima*) where the girls celebrate the happy event collectively.

During the ethnographer Colin Turnbull's fieldwork visit, two young women experienced their first menstruation at the same time, and entered the house together, along with their female friends. Turnbull's (1976: 169) description is enough to refute the view that such 'seclusion' must always and everywhere be a degrading experience:

> Together they are taught the arts and crafts of motherhood by an old and respected relative. They learn not only how to live like adults, but how to sing the songs of adult women. Day after day, night after night, the *elima* house resounds with the throaty contralto of the older women and the high, piping voices of the youngest.

It is a time of gladness, Turnbull continues, not for the women alone but for the whole community. People from all around come to pay their respects,

> the young men standing or sitting about outside the *elima* house in the hopes of a glimpse of the young beauties inside. And there are special *elima* songs which they sing to each other, the girls singing a light, cascading melody in intricate harmony, the men replying with a rich,

vital chorus. For the pygmies the *elima* is one of the happiest, most joyful occasions in their lives.

An aspect of the celebrations is that the girls in the hut have the right to rush out from time to time and chase after the young men. Should a boy or man be caught, he has to enter the hut, whereupon he is teased and is under some pressure to give sexual satisfaction to the girls inside (Turnbull 1976: 171). Clearly, then, this is a very simple form of 'initiation ritual' – a time during which young people of both sexes are made tangibly aware not only of the obligations but also of the rewards of adult sexual life.

Like so many other manifestations of menstrual potency in Africa, the *elima* can influence hunting-luck. Sometimes, during the *elima* there is an injunction against eating meat; 'this seems to be when the *elima* activities are affecting the hunt and the supply of game'. When game is killed, this is seen as a 'gift from the forest', a gift which may be withheld should the forest be displeased. The *elima* is said to 'rejoice the forest', and to make it happy and glad (Turnbull 1966: 134, 161).

Admittedly, this and comparable patterns are nowadays rare. Yet theoretically – in terms of cultural origins and evolution – they surely have as much potential significance as the more oppressive patterns, which need not be regarded as 'basic' or 'original' from an evolutionary standpoint. Other examples of positive or empowering seclusion could be cited, and writing of seclusion in general, Buckley and Gottlieb (1988: 13) decline to rule out the possibility that in many societies at least, 'women themselves may have been responsible for originating this custom. . .'. This was certainly Briffault's (1927) view.

Hunting and 'Ceremonial Chastity'

This book has outlined a model in which women go periodically on an extended sex strike in order to motivate men to hunt. The model stipulates that before and during the hunt, marital intercourse should be ruled out lest it undermine the entire system, threatening in particular the success of the hunt.

It is tempting to relate this aspect of the model to the otherwise inexplicable fact that in many parts of the world, 'ceremonial chastity' is experienced as an indispensable condition of hunting success, while a hunter's contact with a *menstruating* woman is thought of as the gravest possible threat to the chase (Kitahara 1982; Dobkin de Rios and Hayden 1985; Kelly 1986).

Like mother-in-law avoidances, totemic avoidances and menstrual taboos, pre-hunt sex bans are or were sufficiently recurrent features of traditional cultures to have been exhaustively commented upon by early anthropological theorists. For example, Crawley (1927, 1: 65–6) noted the frequency with which men about to go hunting seek to enhance their luck by observing strict taboos, the most constant of which 'prohibits every kind of intercourse with the female sex'. Frazer (1926–36, 2: 191–8) made essentially the same point. Hammond and Jablow (1975: 7), in a more recent cross-cultural survey of traditional women's roles, have confirmed such findings. Virtually throughout the world – and particularly where hunting is a collective activity – hunters keep away from women and all things sexual both prior to and during the hunt. People in western cultures are of course familiar with equivalents: for example, the widespread taboo which prevents a boxer from having sex on the night before a big fight!

Anthropologists have usually interpreted such observations from a male standpoint, accepting native male ideological statements to the effect that women are simply harmful to hunting. But the previous arguments of this book would lead us to suspect that women themselves may have played just as vital a role in setting themselves apart.

In the light of the sex-strike model, women's segregation from direct physical involvement in hunting seems predictable. How could women have maintained the integrity of their strike had they allowed some females to join in long-distance hunting expeditions alongside men? In view of the risks of seduction or rape, it is easy to see how the logic of strike action would have ensured that it was not just some women – for example, those with particularly heavy child-care burdens – who were forced to stay behind, but in principle all women, regardless of their situation or hunting capabilities. The result would have been the 'ideological' exclusion of women from hunting – the exclusion of women simply *because* they were women.

Other considerations – for example the need for women to help as beaters in a communal game-drive – may in practice have led to some relaxation of such rules. But it is noteworthy that here, too, the model fits. In communal game-drives it is not just some women who join the men while others stay at home. The tendency is for the whole community to go hunting, with children also involved. Moreover, segregation is still maintained, with men performing certain tasks – above all, those of actual bloodshed – while women and children perform others. Marital sex during the preparations is never encouraged, despite the sexual excitement and anticipation always associated with a hunt.

In Africa, the Lele of the Kasai (Douglas 1963: 207) will undertake no hunting expedition 'without one night of continence being imposed first on the whole village'. Those directly concerned with the hunt, such as the makers of pit traps, may have to abstain from sex for several months. In Zambia, among the matrilineal Bisa, an informant explains:

We don't have sexual intercourse before a hunt because when we are hunting we are helped by the spirits of dead hunters. These spirits. . . .

have no sexual intercourse. When we have sexual intercourse before a hunt, we get out of tune with the spirits who will help us in the bush. (Marks 1976: 114–15)

An elephant hunt among the Bisa may last for weeks or even months, during which time the hunters' wives, remaining in the village, have to maintain 'behaviour beyond reproach' to ensure success.

Among the Central African Tumbuka, when hunters set off to kill an elephant, after all preparations had been made and sacrifices had been offered to the spirits of the dead,

> The chief hunter charged the villagers who remained that there must be no quarrelling or immorality indulged in within the village. None were to leave their homes to visit other places, but all were to remain quiet and law-abiding lest the game disappear, or turn in anger and rend the hunters. (D. Fraser, quoted in Frazer 1936: 21)

In the case of the Wachamba (also Central Africa), while a hunter was away in the forest his wife at home was bound to observe all the magical restrictions which were incumbent also upon him. She remained alone for weeks. She was forbidden to receive visits from men in her hut. Only her closest relations could feed with her. If she did not observe these restrictions, it was believed that her husband would fall ill or perish in the forest (Frazer 1936: 23). Among the Banyankole,

> when a man was out hunting, his wife refrained from sexual intercourse with other men. . . . She might let no man pass behind her back, but warned him to keep in front of her. Should she neglect any of these precautions, her husband's chances of obtaining game in the hunt would be ruined. (J. Roscoe, quoted in Frazer 1936: 20)

Junod (1927, 2: 62) makes a similar point about the Thonga of Mozambique: 'Old Makhani assured me that incontinence on the part of the wife at home would have as a consequence that the husband would be attacked and killed by wild beasts far away in the desert. . . .'

Such evidence leads us to suppose that evolving early women would not have regarded themselves as in any simple sense harmful to hunting. Sharanahua Indian women regard the periodic 'special hunt' as their own, since it is they who initiate this event and to an extent control it (Siskind 1973a, 1973b; see Chapter 4). In a comparable way virtually throughout the world, women have believed in their sexually controlled influence on the hunt even when distant from the scene.

Ceremonial Chastity and the Menstrual Dimension

An entertaining illustration of the logic we have been discussing – and one which will also serve to introduce the connection with menstrual taboos – is

Nigel Barley's (1986: 110–18) description of a disastrous hunting expedition among the Dowayos, a tribe in the Cameroons, West Africa. In Barley's village, there was one old man who was regarded as a 'true hunter' in possession of the necessary magic. One day, he resolved to direct a new hunt and to co-ordinate the activities of the men:

> The most important thing was that no man should have intercourse with a woman for three days. All agreed to this. The hunter gave them a lecture on the importance of this consideration.

The great fear was that if sex were allowed at such a time, men would quickly lapse into seducing one another's wives, communicating a fatal 'smell' of adultery to each and every hunter:

> A man so infected would be incapable of the simplest shot. His hand would shake, his eyes cloud over. His arrow would miss its mark. Worst of all, dangerous beasts of the bush would home in on him. He would be stalked by leopards and scorpions, and risked an awful death. They would smell him from miles away. He would thus be a menace to everyone.

Among these Dowayos, the chastity rule was difficult to maintain. On the one hand, young men were considered unreliable, while there was little confidence that women of any age category could be counted on to uphold the rule. The older men felt far from secure about their wives' fidelity at the best of times, and suspected that younger, more virile rivals would seize the opportunity presented by the sex ban to cheat, seducing their ever-willing wives in the three days prior to the hunt. To guard against this, some men 'went as far as accompanying their wives down to the water-hole and back. . .' (Barley 1986: 111–12).

All this would be predicted by the model. 'Ceremonial chastity' is not an aspect or derivative form of the sex strike. In the model's terms, it *is* the sex strike.

Even more interestingly – as so often in cultures which practise hunting – among the Dowayos the major terror is of the damage to a man's hunting gear that contact with a *menstruating* woman will cause.

The Dowayos say that hunters' bows can cause women to bleed even if they are merely in the approximate vicinity and even if the women are pregnant. Bows make women miscarry. Such is the fear of the consequent blood contamination that hunters avoid the village's main paths and skulk around on long detours. Should a man meet a woman, he immediately lays his bow down, pointing away from her, and will not speak to her until this has been done.

But the most dangerous women are those who are already menstruating:

Their effluvium is held to 'spoil' the bow and make it useless. The link in Dowayo thought seems to lie in the similarity of the different types of bleeding in each case, hunting or menstruation. *They are sufficiently similar to need to be kept rigorously apart.* (Barley 1986: 112; my emphasis)

For this reason, as part of the pre-hunt ritual of ceremonial chastity which Barley (1986: 112) observed, the men withdrew their weapons from their huts altogether – and hid them well away from the village compound out in the bush.

Notwithstanding such precautions, this particular hunt turned out to be a disaster. After it was over, the men despondently discussed the conclusions to be drawn. 'Everyone was agreed', writes Barley (1986: 118), 'that the hunt had failed owing to the unbridled sexual self-indulgence of almost everyone else'.

In terms of this book's basic argument, we might say that despite the Dowayo hunt-leader's worthy efforts, this had evidently been a 'sex strike' which neither the women nor the men had had sufficient commitment to help one another enforce!

One further example from another culture will help clarify the picture. The Arapesh of Papua New Guinea, according to a classic ethnography (Mead 1941: 421), observe similarly strict taboos:

> A menstruating woman must guard the village from her blood; she must guard her husband, his food or possessions, from any close contact with it, and she must guard herself from her own dangerous state. Consequently, she may not enter a house on the ceremonial level, nor cross the village, nor walk on a good road.

Despite all this, men do actually stay in the same village as their wives even when menstrual blood is flowing. This makes them extremely anxious – and above all worried about the likely effects on their hunting luck. Men explain:

> if we can find game, if we can find pigs in traps and in the rain, if cassowaries fall into our deadfalls, if our dogs catch phalangers, if the yams which we plant stay in the garden and fill the house to the ridge pole, then we say 'This is all right'. But if our yams fail, if our hunting fails, then we go and rid ourselves of the coldness of this woman, we purify ourselves with bark and leaves in the bush, and set the woman afar off, we speak of her as a sister or a mother.

'When it is time to sleep', the same informant continues, 'the woman sleeps in one house and the man in another'. If need be, an Arapesh hunter is prepared to go on treating his wife as a 'sister or mother', the two sleeping in separate houses, for a year or more continuously – until his hunting luck begins to improve (Mead 1941: 421).

Hunting, Menstrual Odours and Game

Writing of North American Indians generally, Driver and Massey (1957: 255) note that the taboos surrounding hunting (see Chapter 3) have never been catalogued or classified. 'One of the most widespread beliefs', however, 'is that menstruating women are offensive to game animals'. In particular, a hunter must take care that his wife 'does not touch any of his hunting gear or drip any menstrual fluid on the meat of previously slain game'.

Taboos of such kinds have long seemed to defy rational explanation. In a variation on the 'menotoxins' theme, a recent tendency has been to link the beliefs with supposedly genuine chemical/biological effects of spilled blood. It is argued that some animals, such as bears, tend to attack women when they can smell their menstrual odours, while these same smells really do frighten more timorous prey animals away (March 1980; Kitahara 1982; Dobkin de Rios and Hayden 1985).

It is probably true that dogs and other carnivores are attracted by menstrual odours, as by other forms of blood. And it has certainly been shown that white-tailed deer show avoidance responses to menstrual blood (March 1980), as well as to blood from men's veins (Nunley 1981). In this context, Kitahara (1982) has argued that menstrual or other blood-taboos may be explained by the fact that 'to a hunting people, it is most important that they can come near game animals without being noticed by them . . .'

Kitahara demonstrates that hunting peoples do indeed tend to have the most stringent menstrual taboos – an important finding in terms of the argument of this book. However, as has been pointed out (Kelly 1986), the theory hardly explains why particularly rigid taboos should apply in north west America to Nootka salmon fishers, Tareumit whale-hunters or Tlingit seal-hunters – marine prey should be in no way affected by female smells.

There are other anomalies. In north-western California, when men returned from hunting, their meat was always taken into the house by removing a wall board instead of through the normal entrance 'for fear that a menstruating woman had dripped fluid in the entrance way'. Expressive of comparable fears was a rule prohibiting menstruating women from eating meat, 'particularly fresh meat' (Driver and Massey 1957: 255). 'Fresh meat', in this context, presumably meant meat with the blood still visible within it. Here, the symbolic connections linking menstrual with animal blood seem evident enough. But references to prey animals' responses to odours do little to explain such ideas. There should surely be no anxiety lest dead meat should flee from menstrual smells.

The odour theorists make no mention of the moon. In view of recent understandings of what constitutes hard science, this may seem unremarkable. In social anthropological terms, however, it is surely a drawback if the paradigm leads us to ignore many of those details of the relevant rituals and mythologies which native informants most strongly emphasise.

Let us turn to the Eastern Chewong, a small Malay group who practice matrilocal residence and live by hunting, gathering and slash-and-burn tapioca cultivation. Here, there is a taboo against giving birth either at full or dark moon; a woman who gave birth at such times, it is said, 'would suffer heavy bleeding'. Numerous work activities are likewise forbidden at full and dark moon, for fear of making the moon itself 'sick', whereupon nothing would grow (Howell 1984: 198–9). The most common colloquial expression for menstruation is 'I don't want meat'; other terms for the condition are 'moon children' and 'moon blood'. The injunction against eating meat is justified on the grounds that 'blood may not be mixed with blood' (Howell 1984: 194). Strict rules compelling returning hunters to give away and share their meat are linked conceptually with gynaecological rules governing the separation of the mother from her baby and separation of the baby from its placenta; in each instance, an act of 'cutting flesh' is involved, with all the dangers inherent in such shedding of blood. The basic rule – in an echo of the 'totemic' logic discussed in Chapter 3 – is that just as a woman should separate herself carefully from her own baby, so a man should separate himself from his kills (Howell 1984: 69–71; 77).

The Chewong case is not unusual. Menstrual blood is in virtually all mythologies associated with (a) the moon and (b) blood from a wound. In hunting symbolism, wounds and bleeding vaginas are frequently juxtaposed, and the one form of blood may be thought to promote the flowing of the other. As we saw earlier, a Kalahari San hunter's association with a first-menstruant may not only fail to damage his hunting luck – treated ritually in the correct way, the blood may actually enhance his luck. Roy Wagner (1972: 69) presents a further example in a report on the Daribi of Papua New Guinea:

> On one occasion Kagoiano had a particularly 'good' hunting dream, in which he was trying to have intercourse with a woman, but stopped when he saw that her genitals were bloody, realising that she was in her period. He explained that 'the blood in the dream is the blood that a man sees on his arrow when he has shot a pig'. Asked whether the penis in the dream is the same as the arrow, he replied that it was.

This belief in the positive import of a menstrual dream fits ill with the theory that hunters avoid menstruants simply because the blood frightens away the game.

A comparable problem is posed by the 'Mistress of Game Animals' – a construct virtually universal in one form or another in the Americas and beyond, although the gender of this personage is variable. The Hopi Indians tell of 'The Bloody Maiden Who Looks After the Animals'. This terrifying mythological woman, having slain a number of hunters who had angered her, appears before the people, 'her face and clothes covered with blood'. Seizing a live antelope, she wiped her hand first over her own genitalia and then over the antelope's face, and let it go after twisting its nose. She then turned to the people who had gathered outside and said, 'After this, you shall have great difficulty in hunting these animals'. (Simmons 1942: 426–8)

By wiping her hand over her own genitals and then over the very nose of the antelope, this blood-stained heroine would seem to be flying in the face of all men's efforts, confirming their worst fears, deliberately causing the game to flee from menstrual odour – and asserting that Womankind's blood in some magical way 'protects' the game itself. In myths of this kind, something more complex than biological reactions to smells is surely involved. An important element seems to be the idea that menstrual blood has a supernatural connection of some kind with hunting blood. It is this supernatural belief which we must attempt to explain.

Alain Testart – the Ideology of Blood

Although menstrual taboos may not be universal, they are so widespread as to suggest their immense antiquity. Their prevalence struck early theorists such as Crawley, Durkheim and Frazer so forcibly that they overcame what must have been very strong Victorian reticences on the subject. 'Blood', as Richards (1956: 19) puts it,

> appears to be the object of a set of emotionally tinged ideas in all human societies. It stands for death, murder, life-giving force or kinship. Menstrual blood with its mysterious periodicity is considered especially terrifying and disturbing, to judge from what we know of primitive ritual.

Developing this idea, my French colleague in Marxist anthropology, Alain Testart (1986), has recently gone so far as to suggest that an 'ideology of blood' can be discerned at the root of all human symbolic-cultural traditions, his view being that humanity's most ancient ideology for some reason originally counterposed two forms of blood – menstrual blood on the one hand, the blood of the hunt on the other. These opposites were felt to attract one another, but the basic, primordial cultural rule was to prevent this – the two blood-forms should never be allowed to mix.

Testart specifies nothing concerning menstruation's cultural-symbolic links with the moon. He makes no claim that his 'ideology of blood' corresponds to a cosmology. His concern is to explain why it is that women are so frequently excluded from shedding blood in hunting. He rejects all appeals to child-care burdens, female body odours or lesser mobility in explaining this, since the rules apply to all women regardless of strength or condition. Neither, he argues, can we explain the sex division of labour by reference to the biological fact that women menstruate. It is only cultural ideology which makes menstrual blood significant in this way (Testart 1986: 87).

The 'ideology of blood', Testart continues, does not in itself imply female inferiority. It becomes a sign of inferiority only when women are in practice socially inferior. In such cases, it functions ideologically to justify keeping women in subordination. But there is no reason to suppose that this is inherent in the nature of things, or inherent in the original ideology. What is universal is only the idea that menstrual blood is *dangerous*, and for that reason, a source of ritual power. Given this ideologically constructed potency, it then becomes possible for either sex to take advantage of it. In certain cases – for example, some northern Australian Aboriginal societies – it is men who monopolise surrogate 'menstrual' power. But other societies are known in which women are felt to be ritually powerful on account of their blood (Testart 1986: 89).

According to the basic ideology, continues Testart, women are not ritually dangerous except in relation to their blood. When avoidance rules affect only menstruating women, we can speak of menstrual taboos. When they affect all women – including menstruants – a consequence is the sexual division of labour. In deciding whether or not women can perform a given role, it is the utilisation of weapons which constitutes the decisive criterion. Whatever else women may be allowed, they cannot be permitted to shed blood (figure 15). Testart lists numerous societies, particularly from the more northerly latitudes, in which it is believed that hunters lose all their luck when they allow a menstruant to come into even the slightest possibility of contact with their hunting gear. Once washed with menstrual blood, hunting implements can never again shed blood of any other kind.

However – insists Testart – to say that women are forbidden to approach men's hunting implements implies discrimination against females. Yet this is only one way of expressing matters. As far as the effects are concerned, it is precisely the same as saying that hunters must keep their weapons well away from menstruating women. This could be conceptualised as protection for women in a vulnerable state. Certainly, it is not the women themselves who are thought to be supernaturally damaged by the contact. The sanction of bad hunting-luck appears in the first instance to affect men, although a failed hunt would of course hit the community as a whole (Testart 1986: 34–7).

In a hunting and gathering society, Testart concludes (1986: 34–42), both sexes regularly come into contact with blood. For a woman, this is her own menstrual blood. For a man, it is the blood he sheds in hunting. Both forms are dangerous – each as much as the other. They must be separated, because ideology fears the unlimited, disorderly flowing out of blood. Thus, one of the most common prohibitions applying to menstruating women is a rule forbidding the eating of meat or the touching of red meat: it is clear (writes Testart) that this food taboo separates the two bloods as surely as does the weapons taboo.

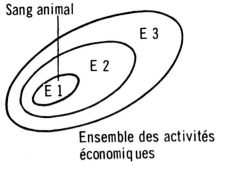

Sang animal

Ensemble des activités
économiques

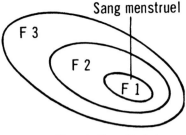

Sang menstruel

Population féminine

Figure 15   The ideology of blood. The set of possible economic activities is trisected, as is the total female population. The figure shows (left) hunting involving bloodshed (E1), subsumed within the wider set of hunting activities generally (E2), subsumed within the set of all economically productive activities (E3). Correspondingly the trisection yields (right) women whilst menstruating (F1), subsumed within the wider set of adult fertile women generally (F2), subsumed within the set of all women, regardless of age or condition (F3). The basic rule is to keep animals' blood and women's blood apart. To achieve this it would suffice, minimally, to exclude just F1 women from just E1 activities. But segregation can be achieved more drastically and with less scope for error by separating any F set up to the widest from any E set. Exclusion of F3 from E2 yields the sexual division of labour. Exclusion of F3 from E1 corresponds to more specific taboos segregating women from contact with spears or other blood-drawing weapons. Exclusion of F1 from E3 would describe women's complete inactivity and seclusion in the bush during their periods. A range of previously unrelated taboos are in this way revealed as variations on a theme (after Testart 1986: Fig. 2).

The Ideology of Blood – a Materialist Explanation

Testart's dismissal of biological and sociobiological findings and his insistence on the independent structure-imparting power of 'ideology' render his fascinating arguments ultimately disappointing. To explain specific, localised ideological constructs by reference to more universal constructs may help us in discerning patterns, but it is not in the final analysis an explanation. If hunter-gatherers perpetuate an ideology of blood, we need to know where this ideology comes from, and why it takes the specific forms that it does.

It is also not clear that Testart has in fact defined his ideology quite accurately. Whilst it is true that menstrual blood and blood from the hunt are often counterposed and kept separate, they are also conceptually confused and combined. Indeed, it could be argued that the taboos depend upon a deeper-level identification of the two kinds of blood.

Suppose that a man were killing a game animal with a menstruating woman in the vicinity. If the hunter for ideological reasons felt obliged to keep her at a distance, it would surely be in part because he perceived a connection. In some way, the danger would be that her blood would manifest itself in the blood of his victim, being in a deep sense 'the same'. The wounded and bleeding game animal would then be 'menstruating'.

We saw this earlier with the 'lucky' dream of the Daribi hunter, who believed he would soon wound a pig with his spear since he had already dreamed of encountering and then avoiding the vagina of a menstruating woman (Wagner 1972: 69). The connection can be illustrated with another ethnographic example, taken this time from David McKnight's (1975: 85–6) description of life among the Wik-Mungkan Aborigines of Cape York Peninsula in Queensland. Here, meat food becomes prohibited from the moment it displays the slightest suggestion of contact or affinity with menstrual blood:

> Any act suggestive of menstrual bleeding makes things *ngaintja* [sacred/ taboo]. Thus if blood from an animal falls on a woman's lap, her father and many other male relatives may not eat it. If a young man carries meat on his back or shoulders . . . so that the blood runs down between his buttocks this, to the Wik-Mungkan, is too uncomfortably like menstrual blood to be ignored.

It is not surprising, then, to learn that when men, having killed a game animal, begin to cut up the flesh,

> they make certain that women, especially their daughters, stand well away. Men will not even take fish from a daughter if she has caught it with a fishing line and pulled the line so that it falls on her lap. If a daughter should accidentally sit on her father's possessions then they are *ngaintja* to him . . . I might add that blood from wounds is also con- sidered to be *ngaintja*, though not to the same degree as menstrual blood.

The direct symbolic identification of menstrual blood with the blood of raw meat is also illustrated by this example from Bernard Arcand's (1978: 3–4) description of the Cuiva Indians of the eastern plains of Columbia:

> Women, fish, and raw meat from all animals share the characteristic of being *asuntané*. This refers to a specific smell and feel: it is a quality attached to the gluey stuff on the back of fish, to animal blood, and to menstrual blood. Women are said to be especially *asuntané* at puberty, when menstruating, and immediately after giving birth. Contact with women during these periods is considered dangerous for men, since it would result in *awapa*, an illness which makes one vomit all one's food. Fear of the same illness is also the explanation Cuiva give as to why men are always quick and careful to wash any animal blood from themselves and why hunters usually leave the preparation of raw meat to women.

Here, then, men seem to actively encourage women's contact with raw and bloody meat, on the grounds that women alone – always in contact with the bloody source of *awapa* – are less in danger of this illness.

The paradoxes are resolved if we adopt a different starting point from Testart's, and take it that women in the first instance assert their periodic menstrual inviolability not for ideological reasons but in order to extract meat from men. We can then see that to indicate non-availability in a language of blood would have been powerfully in women's own interests. It would have been in women's interests not to keep blood separate from blood, but to weave myths asserting that women's and animals' blood-flows attract one another and must conjoin since they stem from the same source.

It will be remembered from previous chapters that in the course of establishing culture, women would have been faced with two closely interrelated problems. One would have been to separate themselves from male company from time to time, inhibiting sexual advances so as to concentrate the minds of the opposite sex on the challenges of hunting. The other would have been to ensure that hunter-males did not cheat them by eating what they had killed out in the bush.

By selecting blood as the basic zero-symbol or indicator of 'taboo', the two problems could have been simultaneously solved. Success would have been achieved to the extent that blood could be equated with blood – that is, to the extent that animal blood could have been perceptually merged or confused with menstrual blood. 'The bleeding feminine condition' writes De Heusch (1982: 168) in his analysis of Bantu myths in Central Africa, 'makes of the patient a wounded game animal'. Lévi-Strauss (1981: 239) at one point in his *Mythologiques* notes the existence of a whole class of North American myths which teach that 'the application of *raw bleeding meat* causes the occurrence of female periods'. Many of these myths confront men with the terrors of being mauled by a savage bear or other carnivore – should a menstruating woman's anger be aroused. We are dealing with variations on a theme.

'The Origin of the Moon's Spots'

Our previous arguments have led us to the finding that earliest fully cultural women could collectively inhibit male sexual advances, signal 'no!' by synchronously bleeding – and use the moon to schedule synchrony-enhancing rituals such as dancing. We have also concluded that men in their periodic hunting exertions were for various reasons able to fit in with this rhythm (Chapter 10). To understand the constraints responsible for the patterns examined in this chapter, we simply have to follow this logic through.

Persistent sexual 'cheating' on the part of females would have been risky because it would have meant getting out of phase, and because menstrual bleeding is not easy to hide. Male cheating would have been detectable in similar ways. Sexual contact with a menstruant can leave a visible mark. Males who cheated by engaging in sex at the wrong time would therefore have risked discovery and exposure. They would have been stained by blood, and to avoid detection would have had to find some way of washing off the blood or otherwise removing it before being seen in public. In practice, in reality, the risks may have been small and the possible solutions numerous. Any man who really wanted to avoid detection ought to have been able to achieve this. But men who wanted to be 'above all suspicion' or who wished to be rid of all guilt or anxiety may have elected to avoid the moral danger with scrupulous rigour. This may have involved strict observances with regard to the dangers of blood contact.

Almost universally, the Indians of North and South America seem to have been aware of some such logic. An extremely widespread myth tells of a man who made love to his sister night after night, visiting her in the dark without letting her know who he was. One day, she decided to smear his face with a dark staining fluid – in some versions, black genipa juice, in others, her own menstrual blood – during the love-making. The next day, the man was seen with his face all stained, and his angry sister was thereby enabled to expose him to the whole community. His crime was written on his face. With help from his mother, the man then escaped into the sky, revealing himself at last as Moon. This celestial being still has spots on his face – spots of dark paint or of menstrual blood (Dorsey 1903: 220) – which tell the whole world of his crime.

The Sharanahua Indian women – who paint their faces with black genipa juice or with red achiote when challenging their menfolk to go on a 'special hunt' (Siskind 1973b: 33, 96, 101, 119) – know this particular story and use it as a basic means of transmitting culture's rules to each new generation (Siskind 1973b: 57). The Peruvian Sharanahua version treats the prototypical man who violates his community's rules as a rapist who is exposed by the indelible 'paint' left on his skin by his victim. Following the incident in which Moon is exposed by his sister, he forces his attentions on many women in succession, so that they all begin to bleed, followed soon afterwards by the synchronised menstruation of the entire community:

> Moon made love to all the women. 'Ari!' they screamed. 'Why does my vagina bleed?'
> Then Moon asked his mother for a black ball and a white ball of thread, which she threw from the house. Then Moon went up the thread to the sky, and all his people watched, and they said, 'My child, my child goes playing to the sky'.
> Then many women, three days after he came, bled. One woman after another, all of them. (Siskind 1973b: 47–9)

This story is thought to be so powerful that women will menstruate merely on hearing it – which explains why under-aged girls are told to cover their ears with their hands during the telling of the final episode (Siskind 1973b: 57).

This story cannot be dismissed as 'mere mythology'. It is sufficiently widespread and invariant to be clearly very ancient. As Josephine Flood

(1983) points out in an Australian context, archaeological information is contained in this kind of evidence no less than in stones, bones, or other more 'material' things. As it happens, this particular tale is unusually valuable because it is representative of what Lévi-Strauss terms a 'vast group' of similar stories which appear in virtually identical forms 'from the extreme north to the extreme south of the New World'. As he mentions this distribution pattern, Lévi-Strauss (1981: 218–19) informs the reader of 'a fact of supreme importance' – that all the myths of the Americas are logically derivable from this one simple tale. 'We might even say', he writes, 'that it constitutes the most plausible initial state for the whole series of transformations. . .', firstly because of its widespread distribution, secondly because it is not the kind of story which can vary to any great extent. In other words, if a single story had to be chosen as the starting point from which all the interlinked myths of the Americas have been derived, this would be a very strong candidate for selection.

There is no need to follow Lévi-Strauss' detailed arguments here, or to try to decide between various possible 'original' myths. The model we are using implies that the interlinked myths of the Americas are similar because they all derive from the same lunar-scheduled 'initial situation', not because certain ancestral myths produced more mythological offspring (in the form of local variants) than did other myths.

Let us take it simply that this particular story could not have survived if men did not understand its basic message – namely that a man risks being suspected of sexual-political 'cheating' if he is blood-stained following sex. This poses a problem. Hunting and butchery are both practices which involve contact with blood. There would be a potential risk of confusion here. A blood-marked hunter might be suspected of having touched or molested a menstruating woman. In any event, morally sensitive hunters might be anxious to avoid even the remotest possibility of such suspicion. Their anxieties would stem not from any conceptual distinction between the two forms of blood but, on the contrary, from an inherent risk of their being confused. To avoid the serious charges levelled at the mythological Moon, then, blood-stained hunters would need to remove such staining from their bodies before returning to female company.

The Ideology of Blood

We are now arriving at the heart of the 'ideology of blood'. It arises out of a dialectical relationship of opposition and polarity between the sexes. On the one hand, women needed to identify their own menstrual blood with the blood of the hunt. They needed to convince men that a violated menstruant would avenge her violator – damaging his hunting luck, perhaps even to the extent of causing him to be killed by an animal during the hunt. Anything which stressed the identity between menstrual blood and hunting blood would have helped in this endeavour, and such symbolic links would quickly have turned into stories about women 'turning into' monstrous spirits or avenging beasts. On the other hand, blood-covered hunters – men who had killed an animal but had not committed rape or any menstrual misdemeanour at all – would have wanted to avoid being misunderstood. Anxious to draw a distinction between one kind of blood and the other, they would have been prompted to deny or at least minimise women's mythological claims.

Let us take women's needs first. For them, what was important was to establish that blood was simply blood. That is, it made no difference where the blood came from: it was conceptually all the same. The blood of murder, the blood of the hunt, the blood of menstruation or of childbirth: it was all in the final analysis just blood. We can speculate on the intellectual processes involved in making this identification. We can describe it as metaphor, perhaps, or as analogy. What is important is that once the confusion or merging had been accomplished an extraordinary result would have been achieved. If the preceding arguments in connection with menstruation are accepted, then no substance could have been equated with menstrual blood without the most potent of consequences in evoking 'respect' or in conveying 'power'.

Once the blood of the hunt had been likened to menstrual blood, a symbolic breakthrough would have been made. At a stroke, women would have achieved a radical simplification of some of life's most pressing problems. No more could men feel at ease about eating an animal raw, out in the bush – even if no one were looking. Each time a group of men killed an animal, its flesh would have seemed to them to 'menstruate'. The men would have *had* to take it home in order to get the flesh cooked, the visible blood removed, and the meat thereby rendered safe to eat. In other words, the same blood symbol through which women temporarily separated themselves from men would have functioned on an economic level as well, temporarily separating game animals from their potential consumers. The equation of blood with blood would have extended women's blood-symbolised sex strike to the world of consumption generally, so that whilst blood of any kind was flowing, abstinence had to be observed not only with regard to sex but with regard to meat-eating, too.

On the other hand, men's interests would have been somewhat different. They may often have needed to claim that hunting blood had nothing whatsoever to do with menstrual blood, being an entirely distinct substance. To have blood on one's hands – men would have needed to establish – does not necessarily make one a murderer or rapist. The blood could be that of a game animal. For men far away from female company, out in the bush or out hunting, there may have been few anxieties on this score – companions would 'know' that any bloodstains must have been acquired in the course of hunting. However, the nearer men came to women, the greater would have been the risk of false accusations or of genuine confusion between the two kinds of blood, and the greater the need to stress the distinction between them.

The strength of this model is that it explains the ethnographic details. It explains not only why men going away to hunt prepare themselves through 'ceremonial chastity' conceptualised particularly as the avoidance of all contact with menstrual blood. It also explains why, on their return, hunters still fear contact between the blood in their meat and menstrual blood. Men who are carrying home bloody chunks of meat will not want this blood to be confused with menstrual blood, and so will do all possible to keep the two kinds of blood apart.

Men could try to avert suspicion by washing themselves or 'sweating' so as to remove all female blood before coming into contact with game animals, and then all bloodstains from the hunt before coming back into contact with women again (we will see in a moment how this may help explain certain details of the Amerindian sweat-lodge tradition). They could attempt it by refusing to approach women for some time, leaving their kills at some point on the periphery of the base-camp area, and insisting that their womenfolk collect the meat. They could do it by insisting that those women who did collect or consume the meat could guarantee that they would not be menstruating at the time (Kelly 1986). And they could do it by refusing any further contact with raw flesh until it had been thoroughly cooked, so that all visible blood within the flesh had been removed.

We would not expect any of this to be directly relevant to hunters' taboos and cooking rules as these have been described in the contemporary ethnographic record. Too much time has elapsed and too many changes will have occurred since the early Upper Palaeolithic. Nonetheless, if such changes as have occurred have always been variations on a theme, the model ought to generate a conceptual structure which illuminates the ethnographic details that have been recorded.

The Amerindian Sweat-lodge Tradition

The Yurok Indians of north-western California, close to the Klamath River, were just one of the very many American Indian groups sharing the institution of the 'sweat-lodge'. In preparation for all important undertakings, Yurok men went into their specially heated lodges to sweat and to train spiritually for ten days – precisely the period of time that women stayed in menstrual seclusion. Elderly Yurok men told the anthropologist Tim Buckley (1988: 204) that men always did this 'during the dark of the moon', which is when women in Buckley's view were probably menstruating. As noted earlier (Chapter 10), women among the Yurok may have secluded themselves and sought spiritual power in large dome-shaped communal menstrual huts (Buckley 1988: 200–4). Like the women in their huts, men in their sweat-lodges maintained strict continence, bathed twice daily and were restricted in their diet to only a few gathered and pre-prepared foods. Moreover, just as women bled menstrually, men during this period 'gashed their legs with flakes of white quartz, the flowing blood being thought to carry off psychic impurity, preparing one for spiritual attainment' (Buckley 1988: 195).

Entering a sweat-lodge – in this culture at least – was, then, a male counterpart of female menstrual seclusion or (to use the terms of the model) the activity of going 'on strike'. Indeed, Yurok women themselves made the connection explicit in stating that their menstrual seclusion house was 'like the men's sweathouse' (Buckley 1988: 190).

We can interpret this ancient tradition theoretically and in terms of our model by saying that if women were on sex strike, then men had to be doing something in that period, too – something which did not involve sex. Over an immense area of America – its distribution map marking a 'vast triangle, the angles of which are formed by Alaska, Labrador, and Guatemala' (Luckert 1975: 142, citing Krickeberg 1939: 19) – 'sweating' prior to hunting was the basic answer that men found. Men would generally sweat just before a hunt, and then again at the hunt's conclusion. Luckert (1975: 145) explains the significance of this by quoting a well-informed Navajo:

> when asked about the meaning of the sweat bath, he acknowledged that one such bath is taken at the beginning; immediately, however, he went on to explain the one which concludes the hunt: 'You do not sleep with your wife with blood on you.'

It would be hard to be more explicit than that.

Blood, Meat and Fire

We have seen that men would have been anxious to avoid suspicion of cheating, and for that reason anxious to avoid being incriminated by the principal symbolic indicator of possible cheating – inexplicable bloodstains. It was also noted that various stratagems to deal with such risks were logically possible, one of these being a refusal to handle raw meat beyond a certain point – abandoning it until it had been cooked by someone else so as to remove all visible blood.

This kind of thinking is well documented almost everywhere in the Americas. Lévi-Strauss (1970: 152) quotes Colbacchini (1919: 28) on the Bororo of Central Brazil:

> They believe themselves to be polluted whenever, for some reason or other, and even while hunting wild animals, they happen to become stained with blood. They immediately set off in search of water in which

they wash and rewash, until all trace of the blood has disappeared. This explains their dislike of food in which the blood is still visible.

Among these Indians, most health practices are connected with the view that the 'spirit' or 'blood' or 'life-force' (the terms are interchangeable) of an animal should never be eaten. 'Meat, for example, is thoroughly boiled to the point of tastelessness to ensure that the slightest trace of blood is removed' (Crocker 1985: 41–2). A similar taboo was widespread in the region. 'Meat, whatever it is', writes Huxley (1957: 84–5) of the Urubu of the Brazilian highlands, 'has to be cooked thoroughly, or the Indians won't eat it – the slightest sign of redness inside, and back it goes to the fire'. Writing of the Eastern Timbira or Ramko'kamekra of the eastern highlands of Brazil, Lévi-Strauss (1969a: 151, citing Nimuendajú 1946: 246–7) notes 'the violent abdominal pains that follow the consumption of roast meat, when it is eaten with fingers stained with blood from the hunt . . . .'.

James Adair (1775: 117) found a variant of the blood taboo among the Indians of the south-eastern United States, seeing it as evidence that the Indians were descendants of the Lost Tribe of Israel:

> The Indians have among them the resemblance of the Jewish Sin-Offering, and Trespass-Offering, for they commonly pull their new-killed venison (before they dress it) several times through the smoke and flame of the fire, both by the way of a sacrifice, and to consume the blood, life, or animal spirits of the beast, which with them would be a most horrid abomination to eat.

These Indians would never eat blood of any kind (Adair 1775: 134).

Similar notions feature prominently in mythology almost throughout the Americas, countless stories identifying culture with cooking-fire and conveying the message that only animal carnivores – not humans – eat their meat still covered in blood. In his *Mythologiques*, Lévi-Strauss (1970; 1973; 1978; 1981) endorses the message of all these myths and beliefs: culture, he argues, was indeed established when men first learned to eat their meat *cooked instead of raw*.

Fire and the Origin of Menstrual Taboos

Apart from its many practial uses, the central *symbolic* importance of fire can now be appreciated in a new way. Perhaps the most important point is that prior to fire's use in cooking, it would have been difficult for women to assert the dangers inherent in blood contact at all. If people habitually ate their meat raw or with visible blood still showing in it, then it would have seemed normal for men to be bloodstained for much of the time, not only out in the hunting grounds but also back in the home. This would have made menstrual taboos difficult to impose. Indeed, to associate blood with ritual pollution or 'taboo' would have been virtually impossible until such time as society could control and negate the bloodiness of meat food. Cooking was the only realistic solution. And if fire was a resource basically under female control, then this whole symbolic system – this 'ideology of blood' to use Testart's term – would have given women further leverage in exerting their power. Since no flesh could be deemed edible until it was cooked, it would have given women substantial control over supplies of meat food.

We can now add a new and important element to the model. It has already been noted that at the time when meat was brought home to be cooked, women ought to have ceased menstruating. If the basic symbolic function of cooking was to remove blood from meat, any excess of menstrual blood in women would have had an anti-cooking effect, negating the cooking process by adding to the presence of blood in the vicinity. Fire and blood, in other words, would have been experienced as antithetical in their effects; consequently, we arrive at an absolutely basic rule – *no menstruating woman ought to have been permitted to cook meat.*

Symmetrical results are arrived at on the level of sexual relations. Men would have brought back meat to the base camp in expectation of sexual rewards. But just as meat could not have been eaten until it had been rendered safe through cooking, so women could not have been approached for sexual relations until they had ceased to signal 'no!' Before sex became permitted, then, women must have signalled that they were ritually safe. They must have washed the blood off themselves, or passed through smoke or fire, or removed all blood or all thought of blood in some other publicly visible way. In some communities, the mere fact of the moon's fullness or of women's involvement with cooking-fire may have been sufficient indication that womankind's 'dark' and 'dangerous' period was now over.

In any event, while menstruating women would have been 'bloody' and in that sense 'raw', women who were safely available as sexual partners ought logically to have been thought of as blood-free or 'cooked'. Put another way, we can say that to be with one's kin – one's 'blood' – would have been to be in a 'raw' state, while conjoining with one's spouse or lover would have involved becoming 'cooked'.

Intimations of a Universal Structure: the Raw and the Cooked

The symbolic logic which applies the 'raw/cooked' opposition equally to women and to meat is familiar as one of the more curious yet widely publicised findings of Lévi-Strauss in his *Mythologiques*. Lévi-Strauss explicitly associates cooking with marriage (1973: 303–4), and shows that '*raw is to cooked as kinship is to marriage*' is a formula discernible not only in American Indian mythology but also in other parts of the world, including within the folklore of certain areas of England and France.

Lévi-Strauss (1970: 334) writes that in France, in the Upper Forez, Isère, Ardèche and Gard areas, women (and sometimes men) who were thought to have remained too long unmarried (that is, to have remained overdependent on their kin) were teasingly reminded of their 'rawness' by being made to eat a salad consisting of onions, nettles and roots, or of clover and oats; this was termed 'making them eat salad' or 'making them eat turnip'. In several areas of England, the penalty was different: the unmarried elder sister of a girl who had already married was forced to dance 'in the raw' — that is, to dance barefoot.

The remedy for such 'rawness', in other cases, was quite literally to be 'cooked'. In the St Omer district of France at the beginning of the nineteenth century, if a younger daughter was married first, 'this was a sad day for her poor elder sister, for at some point during the celebrations, she would, willy nilly, be seized upon, lifted up and laid on the top of the oven, so that she might be warmed up, as the saying was, since her situation seemed to indicate that she had remained insensitive to love'. A similar custom existed during Napoleon III's reign, at Wavrin, in the Lille area (Gennep 1946–58, Book 1, Vol. 2, pp. 631–3; quoted in Lévi-Strauss 1970: 334). English-speakers to this day perpetuate this structure in language: to speak of a woman as 'hot' implies sexual readiness, while 'coolness' of course means the reverse.

Over immense areas of the world, the same logic gave rise to customs comparable with those in France. When women were required, because of their dangerous 'wetness' or 'rawness', to disjoin from society or from men, the fact that they were menstruating or shedding afterbirth blood was emphasised, publicised and even exaggerated. When the aim was, rather, to terminate the period of 'pollution' or 'rawness', the opposite action was taken, and the female flesh concerned was warmed up or 'cooked'. Hence from Cambodia, as well as Malaysia, Siam and various regions of Indonesia, have come reports that a girl during her first menstruation — a phase which had to be accentuated — had to 'go into the shade' and remain out of sunlight to preserve the potency of the supernatural power. On the other hand, a woman who had just given birth — a phase which had to be brought to a close — was 'laid on a bed or a raised grill under which there burned a slow fire' (Lévi-Strauss 1970: 335). Pueblo Indian women gave birth over a heap of hot sand, which was perhaps intended to transform the child from its 'raw' state into a 'cooked person' approachable by society. It was the habit of various Californian tribes to put women who had just given birth into ovens, hollowed out in the ground. After being covered with mats and hot stones, they were conscientiously 'cooked'. The Yurok Indians of California used the expression 'cooking the pains' — a reference to menstrual periods — to refer to all curative rites. 'This rapid summary of customs', Lévi-Strauss concludes (1970: 336), suggests that the individuals who are 'cooked' are those most deeply involved in a physiological process: the newborn child, the woman who has just given birth, or the pubescent girl. The conjunction of a member of the social group with nature must be mediatised through the intervention of cooking-fire, whose normal function is to mediatise the conjunction of the raw product and the human consumer, and whose operation thus has the effect of making sure that a natural creature is at one and the same time *cooked and socialised.* . . .

All this, it would seem, can be put very simply: just as blood imposes sexual and culinary 'consumption' taboos, *so fire is necessary in order to lift them.*

Women and Fire

Women, it was noted earlier, would have gained from promoting male anxieties concerning blood, not for spiritual or religious reasons but because it would have accentuated female control over meat brought back to camp. It would have meant that although men as hunters held a monopoly of access to living game animals, this applied only for as long as the meat was out in the bush. The moment it was brought back, the only way to avoid contamination and possible suspicion would have been for men to relinquish it and wash or otherwise purify themselves. An immediate task would also have been to remove the source of the pollution. This would have required the female recipients' emphatic demonstration that they were not menstruating or about to begin menstruating; it would also have meant proceeding immediately to cook the meat.

Once men's meat had been brought home for cooking, it would have entered the feminine sphere. We can imagine, perhaps, large earth ovens filled with hot stones into which the game was put. To the extent that the blood in the meat was 'like' menstrual blood, the ovens may have been perceived as 'like' immense wombs in which a transformative process was taking place. In the case of a large animal, the cooking may have lasted many hours. The test of whether the meat was finally ready or not would have been a simple one: Was the blood in it still visible? If it was, the oven had yet more work to do. If no blood could be seen, the cooking process had been completed – whereupon eating could safely begin.

The reader will recall that in the early stages of the Upper Palaeolithic, the base camp would have revolved around a fire, with women's control over the domestic space involving particular responsibilities in connection with cooking. Maintaining a fire requires constant vigilance rather than mobility, and it is easy to understand that this would have been primarily the responsibility not of male hunters forever on the move but of females and those males too old, too sick or for other reasons temporarily unable to hunt.

The need to control domestic fire, in other words, would have turned women's relative immobility – a potential disadvantage in other contexts – into an advantage.

The cultural stipulation that meat had to be cooked before it could be eaten functioned to ensure that it was circulated between the sexes. Given female control over cooking (or rather, given the mere fact that the necessary fire remained at the home base, not being readily transportable), it followed that to eat their own kills, men would have had to face the blood-polluted nature of their food. Eating one's own kill would have meant eating meat raw. Getting the meat cooked – obligatory to the extent that blood was to be avoided – implied taking it home, where it came under the influence of the opposite sex. The avoidance of blood, in other words, acted in inhibiting men's consumption of their own kills in the bush.

In this context, the model helps explain a paradox which was noted in this book much earlier (Chapter 8). Why was it so long after the earliest discovery of fire that this resource came to be used systematically for the cooking of meat? Fire was harnessed apparently as early as 1.5 million years ago, yet there is little if any evidence for its use in cooking until over a million years later. How can such an extraordinary delay be explained?

The model would suggest that until women could organise their intervention, the main problem would have been the tendency of males to eat and (in later evolutionary stages) perhaps also to cook meat on a haphazard basis, wherever or whenever an animal had been killed, without following any definite timetable. By contrast, if women were to obtain an adequate share, they would have needed a definite regular schedule: a pre-arranged 'meal time' or 'celebratory feast-time' known to the group's members in advance, and not simply dependent on the particular time and place when a game animal happened to be killed. Imposing the necessary restraints and synchronisation of activities would have been a difficult task to achieve.

The model implies that women solved this problem – just as they solved others that involved timing – by using the moon. It would have been in women's interests to emphasise and perhaps greatly exaggerate the connection between menstruation and the moon. The notion that the period from dark moon onwards inevitably produced menstrual bleeding (Chapter 10) would have given women the leverage they needed. All 'darkness' in the moon – women could claim – was directly 'polluting' in a menstrual sense. It could be claimed that regardless of women's wishes, such blood pollution simply could not be dispelled until the moon itself was full – until it had succeeded in casting off entirely its blood-linked dark shadow. Once women had authoritatively established this ideological/cosmological point, their meat-gaining problems would in principle have been solved. A logical consequence would have been that cooking could not take place before full moon. This in turn would have stopped men from cooking in the bush. Waiting until full moon would have meant delaying cooking activities until the moment of the hunters' return to camp. Such a delay would have guaranteed women access to the meat.

An implication of this model is that long before 'the mealtime' with its cooking-fire became a secular daily event, it was a once a-month ritual event – a special time of celebratory feasting. Large earth ovens or other fires were constructed and efforts were made to schedule the major processes of cooking so that they took place at the most propitious moment for this kind of activity – at about the time of the full moon, or at least as far as possible away from the time of the dark moon. In short, the dark moon made menstrual blood flow. Cooking's purpose, by contrast, was to reverse this flow. Consequently, cooking should occur at full moon.

Put another way, we can say that fire would of necessity have been associated not with darkness or the dark moon but with light, the full moon, marital sex and the sun. This logic finds expression in countless details of ritual and mythology, including the stipulation that a menstruating woman should never cook but should be kept in darkness, safe from all fire including the sun's rays.

Eclipses and 'the Moon's Blood'

The model, in any event, makes certain predictions. Some of these are more testable than others. Some refer us to archaeological inferences, others to already familiar phenomena within the ethnographic record. Menstrual taboos of the kind discussed in this chapter are a prediction of the hypothesis, yet have long been known about. Much the same applies to ritual avoidances of blood in meat. Again, the hypothesis would predict bride-service – the surrender of game to women and their kin, motivated by men's need for social and sexual prestige of a kind which can only be gained by success in hunting. But this, too, has long been a commonplace of hunter-gatherer studies (see Chapter 4). It is more satisfactory when the model predicts something of which we had no previous suspicion. When this happens, the more 'improbable' the prediction, the better. The hypothesis then stands or falls on the basis of an investigation whose outcome is unknown.

A prediction which has just been arrived at is that cooking should occur at or in the days immediately following full moon, but not when the moon is dark. Despite Malinowski's Trobriand Islands finding that in 'all festivities, all enterprises, and on all ceremonial occasions, the climax is reached at full moon' (1927: 206), no anthropologist, to the author's knowledge, has ever suggested that *cooking* is traditionally most propitious at full moon. It is indeed a somewhat inconvenient consequence of the hypothesis, since it is hard to imagine any real human community restricting its cooking activities to within only a certain portion of each month. Contemporary hunter-gatherers are not prominently known to pay the slightest attention to the moon's condition when they need to cook a piece of meat.

However, they do show concern about women's menstrual periods. And a negative test concerning the moon can be envisaged. It would be to see whether the sudden or unexpected *absence* of a full moon would throw the cooking process into reverse. Such an expectation can be formulated more concretely. Were the hypothesis correct, a lunar eclipse should appear in tradition as the sudden and unexpected intrusion of a dark-moon episode into what was supposed to be a full moon. Fidelity to the logic would imply that menstrual blood 'must' be flowing, and that therefore all cooking should cease forthwith.

This expectation is confirmed. Referring to a widespread Amerindian myth linking incest ('excessive' blood unity) with eclipses, Lévi-Strauss in *The Raw and the Cooked* (1970: 298) remarks that the mythological connections also include 'culinary utensils, food, and domestic fire'. In South America, in Guiana, 'the Lolaca and Atabaca Indians . . . were convinced that, if the moon really died, all domestic fires would be extinguished'. In North America, in the lower Yukon region, it is believed 'that a pervasive essence, a maleficent influence, spreads across the earth when an eclipse of the moon occurs, and that if by chance a small particle happens to get inside some utensil or other, sickness will ensue. So, as soon as an eclipse begins, the women hurriedly turn all their pots, pails, and dishes upside down.' The Alsea Indians of Oregon threw out their reserves of drinking water – 'bloodied' by the eclipse. The Californian Wintu 'would throw out all their food, and even water, in case they had become polluted by the blood of the sun or moon'. The Serrano forbade all food, since feasting would only assist the spirits of the dead to 'eat' the celestial body.

Two further examples, both Amazonian, may clarify the nature of the blood in pots and pans. It will be noted that it makes little difference whether the eclipse is lunar or solar: either way, the alignments of both moon and sun are involved in causing the eclipse, and the critical point is that the sudden plunging of earth and sky into darkness indicates the pervasive presence of 'blood':

1

Pirá-paraná mythology says the moon copulates with menstruating women and that during an eclipse of the moon, called the 'dying moon', the moon becomes a small red ball of menstrual blood which comes to earth and fills the house and its objects, (C. Hugh-Jones, 1979, p. 156, on the Barasana)

2

On 24 December 1973, I was startled by a tremendous shout from the men of the village. They had just noticed that the sun was gradually being eclipsed. Dropping all their activities they rushed back to the village in a state of genuine fear and alarm, for Kama (Sun), one of the important male spirits and culture heroes, was 'menstruating'. . . .

Blood from the sun, like menstrual blood, is very dangerous. Each drop can penetrate the skin, causing sickness and leaving moles and blemishes. Quickly the villagers smeared themselves with ashes and manioc flour to ward off the blood. Carrying pots of porridge and stacks of manioc bread, the women threw large quantities of food into the bushes. Contaminated by the blood of the sun, just as a house's food may be contaminated by a menstruating woman, it was no longer fit for human consumption.

In the late afternoon of the day of the eclipse, the villagers scarified themselves with scrapers (*piya*) set with dogfish teeth. Opening long cuts on their bodies, they 'menstruated' so that the sun's blood could flow out. . . . (Gregor 1985, p. 193, on the Méhinaku).

When the moon or sun suddenly becomes dark, then, cooking is inappropriate; people 'ought' to be menstruating – and food ought to be thrown away.

The Model

It is now possible to complete the detailed specifications of the model – corresponding to the 'genetic code', as it were, of the cultural configuration.

Once a lunar month, women enter seclusion. The moon is now dark. At this time, people do not walk out at night, or visit one another, or go hunting. They remain with kin, reassembling as coalitions of kin, men focusing around their 'mothers' and 'sisters', not their wives. Menstrual blood is now flowing, or at least assumed to be, and although a man can be in close proximity to his mother's blood, his wife's is to be avoided.

At dark moon, the blood which flows seems to come from the moon. It is the moon, after all, which brings kin together. It is the clock with which they synchronise their reunion. All symbolic authority in this phase is associated with mothers/sisters, not fathers. All bodily intimacy (for example, in dancing) is legitimate only to the extent that the symbolic authority of blood and of maternity is upheld. Men are of course involved, but the blood contact immediately defines them as 'sons' and 'brothers' in relation to their kinswomen, not fathers, husbands or lovers in relation to affines. This can be put another way by saying that to the extent that men are touched by the 'magic' of blood, their sexuality is washed away, temporarily suppressed or at least confined within the limits of immature, non-fertile eroticism. In essence, men are 'as if' reduced to pre-adolescence, their attitude to their kinswomen's blood being modelled on that of a child to the authority of its mother. This does not preclude physical intimacy or incestuous sexual fantasy, but it does preclude female sexual yielding or surrender to a partner in adult heterosexual intercourse. In short, the sex strike must remain firm.

With sexual energies aroused but not satisfied, both men and women now concentrate their attention on a future goal, channelling all energies into

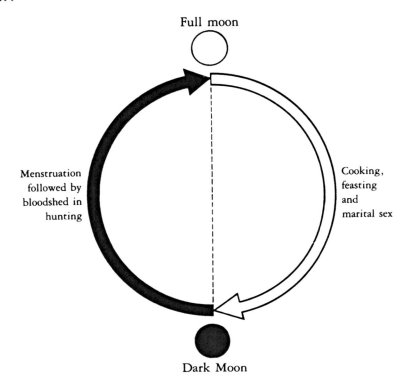

Full moon

Menstruation
followed by
bloodshed in
hunting

Cooking,
feasting
and
marital sex

Dark Moon

Figure 16 A model Ice Age hunting community's ritually structured schedule of work and rest. In addition to daily, seasonal and other periodicities, life normatively alternates to a fortnightly rhythm, switching between a 'production' phase of ritual power (initiated by menstrual onset, continued into hunting, butchery etc. and terminated as raw meat is transformed into cooked) and a corresponding 'consumption' phase of surrender or relaxation (beginning with feasting and celebratory love-making; terminated as meat supplies run low and the next menstrual onset approaches). The thick black line signifies the dominance of blood-relations whilst blood of any kind is flowing. The switch to white at full moon connotes cooking fire's lifting of the taboos associated with 'rawness' or visible blood, allowing feasting to proceed and marital partners to conjoin.

work. Traps are put in place and set, weapons sharpened or made. As the moon waxes, the time for the hunt itself draws near.

Towards full moon, when nights are light, hunting begins. The closer to full moon, the closer to the most propitious time for the kill. Following success, the meat is brought home; fires and earth ovens are prepared; the meat is ceremonially cooked. The killing-to-cooking (blood-to-fire) transition coincides with the transition from waxing to waning moon. Cooking, lunar transition, the removal of blood in meat and the lifting of the blood spell are all symbolised by the same light and fire. The collective, sex-striking community now dissolves: from now on comes feasting, celebration and sex. Couples are left free to enjoy one another's bodies, just as they are

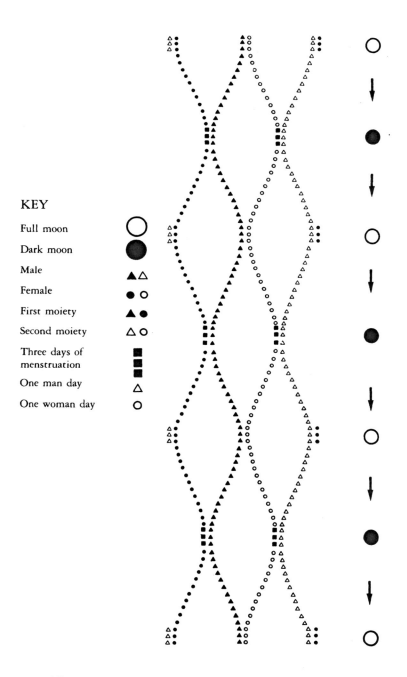

KEY

Full moon	◯
Dark moon	⬤
Male	▲△
Female	●○
First moiety	▲●
Second moiety	△○
Three days of menstruation	■
One man day	△
One woman day	○

Figure 17 A different view of the alternation shown in the previous figure, displaying the model community's division into two exogamous moieties. A succession of repeated cycles is shown, each of 29.5 days, blood-kin conjoining at dark moon, marital partners at full.

free to partake of cooked meat. This lasts for anything up to thirteen or fourteen days – in principle until the time for the polar opposite spell-casting transformation has arrived.

Following a period of pre-menstrual build-up and tension, the power of the strike is once again unleashed. The cooked-to-raw (fire-to-blood) transition occurs ideally at dark moon. The menstrual flow then puts a stop to all feasting and love-making. Now males are reclaimed as sex-strike allies by their mothers and sisters, discipline and solidarity once more prevail over sex – and the cycle is set in motion for a further round (figure 16).

We are left, then, with a picture of two social 'worlds' corresponding to two kinds of time – that of the waxing moon on the one hand, waning moon on the other (figure 17). In one temporal sector, blood relations dominate, marital relations are excluded, meat is raw and meat hunger prevails; in the other, cooking-fires are lit, marital relations predominate and there is feasting on cooked meat. In the first phase, men are essentially 'maternal uncles', 'sons' and 'brothers' to their kin, while women are 'mothers', 'sisters' and 'daughters'; with the transition to the second phase, everyone exchanges partners and roles – to become spouses or lovers to polar-opposite kinds of relatives (a switch-over pictured in Lévi-Strauss' 'bird-nester' stories as a movement between polar-opposite worlds accompanied by an exchange of clothes, gender-roles or 'skins').

The model would define all this as the most elementary possible way of being fully cultural. It implies that at the culminating point of the hominisation process, there was glimpsed the possibility of a harmonious social and ecological logic linking menstrual cycles with the periodicity of hunting expeditions, maternal blood with the blood of game animals, cooking and feasting with sexual enjoyment – and all of these with the periodicity of the moon. So internally coherent and emotionally meaningful did this logic seem that it apparently inspired generations of our ancestors in the course of a human revolution which took millennia to consummate, and whose principles have continued to dominate traditional myths, religious rituals and magical beliefs up into recent times.

Chapter 12
The Reds

Bourgeois society is the most highly developed and most highly differentiated historical organisation of production. The categories which serve as the expression of its conditions and the comprehension of its own organisation enable it at the same time to gain an insight into the organisation and the relationships of production which have prevailed under all the past forms of society, on the ruins and constituent elements of which it has arisen, and of which it still drags along some unsurmounted remains. . . .

Karl Marx, *Grundrisse* (1857–9)

Blood taboos, ritualistic cooking prohibitions and lunar/solar cosmological beliefs, then, are not mere inexplicable manifestations of primitive irrationality. Neither were they invented by men as instruments for oppressing women. They arose out of and expressed a definite mode of production, distribution and exchange. They constitute some of the 'unsurmounted remains', to use Marx's expression, of those ancient institutions of human gender solidarity with which culture began, and which have been 'dragged along' uncomprehendingly by many of us in cultures right up until the present.

In being 'dragged along', however, these institutions have changed. Much has happened to traditions everywhere since culture first originated, and this applies to menstrual taboos as much as to other features. We would not expect to find living ethnographic evidence of people still practising the sex strike in the simple or initial form specified in the model. We are unlikely to find a culture in some forgotten corner of the globe where women still form up in a line, signal 'No sex!' in their own menstrual blood and send men off to hunt. Rather, we would expect derivative forms. The task is therefore to work out on a theoretical basis what evolved forms might logically be possible, attempt to determine the material conditions of these, and test whether our results are consistent with what the contemporary ethnographic record tells us.

Urucú

Cruising through the Bahamas on 15 October, 1493, Christopher Columbus and his crew picked up a lone Indian paddler in a canoe. He was carrying some of the native bread, a calabash of water 'and a piece of red earth made into a powder and then kneaded. . . ' The 'red earth' was in fact a dye made from the berries of a decorative shrub, *Bixa orellana* – familiar under its Portuguese name, *urucú* (Sauer 1966: 56).

Columbus had encountered what is now known to be a key aspect of cultural life in the South and Central American tropics. Among the Méhinaku, along the Xingu – a tributary of the Amazon – the *urucú* shrub with its red berries is grown in gardens, the pods being harvested in June and July. The villagers open the pods in their houses and boil the waxy red seeds in great ceramic pots. A family may be fully occupied for several weeks in the tasks of harvesting, shelling and tending the fires. The result of their labours is several large balls of pasty red dye, which will last throughout the year. It is used to colour masks and, above all, as body-paint. Covering the hair and body with liberal quantities is for the Méhinaku the 'sine qua non of good dress'; it is associated with all ritual occasions. The paint 'has an association with blood in that in a battle it will "attract" an arrow causing a wound' (Gregor 1977: 158–9, 173).

The Asurinis, along another stretch of the Xingu, paint themselves with red *urucú* mixed with oil from babassú palm-nuts, producing a particularly dark shade of red. In this case, their very name – Asurinis – means 'red people' (Lukesch 1976: 33–4). So widespread was such body-painting in the American tropics at the time of contact that, according to the anthropological historian Carl Sauer (1966: 56), it probably explains why Europeans came to refer to all the native peoples of the New World as 'red Indians'.

The Jibaros in eastern Ecuador regard *urucú* paint as 'magical'; the shrub from which the red berries come is a 'sacred tree' (Karsten 1935: 380). The Trio Indians, between northern Brazil and southern Surinam, use *urucú* to cover the whole body as a protection against evil spirits – which 'are unable to see objects coloured red' (Rivière 1969: 34). Female physiological processes are intimately involved in the symbolism:

> Red (*tamire*) is associated with protection against spirits, women (Waraku, the first woman was painted red), fertility, and its application is uniform and without design except on the face. The word to apply red paint is *imuka* which contains the same root (*mu*) as *imuku*, child, *imuhte*, to be pregnant, and *mumu*, blood. (Rivière 1969: 266)

A similar link between 'the first woman', shamanism and *urucú* red body-paint is brought out by Christine Hugh-Jones in her sophisticated structuralist ethnography of the Barasana:

Romi Kumu lives up in the sky and is the first grandmother of us all; she is immortal because she has the sacred beeswax (*werea*) gourd with her. She grows old during the day, bathes at dawn and becomes young and white again. She also renews her red face paint, urucú (*musa*; *Bixa orellana*, used exclusively by women), and takes off a layer of skin with the old paint. This paint is her menstrual blood. Her name means 'Woman Shaman' but she is like a man. (1979: 137)

Among the Urubu of the Brazilian highlands, along the south-eastern limit of the Amazonian basin, numerous myths and taboos concern hunting and hunting luck. There are strict rules prohibiting hunters from consuming their own kills, breaches of which result in *panem* – a kind of impotence associated with loss of hunting luck. Huxley (1957: 145) also discusses 'processes of transformation' – rituals of birth and of death, rites of initiation, the baking of clay pots, the cooking of meat and so on – events which are thought to be dangerously magical and are therefore heavily hedged in with taboos. Having described a number of such transformation processes, he continues:

For the Indians, perhaps the most dangerous of all these processes is that of menstruation, the regular and spontaneous manifestation of the creative power as blood. Blood is the very principle of life, as the Indians acknowledge every time they paint their faces red with urucu, in imitation of it; for that very reason, however, it is dangerous. No Indian will eat half-cooked meat, lest the blood that is still in it should poison him. . . .

Here, in one short passage, all of our origins model's connections – linking menstruation, transformative processes, face painting and avoidance of the blood in raw meat – are neatly made.

An early report on the Toba Indians of the Gran Chaco (Karsten 1926) is equally fascinating. Menstruation is thought to be caused by the new moon – at which time of month a woman is thought to be vulnerable to evil spirits (Karsten 1926: 10–11). On various occasions, women paint their faces bright red with *urucú*. Karsten (1926: 130) was given various explanations for the practice – it was 'to look beautiful', 'to attract the men' and so on – but was not convinced:

As a matter of fact, the truth appeared to be that the Toba women generally paint themselves *at the time of their menses* – no doubt as a prophylactic against the evil spirits whose feared attacks also make them diet during the four or five critical days. (Karsten 1926: 13)

In discussing the Toba and other tribes, Karsten provides intriguing glimpses of a system in which symbolic menstrual blood functions very much as we would expect in the light of our model. For example, describing the Canelos Indians of Ecuador, he notes that men do two things prior to setting off on a hunting expedition. Firstly, they avoid all sexual contact with women for eight days prior to the hunt. Secondly:

> Whether the hunting expedition is undertaken for a feast or not, the Canelos Indian never omits to paint his face red with roucou [*urucú*] before starting. The red paint is supposed to attract animals and birds, and thus to give good luck in hunting. . . . The Canelos Indian says that if he does not paint himself with roucou before going to hunt, he will be unable to kill any game. (Karsten 1935: 163–4)

However, these references to hunters painting *their own* faces appear to be misleading, at least in some important cases. On closer investigation, it turns out that a collective hunting expedition, which may last for anything up to fifteen days, is preceded by a ritual in which the red painting is executed upon the hunters' faces *by an older woman*.

In the following passage (paraphrasing Karsten 1935: 162), we do not exactly see the sex strike as outlined in previous chapters. We are not told of a line of synchronously menstruating women touching or threatening their menfolk with blood before sending them out to fetch meat. But glimpses of this logic — in a description recalling the picket-line of face-painted Sharanahua women discussed in Chapter 4 — can surely be discerned:

> Early in the morning of the day when a major hunting expedition is to start, all the hunters assemble in the house of the Indian who is to organise the feasting which will follow a successful outcome. The hunters' wives bring with them numerous drums, which the men — dressed in festival style — proceed to beat in a slow rhythm, moving in a circle in the middle of the large house. This may continue for about an hour, until the final face-painting ritual begins.
>
> Before leaving the house, the hunters range themselves in a row. An old woman has a gourd ready, containing some *mani* or earth-nuts. Each grain in the gourd is painted red with *urucú*. In another small gourd she has prepared some crude *urucú* with which the hunters' faces are to be painted. The old woman also holds a branch of a certain tree with large soft prickles, which the Indians call *chini papaya*: 'Each hunter in turn steps forward to the old woman, who paints the whole lower part of his face red with roucou and then slightly strikes him on the head, the shoulders, the arms, and the legs with the prickly branch, at the same time saying to him: *sinchita callpángi*, "may you run fast". The hunter thus treated now starts to run away from the house, all the women throwing after him the red *mani* grains. Then the next hunter steps forward to the old woman, to be treated in the same way, then the following one and so forth, until the last of them. After the hunters have left, the women pick up the *mani* grains and eat them.' (Karsten 1935: 162)

We will return to the topic of body-painting and its possible roots in menstrual symbolism later in this chapter. In the meantime, broadening our scope beyond the Americas, let us tackle a long-standing problem in comparative mythology, familiarising ourselves with issues which will deepen our understanding of what *urucú* and similar forms of pigmentation may ultimately mean.

The Myth of Matriarchy

Matriarchy myths are ideological constructs which postulate an 'original' period of 'women's rule'. Such narratives – which are known in many parts of the world – are particularly prominent in those areas in which men seek a monopoly of ritual power through secret male initiation rites. Such areas include much of tropical South America, Africa, Melanesia and Australia. In the societies concerned, men organise an apparent conspiracy against women, using an array of theatrical devices, sound-making instruments, blood-shedding operations and ritual songs, dances and other performances in order, it seems, to intimidate women and separate them from their male offspring as these come of age. The success of these endeavours varies from place to place, but in general the logic which men follow and the myths and symbols used are so stunningly alike in such widely separated regions of the globe that anthropologists have long sought an explanation for the parallels (Allen 1967; Bachofen 1973: 69–201 [original 1861]; Bamberger 1974; Dundes 1976; Gourlay 1975; Hugh-Jones, C. 1979; Hugh-Jones, S. 1979).

Myths of matriarchy, writes Joan Bamberger (1974: 249), have no historical value, and in particular convey no information as to womankind's actual past, present or future in any culture. On the contrary, matriarchy myths are just *patriarchal ideological constructs*. Their function is to justify male dominance 'through the evocation of a catastrophic alternative – a society dominated by women'. In these myths, Bamberger continues (p. 280), womankind 'represents chaos and misrule through unbridled sexuality'. Women are accused of being unable to restrain their sexual appetites. Using the terminology of this book, we can translate this as the accusation that women are unable to maintain any such thing as a 'sex strike'. When it comes to resisting the temptations of sex, women are failures. In the sample of representative myths which I now want to discuss, mythological women leave their legs open or their 'sacred enclosures' unguarded, allowing their privacy to be invaded by men. The conclusion, we will see, is that in the interests of culture, men must organise the necessary sex strike for themselves.

In the myths, woman-dominated society is envisaged not only as excessively sexual. It is seen as a world ruled by mysterious forces emanating in a more general way from nature. These are forces of 'evil', 'witchcraft' or 'medicine' bound up with darkness, wetness and the changing moon (as opposed to the sun) and intimately linked with both reproductive and sexual aspects of female physiology. In a number of myths it is the 'Sun-man' or 'Sun-father' who finally overthrows 'women's rule' (Bamberger 1974: 269, 273).

Few specialists in comparative mythology have doubted that such myths are alleging woman's governance by the moon (cf. Eliade 1958: 154–63; Lévi-Strauss 1978: 221–2, 506). The Oglala Indian saying that woman's power 'grows with the moon and comes and goes with it', women secluding themselves monthly in their menstrual huts 'to keep their medicine effective' (Powers 1980: 62, 57) provides a good example. Beliefs of this kind, while varied in their specific forms, occur virtually throughout the traditional world. Through their bodies and, in particular, through their reproductive organs, women are felt to have a peculiar and privileged mode of access to 'medicine', 'magic' or 'witchcraft' of a kind which is all the more dangerous for being linked with the moon, rooted in nature *and therefore ultimately beyond male cultural artifice or control.*

Against this background, we may examine some typical 'primitive matriarchy' myths, several of them featuring a Women's Lodge or Hut suggestive of a communal menstrual hut:

The origin of the Hain. **Tierra del Fuego: Selk'nam-Ona.**
In the beginning, witchcraft was known only by the women of Ona land. They practised it in a Lodge, which no man dared approach. The girls, as they neared womanhood, were instructed in the magic arts, learning how to bring sickness and death to those who displeased them. The men lived in abject fear and subjection. Certainly they had bows and arrows with which to hunt. 'Yet', they asked, 'what use are such weapons against witchcraft and sickness?'

    The tyranny of women bore down more and more heavily, until at last one day, the men resolved to fight back. They decided to kill the women, whereupon there ensued a great massacre, from which not one woman escaped in human form. The men spared their little daughters and waited until these had grown old enough to become wives. And so that these women should never be able to band together and regain their old ascendancy, the men inaugurated a secret society of their own and banished forever the Women's Lodge in which so many wicked plots had been hatched. (Bridges 1948: 412–3; quoted in Bamberger 1974: 270; slightly abridged)

The essence of this narrative is the allegation that women once 'banded together' in some way connected with a 'Lodge' from which emanated death-dealing supernatural powers.

    The next myth adds to these themes that of a special 'paint' used by women to change their apparent identities. The 'Great Kina Hut' is the hut in which men carry on their rituals today:

The origin of the Kina. Tierra del Fuego: Yamana.

In the beginning, women had sole power. They gave orders to the men, who obeyed just as women do today. The men took care of the children, tended the fire, and cleaned the skins, while the women did no work at all. That was the way it was always to be. The women invented the Great Kina Hut and everything which goes on inside it, and then fooled the men into thinking they were spirits. They stepped out of the Great Hut, painted all over, with masks on their heads. The men did not recognise their wives, who, simulating the spirits, beat the earth with dried skins so that it shook. Their howls and roars so frightened the men that they hid in their huts.

But one day, the Sun-man, whose job it was to supply meat to the women-spirits in their Hut, overheard the voices of two girls while he was passing a lagoon. Curious, he hid in the bushes and saw the girls practising their spirit-impersonations and washing off paint. He confronted them, insisting they reveal their secrets. Finally, they confessed: 'It is the women themselves who paint themselves and put on masks; then they step out of the hut and show themselves to the men. There are no other spirits there.' The Sun-man returned to the camp and exposed the fraudulent women. In revenge the men stormed the Kina Hut, and in the ensuing great battle killed the women or turned them into animals. From that time on, the men have performed in the Kina Hut; they do this in the same manner as the women before them. (Bamberger 1974: 269; citing Gusinde 1961: 1238–49; slightly abridged)

In this myth, men are identified with the sun. The women, by contrast, are associated with a lagoon. When painted, the women inspired terror as they impersonated 'the spirits'. They organised in a fearsome 'hut', but men eventually stormed this, taking it over *and performing in it exactly the same rituals as the women had done before.*

A further myth, from the Méhinaku (whose use of *urucú* was discussed earlier), introduces (a) the theme of flutes and bullroarers and (b) the theme of sexual dominance as expressed in rape. It is narrated by a man:

The origin of the bull-roarer. Amazonia: Méhinaku.

In ancient times the women occupied the men's houses and played the sacred flutes inside. We men took care of the children, processed manioc flour, wove hammocks, and spent our time in the dwellings while the women cleared fields, fished and hunted. In those days, the children even nursed at our breasts. A man who dared enter the women's house during their ceremonies would be gang-raped by all the women of the village on the central plaza.

One day the chief called us together and showed us how to make bull-roarers to frighten the women. As soon as the women heard the terrible drone, they dropped the sacred flutes and ran into the houses to hide. We grabbed the flutes and took over the men's houses. Today if a woman comes in here and sees our flutes we rape her. Today the women nurse babies, process manioc flour and weave hammocks, while we hunt, fish and farm. (Gregor 1977: 255)

In the next myth, women's sacred flutes are associated with the waters of a lagoon. These flutes needed 'feeding with meat' – that is, the women used the flutes to compel men to hunt for them:

The origin of the sacred flutes. Amazonia: Mundurucu.
Three women were walking through the forest long ago when they heard music coming from a lagoon. They investigated and caught three fish, which turned into three sacred flutes. The women played these to produce music so powerful that they were enabled to occupy the sacred Men's House, forcing the men to live in ordinary dwellings. While the women did little but play on their flutes all day long, they forced the men to make manioc flour, fetch water and firewood, and care for the children. The men's ignominy was complete when the women visited the men's dwellings at night to force their sexual attentions on them ('Just as we do to them today').
　　However, the flutes needed feeding with meat. One day, the men – who were the hunters – threatened to withhold what they caught unless the women surrendered the flutes. Frightened of angering the fertility-spirits contained in the flutes, the women agreed, and the men seized the flutes and the power, which they have held to this day. (Murphy 1973: 217–18)

In this myth, the men gain power by organising what may be termed (in the light of the arguments of this book) a male counterpart to women's menstrual 'sex strike' – a collective 'hunting strike'. They then base their power in what was formerly the women's sacred 'House', monopolising now the 'flutes' which 'needed feeding with meat'. In this as in so many similar myths, the implication is that every strategy which women once used against men, men are now justified in practising against women – and in a form as close as possible to the female-inspired original.
　　We now come to a myth which replaces 'flutes', 'bull-roarers', 'masks' and 'paint' with a strange power-conferring garment: a skirt made of fibres stained with the world's first menstrual blood:

The origin of royal dress. West Africa: Dogon.
A woman stole a fibre skirt which was stained with the world's first

menstrual flow. Putting it on herself and concealing her identity by this means, she reigned as queen and spread terror all around. But then men took the fibres from her, dressed themselves in the royal garment, and prohibited its use to women. All the men danced wearing the reddened fibres, and the women had to content themselves with admiring them. (Griaule 1965: 170)

The statement that the woman had 'stolen' the power of menstruation expresses a male stance typical of myths of this kind. While many of the myths state that men 'robbed' women of a power which was 'naturally' theirs, in other cases men use a paradoxical assertion in order, it seems, to escape the implication that male rule must therefore lack legitimacy. They claim that women's power – even when taking the form of the potency of the menstrual flow – had been 'stolen' by women in the first place!

The next myth tells of 'The Origin of the Bull-roarer'; it might have been called 'The Origin of Menstruation', however:

The origin of the bull-roarer. Papua New Guinea: Kwavuru.

Tiv'r, the Originator, was puzzled to hear a faint sound – like that of a bull-roarer – whenever his wife moved. He asked her what the sound was, but she pretended not to know. Eventually, Tiv'r felt sure that it was coming from her vagina, and he commissioned various birds to steal the object responsible. A number of birds swooped down on her while, with bended back and legs spread wide apart, the woman was engaged in sweeping the village. But each time, she frustrated them by abruptly sitting down. Only the parrot got near enough to draw blood: this is why parrots' feathers are red.

Eventually, Tiv'r called upon the little bird, Serekute, and threatened him with death if he failed to obtain the sound-making instrument. Tiv'r shouted to his wife to show a little more rigour in her sweeping, and as she bent down and the point of the bull-roarer protruded from her vagina, the bird swooped down and snatched it away. The woman lay streaming with her first menstrual flow, while Tiv'r hugged the bull-roarer to his breast and declared that henceforth it would belong to man alone. (Williams 1936: 307–8)

Womankind, then leaves her vagina exposed, losing her power along with her blood.

The next myth features a 'sacred enclosure' which seems to correspond to the 'lodges' and 'huts' of other myths. It is similar to the previous story in saying that womankind lost her power when she opened her legs too wide:

The origin of Ida. Papua New Guinea: Umeda.

One day the women – who alone held the secrets of *ida* – were preparing for a ceremony as usual, making and storing the materials, paint, masks etc. in the sacred enclosure. But this time, the men had decided to set a trap for them. They went hunting and killed so many pigs that, when the women had eaten, they lay about in postures of repletion, with their knees spread and their skirts out of place. The men copulated with the women, who 'died' (slept, fainted). While the women slept, the men broke into the sacred enclosure, stole the masks, etc. and began to perform *ida* for the first time. 'We're no good', said the women when they woke up; 'We fell asleep. From now on *ida* belongs to the men'. (Gell 1975: 172)

The image of women lying 'with their knees spread and their skirts out of place' conveys, to use the language of the previous chapters, womankind's abandonment of cultural duty, her surrender of the weapon of the sex strike. The men seize their opportunity to strike-break, taking advantage of the sleeping pickets, invading women's sacred enclosure and in this way stealing the sacred power. Any sex strike from now on will have to be organised by men.

Two more myths in this vein deserve citation. In what follows, it is stated that the flutes – originally women's – had *functioned spontaneously* when still in women's hands:

The origin of the sacred flutes. **Papua New Guinea: Wogeo.**
Two women invented the sacred flutes following a dream. The flutes played of their own accord. But then a man stole the flutes and started blowing into the holes. When the women tried to explain that blowing was not necessary, he kicked them out of the way. 'Very well', shouted the women in anger, 'you males can keep the flutes. But flutes won't sing by themselves again. You decided to blow this one, and that's the way it shall be. And learning what to do won't be easy – no, you'll have to work hard and sweat.' (Hogbin 1970: 101)

My next myth stresses the genital, menstrual associations of the sacred flute, comparing and contrasting female menstruation in huts with male cere-monies in the Men's House:

The origin of the sacred flute. **Papua New Guinea: Gimi.**
A woman kept the sacred flute under her bark-string skirts until, one day, it was stolen by her brother. On putting the blow-hole to his mouth, however, his sister's pubic hairs attached themselves to the man's face: this is why men today have beards. The loss of her flute caused the woman to menstruate for the first time; ever afterwards, she was secluded each month in a menstrual hut. The men, meanwhile, began playing the flute inside the Men's House, and have held power ever since. (Gillison 1980: 156)

Note again how the Men's House is the symmetrical counterpart of the defeated woman's hut. Here as in the myths previously examined, men retaliate against women by building a special pseudo-menstrual hut of their own.

The final myth in this set falls into a slightly different category, since it says nothing about ritual or the transfer of sound-making instruments or ritual adornments to men. Nevertheless, *something* is transferred from female possession to male. The myth was given, writes Lewis (1980: 121), 'in answer to my question why, exactly, the moon was connected with menstruation . . .'

The origin of the moon. West Sepik, Papua New Guinea: Gnau.
A woman caught the moon in her net while fishing in the river. Calling it a turtle, she hid it in her house under a pile of firewood, intending to cook and eat it later. She began to prepare the necessary sago, leaving her house each day with the moon in its hiding-place inside. As she left, she barred her house, and each evening as she returned she refused to let her husband come inside, instead making him eat his sago outside, always outside. He wondered why.
    One day, while the woman was out, her husband peered through a crack in the wall and saw the light of the moon under the firewood. Calling to his brothers in secret, he obtained their help in breaking into the woman's house. They stole the moon. Singing, they pushed it up on a pole until it stuck fast to the sky. At this point, the woman was at work and saw the moon's image reflected in the red-leeched sago washings in her vat. Desperate, she rushed back. Discovering her loss, she cursed her husband. The men hunted by night, killing phalangers and feeding them to the woman until her jaws ached. At last, she made it up with the hunters and demanded no more meat. 'My grandchildren', she said, 'I was cross over my loss. I took all you hunted. From now on, you may eat the phalangers'. (Lewis 1980: 122–3)

This story connects cooking with the moon, and treats woman's 'ownership' of the moon as enabling her *to compel nocturnally hunting men to get meat for her.* Two points deserve mention: firstly, the menstrual connotations of the moon 'reflected in the red-leeched sago washings' of the woman's vat; secondly, the notion that men's capture of the moon and their trick in over-feeding the woman enabled them for the first time *to eat their own kills.* This recalls men's gaining the flutes which 'needed feeding with meat' in the Mundurucu myth.

It is not intended to dwell individually on each myth, or to detail in any depth its specific cultural context. In terms of their logic, such myths are all sufficiently similar to be dealt with, following Bamberger (1974), as a set.
    If it is accepted that the fisherwoman's Moon in the Gnau myth symbolises womankind's lost ritual power, then it may be said that in all these different narratives, the formula remains the same: first, women possess ritual power; then they lose it to men. It seems clear that the 'flutes', 'bull-

roarers', 'masks' and so on are code terms for something which is naturally to be found in womankind's 'lagoon', 'hut', 'enclosure' or 'vagina'. This can be stolen when Woman abandons her menstrual sex strike – when she loses her ability to 'band together' with her sisters in menstrual seclusion, or (to put matters another way) when she leaves her legs apart or her enclosure unguarded. But when the myths speak of this 'something' which is then stolen, what is it in real life to which they refer? Or to put this another way: Granted that women 'in the beginning' probably did not possess *flutes which played music all by themselves*, is there a more realistic, scientific way of agreeing with the myths that ritual in these cultures nonetheless involves robbing women of something which is or was theirs?

Male Symbolic 'Menstruation'

Let us retrace our steps a little and return to the model of origins which this book has outlined.

Menstrual synchrony may have begun as a biological phenomenon, but – if our argument is accepted – it then took on the form of a cultural construct. This would have made it possible for changes to occur quite rapidly and in biologically 'improbable' ways. For example, once blood had begun to be used to signal 'no!' or taboo, and once sufficient levels of collectivity had been achieved, there would have been nothing to stop one woman from smearing herself with another woman's blood. This second woman, then, would have been 'menstruating' in at least a symbolic sense. She could have kept men away just as effectively. Even pregnant, ovulating or menopausal women could have symbolically 'menstruated' when the need arose. And if this were possible, then further departures from biology could also have been rendered feasible. A blood-symbolised sex strike could have been organised even when no woman was really menstruating at all. In theory, women could have used animal blood, the juices from red berries, red ochre – or any other suitably coloured pigment.

Unfortunately for women, this would have opened up yet a further possibility – the potential for a further radical departure from biology. In principle, men, too, could have 'menstruated'. They could have smeared themselves with some pigment *symbolic* of menstrual blood. Alternatively, they could have used real blood – cutting themselves so as to look as if they were menstruating. And if they could do this as a gender group whilst at the same time preventing women from exercising power by comparable means, they could have wrested ritual power away from women in part by wresting from them its symbols. Men could have organised their own 'sex strike', using their own blood, as an answer to what women had been doing.

The idea sounds fantastic. It seems to defy the imagination that men should ever have needed to do this. Yet in association with the myths just examined there is a body of perplexing ethnographic evidence concerning 'male menstruation' which is consistent with the model and would seem to be explicable in no other way.

Examining myths internally and in terms of their mutual relationships – as Lévi-Strauss does – is insufficient as a method of working out their significance (Hugh-Jones, S. 1979). Myths are acted out in ritual, and serve ideological functions in this context. I now want to show that 'male menstruation' is the secret of our set of matriarchy myths, and that such pseudo-menstruation is a means of robbing women of their actual menstrual power. The evidence is to be found in the ritual dimensions and re-enactments of the Gnau, Méhinaku, Dogon, Wogeo, Gimi and other narratives we have just examined.

Gnau men ritually bleed from their penises, but, when asked whether this is 'like' menstruation, reply: 'No, it is not like menstruation' (Lewis 1980; 2). However, in Méhinaku myth and ritual, there is 'evidence of the mutability of gender. During two ceremonies men shed "menstrual" blood by scarifying their bodies and piercing their ears . . . ' (Gregor 1977: 254). Dogon men circumcise their youths, and, in discussing menstrual blood, the ethnographer's informant Ogotemmêli 'compared this blood with that shed in circumcision' (Griaule 1965: 146).

When a Wogeo Islander (Papua New Guinea) has been dogged by bad hunting luck for a period, he soon begins to suspect the cause: it is an excess of sex. For this weakness there is only one remedy – in effect, a male-organised sex strike. It takes the form of an immediate gashing of the penis to make it bleed and thereby remove the 'impurities' arising from contact with women. 'The salutary effects of penile surgery', Hogbin (1970: 91) writes,

> are said to be immediately observable. The man's body loses its tiredness, his muscles harden, his step quickens, his eyes grow bright, and his skin and hair develop a luster. He therefore feels lighthearted, strong and confident. This belief provides a means whereby the success of all perilous or doubtful undertakings can be guaranteed. Warriors make sure to menstruate before setting out on a raid, traders before carving an overseas canoe or refurbishing its sails, hunters before weaving a new net for trapping pigs.

Here, female menstruation prior to a hunt – as specified in our model – appears to have been almost entirely supplanted by its male-controlled surrogate. The Wogeo hunter's 'technique of male menstruation' involves wading out to the sea with a crayfish or crab's claw, until the water is up to the man's knees:

> He stands there with legs apart and induces an erection . . . When ready he pushes back the foreskin and hacks at the glans, first on the left side,

then on the right. Above all, he must not allow the blood to fall on his fingers or his legs. He waits till the cut has begun to dry and the sea is no longer pink and then walks ashore.

The man then wraps his penis in leaves, returns to the Men's House and stays there for two or three days, sexual intercourse being prohibited until the appearance of the new moon (Hogbin 1970: 88–9).

In discussing the Gimi 'Rule of Women' myth, Gillison (1980: 163) turns to the initiation ritual described in the myth:

> clan elders intern one or two of the men at a time inside a 'menstrual hut' or 'flute house' rapidly constructed in a clearing from palm fronds and wild banana leaves. Inside the hut, an older man applies a tourniquet made of peeled banana stems to the upper arm of the initiate and 'shoots' a protruding vein at the inside of the elbow with a miniature bow and obsidian-tipped arrow. As the blood spurts up . . . the men shout threats at the novice, telling him they will kill him if he reveals the secret they are about to reveal to him.

And what is this secret? It is that the initiate whose blood spurts up is symbolically menstruating. The 'secret' is that men are trying in this way to do artificially what women achieve in another way more easily. The novices, having sworn secrecy, are shown the most sacred flutes, which – although in a certain sense symbolic 'penises' – are penises *of a kind originally owned by women*. When they were owned by women, *they took the form of menstrual blood*. The entire ritual, as Gillison (1980: 164) explains, is 'predicated on the "secret" idea that menstrual blood betokens women's original ownership of the penis'.

The myths of the Gimi assert that menstrual potency *left in women's hands* is deadly and destructive, whilst in men's hands it becomes phallus-like and creative. The initiation rite in the forest is designed to transfer the menstrual power of women and attach it to men. 'The rite', as Gillison (1980: 164–5) puts it,

> implies an equivalence between the penis and the creativity of menstrual blood in this sense: *once menstrual blood is taken away from women (by men who menstruate) its phallic power is 'restored'*. Female attributes that are deadly in women become life-producing when they are detached from women and owned by men. Italics in original.

Let me now say what I think these myths really mean. They are expressions of the fact that in all the societies we have been examining, menstrual synchrony is not – or is no longer – the basic ritual organising principle of social, sexual and economic life. For reasons which have yet to be understood, men have learned to supplant and displace women in synchrony's maintenance. This explains both the rites and the myths.

In short, the 'power' which men 'steal' – stated in the myths to be something to do with women 'banding together' – is that of menstrual synchrony and solidarity. Seen in this light, the myths we have examined lose their far-fetched appearance and turn out to make good sense. They reveal themselves, in fact, as uncannily accurate descriptions of sexual-political reality. Because menstrual blood is believed to be supernaturally dangerous, it can be coded as the source of death-dealing 'witchcraft'. Because the blood is 'wet' and resides in the womb it can be coded as 'fish' in a 'lagoon'. Because the cycle is rhythmical and because women's cycles may be synchronised, in part, through dancing, it can be coded as 'music' or 'dance'. Because it secludes women from their husbands – or, from another standpoint, excludes the husbands themselves – it can be coded as establishing Woman's secret 'Lodge', 'House' or 'Hut', which takes womankind to a world apart. Because blood is brightly coloured and because, while secluded, women are no longer playing the role of wives, it can be coded as a 'mask' or 'paint' which effaces one feminine image and replaces it by another. And because menstruation's cyclicity is or can be seen as lunar, it can be coded as woman's prior ownership of 'the moon'.

To these codings and equivalences we may add that if my hypothesis were correct, we would expect women's power to express itself as a form of solidarity, a 'banding together', associated not only with menstrual huts but also with hunting and the obtaining of male-secured meat. As we have seen, these conditions appear to be met.

My origins model would lead us to predict, finally, that *men should be unable to take over and monopolise ritual power of any kind without learning artificially to 'menstruate'*. This, in the instances we have examined, is the case. The myths explain how men establish the Men's House or ritual Lodge as their political answer to women's 'banding together' in their menstrual huts. As the men's counter-revolution is accomplished, male 'menstrual blood' becomes sacred and life-giving, whilst women's becomes polluting and feared, the first symbolising solidarity and power, the second, isolation and exclusion from power.

In a recently published Baruya (Papua New Guinea) matriarchy myth in the same vein as those just examined, the idea that *men steal the power from a woman's menstrual hut* is spelled out in so many words:

The origin of the sacred flutes
In the days of the Wandjinia [dream-time], the women one day invented flutes. They played them and drew wonderful sounds from them. The men listened and did not know what made the sounds. One day, a man hid to spy on the women and discovered what was making these

melodious sounds. He saw several women, one of whom raised a piece of bamboo to her mouth and drew the sounds that the men had heard. Then the woman hid the bamboo beneath one of her skirts that she had hung in her house, which was a menstrual hut. The women then left. The man drew near, slipped into the hut, searched around, found the flute, and raised it to his lips. He too brought forth the same sounds. Then he put it back and went to tell the other men what he had seen and done. When the woman returned, she took out her flute to play it, but this time the sounds which she drew were ugly. So she threw it away, suspecting that the men had touched it. Later, the man came back, found the flute and played it. Lovely sounds came forth, just like the ones that the woman had made. Since then the flutes have been used to help boys grow.

Note that the stolen flute *had been stored by its owner under her skirt in her menstrual hut*. Maurice Godelier (1986: 70–1), who recorded this story, comments:

> The message of this myth is clear. In the beginning, women were superior to men, but one of the men, violating the fundamental taboo against ever penetrating into the menstrual hut or touching objects soiled with menstrual blood, captured their power and brought it back to men, who now use it to turn little boys into men. But this power stolen from the women is the very one that their vagina contains, the one given to them by their menstrual blood. The old women know the rough outlines of this myth and relate it to young girls when they have their first period.

Such stories, then, describe how men – performing the role of strike-breakers – violate women's menstrual space and solidarity, in effect invading women's menstrual huts so as to secure the symbols of blood sanctity for themselves.

So men gain the 'flutes', 'bull-roarers' and 'lodges' – while women are left to menstruate in their little huts. And in this respect, it is not just that my hypothesis is confirmed within the realm of myth. At this point it is as if the characters in the mythical portraits were refusing to stay within the picture frame, insisting on stepping out into real life. Men as they establish and affirm their ritual solidarity set out deliberately and in often painful ways, firstly, to *isolate* menstruating women (both from one another and from their own male offspring) and, secondly, to *menstruate collectively* (whilst conjoining with their offspring) themselves. In this context it seems clear that there are at stake sexual and political issues so burning as to be uncontainable within the confines of Lévi-Strauss' 'myth-making mind'. These are not light, entertaining narratives through which 'the mind' idly 'communes with itself', free of engagement in the practical, political world (Lévi-Strauss 1970: 10). These are *political* myths which codify men's consciousness of and violent maintenance of their own sexual-political supremacy, a supremacy which can be sustained only through an endless process of vigilant suppression, exploitation and *ideological deception* of the female sex.

I asked earlier what could be the explanation for the extraordinary symbolic details of the extremely widespread set of male mythological fantasies concerning an 'original matriarchy'? My model of cultural origins suggests an answer. Men, it seems, have needed to menstruate in collective ritual performances because 'from the beginning' they have lacked an alternative language in which to express ritual power. In those times and places in which real women's synchrony (for whatever reason) broke down, its collapse seemed to threaten the collapse of culture itself. Since women could not synchronise – or proved unable to prevent men from destroying their synchrony – there were basically two alternatives. Either synchrony was lost, along – perhaps – with culture itself. Or culture-heroic men stepped in with their own artificial 'menstrual cycles' and synchronised those.

Menstrual synchrony is touched on or connoted in all of the traditional myths and associated belief systems I have examined here. Often, what is stressed is the idea of harmony between the menstrual cycle and other cycles of cyclical change and renewal. Two case studies – concerning the Fore of Papua New Guinea and the Barasana of north-west Amazonia – may help us to clarify this aspect of menstrual synchrony as a form of ritual power.

The Fore. Eastern Highlands, Papua New Guinea

The Fore case (Lindenbaum 1976: 56–8) illustrates a number of recurrent features: the link between menstrual cyclicity and wider rhythms of renewal, the threat which men may see in this, the 'political inversion' through which men usurp the symbolic potency of menstruation whilst turning real menstruation into a female curse – and finally, the link in male ideology between mastery over nature and men's dominance over women:

> In a sense, female menstrual cycles provide a physiological regularity, like the annual ripening of the pandanus fruit, which is an ecological given. . . . Yet the order in this case poses a threat, since it is a structure provided by women, not men, a phenomenon Fore and other New Guinea groups attempt to neutralize by male rituals of imitative menstruation . . . letting blood from penis and nose.

In this way, 'a political inversion is accomplished; menstruation is dirty and demeaning for women, strengthening and purifying for men'.

Women's own menstruation, given this political inversion, becomes a perpetual suppressed threat. But it is not the only threat: it becomes symbolic of a general threat felt to be posed by nature and the forces of the wild. 'There is a sense of a universe under constraint, of predatory forces purposefully brought under masculine control.' Only with difficulty is mastery of the animal world upheld: myths allow of the possibility that animals might once have gained the upper hand.

But the most precarious victory of all concerns the ownership of the sacred flutes, said to have been once in the hands of women. While the flute myths, stories of male trickery and violence, are myths about the subjugation of women, they are also embryonic statements in the history of the battle of men to control women's bodies. As one Fore man observed: 'Women's menstruation has always been present; men's bleeding, that came later'. (Lindenbaum 1976: 56–8)

The Barasana. North-west Amazonia.

The Barasana case illustrates many of the themes of the preceding discussion; it is particularly valuable for stressing the link between menstrual onset and the onset of the annual rains – a recurrent cross-cultural theme. It is also worth noting how the fairy-tale motif of 'skin-changing' is interwoven with other images of cyclical change.

The initiation-rite known as *He* House is a rite of artificial male collectively synchronised 'metaphorical menstruation' designed to help bring on the rains, which are a 'skin of the universe'. It occurs 'at a time of cosmic skin-change', the time of the onset of the annual rains (Hugh-Jones, C. 1979: 153). Rain, besides being a 'skin', is also the menstrual flow of the most important of all ancestral beings, Woman Shaman, from whom all contemporary shamanic powers derive (p. 156; see also S. Hugh-Jones 1979: 100).

During *He* House, the men apply to their bodies red paint, which 'is identified with menstrual blood' (Hugh-Jones, S. 1979: 184). No woman is allowed to touch this paint; if she does, she 'will immediately start to menstruate; the blood which flows is this paint' (Hugh-Jones, S. 1979: 76). The ritual involves men 'giving birth': in order to do this, they 'must first be opened up and made to menstruate' (p. 132). The boys who are to be newly 'born' must first be put back into a 'womb': they are said to be swallowed by an anaconda (p. 218) and returned to the condition of foetuses (p. 77). This condition is compared to that of 'crabs and other animals that have shed their old shells or skins' (p. 120). *He* House brings about rebirth; it is 'believed to bring about a change of skin' (p. 120), both of the initiates and of the universe, the process being 'associated with the moon' (Hugh-Jones, C. 1979: 156) and modelled on women's menstruation, which 'is an internal changing of skin' (Hugh-Jones, S. 1979: 183).

Women are excluded from the *He* rites, despite (or more accurately because of) being 'naturally' closer to the *He* world then men (Hugh-Jones, S. 1979: 251). The myths tell of how men seized the sacred *He* instruments from Woman Shaman, and punished her and her kind by causing female menstruation (Hugh-Jones, S. 1979: 266). The most coveted object which men tried to steal was a life-giving gourd. However, they were able to gain only an artificial replica of this. Woman Shaman kept and still keeps in her possession the true gourd: it was her vagina, which alone confers real immortality. Men admit that their attempts to achieve rebirth and immortality through the artificial gourd and other paraphernalia are somehow 'false'. 'We were told directly', writes Christine Hugh-Jones (p. 154), 'that *He wi* [*He* house] is like women's menstruation, but that women really do menstruate while *He wi* is *bahi kesoase*, imitation'. Or, as the women say: 'The men make as if they too create children but it's like a lie' (Hugh-Jones, S. 1979: 222).

The magical powers of menstruation, then, derive in part from the blood's perceived connection with wider rhythms of social and cosmic renewal. It is this connectedness – 'harmony' and 'synchrony' are alternative terms – which men appear to envy and attempt to duplicate by artificial means.

Throughout the world, men's 'menstrual periods' were difficult to produce and often, as in much of Australia, involved operations causing intense pain (Gould 1969: 112). On the other hand, provided men were prepared to cut themselves in the requisite way, it would seem that the resultant blood flows had one distinct advantage over women's. Synchrony could be achieved without hormones, without pheromones or without need for the subtle effects of weak nocturnal light. Men could make the blood flow by a mere act of will – simply by cutting themselves at the appropriate times.

All the myths we have been examining make sense in this light. The ideological function of the myth of matriarchy is certainly, as Bamberger (1974) says, to justify 'men's rule'. But it does this by legitimising the otherwise inexplicable and certainly unnatural fact that today men 'menstruate' in order to exert ritual power. The widespread recurrence of seemingly conspiratorial secret male initiation rites testifies to this process. All such rites involve male self-mutilation and/or bleeding as an 'answer' to women's more natural blood-making and reproductive powers. All such rites involve men 'giving birth' to their own kind on the grounds that women cannot do it in accordance with the proper rhythms or in the ritually correct way. The myth of matriarchy in its countless versions legitimises this male sexual-political counter-revolution in pseudo-historical terms, constantly reiterating, as Bamberger (1974: 280) puts it, that 'women did not know how to handle power when they had it'. Women did not know how to handle menstrual potency when they had it, and so men have had to appropriate it for themselves.

Ochre in Prehistory

Radio-carbon dating of human blood discovered in red pigments drawn on ice age rock surfaces in Australia – particularly in Laurie Creek in the Wingate Mountains, Northern Territory (see references in Bahn 1990) – has revealed many of these paintings to be among the world's earliest – some of them more than 20,000 years old. Where traces of this kind exist, archaeology may help add to our understanding of the mythological patterns we have examined and the historical processes which gave rise to them.

Ochre is an ill-defined term referring to various natural rocks and clays, most of them containing iron and usually of reddish colour but varying from pale yellow to deep orange or brown. Indications of ochre's use as a pigment have been found at archaeological sites dating back – according to some claims – to as early as 250,000 years ago. Although it was once argued that *Homo erectus* at still earlier dates regularly used ochre pigments, most of these claims are now discounted (Butzer 1980). Some Neanderthal groups may have begun to use ochre in burials and for ritual purposes, but there is good evidence for this only from about 70,000 years ago.

It is not until the emergence of the Upper Palaeolithic that crayons, painted bones, shells and other ochred objects become abundant, although it appears that even as recently as 30,000 to 35,000 years ago many communities may not have been ochre users. One writer has pointed out that most prehistoric burials are in fact without ochre (Wreschner 1980: 632). However, this does not mean that such communities used no pigments. Many of the colorants used in the past – whether for treating skins, for body-painting or for other purposes – would have been biodegradable substances such as berry juices and extracts of roots, bark, leaves and so on. We tend to concentrate on 'ochre' simply because it has survived in the archaeological record.

It was noted in Chapter 9 that when modern humans first spread across Europe between 40,000 and 32,000 years ago, it was on the basis of a tradition known as the Aurignacian. It is worth quoting the French prehistorian André Leroi-Gourhan (1968: 40) as he comments on one striking characteristic of this earliest modern pan-European tradition:

> The use of ocher is particularly intensive: it is not unusual to find a layer of the cave floor impregnated with a purplish red to a depth of eight inches. The size of these ocher deposits raises a problem not yet solved. The colouring is so intense that practically all the loose ground seems to consist of ocher. One can imagine that with it the Aurignacians regularly painted their bodies red, dyed their animal skins, coated their weapons, and sprinkled the ground of their dwellings, and that a paste of ocher was used for decorative purposes in every other phase of their domestic life. We must assume no less, if we are to account for the veritable mines of ocher on which some of them lived. . . .

Later in the Upper Palaeolithic, graves were richly ochred and whole caves painted red – suggesting, as one writer has put it, 'the magic making of life deep in the earth, as though in the menstruous womb of a woman' (La Barre 1972: 395).

Leroi-Gourhan, in the passage on ochre use just quoted, is referring only to the Aurignacian peoples of Western Europe and particularly France. But in European Russia and in Siberia, comparable patterns are found. Quantities of ochre have been recorded at many sites; for example, about 10 kg was found in a dwelling made of mammoth-bones at Mezin in the Ukraine. It was also used in quantity in many burials. Paint made from mixing ochre with other materials was widely used. Mammoth-bones from Mezin were painted with red-ochred lines and zigzags; at Kapova Cave, similar paint was used to outline representations of animals. Colouring materials, usually ochre, may also have been used in dressing skins, as is suggested by ochre traces on bone burnishers. Richard Klein (1969: 226) in a survey of Soviet archaelogists' work writes of the 'extraordinarily large amount of red ochre found in many of the Kostenki-Borshevo sites'; these are the sites discussed earlier (see pp. 322–4), many of which indicate collective living in large dwellings, with female figurines buried in pits in the floor.

Views on the significance of ochre are basically of two kinds. First, there are the 'symbolic' interpretations, typically seeing ochre as meaning 'ritual potency', 'danger' or 'life blood', its use in burials being interpreted as an attempt to establish the grave's sanctity, to deny the finality of death or to ensure resurrection. Secondly, there are those sceptics who question all such speculations and who believe that ochre may have had some much more prosaic, utilitarian significance, any ritual or symbolic connotations being secondary.

A representative of the first school of thought is Ernst Wreschner, a palaeoanthropologist at the University of Haifa who has made a special study of the whole subject. Wreschner (1980) freely uses ethnographic analogies in his speculations on the prehistoric significance of ochre.

The symbolic systems of Upper Palaeolithic hunters, Wreschner writes (1980: 632), 'seem to revolve around fertility and procreation, death-life, and the cycle of the seasons'. In recent nonliterate societies, he continues, 'red is closely connected with reproduction, with "mothers", with blood, and with rituals and symbolism related to life and death'. In Central African Ndembu rites of the river source, according to Wreschner, red clay represents the blood of the 'mother' (1980: 633, citing Turner 1969: 53–69). The relationship between ochre, blood and 'mothers', continues Wreschner, 'is signified by the Greek *haemal haima* (as in haematite), which means "blood"', and is related to the basic Indo-European root MA which means 'mother'. Citing the Africanist Victor Turner (1967: 172), Wreschner observes that 'the womb is in many cultures equated with the tomb and both associated with the earth, the source of fruits. It is believed that ores grow inside the earth like an embryo in the womb.'

Finally, Wreschner (1980: 633) mentions prehistoric burials on the island of Malta – burials in which the corpses were not only heavily ochred but provided with bowls of additional ochre set alongside them. 'The placing of a bowl of ochre in the grave', comments Wreschner,

> recalls the Maori legend of the woman who went to the netherworld and
> found there a bowl of red ochre; she ate the ochre, became strong again,
> and was restored to life.

In a commentary on Wreschner's 1980 article, Bolton (1980: 634) notes the
salience of red as a colour-term in folk-tales from all over the world, and
comments that cross-culturally, 'red connotes potency more than any other
colour does'. Bolton suggests that red colouring was used by prehistoric
peoples in their mortuary rituals in order to express 'defiance of death'.

    However, there is another view. Most prehistorians believe that Middle
and Upper Palaeolithic peoples often ochred bones, corpses and also living
bodies, but the cave-art specialist Paul Bahn (Bahn and Vertut 1988:
69–70) argues that even if we accept this consensus, the practice may have
been functional and utilitarian rather than ritual/symbolic. Ochre, notes
Bahn, can be used in cauterising and cleaning injuries, in warding off the
effects of cold and rain, and as a protection against mosquitoes, flies and
other disease-carriers. Moreover, ochre is useful in the treatment of animal
skins because it preserves organic tissues, protecting them from putrefaction
and from vermin such as maggots. 'It is probably this kind of function', he
writes of the European Upper Palaeolithic data, 'which explains the impregnated soil in some habitation sites and the traces of red mineral on many
stone tools such as scrapers'. Similarly, he continues (citing Audouin and
Plisson 1982), 'red pigment may have been applied to corpses not so much
out of pious beliefs about life-blood, as is commonly assumed . . . but rather
to neutralise odours and help to preserve the body'.

The many theories resting on a utilitarian function for ochre use may seem
healthily sceptical and sober, but ultimately they fail to satisfy our curiosity. Such narrowly functionalist-utilitarian arguments would seem to rob
early humans of ritual or aesthetic sensibilities. Those who argue along such
lines make evidence for ochre use seem unconnected with the origins of art,
ritualism, personal adornment or symbolic culture more generally. Ochre, it
is said, was used by this group to ward off mosquitoes, or by that one to keep
away the maggots. This whole approach is surely undermined by the
evidence that as ochre use intensifies, it is found in archaeological deposits
which also testify to a sudden flowering of interest in pierced shells, teeth
and other objects clearly intended as personal adornments (White 1989a,
1989b; Wreschner 1980: 632; Masset 1980: 639).

    Beyond this, it seems odd that a variety of chemically different clays
sharing little more than the fact that they are reddish-coloured (Butzer 1980)
should turn out to be equally good at repelling mosquitoes, neutralising
odours or cauterising wounds. What is it about redness which has such

consistent chemical effects?

Finally, the utilitarian, anti-symbolic approach shares with its symbolic counterpart a basic weakness. Each camp's arguments seem ultimately aimless and anecdotal, failing to engage effectively with any wider context of evolutionary or palaeoanthropological theory. In contrast to the study of tools, discussions concerning the significance of ochre have unfortunately remained a backwater of palaeoanthropological debate.

The model of origins presented in this book has a ready-made theoretical place for ochre. This is because it has a place for the symbolism of blood. The term 'ochre' is in fact almost meaningless, since it has been used by archaeologists to describe a wide variety of ferruginised shales or sandstones, haematitic or limonic concretions and pastes made from sesquioxide-rich clayey or sandy soils (Butzer 1980). Just about the only thing held in common by these variegated soils, clays, pastes, sands and rocks is the fact that they are orange, reddish or brown in colour – or can be made so by heating them to a high enough temperature. It is the colour category, then, which seems significant – not the precise chemical composition, which may vary from place to place.

Our model of cultural origins would lead us to expect a certain extremely ancient cultural attitude towards redness. Early kinship coalitions should have valued blood as a means of signifying their shared identity and power, while menstrual blood in particular should have signified a state of ritual sanctity or inviolability ('protection from evil spirits'). Women who were covered in blood should have regarded themselves as shielded from sexual violation or other harm by the symbolic effects (conceptualised, we might suppose, as 'the magic') of this blood.

From this, we might go on to predict that evolving humans in diverse circumstances would have experimented with symbolic elaborations on the theme. On occasion, coalitions may have had no menstrual blood, or they may have had to make a small amount go a long way. After all, as earlier noted, women may have been pregnant or nursing for much of the time, and for this and other reasons menstruation may, on a physiological level, have been quite a rare event. Studies have shown that menstrual flows can be sparse and infrequent in contemporary hunter-gatherer and other non-western cultures, particularly where nutrition is poor (Harrell 1981). The implication is that even though the evolving human female may have been losing more blood than any primate female had done before, it was still not always enough to serve the sex strike's symbolic purposes.

Of course, women could have insisted that even the most microscopic speck of blood could still pollute a man who violated their space, or that even a single menstruant amidst a hundred women sufficed to pollute/protect them all. Women might well have discovered the value of exaggerating such things almost indefinitely – until it was established that blood could pollute a man 'magically' even when it was totally invisible to anyone. The mere fact that the moon was dark or in the culturally 'correct' phase for menstrual bleeding (Lamp 1988; Buckley 1988) could also have been taken as sufficient. Certainly, there is enough ethnographic evidence for this kind of thing – evidence to suggest that by magnifying the imagined powers of eclipses or the supernatural dangers of menstrual blood, cultures have allowed miniscule or even non-existent quantities of the real substance to serve virtually unlimited ritual and symbolic purposes. Indeed, this is a useful aspect of the model: it helps to explain why eclipses should be so greatly feared (Lévi-Strauss 1970: 298) and why menstrual blood should be regarded in cultural traditions as so 'contagious' in its magical effects (Briffault 1927, 2; Delaney et al. 1977; Buckley and Gottlieb 1988). The cultural construct of 'contagiousness' is simply a means of making meagre quantities of menstrual blood go a very long way.

But despite this, it is reasonable to suppose that on many occasions, humans would have experienced the need to make visible the source of the 'magic'. The strike itself may have seemed in this context somewhat demanding of blood. If my hypothesis were correct, we might expect cultures to have evolved artifices serving to amplify the visual impact of women's blood. Real menstrual blood dries, flakes and turns almost black rather than red within a few hours. If women wanted to declare themselves defiantly 'powerful' for longer and longer periods, and wanted to express this in some visually unmistakable way, they may well have felt the need to augment their blood with something which stayed red for longer and did not quickly flake. Could red juices, ochre, or mixtures of ochre with blood and/or animal fat, have fulfilled such a function? And – assuming that this is accepted as a theoretical possibility – is there any way of testing this idea?

As anatomically modern humans moved into Western, Central and Eastern Europe, we witness 'a rapid spread of ochre customs' (Wreschner 1980: 632). Over a hundred ochre-bearing sites have been excavated, including twenty-five ochre burials, spanning the whole Upper Palaeolithic period (Wreschner 1980: 632). As the first modern humans spread across the globe, Australia was reached remarkably early, and it is intriguing to discover that here, too – as was later to happen when the first humans penetrated into North America (Wreschner 1980: 633) – the very first immigrant waves apparently shared traditions in which ochre was of central importance.

The Australian evidence is particularly interesting. In 1968, the geomorphologist Jim Bowler was attempting to establish the pattern of climatic change over the last 100,000 years in western New South Wales when he uncovered some burnt human bones, hearths and tools dated to about 26,000 years ago. There was also a quantity of ochre in pellets, which must have been brought from at least 10 km away. The context was a ritual cremation of a woman. In 1974, Bowler discovered a skeleton of a tall man who had been laid in a shallow grave on his side with his hands clasped. 'The bones and surrounding sand were stained pink; the pink colour, derived from ochre powder that had been scattered over the corpse, clearly defined the size and shape of the grave' (Flood 1983: 46). This burial took place about 30,000 years ago. Both these finds of ochre were made close to the edge of what used to be a large lake – Lake Mungo.

In fact, at Mungo red pigment was in use still earlier, for lumps of ochre and stone artefacts were found deep below the ashes of a fire lit 32,000 years ago. Similar lumps of pigment, some showing signs of use, have been found in Pleistocene levels in other sites – such as Kenniff Cave in Queensland, Cloggs Cave in Victoria, Miriwun in Western Australia and several rock shelters in Arnhem land. Ochre 'pencils' with traces of wear have been found in layers in Arnhem Land, in northern Australia, dating to 18,000 and 19,000 years ago, and perhaps even 30,000 (Bahn in Bahn and Vertut 1988: 29, citing Chaloupka 1984; Murray and Chaloupka 1983–4).

What makes this Australian evidence particularly interesting is not only its extreme antiquity. It is the fact that contemporary Aboriginal attitudes to ochre can assist us in interpreting these archaeological finds.

We have no way of knowing what red ochre meant to the prehistoric Australian Aborigines who used it. Contemporary Aborigines associate it with blood. Whilst this may not be a universal association, it is extremely common; it is also not unusual for the association to be *specifically with that most ritually potent of all categories of blood – menstrual blood*.

Sometimes, as we will now see, myths which explain the origin of much-valued ochre deposits tell of matriarchal ancestral power, all-female forms of solidarity – and explicit menstrual synchrony. Groups of mythological women are said to have danced or practised ceremonies together, synchronised their periods as a result – and from their blood produced the ochre which is now mined for use in ceremonies.

Blood, Ochre and Ritual Power in Aboriginal Australia

'The deposits of red ochre which are found in various parts of the country', write Spencer and Gillen (1899: 463–4) in their classic account of Aboriginal Central Australia,

> are associated with women's blood. Near the Stuart's Hole, on the Finke River, there is a red ochre pit which has evidently been used for a long time; and tradition says that in the Alcheringa two kangaroo women came from Ilpilla, and at this spot caused blood to flow from the vulva in large quantities, and so formed the deposit of red ochre. Travelling away

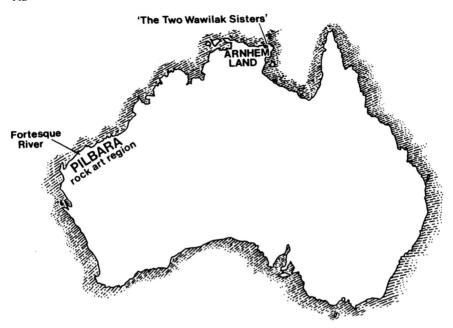

Figure 18 Map of Australia. Rock-engravings from the Pilbara region (see Figs 19, 21) often depict pairs of dancing women reminiscent of the heroines of the Wawilak myth recorded half a continent away. Little is known of the engravings' meanings, but at Pirina, some fifty miles upstream along the Fortesque River, rock-art specialist Bruce Wright (1968: 25) followed his Aboriginal guides as they looked among rocks in the flowing water, 'searching for certain eroded marks which they had been told had ritual significance'. They later showed Wright 'a circular mark, said to represent the moon, and a slightly raised natural platform, said to have been worn smooth by the dancing feet of the girls participating in the ceremonies'.

westward they did the same thing in other places.

In much the same way, again in Central Australia,

> it is related of the dancing Unthippa women that, at a place called Wankima, in the eastern part of the Arunta district, they were so exhausted with dancing that their organs fell out, and gave rise to the large deposits of red ochre found there. (Spencer and Gillen 1899: 463–4)

Myths and rock-art images from other parts of Australia repeat such motifs with some insistence. In the Pilbara region of Western Australia, a number of rock-engravings appear to show women who are dancing together, usually in pairs, simultaneously shedding what looks like menstrual blood and, in some instances, becoming conjoined or encircled by the consequent flows (figures 18, 19, 21). We will examine a well-known Arnhem Land myth in a similar vein – the Yolngu people's story of the synchronously menstruating Two Wawilak Sisters – in Chapter 13.

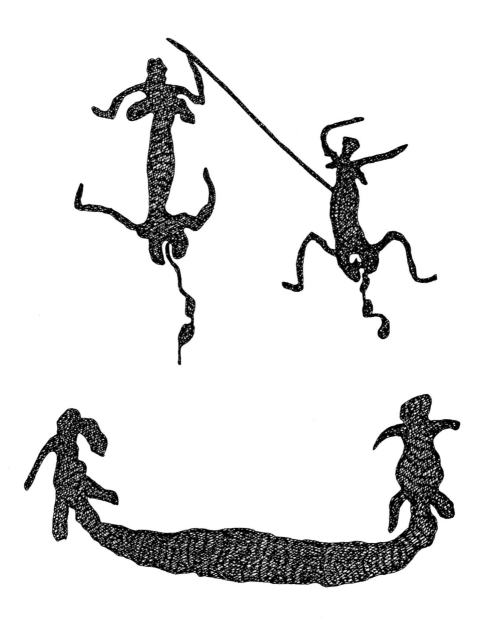

Figure 19 Pilbara rock-engravings. Age uncertain but probably recent. *Top*: Upper Yule River. Figures dancing, with vaginal flows. *Bottom*: Cape Lambert. One of many Pilbara scenes of figures linked by genital streams. Here, both figures may be female and the stream conjoining them a shared menstrual flow (redrawn after Wright 1968: Figs 112, 845).

There are further echoes of such themes in myths and songs concerning the awesomely powerful ancestral *alknarintja* women of Central Australia:

> They are menstruating.
> Their flanks are wet with blood.
> They talk to each other.
> They make a bull-roarer. . . .
> They are menstruating.
> The blood is perpetually flowing. (Róheim 1974: 138–9)

In any Aranda myth, an *alknarintja* may be recognised by the fact that she is constantly decorating herself with red ochre, is associated with water and is 'frequently represented as menstruating copiously' (Róheim 1974: 150). Such women are 'like men' in that they possess bull-roarers and other symbols of primordial, culture-creating power – power which is nowadays reserved for men. They also have solidarity – evoked in one song through the image of a clump of bushes 'so thick and so pressed against each other that they cannot move separately' (Róheim 1974: 144).

The central Australian *alknarintja* women, while not characterised as on 'sex strike', are known as 'women who refuse men'. The name *alknarintja* means, in fact, 'eyes-turn-away'. From another song come these lines:

> They say, 'I won't go with you'.
> 'I will remain an *alknarintja*'.
> They whirl their bull-roarers.
> They stay where they are. They sit very still.
> The man wants them to say, 'I will go with you'.
> But they remain where they are. (Róheim 1974: 141–2)

Interestingly, an informant told Róheim (1974: 122–3) that 'all women become *alknarintja* when they are very small, i.e. they begin with an attitude of avoiding men'; it is only in later life that the 'resistance' of young women is broken and they lose their 'original' power.

Arnhem Land: Ochre, Blood and Dance

In north-east Arnhem Land, among the Yolngu (formerly known as the Murngin), menstrual synchrony is an acknowledged ritually potent possibility. Women tend to seclude themselves in groups, and among their pastimes on such occasions is the making of string-figures or 'cats' cradles' (as they are termed in English). Men are not supposed to see these. At Yirrkalla, such string-figures depict many things – particularly game animals, but also female reproductive events such as 'birth of a baby'. One conventional subject for a string-figure is 'menstrual blood of three women' (figure 20). Ethnographic reports do not explicitly document menstrual synchrony, but 'menstrual blood of three women' is surely not a conventional topic which

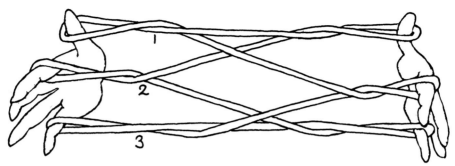

Figure 20   Yolngu (north-east Arnhem Land) women's string-figure: 'Menstrual blood of three women' (redrawn after McCarthy 1960: 466). An associated myth states that string-figures were invented by Two Sisters who in a ritual act 'sat down, looking at each other, with their feet out and legs apart, and both menstruated'. They then put string loops made of one another's menstrual blood around their necks. Note how this concept of genitally derived, all-encircling 'loops' finds apparent echoes in the Pilbara images shown in Figures 19 and 21.

would occur to women unless they were familiar with this potentiality (McCarthy 1960: 466).

Numerous myths from the region confirm the apparent ordinariness of synchrony, including a story which explains the 'origin of string-figures' themselves. According to this myth, Two Sisters invented string when they went on a long journey. Towards the end of this, they 'sat down, looking at each other, with their feet out and legs apart, and both menstruated'. The story identifies 'string' as inseparable from these sisters' menstrual flows. Having sat down and bled together, the women continued with their ritual: 'Each one made a loop of the other one's menstrual blood, after which they put the string loops around their necks.' This led to their being 'swallowed by a Snake' (McCarthy 1960: 426). Certain of Wright's (1968) rock-engravings – despite coming from a very different part of Australia – suggest women's or kinship-groups' encirclement by 'loops' of menstrual blood (figure 21).

Other myths from northern Australia feature various water-loving 'daughters of the Rainbow' or 'daughters of the Rainbow-Snake', such as the 'Mungamunga' girls. In one song from the Na:ra, a man called Banangala 'comes over and wants to copulate with the Mungamunga, but they are menstruating. They each say to him, "I've got blood: you wait for a while"' (Berndt 1951: 164). Another song from the same area concerns two men who encounter a group of Mungamunga by a lagoon: 'No sooner do they seize a Mungamunga and put her on the ground, ready for coitus, than she slides away, jumps up and runs down to the lagoon, and dives into its water; then she emerges and joins the rest' (Berndt 1951: 174). These women, then, have two ways of avoiding sex with a man: menstruating, or 'diving into the water'.

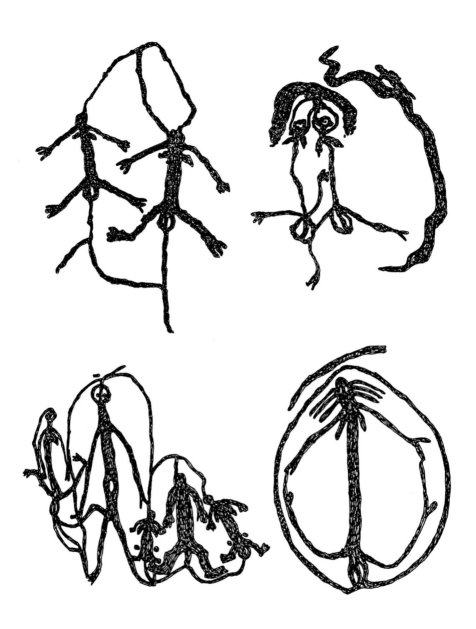

Figure 21 Pilbara rock-art (Upper Yule River). *Upper left*: dancing, genitally linked females (Wright 1968: Fig. 105). *Right*: similar scene; linking streams absent, possibly replaced by overarching shared ritual ornament (rainbow?) and nearby snake (Wright 1968: Fig. 383). *Lower left*: three females, two males, all genitally connected (Wright 1968: Fig. 11). If this echoes previous themes, these figures are linked not maritally but as blood kin, the streams denoting blood potency as a source of within-group oneness and ritual status. *Lower right*: female encircled by her own flow (Wright 1968: Fig. 85; all figures redrawn).

All over northern Australia, when mythological women in groups 'dive into the water' to escape a man, it is clear that menstrual solidarity is the logic at the basis of the motif. The Alawa Aborigines of western-central Arnhem Land say that on entering the water, the Mungamunga girls become merged in the corporate identity of their 'Mother', the 'Kadjari'. They only recover their separate identities once again when this Mother figure emerges from the water and 'stands on the dry land' (Berndt 1951: 189–90).

Since 'entering the water' or menstruating is a kind of 'death' to marital life, it can be used symbolically to stand for other kinds of death. This is a positive, immensely hopeful symbolic equation, since menstrual bleeding leading to 'death' is for a woman not permanent. It is followed quickly by her emergence from seclusion – a kind of 'resurrection'.

Mortuary ritual among the Yolngu involves painting the corpse with red ochre. Howard Morphy (1977: 318) explains the symbolism of this: 'the red ochre painted on the body during mortuary ceremonies is said to be (or to signify) the menstrual blood of female clan ancestors'. As if to accentuate this symbolism, women during the period of mourning cut their heads so as to bleed. The resulting blood – like the ochre on the body itself – is symbolic of menstrual blood (Morphy 1977: 318).

This and other evidence shows how mortuary ritualism among the Yolngu is assimilated to menstruation and a 'return to the womb'. The flowing of 'menstrual' blood and the red-painting of the corpse both help to make this point. We can appreciate how all this helps to soften the impact of death. Menstrual bleeding is known to be only a 'temporary death' – like that of the moon each month. Similarly, if the grave is 'blood-filled' – if one is inside a womb rather than just dead and in the ground – birth or 'rebirth' is the inevitable next stage.

Recalling my survey of ochre use in ice age burials, it seems significant that so many Aboriginal ceremonies are 'birth' or 'rebirth' rituals which can also be used to bury the dead. Time in the Aboriginal view is cyclical and therefore ultimately reversible; birth and death are seen in ritual terms as cyclical transformations and inversions of one another. Each presupposes the other, and therefore the same rites apply. As Morphy (1984: 31) puts it, most Aboriginal rituals 'concern both initiation and fertility, the living, and the dead, and contain themes and events which cut across myth, moiety and context'.

In one Arnhem Land group, the Gunwinggu, the *lorgun* is a combined circumcision and mortuary ritual; it 'is held when the moon is waning', its basic myth telling of how the Moon decided to die and come alive again, whereas a certain Pigeon-man foolishly ignored the Moon, deciding to die and stay dead – thereby for the first time introducing to humanity the calamity of non-lunar (i.e. non-reversible) death (Berndt and Berndt 1970: 133). Versions of this myth are known all over Australia (Knight 1985), as indeed over much of Africa and the world. Their sad message to humanity is that if only we had known how to listen properly to the Moon, we might have retained the secret of its immortality to this very day.

I have cited some evidence linking Aborigines' traditional use of ochre with menstrual symbolism. Admittedly, not all female ancestral beings in Aboriginal mythology are depicted as synchronously menstruating, not all red body-paint is symbolic menstrual blood, and not every traditionally used ochre deposit in Australia is linked in myths explicitly with such blood. Yet such themes are common, and the fact that ochre *can* be conceptualised in this way has obvious significance for the argument of this book. The theory that ochre is in the first instance a substitute for human blood has – over all other theories – the additional advantage of simplicity. The model of cultural origins presented here does not require us to assume some additional factor in order to explain why early Australians were using blood-like substances to cover corpses or as body-paint. Given menstrual synchrony, and given women's need to mark themselves strongly with blood – perhaps often having to make a little blood go a long way – the logical principle behind the use of ochre in body-painting is already accounted for.

Chapter 13
The Rainbow Snake

It is, in reality, much easier to discover by analysis the earthly core of the misty creations of religion, than, conversely, it is, to develop from the actual relations of life the corresponding celestialized forms of those relations. The latter method is the only materialistic, and therefore the only scientific one.

Karl Marx, *Capital* (1887)

In Australia as elsewhere, the end of the ice age brought with it a wave of extinctions of the very large game animals on which hunters had probably to an extent depended since the earliest occupation of the continent. The giant marsupials, Flood (1983: 147) points out, would have been relatively slow-moving, vulnerable to human hunters until they had learned to adopt defensive strategies. It may be significant that in the areas where the earliest occupation has been found, such as the Willandra Lakes and Perth region, the megafauna apparently disappeared earliest. Megafauna are absent from both Koonalda and Allen's Caves on the Nullarbor Plain. Since occupation of these caves had begun by at least 20,000 years ago, the megafauna may already have been extinct in this arid region by that time.

Those giant creatures that survived the initial impact of man the hunter, continues Flood (1983: 147), seem to have met their end during the Great Dry at the end of the Pleistocene. Because of their size, all of these animals would have needed to drink copiously at waterholes, and would have died of thirst as the lakes and other water sources dried up (Flood 1983: 155–261, citing Gillespie *et al.* 1978; Horton 1976, 1979; Horton and Wright 1981). Some – such as the red kangaroo – managed to adapt. Others escaped extinction by evolving to smaller sizes. The rest died out completely. The period from about 25,000 to 15,000 years ago was a time of stress: stress from diminishing water supplies, from desiccation and the loss of vegetation, and – perhaps most significantly – from the fires and hunting activities of human predators (Merrilees 1968). Most of the very large animals appear to have become extinct as early as 20,000 years ago. Wooded areas near the coast probably acted as refuges, which would account for the large animals' apparent survival there longer than in the arid inland regions.

Humans arrived in Australia somewhere between 40,000 and 50,000 years ago, probably at first keeping to coastal regions and river valleys but penetrating long before the end of the ice age into every major ecological zone including the extremely arid centre (Smith 1987). It would be an oversimplification to assert that the earliest modern human intruders into Australia made straight for the very largest game animals and drove them to extinction, although this theory has been vigorously proposed (Martin and Wright 1967; Merrilees 1968). In almost all of the hundreds of archaeological sites known in Australia, the bones of small animals predominate markedly (Flood 1983: 155). As suggested earlier (Chapter 8), it seems probable that the earliest migrants were adapted to shoreline riverine foraging concentrating on fish, aquatic or other plants and small-to-medium-sized game, and that specialized big game hunting within the more arid interior regions did not develop until later. Women with their gathered resources may at first have been relatively autonomous; from earliest times, menstrual synchrony in many regions could have been directly related to the pull of the moon through the tides.

Although neither large collective groups nor a specific focus on hunting megafauna can be documented archaeologically, nevertheless some sites — such as the so-called 'Mammoth Cave' in Western Australia — do show evidence of what seems to be the deliberate breaking, cutting and burning by humans of megafaunal bones over 37,000 years ago (Flood 1983: 154, citing Archer et al. 1980). And even if humans in most regions were never primarily reliant on megafauna for their food, human activities may still have altered the ecosystem in unfavourable directions precipitating major social changes as relative scarcity ensued.

Humans' use of fire in grass-burning and in driving game almost certainly had profound consequences. Despite the value of light burning once the vegetation had adapted (Hallam 1975), fires would often have got out of control, raging over vast areas during dry periods. It was this which must have led to the relatively recent supplanting of fire-sensitive shrubs and trees by fire-resistant eucalypts over much of the continent. The early giant marsupials were browsers, needing large quantities of foliage, and it seems likely that many of the trees and plants they ate were drastically reduced by human use of the fire-stick. In addition to the consequences for megafauna, the effects on all game as well as on other resources may have been quite severe.

In any event, for whatever reasons, we know that in many regions desiccation occurred, numerous inland lakes and river systems dried up — and formerly lush rain forests, woodlands and grasslands turned to almost barren deserts. As hunting conditions changed and in many regions became more difficult, humans would have had to adapt.

It would be beyond the scope of the present work to trace the global consequences for menstrual synchrony of the ecological and other changes associated with the ending of the last ice age. Even were we to limit ourselves to Australia, much research would be needed to document the relation between the extinctions and other processes just touched upon and the origins model which has been proposed. However, if the argument for menstrual synchrony in ritual traditions is accepted, we can take it that the Aborigines' myths are in essence correct. Women once manifested synchrony, and then lost it. Whether this loss occurred recently, at some time during the glacial period or even – as is theoretically possible – prior to the earliest Australians' arrival in the continent is not a question that has previously been asked, and so any answers suggested here can only be tentative. But it seems likely that wherever game became scarce, the temptation would have been to chase after prey animals whenever they were encountered – regardless of what women or the moon were doing. Women, moreover, may have been forced to disperse for much of each year in relatively small, loosely organised bands or family units, isolated from one another as they attempted to maximise their foraging success by covering wide areas. And then, as spatial distances meant that synchrony of the old kind was partially or seasonally lost, people would have found it more and more difficult to preserve intact the ancient blood-encoded system of life-preserving cultural rules.

The Rule of Men

With women's solidarity for economic reasons declining, it may have become increasingly difficult to prevent male power from supplanting it in its cultural functions. Sexism alone would not be an adequate explanation here. Whilst men's mythological allegations concerning primordial female wrongs were no doubt politically motivated, it may have been true that women were unable to maintain sufficient synchrony under conditions of relative scarcity, and that without male intervention to sustain synchrony on another level, all ritual structure would simply have been lost. It would certainly seem that throughout Aboriginal Australia, if ritual traditions have been preserved across the millennia, this is thanks not only to women's own commitment (Bell 1983) but also to the extraordinary resolve of initiated men who knew the immensity of the responsibilities placed upon them. Jealous guardians and custodians of their cultural DNA, these men knew that in accordance with some mysterious primordial design, women's world-creating secrets had been placed in their trust. They did not betray this trust. It is thanks to this fact that anthropology, palaeoanthropology and – through such sciences – knowledge-seeking humanity as a whole can make contact with such traditions today.

Yet on another level there was political deception and manipulation –

however unavoidable this may have been. Women not only lost power, it was actively taken from them. An open male counter-revolution – a blatant violation of women's menstrual space – would have been difficult to impose. Naked licence to violate sacred taboos would have risked the destruction of all order as society became threatened with incest, violent conflict and rape. But if men could progressively subvert and usurp women's power through the use of women's own sexual-political symbols, preserving women's blood sanctity even whilst detaching its creativity from women's own bodies, success might have been achieved. Men could turn the symbolic potency of menstruation into a force opposed to women themselves. They could override women's real, physical menstrual solidarity and yet preserve it on an abstract structural level. In short, the whole complex configuration of blood-encoded cultural symbolism could be transferred intact from women's bodies to men's, leaving it as little altered as possible on the level of form.

It was an early version of what was to become an age-old technique. Subtle subversion, rather than explicit negation, would seem to be how most successful counter-revolutions in human history have been achieved. All is utterly changed – yet ostensibly all stays the same. Even when counter-revolutions involve flagrant violence and – at first – naked illegality, it always makes political sense for the new rulers to clothe their usurpation as quickly as possible with the banners and slogans of the very movement they have just overthrown. It may seem an astonishing story. But looked at in this way, the otherwise baffling ritual and mythological details of Australian Aboriginal ethnography do at least seem to make some kind of sense.

The Floods

The end of the ice age in Australia was a period of dramatic change. Rising temperatures dried up the lakes of inland Australia; rising seas at the same time drowned vast areas around the coasts. Within a few thousand years, about one seventh of the land mass of Greater Australia had been inundated, and there were times when the seas would have been encroaching on tribal territories and submerging them at a rate of about 100 km per generation, or 5 km a year. It is thought that the sea rose fairly rapidly until about 7,000 years ago, and then more slowly until the present level was reached about 5,000 years ago. The land bridge across the Torres Strait was finally drowned about 6,500 years ago, separating Australia once and for all from New Guinea.

Many Aboriginal myths appear to reflect these events (Campbell 1967). From Gippsland in the east to the Nullarbor Plain in the west, southern coastal Aborigines retain clear memories of a distant past when sea levels were lower and the coast extended further south than at present. To take only some among many impressive examples, the Yarra and Western Port tribes recollected a time when the present Hobson's Bay was a kangaroo hunting ground:

They say 'plenty catch kangaroo and plenty catch possum there' and that 'the river [Yarra] once went out to the Heads, but that the sea broke in and that Hobson's Bay which was once a hunting ground, became what it is'. (Quoted in Campbell 1967: 476)

The Aborigines possessed this information long before Europeans knew anything about the rise in sea levels which accompanied the end of the ice age. Likewise, the separation of Kangaroo Island from South Australia, which is now known to have occurred about 10,000 years ago, is remembered in the legend of Ngurunderi drowning his wives as they fled across on foot (Flood 1983; 180, citing Isaacs 1980: 108).

From Mornington Island on the northern coast come legends of the seagull woman, Garnguur, who pulled her raft backwards and forwards across what was then a peninsula to form the channels that now separate the island from the mainland. Elcho Island was similarly severed from the mainland when the Djankawu brother tripped and accidentaly pushed his stick into the sand there, causing the sea to rush in. The narrow seas between Milingimbi in the Crocodile Islands and the mainland were made by the Creation Shark. These and numerous other stories, the archaeologist Josephine Flood (1983: 180) comments, 'are so detailed and specific that there can be no doubt that they recall events thousands of years ago'. Support for the notion that myths can preserve genuine historical memories comes from an extraordinary finding – Aborigines in many coastal regions allegedly possess mythologically encoded *accurate mental maps* of territorial contours which were submerged as the world's sea levels began rising between ten and fifteen thousand years ago (Flood 1983: 179–80).

In addition to the legends about floods, there are many stories about giant mythical beings of the Dreamtime. Some of these quite possibly enshrine memories of the gigantic game animals that roamed Australia in the early days of human occupation of the continent. Flood (1983: 147) cites one especially dramatic story from western New South Wales. It tells of an ancient community's life-and-death battle with a tribe of giant kangaroos.

The first Australians would have migrated along the coastal regions of a continent extraordinarily rich in fish, protein-rich grubs and nutritious plant foods in lush, well-watered riverine and lakeside regions. As they moved inland, they would also have become familiar with an abundance of large animals such as has never since been known. Among these would have been the world's largest ever marsupials – the *Diprotodons*, wombat-like browsers the size of a rhinoceros. Early Aborigines would likewise have met giant wallabies, *Protemnodon*, which were larger in size than the largest living kangaroos. There would also have been genuine kangaroos of huge size, such as *Macropus titan*, *Sthenurus*, and *Procoptodon goliah*, a massive creature 3 m tall with huge front crushing teeth for feeding on shrubs and trees (Flood 1983: 148). If ice age Aborigines were actively hunting huge creatures such as these – and there is increasingly solid evidence that they were (Flood 1983: 147–59) – then we can imagine a single kill sometimes providing enough meat to feed a sizeable community for days on end.

Such abundance would have had profound social consequences, for as Flood (1983: 250) points out, it would have given the Aborigines ample amounts of leisure time. In fact there is every reason to suppose that under such conditions, collective hunting would have been regularly and predictably successful, as a consequence of which people would have been in a position to adopt something very like the 'slow' rhythm of hunting-versus-rest which was outlined in Chapter 10. Abundant gatherable food and very large game would have made it possible to 'slow down' to a leisurely two-week-on, two-week-off rhythm in which strenuous hunt-related rituals and activities alternated with pleasure-seeking, relaxation, singing, dancing, storytelling, feasting and sexual enjoyment. Abundance, in other words, would have made it realistic in many areas to approximate closely to the 'pure' model of lunar-scheduled production/consumption on the basis of which the human revolution had been consummated in an earlier period. Only later, with increased desiccation, population pressures in certain areas and/or the extinction of many large species of game, would such ideal conditions for synchrony have begun to change.

All this might help explain why Aboriginal legends so frequently depict the world as having been created by the Moon, by a Great Snake or by an All-Mother or other semi-human immense entity who combines lunar/tidal features with snake-like, mother-like and/or rainbow-like ones (Hiatt 1975b; Buchler and Maddock 1978). Among the Lardil Aborigines on Mornington Island, for example, Gidegal the Moon features in myth as 'the main boss' at the first male initiation ceremony; he has a special association with fish, and travels along rivers and across the sea (Trezise 1969: 43–4). In Central Australia, an Aranda myth tells of how Moon was the original custodian of all women. Having tried for himself females of all the different subsections, he decided to renounce them and distribute them in the correct order among men:

> To a Kumara man he gave a Bulthara woman, to a Purula a Panunga, to an Apunngarti an Umbitjana, to an Uknaria a Thungalla. The moon man led the lubras out one by one to the proper men, and told them always to marry straight in that way, and not to take wrong lubras. (Spencer and Gillen 1940: 412–13)

In South Australia, the Dieri believed 'that man and all other beings were created by the moon . . .' (Gason 1879: 260). Whilst the moon's involvement in cultural creation is a recurrent theme, the sun is never given such a mythological role. It seems possible that the myths enshrine memories of a time when kin relations and all social life were indeed, and on quite a mundane level, regulated in accordance with a cyclical logic responsible for the changing phases of the moon, for female menstruation, for human fertility and for all health and hunting success.

The Rainbow Snake

Almost all over Aboriginal Australia, 'divinity' or 'ritual power' is conceptualised as (among other things) an immense Rainbow which is simultaneously a Snake (Radcliffe-Brown 1926, 1930; Mountford 1978). Europeans frequently refer to this mythological creature as 'the' Rainbow Snake, as if it were a definite personage. But most myths themselves are less clearcut and consistent in specifying the identity of this being. The Euhalayi Aborigines traditionally ascribed immense power to Bahloo, the Moon, but also thought of this creature as the guardian of a sacred waterhole filled with supernaturally powerful 'Snakes' (Parker 1905: 50). Other Aborigines in coastal regions associated the 'Snake' with the tides (Memmott 1982: 174). The variations are endless, leading us to suppose that what all these myths are referring to is not really a 'thing' at all, but a cyclical logic which lies beyond and behind all the many concrete images – moon, snakes, tidal forces, waterholes, rainbows, mothers and so on – used in partial attempts to describe it. Maddock (1974: 121) suggests 'that what is called the Rainbow Serpent is but a visually striking image of force or vitality, a conception that cannot adequately be given figurative expression'. As evidence, he cites the Dalabon term *bolung*, which signifies not only 'rainbow', 'snake' and 'the mother of us all' but also 'ambiguity in form, creativity, power and time long past' (1974: 122–3). The reality in mind 'cannot be more than partially and misleadingly conveyed in visual and psychological images like rainbow or snake or mother'. In fact, Maddock concludes, no ready-made western concept or expression can hope to convey the notion of what is meant.

In all native accounts, the Rainbow Snake is paradoxical to the core. The great copper python Yurlunggur of the Yolngu 'is both in the heavens . . . and in the subterranean depths' (Warner 1957: 386). 'He is the highest in the sky and the deepest in the well' (Warner 1957: 255n). Although 'he' may be male, he is both 'man and woman' (Warner 1957: 383). The Rainbow Snake Kunmanggur, say the Murinbata, is bisexual: 'Even those who asserted the maleness of Kunmanggur said that he had large breasts, like a woman's' (Stanner 1966: 96). 'It is as though paradox and antinomy were the marrow in the story's bones', comments Stanner (1966: 100) on the basic Kunmanggur myth. Eliade's (1973: 115) cross-cultural surveys of this monster are among the best: he writes that the Rainbow Snake in Australia is able to relate 'to women's mysteries, to sex and blood and after-death existence' because 'his structure has permitted [him] to unite the opposites . . . '

For Maddock (1978a: 1), rainbows, snakes, sisters, and related images are 'a host of fleeting forms in and through which a fundamental conception of the world is expressed'. As a first approach to an understanding of the Dalabon (central Arnhem Land) term for rainbow snake, *bolung*, he suggests that we should 'lay stress on the cyclicity embedded in the concept and . . . draw attention to the role of cyclical thinking in Aboriginal thought generally' (1978b: 115). Other specialists have stressed the centrality of cyclicity in all Aboriginal thought:

> The aborigines are not interested, as we are, in the episodes of the past. The important things to them are the cycles of life: the development of the individual from infancy to old age; the path of the initiates from ignorance to knowledge; the yearly round of the seasons; the movements of the celestial bodies; and the breeding time of the creatures. These cycles are full of meaning to the native people, but to them the remote past, the present and the future are and will be changeless. (Mountford 1965: 24)

Or again:

> Although no Yolngu person has explained it in precisely this way, it seems to me that Yolngu perceive time as circular, so that from any particular time, what is past may be future, and what is future may be past. (Williams 1986: 30)

Stanner (1956: 60) confirms that Aboriginal 'social time' is 'bent' into cycles or circles, each cycle being in essence 'a principle for dealing with social inter-relatedness'. He adds that this *social* cyclicity is integral to the concept of 'the Dreaming', a concept usually inseparable from 'Rainbow' and/or 'Snake'. Certainly it is the case that Aboriginal paintings and depictions of Snake/Rainbow/Dreaming mythic powers and personages recurrently take the form of circles, concentric circles and curvilinear motifs of all kinds, often in association with women's bodies (figure 22).

So what precisely is this cyclical 'power' or 'Snake' which has been seen as 'a principle for dealing with social inter-relatedness'? It has been argued here that culture was created by menstrual solidarity. If this idea were correct, we might expect hunter-gatherer cultures – or more particularly those mythico-religious aspects of such cultures which represent long, unbroken traditions – to have preserved information telling us of these origins, at least on some level. Such knowledge has not to date been documented ethnographically, anywhere in the world. What we do know is that in Australia, Aboriginal thinkers attribute the origins of their world to the Rainbow Snake.

Let us suppose, for the sake of argument, that such Aboriginal thinkers are in some sense correct. In the light of my thesis, there would only be one way in which they could be correct. The term 'Rainbow/Snake' would have to be Aboriginal Australians' way of referring to menstrual solidarity itself.

It is a risky hypothesis, but fortunately one which we can rigorously test. If it were correct, one would expect *everything which can be said of menstrual*

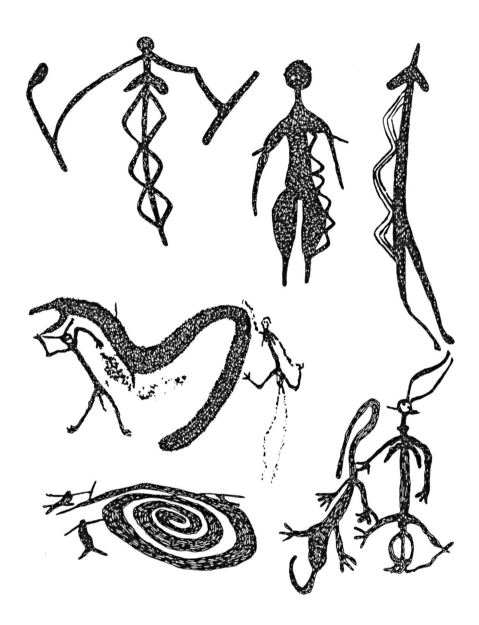

Figure 22 Upper row: serpentine forms and women. Cave paintings; Oenpelli region. Arnhem Land (Mountford 1956: 167, Fig. 49). *Middle and lower:* Pilbara rock-engravings. *Centre-left:* Upper Yule River, male figure with head-appendages, snake and apparently menstruating female (Wright 1968: Fig. 372). *Bottom left:* Black Hill Pool. Three men with coiled snake (Wright 1968: Fig. 648). *Bottom right:* Upper Yule River. Menstruating (?) figure and reptile (Wright 1968: Fig. 80; all figures redrawn).

solidarity to be equally applicable to 'the Snake'. Menstrual solidarity as specified in the previous chapters on the one hand, *and "the Snake" as specified by the Aborigines themselves on the other*, should correspond with one another at every point. The 'Snake' should therefore not be a physical reptile at all but something in zoological terms quite strange. Neither should it correspond in any simple way with the tides or moon, or with the sun's light as refracted through raindrops to form a rainbow. It should be 'like' the tides, and 'like' a rainbow — but it should also be more than these things. In conformity with the model it should be cyclical, alternating continuously between opposite phases or states, blood-linked, linked in particular with *synchronised* menstruation, identifiable with the blood of game animals, responsible for the 'sacredness' of menstruating women and of game animals alike, associated with the moon and therefore in coastal regions with floods and the tides — and conceptualisable as 'like a Mother', although this personage would have to be a collective mother rather than an individual.

Like menstrual solidarity — or indeed like any powerful social movement or force — it should 'carry away' or 'engulf' those falling under its spell. Assuming that menstrual blood were thought of as 'wet' rather than 'dry', this action should be depictable as a snake-mother's or rainbow's drawing of women into a watery world. In terms of detailed mythological imagery, such 'swallowing' episodes should be associated with pools, streams, marshes, rains, storms, wet season, and so on, while the 'regurgitations' should be linked with dryness (fire, dry earth, sun, dry season etc.). 'Dry' swallowings and 'wet' regurgitations would of course disprove the hypothesis completely.

If the hypothesis were correct, we might expect synchronously cycling women to be thought of as 'snake women', with half of their being or their time spent in a 'wet' element or phase, and half in the 'dry'. Meanwhile, so-called snakes would turn out to be human mothers. They should menstruate, give birth to human offspring, copulate with human partners. Where snake copulation is concerned, there should be strict rules which, however, should be the reverse of those applying in normal life. Menstrual withdrawal in the real world is a retreat from exogamous sex into 'one's own blood'. No union with a snake, therefore, should have the characteristics of exogamous marriage. Only intense kin-to-kin intimacies ('incest') should be allowed. 'Correct' or exogamous marriages between women and snakes would disprove the hypothesis.

If snake power coincided with the specifications of the menstrual sex strike, it should have further finely delineated characteristics. It should come on in the darkness of night, and disappear under the bright light of the midday sun or of the full moon. It should be felt to emerge whenever blood began to flow, and should fall away again towards the time when cooking-fires should be lit. Under its spell, it should become impossible for anyone to cook: all meat should resist fire, conjoin with blood or water ('anti-fire') and stay raw. Moreover, the power should punish those who attempt to eat their own kills or cook their own meat secretly out in the bush. It should correspond, in other words, to what in other parts of the world is known as the Guardian Spirit of the Game Animals, or the Master or Mistress of Game. Were myths to depict cooking as occurring whilst a Rainbow Snake were present, the hypothesis would be disproved.

It should be impossible for humans ritually to embody this power without menstruating. This should make women the 'natural' or 'original' custodians of such power. It should be impossible for men to monopolise or give expression to this power independently of women – unless by some artifice it became possible for men to 'menstruate' synchronously themselves. If men *were* to monopolise snake power at women's expense, despite all the obvious difficulties, they would have to prohibit menstruating women from associating with one another. Then, to enhance hunting luck and general health and well-being in something resembling the traditional ways, these men would have to organise a 'menstrual' sex strike of their own. To be consistent in supplanting women's roles, moreover, men would have to go so far as to 'give birth', sit at a symbolic 'home base' and receive gifts of meat for themselves and for their dependants.

Throughout Australia, ritual power manifests itself in forms which confirm these expectations. 'The Snake' – overwhelmingly the dominant image in most Aboriginal iconography – is identified mythologically as a rainbow-like, blood-red, mother-like, marriage-negating, tribute-demanding cyclical force which has the characteristics which we would expect, down even to some of the smallest details.

In the coastal regions of the Northern Territories and of Western Australia – the regions about which we are best informed – the 'rainbow-snake' is associated with the tides (Memmott 1982), with feminine wetness and with blood. One of its recurrent names is 'Muit'. According to von Brandenstein (1982: 58), this name derives from a Kariera (Western Australian) root meaning 'blood & red & multi-coloured & iridescent'.

In north-east Arnhem Land, during the darkness of night, when Yolngu neophytes are shown the snake for the first time, it is in the form of two immense white 'Muit emblems' consisting of padded poles 'with the rock pythons painted in blood on the white surfaces gleaming in the light of the many fires' (Warner 1957: 304). 'The Snake' in this context appears in the form of two alternating, zigzagging lines of blood. The Wik-Mungkan of Cape York confirm the link with menstruation: the Snake is that force which is 'responsible for women menstruating' (McKnight 1975: 95). Seeing the red band in a rainbow, Wik-Mungkan Aborigines say 'Taipan the-rainbow-snake-has-a-"sore inside" i.e. has her menstrual pains' (McConnel 1936: 2: 103).

The Myth of the Two Wawilak Sisters

We have already encountered a Yolngu myth telling of how two world-creating females 'sat down, looking at each other, with their feet out and legs apart, and both menstruated', following which each put a 'loop' of the resultant blood around her partner's neck (McCarthy 1960: 426). In this version of the story of the Two Wawilak Sisters, the narrative immediately repeats the climactic episode of blood-encirclement in a different way by saying that the sisters were 'swallowed' by a 'Snake' (McCarthy 1960: 426). A related myth ends by describing how two unnamed sisters 'decided to go into the waterhole and become a rainbow'. Note that they *decided* to do this. It was neither an accident nor a calamity, but a deliberate act. It is explained: 'They wanted to be a snake, like the rainbow, when she is standing up in the waterhole and makes lightning' (Groger-Wurm 1973: 120).

Now, we might ask: Why, in this myth and its countless variants, should two women *want* to 'enter a waterhole'? Why should they *want* to 'become a rainbow', 'make lightning' or get themselves 'swallowed by a snake'? What is really going on in all this?

'Becoming a rainbow' is a reference to the menstrual blood-spell. The rainbow-like 'Snake' — always described in Arnhem Land mythology as water-loving, odour-detecting, woman-encircling and, above all, as blood-loving — is nothing other than the combined symbolic power of women's 'floods' or 'flows'. The fact that the same creature is also identified with tidal movements or monsoonal storms and floods (Memmott 1982; Warner 1957; Lévi-Strauss 1966: 75–108) does nothing to contradict this interpretation — for such 'floods' themselves are in native terms conceptualised as blood-streaked to the extent that they are powerful at all.

We see the blood/flood/snake/rainbow chain of associations endlessly confirmed in all the fine details of Yolngu myth and ceremonial performance. By their ritual dancing around the Snake's sacred waterhole, the mythological Two Sisters are said to have actively conjured up floods and storms *as they combined their blood flows*, the great female 'Rainbow Snake' emerging from its waterhole precisely as blood *streams from the dancing women's wombs*. So accurate is this correspondence that when the blood stops, so does the Snake. When the blood flows out again, so the Snake flows with it. As we read in Berndt's (1951: 22–3) version:

> So the *wirlkul* [younger sister, non-bleeding] began to dance, to hinder the Snake's progress. . . . The Julunggul [Rainbow Snake] stopped in her course, and watched the dancing. But the girl grew tired, and called out: 'Come on, sister, your turn now. I want to rest.'
>
> The older sister [*gungman*, bleeding afterbirth blood] came from the hut, leaving her child in its cradle of soft paperbark, and began to dance. But her blood, still intermittently flowing, attracted the Snake further; and she moved towards them.

'Come on, sister', cried the *gungman*. 'It's no good for me; my blood is coming out, and the Snake is smelling it and coming closer. It's better for you to go on dancing.'

So the younger sister continued, and again Julunggul stopped and watched. . . . In this way, the Wauwalak took it in turns to dance; when the younger sister danced, the Snake stopped; but when the older one continued, she came forward again. So the younger girl danced longer than the other, and as she swayed from side to side the intensive activity caused her menstruation to begin; then the Python, smelling more blood, came forward without hesitation.

The Rainbow Snake in northern Australia comes on when genital blood starts to flow, sometimes 'swallowing' whole communities into its domain; it retreats in face of the dry season or fire, releasing its victims at this point from its sway (Mountford 1978: 23). It is explicitly described as the guardian spirit or 'headman' of all the game animals (Berndt 1951: 21). Consistently with this role, when a man tries to cook or eat his own kill secretly in the bush, it may well be the Rainbow which swallows up the flesh-abuser in punishment (Berndt and Berndt 1970: 44). A consistent theme, moreover, is that those identified with the Snake can expect tribute in meat and other resources. Older initiated men who supply younger men with ritual secrets expect such tribute in exchange. And mythology states that before women were robbed of the magic emanating from their vaginas, they, too, could use their menstrual power to extract meat from men. It was only when women were deprived of their 'dilly bags' – symbolic vaginas – that such roles were reversed, women thenceforward having to grind cycad nuts to sustain men in the performance of *their* great ceremonies (Berndt 1952: 232–3; Warner 1957: 339–40).

The Secret of 'the Snake'

The myths of northern and much of western Australia agree that snake power is 'women's business' in origin. Despite its often ambiguous gender, the Rainbow Snake – as people say in north-east Arnhem Land – was first conjured up when two 'incestuous' Sisters became so intimate with one another that their blood-flows came on together, pouring into a nearby sacred waterhole. In some versions of the tale of the Two Wawilak Sisters (Berndt 1951; Chaseling 1957; Warner 1957), a baby was born at the same time, the afterbirth blood of one sister mingling with the menstrual flow of her partner.

Let us briefly follow this extraordinary story through (see also Berndt and Berndt 1964: 212–13; Berndt, R. M. 1976; Berndt, C. H. 1970: 1306; Kupka 1965: 111–21; Mountford 1956: 278–9; McCarthy 1960: 425–7; for a survey and comparison of the different published versions, see Knight 1987: 235–54). In the following abridgment, Warner's (1957: 250–9)

version (1) provides the basic story-line, with additional information taken
from (2) Berndt 1951; (3) Robinson 1966: 37–43; and (4) Chaseling 1957:
139–46:

The story of the Two Wawilak Sisters

At the beginning of time, two sisters were travelling across the landscape,
conferring names on the features of a previously unnamed world. One
carried a child, the other was pregnant. They had both committed incest
in their own country, the country of the Wawilak. Carrying spears and
other symbols of masculine power, they carried food and hunted game
animals, prophesying that everything they collected would soon become
marreiin (sacred/taboo).

At last, having traversed many countries, they arrived at a waterhole in
which, unknown to them, dwelt the great Rock Python or Rainbow
Serpent, male in some versions (1, 3, 4), female in others (2). This
Serpent was a kinsperson to the Sisters. As the pregnant sister felt she was
about to give birth, the other sister began to help her. They camped by the
waterhole and lit a fire on which to cook their gathered food and game.

As the sister, helped by her companion, began to give birth, afterbirth
blood began flowing into the sacred pool, polluting it and arousing the
Snake. A rain cloud, lightning flashes and a rainbow (version 3) appeared
in the sky: the Serpent was emerging in anger from its hole, unleashing
the season of rain, floods and storms. The night was dark except for the
thin curve of the moon (3). As the women's genital blood flowed, all
cooking-fire became suddenly ineffective. The animals and plants which
the women had hunted/gathered refused to cook, jumped up alive from
the fire on which they had been placed – and dived 'like men' into the
nearby blood-streaked waterhole. The well-waters began to rise.

'Go away! Go away!', the sisters cried, as they became aware of the
immense Snake in the sky. Seized with fear, they danced to make the
snake go away. But the dancing only brought on the second sister's
menstrual flow, attracting the Serpent still more. The waterhole began
overflowing, flooding the dry land all around.

Now, filled with foreboding and despair, the sisters fled into the little
parturition hut/menstrual hut they had built. But at this point, inside the
hut, they were both shedding blood, and as they sang out the words
'Yurlunggur and menstrual blood' – the most taboo and potent of the
songs known to them – the angry Serpent thrust its nose into the hut and
swallowed the women and their children alive.

Black clouds now blotted out the sky, and rain crashed down in a
terrible storm. As the waters enveloped the women and their babies, they
bled still more (1) and began undergoing a change of name (2), moving
into another realm beyond death. At this point, the Two Sisters had
turned into or become the Snake. In a voice of thunder, the great Snake

roared. This 'was the spirits of the two sisters who were speaking out of his mouth. "We are here now", the sisters said. "The snake has eaten us. We are the Marraian, the sacred knowledge of Wittee [the Snake]. Our spirits talk through him for another country "' (3). As the Snake became erect 'like a tree', its head stretching high into the clouds, the Sisters in this way continued to give names to the world. Snakes from neighbouring countries joined in the roaring and name-giving, and all together inaugurated the great rituals which today bind in solidarity tribes from far and wide despite their linguistic differences.

The sisters' symbolic 'death' or Snake-identity, however, was only a temporary phase in a larger cycle. Soon the upward movement had passed its peak. The sisters' incestuous intimacy was now publicly exposed, attacked and disowned. At this point, the floods subsided, the land dried out, the 'Snake' came crashing to the ground, splitting it open – and out from its coiling skin came two women with their babies, now once again in possession of their separate identities, 'regurgitated' on to an ants' nest to be bitten by meat-ants and thereby 'resurrected'. After a brief spell of life, the victims were swallowed again and then finally regurgitated to turn to stone – the form in which they can still be seen to this day.

It will be appreciated that the logic of this myth conforms neatly with the cyclical structure of alternation between two 'worlds' at which we arrived at the end of Chapter 11.

North-east Arnhem Land: a Humanised Landscape

Aborigines in north-east Arnhem Land model many of their most important rituals on the events described in this myth. Whether the rituals are categorised by Europeans as 'mortuary rituals', 'increase rites' or 'initiation rites' makes little difference – essentially, the logic of the ceremonies is the same. The basic idea is always some variation on the theme of rebirth, whether of the dead, of game animals, of young men undergoing initiation – or of nature and the cosmos as a whole.

Religious life in this region 'centred on procreation, on the renewal of human beings and of the natural species, and on the continuity of family and community life through mythic intervention and guidance' (Berndt 1976: 4). The menstrual ritual of the synchronising Wawilak Sisters is believed to have given rise to all cyclicity, all alternation, all movement between opposite phases and states. Even when men put this in typically negative terms, their awe in the face of mythic Womankind's alleged accomplishments shines through: 'The cycle of the seasons with the growth and decay of vegetation, copulation, birth and death of animals as well as man, is all the fault of those two Wawilak Sisters' (Warner 1957: 385). Had the Sisters not menstruated into the Snake's pool, there would have been no birth and no death, no male and no female, no wet season and no dry. 'After they had done this wrong', however, 'they made it the law for everyone'.

Menstruation is 'wrong'. It is 'negative', like the rainy season, or like death itself. But – like death – it is part of the necessary scheme of things. As Warner (1957: 404) puts it, the 'swallowing' of the earth by the rainy season 'is known to be caused by the wrong actions of the two Wawilak women' in 'profaning' the Snake's sacred waterhole with their blood. This is not considered an unmixed calamity, because the rain and water bring the plants and bulbs and flowers which are consumed directly by man or provide pasturage for kangaroo, opossum, and other animals eaten by man. In other words, the Yolngu see the Snake's swallowing the women and animals – that is, the flood's engulfing of the world – as necessary and part of the scheme of things, 'and their testimony clearly demonstrates the causal relation between the actions of the Wawilak women and the seasonal cycle' (Warner 1957: 404).

The wet season, then, is 'death'; the dry season, 'life'. But death is the precondition of life in the scheme of things which the Two Sisters established. Menstruation implies seclusion. Just as the floods of the rainy season make travel difficult or impossible, marooning small bands of Aborigines in isolated close-knit groups (Warner 1957: 378–404), so women's own 'floods' mean relative immobility, food taboos, hunger and intense kinship dependency with little social exchange. Women are as if 'swallowed up' in their own blood. But this withdrawal into the self is a necessary retreat, for it is an accumulation of inner strength, like sleep. The skies darken, the eyes close, the withdrawal into the 'Dreamtime' begins. The rains fall – triggered, in ritual conceptions, by women's own blood (Berndt 1976: 68) – and dark clouds blot out sex, feasting and adventure as they blot out the sun. Seasonal cyclicity, in other words, is conceptualised entirely in menstrual terms, being thought, as Warner (1957: 397) puts it, to 'lie within' the menstrual cycle as 'a part of the process of reproduction'.

In the love songs of Goulbourn Island, men are depicted as having incestuous, intra-clan or intra-moiety intercourse to help women bring on and synchronise their menstrual flows – blood-flows which are thought to be essential in triggering the onset of the annual rains. 'North-eastern Arnhem Landers', as Berndt (1976: 68) writes,

> saw this as an observable progression of inevitable events: coitus among the palms; the onset of the menstrual flow; the attraction of the clouds; the arrival of the Lightning Snake, drawn by the smell of the blood; and finally the coming of the monsoonal season.

Note here that the Snake is not 'angered' by menstrual blood – on the contrary, it is 'drawn' by its 'smell'. In such coastal songs, the connection between menstrual blood and monsoonal rain is conceptualised through images in which the blood pours down from women's vaginas into each major 'Vagina Place' of the land itself – the life-giving waterholes, streams and inlets on which fertility depends – and flows thence into the sea, and into the clouds that rise from the sea, returning later transformed, in the shape of the dark monsoonal storms and floods which 'swallow' the earth (Berndt 1976: 100–1).

In this scheme of things, human and natural cycles of renewal are mutually supportive and sustainable through the same rites. The skies and the landscape are felt to beat to human rhythms. Everything natural, in other words, is conceptualised in human terms, just as everything human is thought to be governed by natural rhythms. 'Physiographic features of the countryside', as Berndt (1976: 7) puts it, were traditionally 'likened to male and female genitals', so that imprints in rock told of a mythic act of coitus, a sacred waterhole was a vagina, a shining white substance on a rock surface seemed like semen. Berndt (1976: 12) phrases this in his own way by commenting that the Aboriginal intellectual 'projected his own belief system on to the environment in which he lived. He saw within it the same forces operating as he identified within his own process of living'. But 'projection' is, perhaps, an inadequate term. If synchrony of the kind this book has described was at one time central to Aboriginal life, it would seem that rhythmic nature was projecting her logic into a listening human culture as much as the other way around.

There seems no reason to discount the Aborigines' own belief that in their rituals they were drawing upon natural rhythms and harmonising with them to the advantage of their relationship with the world around them. It was not that man was dominating nature; but neither was it that human society stood helpless in the face of nature's powers. Rather, human society was flexible enough and sensitive enough to attune itself finely to the rhythms of surrounding life, avoiding helplessness by replicating internally nature's own 'dance'. Nature was thereby humanised, while humanity yielded to this nature. If the hills felt like women's breasts, if rocks felt like testicles, if the sunlight seemed like sexual fire and the rains felt like menstrual floods, then this was not mere 'projection' of a belief system on to the external world. This was how things felt – because, given synchrony and therefore a shared life-pulse, this was at a deep level how they were.

Rebirth, in any event, is or was achieved in northern Australia by organising symbolic death so that it took the form of self-dissolution into the corporate identity of 'the Snake' – a self-renunciation explicitly likened to an 'incestuous' return to 'the womb'. This was followed in due course by ritually induced self-recovery or 'resurrection'. For all this to work properly, it was necessary to ensure only that the voluntarily accepted 'death' was menstrual, on the model of women's temporary 'death' each month.

A similar logic seems to have prevailed over much of Australia. Far from Arnhem Land, when the Berndts (1945: 309–10) observed an initiation ritual in the Ooldea region, South Australia, ten men opened the blood-letting phase when they stood up, built a fire, broke off some sharp acacia thorns and pulled at their penises to enlarge them:

> Then holding a thorn in the heat of the fire for a few seconds, each pierced
> his penis incisure; the sound of the thorns puncturing the skin could be
> clearly heard. The incisure when pierced several times bled freely, the flow
> being accelerated by pressure of the hand. The blood was sprinkled on the
> thighs of the men, either by holding the penis at each side and letting it
> drip, or by moving so that the bleeding penis flopped from side to side, or
> upwards and downwards, the blood touching the lower buttocks and
> loins.

'The actual initiation', write the Berndts (1945: 308n), 'was held during the
period of the new moon'.

'Inside' and 'Outside' Meanings

In addition to its other features, the story of the Two Wawilak Sisters is a
myth of 'primitive matriarchy'. That is, it explains how women once
monopolised ritual power, but then lost it. In fact, like all matriarchy
myths, it is on one level little more than a male attempt to justify politically
the far from self explanatory fact that menstrual power is nowadays exercised
by men.

In Warner's (1957) version, the narrative ends by describing – almost as
an afterthought, it seems – how two ancestral men appeared at the Rainbow
Snake's sacred waterhole some time after the events described in the main
body of the story. They found some of the Two Sisters' blood, carefully
collected it in containers and went to sleep. Warner's (1957: 259) version
ends:

> The sun went down. They left the blood till morning. They slept, and
> while they were in a deep sleep they dreamed of what the two women sang
> and danced when they were trying to keep Yurlunggur from swallowing
> them. The Wawilak women came back as spirits and taught the two
> men. . . .
>
> The two sisters said to men 'This is all now. We are giving you this
> dream so you can remember these important things. You must never
> forget these things we have told you tonight. You must remember every
> time each year these songs and dances. You must paint with blood and
> feathers for Marndiella, Gunabibi and Djungguan. You must dance all
> the things we saw and named on our journey, and which ran away into the
> well.'

All the songs, dances and blood-shedding operations through which the
women had conjured up the Snake were carefully described, so that the men
could bleed and thus get themselves ritually 'swallowed' in the same way.

The men succeeded in memorising the details. Having woken up, they cut themselves, bled, synchronised their flows with one another, got themselves swallowed, 'died' only to 'come alive' again – and resolved never to forget the secrets they had learned. 'We dance these things now, because our Wongar ancestors learned them from the two Wawilak sisters.' Such rituals – Yolngu Aborigines insist – have been faithfully preserved by men to this very day.

I have stated that 'the Snake' in the Wawilak myth is in fact the symbolically constructed menstrual synchrony of the heroines. But there is an apparent difficulty for this interpretation. It is that 'the Snake' – far from representing women's own menstrual solidarity and power – is in the most familiar versions depicted as just the opposite. The monster is said to have been outraged by menstrual pollution, and to have punished the Sisters responsible for it.

It must be conceded that outsiders and the uninitiated throughout northeast Arnhem Land are encouraged to view being 'swallowed by the Snake' as a calamity – a punishment suffered by the Two Sisters for their 'wrong' in having 'polluted' the Snake's sacred waterhole. Certainly, it always suited the structures of Aboriginal male dominance to depict the 'Snake' as the Two Sisters' – and hence all women's – mortal antagonist. In this context, to be 'swallowed' by the Rainbow Snake is simply to be killed.

In conformity with such 'outside' interpretions of the basic myths, reproductively potent women in much of Arnhem Land – as the following passage on the Gunwinggu shows – are warned to keep away from one another and from waterholes precisely lest they become 'swallowed' by 'the Snake':

> When a woman is pregnant . . . she should keep well away from pools and streams, for fear of the Rainbow – other women should get water for her. Babies are especially vulnerable to attack from the Rainbow. In rainy weather, or if she goes near water, a mother should paint herself and her baby with yellow ochre or termite mound. And a menstruating woman should not touch or even go close to a pregnant woman or a baby, or walk about in the camps, or go near a waterhole that other people are using. Traditionally, she should stay in seclusion, with a fire burning constantly to keep the Rainbow away. (Berndt Land Berndt 1970: 180)

But although all this may at first sight seem to present a problem, in fact it is exactly what we would expect. What we are witnessing is not a primal scene or pristine construct free of the ravages of time. The Rainbow Snake as it actually exists is a secondary, derivative construct. Its functions are political, and bent to the service of contemporary forms of power. By means of this construct, women are prevented from experiencing their reproductive powers as sources of collectivity or strength. Just as women produce male babies who are eventually turned (through initiation ritualism) into their oppressors (Bern 1979), menstruating women are in effect alienated from the power of their own blood. As they recoil from the menace of 'the Rainbow' or 'Snake', they are oppressed by and made to fear the consequences of what is in reality their own extraordinary potential for synchrony and ritual strength.

Alain Testart (1978: 113) describes the relationship between the Rainbow Serpent and menstrual blood in Australian Aboriginal mythology as 'an association of opposites linked by their very contradiction'. But in this case as in others, a dialectic of paradox is in operation, clarifying that the seeming polar 'opposites' – the menstrual flow on the one hand, Serpent on the other – are at a deeper level one and the same. 'They sang blood because that is what brought the snake when Yurlunggur came', an informant explained to Warner (1957: 270), referring to the Wawilak Sisters whose dancing and menstrual bleeding generated the Serpent at the beginning of time. But were not the Sisters, in 'singing menstrual blood', attempting to *stop* the Serpent from swallowing them up? What is really being suggested here?

The truth is that two opposite messages are being transmitted at once. One is that the 'dancing' and simultaneous 'bleeding' of the Sisters were futile activities in that they had the opposite effect to the one which was desired. *Despite* 'singing menstrual blood' and *despite* dancing frantically (in a way which induced the menstrual flow: Berndt 1951: 22–3), the Sisters found themselves being swallowed by the Snake. Everything the Sisters did – singing menstrual blood, dancing menstrual blood – was precisely and with unerring accuracy *the wrong* thing to do if they wished (as the myth says they wished) to avoid becoming engulfed.

But this leads us to the opposite implication of the myth – that the Serpent was conjured up not *despite* the Sisters' dancing and singing, but *because* of them. We have seen already that 'the Serpent' flows from its deep hole in precise proportion as the Sisters' blood flows from the vagina, even to the point of stopping and starting in time with the flow (Berndt 1951: 22–3). It was when the two sisters were *bleeding together* that two things simultaneously happened: (1) they entered their little menstrual/parturition hut together; (2) they were swallowed by 'the Snake'. The implication is that it was the generalised 'wetness' and combination of their blood-flows – the connection of womb-with-waterhole or womb-with-womb – which constituted the force carrying off the Sisters to 'the other world'. This would be consistent with Hiatt's (1975b: 156) suggestion that, in Aboriginal 'swallowing and regurgitation' myths generally, the ingesting and regurgitating organ is really an immense vagina or womb.

It might be objected: 'But if "the Snake" is really nothing other than the combined "flood" or "flow" of the women, why is this message so effectively concealed? Why is "the Snake" depicted as a force alien to the women themselves?' At the story's reproductive and dramatic climax, the Sisters become 'as one'. They enter a birth hut/menstrual hut together, both connected by a shared flow of blood. If this is really a shared 'return to the womb', conceptualised as a journey to the sky, why depict it as the trauma of being 'swallowed' by an alien, monstrous 'Snake'?

In penetrating beneath the surface of sexual-political constructs of this kind, the first thing to appreciate is the total contradiction between what men say to women or outsiders, *and what they say in secret among themselves*. It is clear that to those with 'inside' knowledge, the 'outside' interpretations of the basic myths are superficial in the extreme. Not only are these readings known to be mistaken. They are well understood to be *precise mirror-image inversions* of what initiates eventually come to understand.

In the case of the Wawilak myth, the nub of the story is the episode in which the Two Sisters supposedly 'pollute' a waterhole said to be 'sacred'. This is a conventional enough idea: women in real life are often told not to approach sacred waterholes on account of their polluting blood. This blood, it is said, 'angers' the Snake which dwells within the waters. Yet initiated men know a paradoxical secret – namely that if the waterhole of Yurlunggur the Great Snake is sacred at all, it is actually *because* of its having been 'polluted' in this way. 'From its association with that blood. . . .', as Berndt (1976: 70) notes, 'the water itself becomes sacred'. Moreover, the Snake is not simply hostile to women's blood. It is aroused by this blood and in fact needs it in order to be summonsed up from the depths. 'There is the suggestion', comments Berndt (1951: 22n), 'that the snake found the blood attractive'.

Again, the 'Snake' in the Wawilak myth is supposed to have 'punished' the Sisters by 'swallowing' them. But initiated men know that for the two Sisters to have been 'inside the Serpent' would have been no calamitous encounter with an alien being. The Snake would have been the women's kin. To be engulfed by its power would have been to feel an immense sense of *kinship solidarity and strength*. In fact, the myth makes no sense unless this point is acknowledged, for why else would the Sisters have wanted to pass on to future generations their precious knowledge? If all that happened to them was a disaster, why would passing on the secrets have seemed so vital? Why should men in subsequent generations have *wanted* to learn from the Two Sisters how to preserve, symbolically, that supposedly polluting blood?

But it is in the ritual domain that the deeper meanings emerge most incontrovertibly – which explains, of course, why the innermost secrets of such rituals had always to be kept carefully from women. To those with 'inside' knowledge (revealed only gradually through the various stages of initiation), to be 'swallowed by the Serpent' is no disaster at all. On the contrary, to be so engulfed is to feel an immense sense of collective solidarity and power. Throughout Aboriginal Australia, there is no way to generate this serpent power other than by bleeding. We are here discussing what in

Arnhem Land Donald Thomson (1949: 41) called 'the solidarity (the *marr*) of a group, members of which are bound together by the sharing of a special bond'. The highest expressions of this collective 'reproductive power' — which may in adjacent regions be termed *ungud, wondjina, bolung* and so on (Maddock 1978a, 1978b) — is found in the physical intimacies of ritual life, when men share even the warmth of one another's life-blood itself, smearing blood over one another from penis or arm. In the course of male initiation rituals (designed to sustain the reproductivity of both human and natural realms), men shed large amounts of blood, dipping their hands in each other's streams, fondling each other's bodies and becoming generally immersed in the flow of both affection and blood. In north-east Arnhem Land, men use the Wawilak myth *both* to discourage women from doing any such thing *and* to justify the fact that men alone are today permitted to immerse themselves in one another's 'menstrual' flows.

The Djungguan

Let us return to Warner (1957: 274–8) as he describes 'the principal interclan circumcision' ceremony of the Yolngu. This is the *Djungguan* ritual re-enactment of the Wawilak Sisters myth.

On the day before the circumcision, a blood-letting ceremony takes place in the old men's camp. The blood is to be used as an adhesive to hold the birds' down and native cotton to the dancers' bodies. Before a man offers his blood for the first time Yurlunggur — a trumpet symbolic of the Snake — is blown over his body. Then the old men sing over him. Meanwhile, his arms are tied near the wrist and shoulder with stout cord. A stone spear head is broken and a flake of it used to make a half-inch cut in the lower arm. The leader rubs the man's head with his hand while another cuts his arm. The totemic emblem is blown against the wound:

> The blood runs slowly, and the rhythm of the song is conducted with equal slowness. In a second or two the blood spurts and runs in a rapid stream. The beat of the song sung by the old men increases to follow the rhythm of the blood. The blood runs into a paper-bark basin. . . . (Warner 1957: 276)

The next man opens a hole from yesterday's giving and the blood pours forth in a stream. It runs quickly, and the rhythm of the song is at a fast tempo. 'There is much smiling among the men and an occasional *"main-muk, main-muk* (good, good)". ' A third man pulls off an old scab from his arm and the blood pours forth in a larger stream than that of the others. The trumpet continues to blow. Several men proudly exhibit their arms, which show five and six cuts that have been made during previous ceremonies. An informant explains the meaning of the blood:

The meaning is like this: suppose you and I have come a long way and we reach a good camp and our people have one house empty and it is a good place for us and they take us in and put us in it. We get in that house and have a good sleep and no one can hurt us because we have friends. That blood is just like that. It makes us feel easy and comfortable and it makes us strong. It makes us good. (Warner 1957: 277)

In being enveloped with a coating of blood, the men are being 'swallowed' by 'the Snake'. *The snake is always defined as kin.* And *this* — this sensation of 'belonging', of being 'at home', of being with kin — is what it feels like to be 'swallowed'. Whatever the myths told to frighten uninitiated outsiders, the men are quite adamant that being 'inside the Serpent' is what sacredness and strength are all about. Whereas the mythological Sisters are alleged to have been afraid of the impending disaster of being swallowed by the great Serpent, the real secret is that the men actively court this 'disaster', which they bring upon themselves by 'menstruating' precisely as the Sisters had done:

Native Interpretation. – The blood that runs from an incision and with which the dancers paint themselves and their emblems is something more than a man's blood – it is the menses of the old Wawilak women. (Warner 1957: 278)

Hence Warner (1957: 278) was told during a ceremony:

'That blood we put all over those men is all the same as the blood that came from that old woman's vagina. It isn't the blood of those men any more because it has been sung over and made strong. The hole in the man's arm isn't that hole any more. It is all the same as the vagina of that old woman that had blood coming out of it. This is the blood that snake smelled when he was in the Mirrirmina well. This is true for Djungguan and Gunabibi.' – 'When a man has got blood on him [is ceremonially decorated with it], he is all the same as those two old women when they had blood. All the animals ran away and they couldn't cook them.'

When the trumpet blows over the man giving his blood, it is the Snake risen out of his well to swallow the women and their two children 'because he has smelled the menstrual blood of the older sister'. Several well-informed men told Warner: 'When Yurlunggur blows over them when they cut their arms it is like that snake comes up and smells that woman's blood when he is getting ready to swallow them.'

All this, Warner (1957: 278) comments, 'means that the man who is giving his blood for the first time is being swallowed by the snake and is at the moment the old woman'. It follows that although ostensibly the Wawilak Sisters met disaster in being 'swallowed' by the 'Snake', the 'inside' meaning of all this is just the opposite. Men eagerly repeat the 'wrong' of the Sisters' intimacy and menstruation in order to be 'swallowed' themselves.

Dancing, singing, holding and fondling one another, they let flow their own blood in a rhythm which — to the accompaniment of singing to the same beat — conjures up 'the Serpent' and engulfs them all in feelings of profound security, warmth, solidarity and strength.

Myth, Social Conflict and Contradiction

The various seemingly conflicting and irreconcilable messages of the Wawilak myth, then, revolve around the ambiguity inherent in the identity of the Serpent itself. One reading is that this Snake is 'that which controls women' in the sense not of menstrual cyclicity but of male dominance over the female sex. It is therefore a phallic symbol within a context of male rule and possible rape. The Two Sisters pollute a male sacred site and are sexually punished as a result. This is certainly the story which the women are supposed to swallow, and it is also the message which most social anthropologists appear to have accepted more or less at face value. The great Snake, as Warner (1957: 387) puts it, 'is a ritualization of the male section of society, and the Wawilak sisters who by their uncleanness have provoked the snake (men) into swallowing them are the unritualized or profane sections of the tribe, i.e., the women and uninitiated boys'. Lévi-Strauss (1966: 91–4) accepts this reading in its entirety, and it is generally the case that the Rainbow Serpent in Aboriginal Australia as such has been interpreted as a 'penis-symbol' (for a survey of interpretations see Maddock, 1978a). The Serpent in our myth — which advances upon the Sisters even as they cry 'Go away!' — appears therefore as an immense phallus which rises up into the air and falls, rises and falls, punishing the women for their crime in a cosmic act of rape. Even Berndt (1951: 21), in whose version the Serpent is definitely female, insists: 'The fact that a female snake eventually swallowed the Two Sisters does not affect its role as a Penis symbol.' But the words of Berndt's Aboriginal informants themselves are perhaps more interesting, for according to them the Sisters, in being swallowed by the Serpent, are 'like a penis being swallowed by a vagina, *only we put it the other way around*' (Berndt 1951: 39, my emphasis). The monster is, then, an immense vagina — yet this knowledge is tampered with. The all-*swallowing* organ, however improbably, is said to be a penis. Things are exactly inverted for the benefit of those on the 'outside' of the circle in which the essential secrets are known.

We know that the Serpent rose out of its well and reached up straight into the sky having 'swallowed' the Sisters. But is the experience of being swallowed 'like' that of being drawn back into the womb — transported to the world beyond — or 'like' that of being raped? Was the Snake at that point 'big' because it was a womb filled with human flesh waiting to be born — as Berndt (1951: 25) suggests when he writes: 'the female Julunggul is big (as if she were pregnant) from having swallowed the Wauwalak'? Or was its immense size that of a penis in an erect state? Berndt insists that despite the

Snake's femaleness, she 'symbolises a penis'; 'her entry into the hut "is like a penis going into a vagina". The whole process of swallowing is interpreted by natives as an act of coitus' (1951: 25). Yet it seems pointless to try to settle on just one of the two diametrically opposed possible interpretations of all this when clearly the ambiguities and conflict between meanings was essential to what the Aboriginal elders were attempting to achieve.

It seems that the essential function of the myth is precisely to convey opposite messages to 'opposite' sections – uninitiated and initiated – of society itself, so that the contradictions in the myth express faithfully the essential contradictions buried in the social structure. Everything in the myth is 'turned the other way around', inverted with respect to its inside or secret meaning, because deception of the uninitiated is essential to the maintenance of male ritual rule. Maddock (1974: 146–52) uses the term 'rites of exclusion' to describe such myths with their associated rituals. It is not simply that women are not needed in the ceremonies, but that their spiritual exclusion should be accentuated by their being brought into the closest possible contact with secrets of whose significance they must be kept unaware. In many Arnhem Land secret/sacred ceremonies, women actually see the forbidden sacred objects, but fail to realise that they are seeing them, since the messages they have been given by men are wholly incorrect. Maddock (1974: 151) comments that if the 'original psychology' of such rites were to be reconstructed, 'it might be found to consist in a deep feeling that it is unsatisfying merely to keep women ignorant, that it is preferable to flaunt in women's faces the things of which they are kept ignorant'. My suspicion is that the old Aboriginals rather enjoyed deceiving anthropologists in the same way.

In the myth of the Two Wawilak Sisters – whose story-line is familiar to both sexes – women are having flaunted in their faces information of vital importance to them. They are able to hear a narrative telling of their own immense culture-creating power. Yet all the time, they are kept as far as possible unaware of the *significance* of what they both see and hear. As the primordial potency of menstrual synchrony is both shown to women and yet made terrifying in their eyes, men set about alienating the value of Womankind's blood-making and child-bearing capacities – even to the point of claiming that the production of babies is in some sense valueless when performed by women, yet of immense culture-creating value when symbolically acted out by 'child-bearing' men.

In the Wawilak myth, it is incest (a 'return to the womb') associated with the ultimate symbol of kinship connectedness – 'blood' – which generates the 'wet' season of rain and storms. The two great wrongs – incest and blood-spilling – are merely different aspects of one and the same sin of excessively stressing blood connection, and it is this which brings on the rains. Lévi-

Strauss (1973: 379–81) shows how, in myths from America to Japan, such
'excessive longing for conjunction with the family' has the same effect,
bringing on rain and the anger of the rainbow in various forms. The
Wawilak myth describes a journey to the sky followed by a return journey,
the result being men's ritual power to re-enact such trips, thereby ensuring
the coming of the annual rains. The men re-enact (a) the Sisters' 'incest' and
(b) their letting loose of 'floods'.

The 'bird-nester' myths of *Mythologiques* fall within the same transformation group, for the hero who (like the offspring of the Wawilak Sisters)
becomes temporarily stranded in the sky (just as boys during initiation are
temporarily secluded from this world) is invariably guilty of some 'excessive'
longing for conjunction with a female relative, as a result of which he
generates seasonal periodicity with its rain and storms (Lévi-Strauss 1970:
35–7). This hero is a 'crying child' or an 'orphan' – one who feels cut off
from his mother and the feminine world and insists on being rejoined (Lévi-
Strauss 1973: 379–81). Crying babies and orphans seem to have a similar
effect in western Arnhem Land as elsewhere in the world: they conjure up
fears of excessive maternal desire, and with these, fears of 'floods' and the
anger of 'the Rainbow'. The myths tell of babies whose cries trigger floods
and storms – presaged by the appearance of a rainbow – which drown whole
communities. 'The combination of Orphan and rainbow', the Berndts (1970:
21) remark in this context, 'appears throughout the whole region'. The
implication is that the Rainbow Snake is generated or constituted by (a) the
too-close attraction between babies and their mothers (precisely the bonds
that male initiation rites strive to cut) and (b) the 'excessive' closeness of
reproductively potent women themselves. In western Arnhem Land, a
woman who is pregnant, menstruating or carrying a child is told *not to go near
other women*, particularly if there is water nearby, for fear of generating the
Rainbow (Berndt and Berndt 1970: 180). The effect of such taboos is, of
course, to atomise women in their experiences of reproductive power.

What is it which makes the moral legislators (almost exclusively male) in
Aboriginal Australia insist that when women give birth to babies, they
should do so alone? This rule is not always strictly enforced (see for example
Hamilton 1981: 27), but almost everywhere it seems to coincide with what
men regard as the ideal. Men should 'give birth' collectively; each woman
should have to do so alone. Ryan (1969: 46) reports the following isolation
rule from a Queensland (Bulloo River) tribe:

No woman must see a baby born except her own, and nobody except the
mother of the child must be present at the birth. When a woman knows
she is to have a baby, she goes away to a place she has picked for that
purpose and there she makes a large fire so as to have plenty of ashes to
clean herself and the baby when it arrives. After the baby is born she
returns to the camp and then it can be seen by all. She must have no help
or aid from anyone. . . .

In this tribe, too, male 'childbirth' – the initiation process through which boys are 'reborn' – is a decidedly collective affair, in starkest contrast with what women are supposed to be allowed (Ryan 1969: 14–15). The logic at work is everywhere the same; so it seems that when the Wawilak myth depicts the closeness of the two Sisters as the birth process begins, a definite point is being made:

> The two women stopped to rest, for the younger felt the child she was carrying move inside her. She knew her baby would soon be born. Yeppa [sister], I feel near my heart this baby turning', she said. The older one said, 'Then let us rest.'
>
> They sat down, and the older sister put her hand on the abdomen of the younger sister and felt the child moving inside. She then massaged her younger sister, for she knew her labor pains had commenced. The baby was born there. (Warner 1957: 251)

These mythical women bleed and give birth displaying affection and solidarity with one another, not in lonely isolation. They are in tune with the immense powers vested in one another's physiologies and blood. Is is not these powers which are thought 'too dangerous' by men, and which men's taboos and initiation rites are designed simultaneously to suppress in women, to alienate and to usurp?

Giving birth – where men are concerned – is not just one among other collective activities from time to time performed. It is the most collective, solidarity-engendering of all activities – far more so than hunting ever is.

Male childbirth needs women, but only in a negative sense – for in changing a pubescent child's name and 'killing' it prior to rebirth, the mother's contribution is acknowledged only to be negated and supplanted. The process typically involves seizing frightened young boys from the arms of their mothers in the women's camp and then carrying them off to be 'swallowed by the Snake' within the men's sacred ground. There follow procedures such as cutting the boy's flesh, anointing their bodies with 'menstrual' blood, placing them in a pit or other encircled space symbolising an immense womb or women's hut, blindfolding them, declaring that the Snake/Mother/Rainbow has now swallowed them – and finally, releasing them back for their mothers to see, now covered in red ochre and/or blood and 'reborn'.

An example is the Karwadi initiation ritual of the Murinbata of Western Australia. Here, body-painting with blood is practised on young boys who enter into a symbolic womb. Men stand before the boys holding containers of blood, which is said to be 'the blood of the Mother' (Stanner 1966: 7). They smear the youths 'from head to foot with the blood: eyes, ears, nostrils, lips and nose are all liberally covered. . . ' Eventually, the boys emerge from this ordeal 'reborn'. This ritual, it is said, was originally performed by 'the Mother' herself, until men sadly had to kill her and take her place with artificial replicas of her bloody presence (Stanner 1966: 40, 43, 63).

Among the Ma:ra Aborigines, boys undergoing initiation are symbolically 'swallowed' into the womb of an ancestral 'Mother' called Mumuna. At the end of the ceremony, the initiates are revealed to their mothers – who see them covered from head to foot with a paste made from earth, blood and red-ochre. As the 'blood-covered' boys shine in the sun, the ritual leaders call out: 'Look at the colouring they have on their bodies: they are smeared with the inside liquids of Mumuna's womb!' (Berndt 1951: 160).

Before being allowed to eat normal food or return to female company, the newly reborn and hence 'raw' boys typically have to be 'cooked' – that is, they must have smoke blown over them, or they are made to jump over flames or stay uncomfortably close to a fire. In northern Australia as elsewhere in the continent (Elkin 1938: 167–8), this concluding 'fire' phase of each blood-letting ritual – consistently with the model – signals the removal of blood pollution, the retreat of the Snake, and the simultaneous lifting of the blood-linked taboos which for a period of days or weeks had previously outlawed all cooking, feasting and marital sex (Warner 1957: 324, 328–9). 'The rainbow serpent', as Mountford (1978: 23) puts it, 'is essentially the element of water, and any sign of its opposite element – fire, even fumes of smoke – is sufficient to drive this mythical creature back to its home under the water'.

The Delineation of Sisterly Power

The 'Snake', we can now see, is a way of describing women and their offspring in such rhythmic intimacy with one another that they feel as if they are 'one flesh', 'one blood' – or one immense 'Mother'. As the Central Australian (Aranda) songs of the *alknarintja* put it, such ritually potent women resemble a clump of bushes 'so thick and so pressed against each other that they cannot move separately' (Róheim 1974: 144). With their blood-flows conjoining, they form into a single flow or stream – its elements as harmoniously conjoined and as inseparable as those of a snake. The Two Sisters who in northern Australian myths 'turn into a rainbow' or are 'swallowed by a Snake' are in reality doing something simple, yet magical enough in its own way. They are entering the 'wet' phase of their menstrual cycle and becoming engulfed in their own blood-derived unity with one another. Like water-women diving into a river, they are being 'swallowed up' in a collective medium transcending the body boundaries of each. It is as if the blood at this point were acting as a snake-like 'skin' embracing them all.

Whenever an out-of-phase woman is brought back into synchrony, it is as if her 'water-sisters' were claiming her back into their realm. A myth from Arnhem Land describes one such process of reclamation. A 'lost' Sister shakes off the man who had led her astray; she returns at last to her true watery element of sisterhood:

And when she drank, all the Murinbungo, the water-lubras, rose up out of the billabong. They had long streaming hair and they called out to her: 'O, sister, where have you been? We cried for you. Come back to us, sister'. The water-lubras reached out their arms to her. They pulled her down to them in the water. (Robinson 1966: 61–6)

These women – 'daughters of the Rainbow' – are indeed 'like a snake', for no creature on earth more closely resembles a river or flow, or can coil itself into so many repeated cycles. And women are indeed 'like a rainbow' – because the blood-flow is not mere physical blood. As the symbol of the sex strike, it carries women as if from world to world. Under the blood's spell, women move from their 'dry' phase to 'the wet', from 'the cooked' to 'the raw', and also from marital life to the world of seclusion and blood unity – just as the rainbow leaps cyclically between sunshine and rain, dry season and wet, earth and sky.

In Aboriginal Australia, then, the 'Snake' is nothing other than women's culture-creating, menstruation-synchronising dance. 'A dance ground is a snake's body', writes Warner (1957: 274) as if in confirmation, 'and it is usually thought of as having the women and children inside it'.

But although mythology knows that 'the Snake' and women's 'dance' are one and the same, male initiation ritualism, as we have seen, inverts all this, attempting to exclude women from their own dance, which must now be monopolised by men. Aboriginal men who dance themselves into a 'Snake' know that they first learned to do this when they 'stole' women's secrets long, long ago in the mythological past – and they know it with quiet confidence because such things do not change, and *they are still doing it today*.

To bring out the ultimate paradox which all this involves, let us conclude this chapter by checking once again with the ritual that re-enacts the Wawilak Sisters myth.

Just before the Yolngu Kunapipi ('fertility/initiation') ceremony begins, Yurlunggur or Julunggul the Snake is heard roaring some distance away; she/he can smell blood. The 'weird sound' of the bull-roarers, Warner (1957: 270) comments, is 'a kind of bellowing roar . . . like that which one imagines a wounded dragon would make'. The terrified boys due to be snatched from their mothers and 'swallowed' have been smeared with red ochre and arm-blood. The snake-like dancing procession of men carries them away, taking them to the male sacred dance ground, whose 'inside' (secret) name is 'the Mother's uterus'. At the same time, however, the dancing men come up to the boys' mothers and female kin, surrounding them. Pointedly, the men refuse to 'swallow' these. Berndt (1951: 42) comments:

The dancing men symbolise Julunggur surrounding the women (the Wauwalak in their *murlk* [hut]); but these are not swallowed, because none are menstruating or have afterbirth blood. 'The men dancing around are smelling, but they smell no odour of blood'.

So when the dancing men approach the women and children, they *discriminate* against the women and girls, resolving to swallow only male offspring, on the paradoxical grounds that their womenfolk are *not bloody* whereas their sons are. We have, then, the insistence that present-day women – in contrast to their mythological ancestresses – at the crucial moment neither menstruate nor smell of blood, and therefore must be excluded from the heart of the ritual. Meanwhile, men and boys can be swallowed because they do menstruate and do smell of blood. The dialectical inversion is complete.

Yet if anything is truly extraordinary about these rituals, it is the extent to which the men are aware of what they are doing. They seem to be consciously tricking the women, who in turn seem to be colluding, to some extent, with a certain collective awareness of what is going on. The sexes are contesting their respective rights to a power whose basic nature is understood. They are struggling for 'the Snake', and both sides know in essence what this means. Sometimes the women are permitted to gain the upper hand, while more often they concede victory to the men. But at Yirkalla, in the lush, game-rich region of north-east Arnhem Land which is the Yolngu people's home, women's solidarity is still very strong, menstrual blood is regarded as 'sacred' in a strikingly positive way, and the struggle for 'the Snake' is therefore a very real, living sexual-political fight.

Two or three nights before the finale of the Kunapipi at Yirrkalla, after the boys have passed through 'the core of their Kunapipi experience' (in being swallowed into the Uterus of 'the Mother') all the women dance into the men's sacred ground. Some are painted with red ochre, and decorated 'to dance for coitus' (Berndt 1951: 50). This is 'incestuous' coitus; it must embody the blood unity which is 'the Snake'. It is the women themselves who now hold the power, invading the men's 'sacred' ground and forming themselves into a 'Snake' of their own. The women have their own secret name for this Snake, with which they are supposed to deceive the men, and as they call out this name ('Kitjin') they warn the men not to get too near 'or your bellies will come up like pregnant women'. The men sit down quietly, with heads bent.

It is only once this snake power of the women themselves has been established that the conditions are felt appropriate for the climax of the ceremony – collective and 'incestuous' sexual intercourse within the dance-ground or symbolic 'womb'. Following this genuine, flesh-and-blood 'return to the womb', the initiates are removed in imitation of childbirth from a large menstrual hut/parturition hut representing that in which the Two Wawilak Sisters were swallowed at the beginning of time. Berndt's (1951: 55) male informants observe, in words which seem to display astonishing consciousness of the fact that all this is something which women should really be doing:

> But really we have been stealing what belongs to them (the women), for it is mostly all woman's business; and since it concerns them it belongs to them. Men have nothing to do really, except copulate, it belongs to the women. All that belonging to those Wauwalak, the baby, the blood, the yelling, their dancing, all that concerns the women; but every time we have to trick them. Women can't see what men are doing, although it really is their own business, but we can see their side. This is because all the Dreaming business came out of women – everything; only men take 'picture' for that Julunggul [i.e. men make an artificial reproduction of the Snake]. In the beginning we had nothing, because men had been doing nothing; we took these things from women.

It is one of the severest indictments of twentieth-century anti-evolutionist anthropology that its models have led ethnographers to dismiss such profound Aboriginal insights as scientifically valueless.

Chapter 14
The Dragon Within

> . . . and these petrified social conditions must be made to dance by
> singing their own melody to them.
> Karl Marx, *Contribution to the Critique of Hegel's Philosophy of Right*
> (1843–4)

The rainbow-snake complex as a rock-art motif extends back in northern
Australia for at least 7,000 to 9,000 years, making it 'probably the longest
continuing religious belief documented in the world' (Flood 1989: 293).
Several authorities (Chaloupka 1984; Lewis 1988) have suggested that the
post-glacial sea rise between about 9,000 and 7,000 years ago inspired many
of the images; floods and tidal waves may have been conceptualised as an
immense 'Snake' submerging much of the Aborigines' former land. Many
contemporary Aborigines in coastal regions still see 'the Snake' in something
like this way. The Great Snake Thuwathu of the Lardil tribe, Mornington
Island, for example, 'only emerges on a high tide' (Memmott 1982: 171).
Until recently on this island, menstruating or otherwise reproductively
potent women had to be especially careful; their bodily processes could easily
conjure up a flood which would risk drowning everyone. 'Babies were
therefore not carried over tidal estuaries when groups were moving along the
coast' (Memmott 1982: 174).

Lewis (1988: 91) sees the extremely ancient image of the Rainbow Snake
in animal-headed form (that is, with prominent 'ears') as a composite
construct, its various body-parts connoting the totemic affiliations of the
different local groups which came together for ritual performances (figure
23). 'Given the demonstrated continuity of composite Rainbow snakes in the
art', he adds, 'I believe it is reasonable to hypothesise that the early rock
paintings of this being document rituals that fulfilled a similar function to
the rituals of the present time' (Lewis 1988: 91). Just as recent Rainbow
Snake rituals embody the widest possible levels of inter-regional solidarity,
so the ancient ones functioned to offset the social tensions and fragmentation

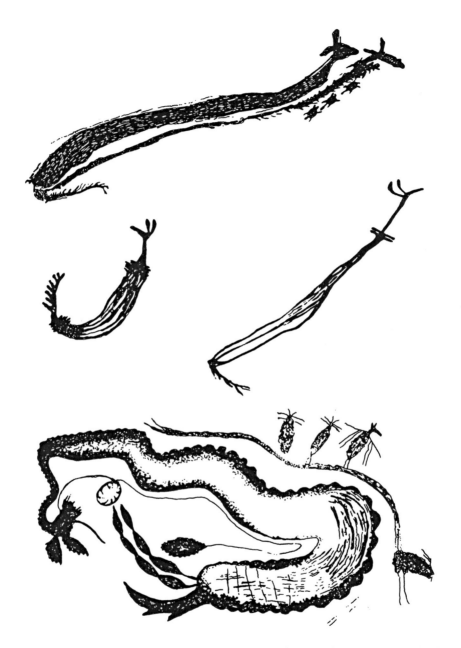

Figure 23 Arnhem Land rock-paintings of Rainbow Snakes with kangaroo-like heads. Colour: dark red. Age: about 7,000–8,000 BP. *Upper*: Deaf Adder Creek headwaters (Lewis 1988: Fig. 122). Two snakes with ears, and three turtles. *Middle*: Stag Creek (Lewis 1988: Fig. 123). Snakes with ears and crocodile tails. *Lower*: Jim Jim Creek (Lewis 1988: Fig. 121). Complex composite Rainbow Snake with ears and crocodile tail, surrounded with bird, yam and flying fox designs (all figures redrawn).

threatened as coastal Aborigines were forced to retreat inland into areas already occupied and perhaps overpopulated by long-settled residents.

Although it would explain only certain aspects of the mythological motif, Lewis' interpretation can readily be integrated with our model. *The Snake is an image of human solidarity.* In Lewis' (1988: 91) words, 'the Rainbow snake symbolises the possibilities of alliance among clan groups; it is a means of inclusion, a counter-balance against tensions that tend to fragment larger social groups'. Humans have always harnessed aspects of the natural order to the requirements of the moral order – ascribing sickness, storms, hunting failures and so forth to the anger of 'the spirits' or 'the gods'. Aboriginal ritual authorities under changing social conditions may well have attempted to make use of post-Pleistocene floods in a similar way, drawing on traditional linkages between lunar/tidal rhythms and 'the Snake' whilst arguing that particularly disastrous flood-tides came as punishment for allowing the obligations of solidarity to be abandoned.

But of course, the model of cultural origins advocated in this book would lead us to trace the underlying abstract logic of the Rainbow Snake (although not necessarily its imagery) much further back into the Aborigines' past – indeed, right back to their first entry into Australia. The model would imply that shoreline-foraging Aboriginal women from earliest times phase-locked with the tides, and correspondingly conceptualised themselves as immersed once a month in a 'flood' of blood-symbolised togetherness transcending the individuality of each participant. In their monthly menstrual immersion or sex strike – as in any strike – the participants would have felt their separate identities being transcended in that of the great kinship coalition which together they formed. As time passed, this entity would have become conceptualised through a variety of different images, no one of which would in itself have seemed adequate to symbolise the experienced reality in its full richness and complexity. 'Mother', 'All-Mother', 'Rainbow' and many other images would all have been tried. We know, however, that one of the most recurrent iconographic motifs came to be that of an immense sea-, river- or lake-dwelling 'Snake'.

An International Myth

Not only can 'the Snake' be assumed to extend back to the first entry of modern humans into Australia. Its centrality to world mythology (Mundkur 1983) implies that it is older still. Mountford (1978: 23) notes that versions of the Rainbow Snake myth 'appear to belong to all peoples, irrespective of time and race'. Ancient Hebraic patriarchal mythology is familiar with supernaturally potent snake imagery in association with female 'evil'. In the myth of Genesis, it was when the Serpent tempted Eve to 'taste the fruit of the Tree of Knowledge of Good and Evil' that humanity first realised *the distinction between the sexes* (Leach 1961b). Equally familiar to Bible-readers is a story about being swallowed and regurgitated by a whale, and another narrative about a primaeval flood, the guardianship of animals in and through this flood, a pan-human watery 'death' followed by 'rebirth' – and a covenant between God and humankind written across the skies in the shape of a rainbow (Gen. 9, 12–17; see Dundes 1988).

Even under a stricter definition, 'The Rainbow Snake', 'Great Sea Snake' or 'Water Snake' is not just Australian. Astonishingly similar beliefs concerning an immense, visually striking, water-dwelling snake linked with the rainbow are widespread in tropical and subtropical regions in the Far East, Africa and the Americas (Blacker 1978; Forge 1966: 25, 29; Hugh-Jones, C. 1979; Hugh-Jones, S. 1979; Huxley 1962: 188; Loewenstein 1961; Mead 1933, 1941; Reichel-Dolmatoff 1968: 79; Schafer 1973; Werner 1933). Even far from the tropics, Celtic mythology once filled all deep lakes and inlets with watery snake-like beings – the Loch Ness Monster being nowadays the best known. Comparable traditions extend even further north. Monsters such as the dragon-like *palraiyuk* and the 'man-worm' of the Bering Sea Eskimo show that mythical serpentine creatures can survive even when transported to arctic habitats which in reality are uninhabitable to reptiles of any kind (Borden 1976: 441).

Africa

Among the Central African Luba, 'the rainbow, *nkongolo*, is formed by two snakes coupling in the sky' (Reefe 1981: 24). 'Nkongolo' is also the name of the first ritual ruler of the Luba; de Heusch (1975; 366) notes how Luba origin-of-kingship myths turn, at certain points, on 'the transformation of the image of the rainbow into that of a continuous stream of menstrual blood. . .'

The Mbuti of the Ituri Forest, Zaire, tell the story of a couple crossing a stream on what they thought was a fallen tree: they were carried down under the water by *Klima* – 'the dead tree which was really the rainbow which was really a water animal' (Turnbull 1959: 56). Comparable 'water animals' are central to the mythology of almost all known sub-Saharan African hunter-gatherer groups, and are prominent in much prehistoric rock-painting. Curiously – just as in ancient northern Australian rock-art – these snakes are often depicted with prominent 'ears' (figure 24a). Brincker (1886: 163; quoted by Schmidt 1979: 209) writes of the boa-constrictor associated with the mythical snake *ondara* of the Herero: 'It is said to have two "flaps" at the head, similar to goats' ears with which it makes a noise'. Such noise-making, big-eared creatures, whether in real life or in rock-art, are known as 'rain snakes'; in some regions they merge into images of the more generalised 'rain-animal', 'rain-eland' or 'rain-bull' with its crescent 'horns' (Schmidt 1979). This 'eland' or 'bull' is central to rain-making magic and may be 'accompanied by rainbows, lightning, fishes or snakes' (Pager 1975: 45). The

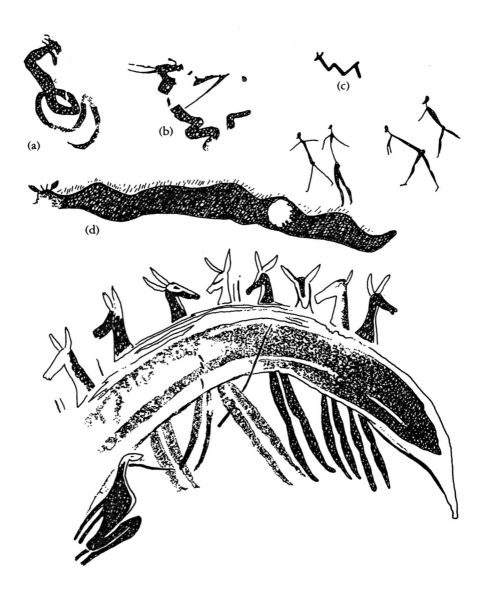

Figure 24 San paintings from rock shelters in the Ndedema Gorge, Drakensberg Mountains, Natal. *Upper*: snakes with antelope heads, horns and/or ears (Pager 1972: Fig. 377). Locations: Van der Riet Shelter (a); Sebaaieni Cave (b); Junction Shelter (c); Bemani Shelter (d). *Lower*: a row of antelope heads above a rainbow, while human legs protrude below and an 'ales' (flying magical antelope) crouches nearby. The scene probably relates to the shamanic experience of metamorphosis through dance and trance (Pager 1972: Fig. 384; all figures redrawn).

connection with rainbows (figure 24) is recurrently stressed (Schmidt 1979: 209–20). Schmidt (1979: 220) argues that the *eland* originally lay at the core of what she terms the 'trickster/moon/lightning/rain/fertility/life/eland/ horns' symbolic chain which was central to the ancient southern African hunter-gatherer cultures. 'The mythical *likongoro* of the Okavongo', she writes, 'whose name could also be translated as "rainbow", resembled, when in the water, a horned snake, but outside – a kudu!' Linking this with images of antelope-headed snakes in rock-art, she goes on to suggest that the serpents with 'horns' or 'ears' belong in the same category; among the Sandawe, she notes, ' "the word for 'ears' . . . and 'horns' . . . may both be used to describe the horns of the moon" ' (Schmidt 1979: 220, quoting Ten Raa 1969: 41). (Even in European Christian traditions of demonology, it might be added, 'the Serpent' is a creature who has been depicted by artists fully equipped with cloven feet, horns and a head remarkably like that of a goat).

A snake is liquidly 'flowing' in its movements – flowing as no other animal can be. But in southern Africa as elsewhere, there can be no doubt that 'the Snake' signifies 'that which flows' in a much wider symbolic sense, including streaming water, torrents of rain, rivers – and above all, *blood*, whether animal or menstrual. All of these phenomena equally are manifestations of the underlying abstract entity, 'that which flows'. Etymology in some instances seems to confirm this. In the Khoekhoe language, for example, the words for *'snake'* – /aub – and 'fountain' – /aus – are etymologically almost identical, the difference being that the first ends with the feminine suffix, −s, while the second takes its masculine counterpart, −b. Sharing the common root, /au, both terms originally meant 'the flowing one' or 'the flow-er'. Animal or human blood is 'the flowing one' in a similar sense; in Khokhoe, the colour red, /ava, takes its origin from /au, to bleed; hence /ava or /aua, blood-like, blood-coloured – i.e. red (Hahn 1881: 79).

'The Snake', in short, corresponds to the same symbolic blood construct as has been central to this book's argument up to this point. It is blood, namely, to the extent that its outflowing links menstruants with raw or living animal flesh, preventing hunters from immediately appropriating their own kills. Without this paradigm, in any event, it would seem difficult to explain formulations such as the following, which encapsulates the San belief system which we have been discussing: 'A special snake lives between the horns of all eland, and before eland meat can be consumed, it has to be "purified" of the venomous juices it contains' (Vinnicombe 1976: 233).

In accordance with the same logic, we find that over much of southern Africa, rain animals and first-menstruants merge into one another. Depending on the precise region, either one or the other may be led out into the bush to attract rain. When it is an animal, it is killed so that its rain-making blood, uterine fluids or urine can bring on the rains. When it is a girl, she only has to menstruate (Schmidt 1979). Among the !Kung of the Kalahari, the construct which I am here terming 'menstrual potency' – child-making, rain-making, culture-establishing blood-magic – is known as *now*:

> With childbearing for women and with killing the great antelope for men . . . the *now* has a . . . complex effect. In these cases the *now* of the hunter interacts with the *now* of the antelope, the *now* of the woman interacts with the *now* of the child newly born, and when the blood of the antelope falls upon the ground as the antelope is killed, when the fluid of the womb falls upon the ground at the child's birth, the interacting of *nows* takes place, and this brings a change in the weather. (Thomas 1959: 162)

Equally instructive is a G/wi version, in this case more directly menstrual. The female subject has just emerged from her first menstrual seclusion:

> the girl is grabbed by the younger women of the band and rushed out, away from the small group of grass huts which is the village. Shouting and laughing they run her in a circle and then back into her hut. This is a 'rainstorm' and the noise is excitement and joy at 'getting wet'. (Silberbauer 1963: 21)

Hahn (1881: 87), writing rather earlier, found an even richer Khoekhoe variant:

> The girl or girls who have become of age must, after the festival, run about in the first thunderstorm, but they must be quite naked, so that the rain which pours down washes the whole body. The belief is that they will get fruitful and have a large offspring. I have on three occasions witnessed this running in the thunder-rain, when the roaring of the thunder was deafening and the whole sky appeared to be one continual flash of lightning.

Just as menstruating girls throughout the region symbolically *become* 'wet' whilst simultaneously *turning into* an eland or other game animal, the Khoekhoe link this rain-attracting, menstruation-linked, thunder-and-lightning-generating magic to an aquatic 'snake' which, according to one classical authority, was ' "so large that when its head is resting on the north bank of the Orange River, its tail is still on the south bank" ' (quoted in Carstens 1975: 90; see also Hahn 1881; Schmidt 1979). The Griqua tell how the 'Great Watersnake' of the Orange River catches pubescent girls to become 'his' wives; this is puzzling, however, because the snake is actually called Keinaus – that is, it is in this case given the *feminine* ending –*s*! (Schmidt 1979: 211). Indeed, there are many other indications that this particular creature has failed to undergo so extreme a political inversion as is common in Australia and elsewhere in the world. *It is still on the side of women.* Among the Khoekhoe:

The Big Snake is hated by all males, towards whom it is equally unfavourably disposed, and it is said to become angry at the sight or smell (especially the latter) of a male. Moreover, the snake when angry is believed to give off a smell which is lethal to all males, and it spews a deadly venom. On the other hand, women are believed to fall in love with the Big Snake, which is also said to have fallen in love with certain women, some of whom are alleged to have had sexual intercourse with it and conceived children. (Carstens 1975: 90).

This easygoing, intimate relationship between women and their 'Snake' – whose deadly 'smell' or 'venom' suggests, of course, women's own husband-repelling blood – may be linked to the fact that among the Khoekhoe, as among other San herders and/or hunter-gatherers, 'there seems to be . . . possibly a slight *female* dominance in the husband/wife relationship' (Barnard 1977: 6). Hahn (1881: 19) makes a rather stronger statement:

In every Khokhoi's house the woman, or *taras*, is the *supreme ruler*, the husband has nothing at all to say. While in public the men take the prominent part, at home they have not so much power even as to take a mouthful of sour milk out of the tub, without the wife's permission.

But we may end this section by recalling a still more instructive Snake-Woman, first touched on in Chapter 4. Menstruation is not central in this particular account. But flowing water, a python-linked sex strike and the repulsion of husbands is.

Among the Igbo in Eastern Nigeria, in the Idemili local government area, the Idemili stream is said to be a python or water spirit and is addressed as 'Mother'. All creatures in it are sacred and must not be killed, the python-goddess forbidding the spilling of her blood. Her shrine is located nearby, guarded by a priest who is 'female' in that he has to tie his wrapper like women do, not loincloth fashion, like men (Amadiume 1987: 53–4).

This shrine priest was important, but 'the favoured one of the goddess Idemili and her earthly manifestation' was the Agba Ekwe, an authoritative woman who headed the Inyom Nnobi or 'Women of Nnobi'. This was in effect an ancient, traditional 'trade union', whose multiple 'eyes' were those of all its members as they watched for, reported and retaliated against sexual misbehaviour or violence. Anyone – male or female – who angered a group of women would risk being told by them that they might soon see, with their own eyes, 'how the python basked in the sun'. 'The python', Amadiume (1987: 68n) explains,

is known to loathe the sun, consequently it usually lies in the shade of bushes, under trees or in caves. Only as a result of acute hunger does it appear in the sun. When it does, it appears full of rage, becomes entangled and suffocates and swallows anything within sight, human or animal. It then returns to the shade and lies there for months, digesting its victim. During this period it is the most harmless creature in the world!

The meetings of the Women's Council were held in private; great secrecy surrounded them. Like some dragon guarding her treasures and secrets – or like a modern strike committee in the midst of a bitter dispute – the Inyom Nnobi ensured that any women's representative who broke ranks and betrayed her sisters by revealing their discussions would be ostracised by all. 'The men were said to be uneasy every time a Women's Council was called, since they were unaware of what would be discussed, or what the women might decide to do' (Amadiume 1987: 67).

All this gives us a wonderful glimpse into the identity of that Snake-linked 'monster' whose secrets were eventually 'stolen' by men in the many traditional myths about a 'primitive matriarchy' studied in Chapter 12. The Inyom Nnobi clearly was 'the python' or physical manifestation of 'the Goddess'. In a real way, this 'python' *did* 'swallow up' or 'seize' women and babies from men. *Its basic weapon was that of the strike.* When women throughout the community were ordered by the Inyom Nnobi to strike, 'all domestic, sexual and maternal services' were withdrawn, women carrying only suckling babies as they left their husbands *en masse* (Amadiume 1987: 67). Among the typical offences provoking such action, two are worth singling out. If anyone either (a) sexually molested a young girl while she was travelling along a bush path or (b) killed a python, it was regarded as an assault upon *all women* and therefore an affront to the goddess herself. She withdrew the female flesh which it was her responsibility above all to protect. Although varying levels of action were resorted to, all-out, community-wide strike action against *all men* was the time-honoured response if all else failed (Amadiume 1987: 122). It is perhaps worth noting – as we grope towards an understanding of the world's dragon-legends – that only an extremely ruthless and violent 'dragon-slayer' could have coped with such many-headed potency as this.

America

In parts of the New World, particularly in South America, the parallels with Aboriginal Australian ritual and mythology seem closer than in the Igbo or southern African cases: masculinist sexual-political inversions have followed a more familiar course – leading, often, to Australian-American identities which become quite astonishing. They extend to almost identical matriarchy myths, to the use of bull-roarers, to male symbolic menstruation – and to the concept of a rainbow-like 'Snake' which has a special, *now supposedly 'dangerous'* affinity with menstruating women.

'The conception of the rainbow as a large water serpent', writes Métraux (1946: 40), 'is widespread in South America'. Métraux documents the belief among the Arawak, Arekuna, Caxinawa, Ipurina, Carajá, Cocama, Chiriguanao, Guaraní, Bororó, Lengua, Vilela, Inca and Araucanians – a conservative list, since the belief undoubtedly spread much further. 'One of the most formidable demons known to the Indians', wrote Karsten (1935: 220) of the Quechua-speaking tribes,

> is the huge water boa, called *amárum* . . . It is the original source of witchcraft and the souls of sorcerers specially are believed to take up their abode, temporarily or permanently, in this monster. Now, in the imagination of the Indians the rainbow (*cuichi*) is nothing but a huge boa in the air or, as they generally express it, the rainbow is the 'shadow of the boa'.

One superstition held about this phenomenon, continues Karsten, is that it makes women pregnant: 'When the rainbow appears, therefore, the women who are menstruating ought not to go out lest an accident of this kind should happen to them.'

In the Andes, Aymara speakers share similar beliefs with the Quechua. 'Serpents are thought to be attracted by menstrual fluids, and they may pursue menstruating women, entering them through the vagina while they sleep or when the have become inebriated' (Bolton 1976: 441).

Myths from the Gran Chaco tribes – such as the Toba and the Pilagá – describe how incautious young menstruants, disobeying their seclusion rules, provoke floods unleashed by 'the Rainbow', and as a result are drowned along with their entire communities (Métraux 1946: 29–30). Likewise, the Amazonian Waiwai have a complex set of beliefs according to which all women are in some original sense the great water-snake's property. Men's wives belonged once to 'the Anaconda-people', a snake-like community consisting of water-boas, large fish and similar creatures who live at the bottom of rivers, but can assume human form when they surface from time to time. All women are the kin of these Anaconda-people, who exercise a constant claim over men's wives as a result. The first human husband is said to have seized his water-dwelling wife from the Anaconda-people without paying them the proper bride-price. 'They therefore want bride-price or a woman in exchange . . .' (Fock 1963: 31). The Anacondas, in other words, constantly and *legitimately* attempt to reclaim the female flesh which is theirs. Young women are particularly at risk of being reclaimed should they *look towards the river whilst undergoing their first menstruation ritual* (Fock 1963: 48).

This is important, because it allows us to make the necessary links with the Nigerian strike-organising python-goddess Idemili discussed earlier – affording a rare glimpse into the logic behind all those many myths, throughout the world, which tell of a watery Snake's primordial periodic power over women, and its 'cruel demands' for what men choose to interpret

as the 'sacrifice' of marriageable young maidens. What the Women of Nnobi
would have thought of as a young maiden's withdrawal from sexual circulation by her gender group is experienced by men as a tragic waste of a
desirable maiden who could have been sexually enjoyed! Interestingly, the
Waiwai themselves have just such a myth. It concerns a gigantic Serpent
who once used to kill all who approached:

> After it had been appealed to, it agreed to kill no more provided the most
> beautiful woman in the tribe was sacrificed to it. She was then cast into a
> lake on the north slope of the Acarai mountain, which was the abode of
> the serpent. Here she still lives. The serpent, satisfied, no longer molests
> the Waiwai. (Fock 1963: 53, citing Farabee 1924: 174)

The World-dragon

Most of us have been brought up since infancy in vague familiarity with
legends of this kind. Images of a lake-dwelling, winged, fabulous, woman-
devouring, kingdom-ruling, tribute-demanding 'Snake' have come down to
us as the central motif in countless fairy-tales which still have the power to
enchant — many of them translated from the mythologies of Tibet, China,
Japan, India, pre-Columbian Central America, the Middle or Near East, pre-
Christian Europe or some other corner of the globe. In most translations, the
monster has been given its properly recognisable, heraldically fixed form.
The name traditionally used by folklorists to refer to this extraordinary,
blood-loving, weather-changing, coiling magical monster is, of course — 'the
Dragon'.

Just as 'the Seven Sisters' are found in mythology throughout the world,
often connoting seven women who retaliate against their lazy or cruel
husbands by rising up into the sky to become the Pleiades (Buckley 1988:
200, citing Harrington 1931: 142–5, Reid 1939: 246–8; Hahn 1881: 74),
so the *seven-headed dragon* is an international motif. Here is a Japanese version:

> A man came to a house where all were weeping, and learned that the last
> of seven daughters of the house was to be given to a dragon with seven
> heads, which came to the seashore yearly to claim a victim. The man
> changed himself into the girl's form, and induced the dragon to drink
> sake from seven pots set before it. He then slew the drunken monster.
> (Ingersoll 1928: 65, 6)

Naturally, the hero then married the maiden himself. From the end of the
dragon's tail, he 'took out a sword which is today the Mikado's state sword'.
The ritual power of the divine ruler, then is the usurped or stolen power of
'the Dragon'.

This, too, is a common theme. The ancient divine kings and emperors of
most of the world were according to Elliot Smith (1919: 76–139), identified
with dragons whose blood-making and rain-making powers were associated

with the tides, floods and potencies of the moon. Solidarity in its original forms was of course turned on its head by these often-violent patriarchal rulers. But as in the case of male initiation rites throughout the world, so when divine rulers were being enthroned or empowered, trickery of the kind depicted in the myths was the order of the day. The Japanese dragon-slayer, as we have just seen, *dressed up as a woman*. Secluded from the sun and carried above the ground, he and similar divine kings and priest-kings were treated *as if* they were menstruants whose rain-making and other magical powers needed preserving for the good of the realm (Frazer 1900: 3: 204). The Chinese emperor Yao was said to be 'the son of a dragon'; several other Chinese rulers were metaphorically called 'dragon-faced' (Ingersoll 1928: 100). In all these cases, solidarity's symbols – the 'Dragon' foremost among them – had been politically usurped and then used *against* the very forces from whom they had initially been derived. All those rulers who sought 'The Mandate of Heaven' – claiming to root their power not in earthly sources but in patterns written in the skies – were stealing an authority which was never legitimately their own. The notion of divine rule 'in harmony with the celestial spheres' stemmed ultimately from Womankind's time-honoured reliance on the moon as the source of her synchrony and therefore of her power. Whenever and wherever men have claimed to possess any such mandate, it has been a deception and usurpation. The first representatives of ritual or 'supernatural' authority were menstruating women. The first 'mandate of heaven' was the legitimacy won by women when – in some ways like their distant descendants in the Paris Commune of 1871, or more recently in Tienanmen Square on that night of the dark moon in June 1989 – they wrote out culture's rules in their own blood.

A seven-headed dragon is central to mythology in Cambodia, India, Persia, western Asia, East Africa and the Mediterranean area. In parts of Scotland, the seven-headed sea monster comes 'in a storm of wind and spray' (Elliot Smith 1919; cited in Ingersoll 1928: 105). But if we now disregard the precise number of heads – seven, a hundred, a thousand or more – the monster becomes still more international. In most of the world's great patriarchal foundation myths – Perseus and Andromeda, Heracles and the Hydra, Zeus and Typhon, Marduk and Tiamat, Indra and Vritra, St George and the Dragon and so forth (Fontenrose 1959) – a coiling, wet, reptilian, blood-red, fire-breathing 'plumed' or 'winged' Serpent with its multiple heads and all-seeing eyes carries off marriageable maidens to the world beyond men's reach, doing so periodically and to the accompaniment of flood tides and storms. Woman are considered to be in need of male rescue from this fate, a task which is accomplished by the patriarchal hero only after an immense struggle in which the cords or coils binding the earth to the heavens are cut and the magical potencies of the dragon – including above all its powers over women – are triumphantly stolen for the benefit of mankind.

These potencies have everything to do with the dragon's ability to produce blood: the many-headed water-dwelling Hydra is typical in that its 'heads' sprouted up wherever its blood flowed, so that merely cutting off a head achieved nothing – the bleeding stumps had to be cauterised with fire (Kerényi 1959: 143–4, citing Apollodorus Mythographus 2.5.2). In Aboriginal Australia, too – where the Rainbow Snake is often said to be the source of women's menstrual flows – it is only when men can surround and isolate menstruating flesh with *fire* that they feel safe from the dangers that the Serpent represents. Everything which uncontrollably 'flows' threatens to summon up the evil; the way to keep it down is to use fire to dry up the world-threatening blood (Berndt 1970: 180; Mountford 1978: 23–4). The atomisation of menstruating womankind and the chopping up of her Serpent into isolated, impotent bits of flesh can be seen to be one and the same.

In his scholarly treatise on the explicitly lunar-menstrual 'Tsuni!-Goam: The supreme being of the Khoi-khoi', Hahn (1881: 79–80) extends his argument from southern Africa to what he calls 'the whole realm of Indo-European folk-lore and mythology'. Everywhere, he writes, legends of dragons and serpents have their origin on the banks of lakes and rivers:

> We refer to Hercules, who killed the Lernaic Hydra. Apollo kills Python close to a fine flowing fountain. . . . At the fountain of Ares watched a dragon, who refused water to Kadmos and his followers. In Switzerland, if rivers break down from the mountains after a thunderstorm, the people say: 'a dragon has come out'. In Denmark Müllenhof found a legend, that in the spot where once a Lindwurm's (i.e., a dragon's) tail was to be seen, now a brook is winding'. Beowulf kills the dragon who lives in the lake. Acheloös, the River-god, became a serpent when Hercules fought for Deîaneira. Siegfried kills the dragon in the cavern on the Rhine; and many more instances too numerous to mention.

In most instances, the dragon-slayer confronts the Snake in order to wrest from its clutches the maiden caught up in its embrace.

The Wawilak myth central to Chapter 13 is therefore significant precisely because it is not unique. Its value resides in the fact that it is just one of the more beautiful, exhaustively recorded and complete dragon legends known to us – complete because recorded unusually fully in the context of its *basis in ritual*. But what is interesting is that wherever in the world it is found, 'the Dragon' remains true to itself. Like this book's central construct of 'sex strike' or 'blood', it is always a male-dominance-threatening 'stream' or 'flow' (Hahn 1881: 77–8), the principle of alternation and opposition, the dialectic itself incarnate. It is water which retreats before fire, animal which reveals itself as human, a snake which nonetheless flies, female which is also male, death which is also life. Taller than the tallest tree, itself often coiled around the 'world-tree', immense and brilliant as the rainbow – it carries those who ride it between life and death, marriage and kinship, fire and water, sunshine and rain.

Such adventures are the stuff of Lévi-Strauss' 'bird-nester' myths, which are dragon myths in yet another form. The heroes of these strange narratives are 'incestuous' boys who in their hunger for their own kin are often linked with the moon (1981: 350), and are invariably 'secluded' in some menstrually suggestive way. These boys, as they go hunting for eagles' eggs or for macaws' brilliant red feathers up in the sky, become men in the manner of Yolngu youths. Painted in blood (or a substitute such as faeces), they are engulfed in 'rawness', 'rottenness', 'stench' and 'temporary death', and — ritually secluded from ordinary society — are as if stranded in the sky. After their experience of symbolic 'death', they then return to earthly life safely — now in possession of immense weather-controlling, rain-making, healing and other magical powers.

The Yolngu ritual participants who act out the Wawilak story go to the sky in a Rainbow Snake's womb, which therefore takes the place of the red-feathered, bird-bedecked, blood-or-faeces-bespattered, magically growing, man-eating 'trees', 'cliffs' and other strange vehicles which take youths to the sky in Lévi-Strauss' 'bird-nester' tales. When the Navaho bird-nester Nayenezgani wraps himself in the blood-filled intestines of 'the Horned Monster', pricking himself so that the blood covers his body and using the monster's stomach as a 'mask', he is re-entering a symbolic blood-filled womb and *thereby* entering the other world. His narrow escape from being eaten alive, and his subsequent adventures in vanquishing such terrifying monsters as 'Snapping Vagina' and 'Overwhelming Vagina' (Haile and Wheelwright 1949: 73–4) help confirm that the usurpation and simultaneous political inversion of women's menstrual powers is what such dragon-slaying or monster-vanquishing initiatory experiences are really all about. Today's gods and goddesses become tomorrow's demons and monsters. In voices of lightning and thunder, storms and floods of blood, women once gave awesome expression to 'the anger of the gods'. It was these empowered forces which had to be defied before patriarchy could be safely enthroned.

We have seen that women, in shedding their own blood, seem to die, but that this kind of death is only temporary. Instead of continuing until death, the blood-flow seems to be set in reverse, so that women return from watery seclusion back once again into marital life with its sex, cooking, consumption and other pleasures. Women resurrect themselves monthly, just as does the moon, and all animal life is thought to renew itself at the same time.

The drying up of the flow and the kindling of domestic fire appear in the myths as this reverse movement: from seclusion back to ordinary life, from 'sky' to 'earth', from 'death' to 'new life'. The 'swallowed' flesh is 'regurgitated' once more. The 'bird-nester' descends gently to earth and 'wakes up'. It is this kind of experience — a male usurpation of the periodicity of the menstrual flow — which is undergone by boys during initiation rites all over the world. For men to carry the burdens of these menstrual rhythms has been no easy thing, but the myths of much – perhaps all – of humanity testify that it can and has been done.

Mythologiques Regained

The early chapters of this book focused on Lévi-Strauss' 'exchange of women' theory, on his treatment of 'totemism' and on related themes. Although many 'totemic' and other aspects of ritual and mythology have now been re-evaluated in the light of our model, it may still seem that the net result has been to pose more problems than have yet been answered. In returning to the work of Lévi-Strauss, let us see if we can tie up the remaining loose threads. *Mythologiques* poses the most perplexing intellectual challenges; consequently, we will confine ourselves to the four volumes of this work.

Although this is not the place to give a full or in any sense adequate description of Lévi-Strauss' findings in *Mythologiques*, it does seem important to recall that linkages between daily, monthly and seasonal forms of periodicity are a central unifying theme of the myths collected together and analysed with unprecedented thoroughness by the founder of structuralism in *Mythologiques*. The myths discussed in volume 3 – *The Origin of Table Manners* (1978) – explicitly centre around periodicity in lunar and menstrual forms. While many of the narratives analysed in the other three volumes seemingly relate to different themes, Lévi-Strauss shows that the stories are in reality transformations of one another, so that the logic underlying them can be seen to be ultimately the same.

The myths, according to Lévi-Strauss, are generated by logical and sociological problems. These are varied, but relate essentially to difficulties encountered in attempting to preserve the coherence of certain mental structures – logical thought processes – which in turn are tied up with the maintenance of certain sexual, economic and other social taboos and regulations. Those collectivities preserving, reworking and telling the myths seem to feel threatened with various forms of cultural chaos and structural collapse. Social contradictions are conceptualised in formal terms on the logical plane, appearing as logical contradictions which the myths attempt to sort out.

To the extent that the myths, taken collectively, have a surface ideological message or aim, it is the achievement of moderation and balance in all things – the definition of what is 'excessive' depending, of course, on the conceptual system being used. Models of balance and harmony in social life are shown against a backdrop of various expressions of extremism or excess. At the core of the collective concerns are male anxieties (female ones are not equally represented) of a sexual kind.

In this respect, men's fears essentially concern women. Women can be 'too clinging' or 'too distant', 'too near' or 'too far', 'too hot' or 'too cold', 'too seductive' or 'too shy' and so on. The various extreme possibilities are pictured by means of metaphorical techniques in which a 'distant' woman becomes, for example, a constellation of stars in the sky, or a 'too clinging' woman becomes a limpet-like clinging frog. In addition to metaphor, the full range of expressive techniques known to literature and song are employed.

The first of Lévi-Strauss' four volumes, *The Raw and the Cooked* (1970), selects myths dealing with the function of cooking-fire as something which transforms raw, bloody and hence tabooed meat into edible food. Normally, raw meat – characteristically thought of in the native (or native/Lévi-Straussian) paradigms as 'very wet' – should be transformed into cooked meat, which is properly 'moist' or 'moderately dry'. If men's alimentary needs are to be met, two extremes have to be avoided in this respect. On the one hand, if there were no fire at all, the meat with its blood would go 'rotten' – this being the most extreme form of the category 'very wet'. On the other hand, if there were too much fire, the meat would become 'burnt', the most extreme form of the category 'very dry'. There is a need, therefore, for *both* fire *and* the negation of fire. This combination of opposites finds its embodiment in the ideal of 'domestic fire' – fire which does not burn endlessly or uncontrollably but is kept instead within strict temporal and spatial bounds. In the 'key myth' with which *The Raw and the Cooked* begins, such fire is bounded safely by the 'very wet' – in this case not (or not explicitly) by menstrual blood, but by the torrents of a rainstorm. This storm is magically controlled by the hero of the myth – an incestuous 'bird nester' whose weather-changing powers are granted to him when he is eaten alive from the waist down and made to suffer acute anal incontinence (a version of male surrogate 'menstruation') while stranded in the sky. The rain extinguishes all fires in the world with the exception of just one (Lévi-Strauss 1970: 37, 137).

The myths use an elaborate series of codes in order to link up the twin dangers of uncontrolled fire on the one hand and the absence of fire on the other, with some formally homologous dangers presented in connection with men's sexual needs. The logic behind these connections, reduced to the simplest form possible, seemingly runs as follows:

1. Whereas men's hunger relates them to animal flesh, their sexual desire relates them to female human flesh.
2. Human female flesh presents itself to men in accordance with a logic of alternation which is shared by animal flesh as well. For example, like animal flesh, female sexual flesh should alternate predictably between the states of 'very wet' (bloody, raw) and 'suitably moist' ('cooked' to a moderate extent – i.e. transformed so that all visible blood is removed, but without being 'burnt' or 'dried up').
3. The agent of such transformation in the case of both human female

and animal flesh is 'cooking-fire'. In the case of human female flesh, the 'cooking-fire' which stops the flow of blood may also be conceptualised as internal to the woman.

4. The 'cooking-fire' inside a woman's vulva – the invisible physiological mechanism responsible for doing to female flesh what cooking-fire does to meat – is theoretically liable to malfunction. In such a case, women's menstrual flows might either (a) last indefinitely (the flesh moving from being 'very wet' to a state of 'rottenness') or (b) never come at all (the flesh becoming 'dried up').

5. Translated from the 'sexual code' into the 'alimentary code', these dangers beome: (a) the complete absence of cooking-fire, so that nothing can prevent all meat from becoming 'rotten' and (b) uncontrolled fire, so that everything gets burned up.

Whilst concerned with avoiding the extremes of 'the rotten world' on the one hand and 'the burnt world' on the other, the stories in fact bind these alternatives intimately within a dialectic of 'the near' and 'the far', 'the high' and 'the low', 'the inside' and 'the outside' and so forth. And the choices and extremes are expressed in a variety of different codes, one of the most central being 'the astronomical code', which describes conjunctions and disjunctions between 'wet' and 'dry', 'animal' and 'human' forms of flesh in terms of cosmic conjunctions and disjunctions involving earth, sun, moon and other celestial bodies.

In the astronomical code, uncontrolled cooking-fire is typically represented in terms of the sun's conjoining with the earth and burning it up in a universal conflagration. The complete absence of fire – associated with an unending blood-flow – is depicted through the image of universal darkness and a flood which submerges the entire world. The correct balance is depicted with the help of the moon, which should be the right distance from the sun, just as the sun should be the right distance from both moon and earth. This correct distance is conceptualised both spatially and in terms of periods of time: neither spells of sunlight nor periods of darkness and floods should last 'too long', nor pass 'too quickly'. Since everything is interlinked, it is by controlling carefully both menstrual periodicity and fire – or, in other words, *women*, who are the custodians of both – that such cosmic catastrophes are averted. Fire and the menstrual flow are the elements which, properly controlled, act to mediate between the cosmic poles of which the universe is composed, keeping them always the right distances apart in terms of both space and time (Lévi-Strauss 1970: 64, 137, 139, 289, 293–4; 1973: 115, 165, 303–4, 471; 1978: 77–9, 83, 109–12, 126–7, 143, 185–90, 221–5, 500–6).

The second volume of *Mythologiques*, *From Honey to Ashes*, selects myths which clarify the basic logic by showing it up against a background of contrasting terms associated with the concept of 'cooking'. Honey is a substance which, without being cooked at all, is already highly edible – as if it had been 'cooked' already by the bees. Tobacco-smoke, on the other hand, can only be consumed in an opposite fashion – after the tobacco has been not merely 'cooked' but truly 'burned'.

A central figure in this second volume is the 'Girl Mad About Honey' – a woman whose appetite for sweetness is associated with (a) the full moon and (b) her 'excessive' sexual desires. These myths from the Chaco region place the blame for the fact that men 'had to' overthrow the Rule of Women on the seductive behaviour of this girl (1973: 286). She is incapable of observing sexual self-restraint; consequently she – and all women through her – must cede this culture-preserving responsibility to men. She is the symmetrical inversion of the woman whose menstrual period never ends. Instead of representing permanent sexual disjunction (floods, darkness, 'the rotten world'), she represents permanent 'honeymoon' (coded as light and fire – the girl is 'dry' in the sense of being always 'thirsty', and is in some versions 'the daughter of the Sun').

In connection with all this, perhaps the most important point Lévi-Strauss makes is a sociological one. Unlike raw meat, honey is *not* taboo to the person who finds it. The fact that it does not need to be cooked is inseparable from the fact that it does not need to be *exchanged*:

> the heroine who is mad about honey is giving in to nature: she covets honey in order to eat it straight away, thus diverting it from its cultural function as a mediator of matrimonial exchanges. (1978: 271)

In effect – and herein lies the real danger of honey – this is to short-circuit the system of wider solidarities and exchanges on which cultural life depends. Culture crucially *depends* upon periodic gender segregation. As Lévi-Strauss (1973: 412) puts it – endorsing in this respect something like the origins model central to this book – 'the power of nature conjoins the sexes to the detriment of culture', whereas

> the power of culture disjoins the sexes, to the detriment of nature which prescribes their union; temporarily at least, family links are broken in order to allow human society to be formed.

If the 'honey' myths express concern over cultural collapse, it is because

> in native thought, the search for honey represents a kind of return to nature, imbued with an erotic appeal transposed from the sexual to the gustatory register, and which would sap the very foundations of culture if it lasted too long. Similarly, the custom of the honeymoon would be a threat to public order if husband and wife were allowed to enjoy each other indefinitely and to neglect their duties towards society. (1978: 413)

The final sections of *From Honey to Ashes* are about 'instruments of darkness' designed to counteract risks of this kind. They do this by making loud noises, interrupting love-making and keeping the sexes apart at least for certain periods of time.

Din and Stench

The themes brought together in Lévi-Strauss' chapter of this title (1973; 361–422) include:

discontinuous noises designed to disjoin the sexes;

the rattles, clappers and other instruments which make such noises, for example the Bororo *parabára*;

the extinguishing of all lights and fires;

the stench of 'the rotten world';

the 'long night';

menstrual blood.

The connections are suggested already in a passage by Lévi-Strauss (1973: 373) early on in this chapter. The Tucuna Indians, one of whose myths put him on the track of the Bororo *parabára*, 'knock sticks together in one set of circumstances at least':

It is well known that these Indians attach great importance to the puberty rites for girls. As soon as a girl detects signs of her first period, she takes off all her ornaments, hangs them in an obvious place on the posts of her hut and goes off to hide in a nearby bush. When her mother arrives, she sees the ornaments, realizes what has happened and sets off to look for her daughter. The latter replies to her mother's calls by striking two pieces of dry wood together. The mother then loses no time in erecting a partition around the young girl's bed and takes her there after nightfall.

The clapping noise made when two sticks are knocked together – perhaps the most simple conceivable use by a girl of her 'instruments of darkness' – is triggered, in other words, *by the onset of menstruation*. It leads to the erection of a partition for the young woman's seclusion. It is as if discontinuous noises were the acoustic mode of existence of the menstrual flow, generating *disjunction* in the same way.

Lévi-Strauss goes on to discuss the 'instruments of darkness' used in Europe from the twelfth and thirteenth centuries. These were hammers, hand-rattles, clappers, castanets and similar instruments which replaced the chiming of church bells for one short period in every year – for the three days, from Thursday to Saturday, before Easter Sunday in Holy Week. Three days is, of course, at least conventionally and symbolically, the duration of the temporary 'death' of the moon – and therefore by association of a menstruating wife with respect to her husband. In the case we are discussing, however, the 'temporary death' which is marked and respected is that not of a lunar deity or menstruating woman – but of Christ. Lévi-Strauss (1973: 405) suggests that 'the instruments of darkness may have been intended to represent the marvels and terrifying noises which occurred at the time of the death of Christ'. In Corsica, various percussive devices were used: the beating of the altar and benches in churches, the smashing of planks with clubs and the use of hand-knockers, clappers and hand rattles of various types. In France, metal pots and pans were beaten, and wooden clogs were used to hammer the ground. The Church itself seems to have been generally opposed to such noise-making activities, and tried to restrict them. Lévi-Strauss traces their use back to neolithic or even palaeolithic times.

The reasons for associating a magico-religious three-day period of 'darkness' and 'death' with 'the very wet' should need no elaboration, so it comes as no surprise to find that the period coincides with the ritual *extinguishing of all fires*. Just before Easter, in mediaeval Europe, all candles and fires were extinguished and then lit afresh on Easter Sunday, when the Lenten fast was also ended and church bells were permitted to ring out again (Lévi-Strauss 1973: 408). Something similar used to happen in China, as Lévi-Strauss (p. 406) shows by quoting a passage from Frazer (1926–36, 10: 137):

> In China, every year about the beginning of April, certain officials called Sz'hüen used of old to go about the country armed with wooden clappers. Their business was to summon people and command them to put out every fire. This was the beginning of the season called Han-shih-tsieh, or 'eating cold food'. For three days all household fires remained extinct as a preparation for the solemn renewal of the fire, which took place on the fifth or sixth day after the winter solstice. The ceremony was performed with great pomp by the same officials who procured the new fire from heaven by reflecting the sun's rays either from a metal mirror or from a crystal on dry moss. . . .

This ritual was of great antiquity, dating in China from at least 2,000 years before Christ.

Apparently the aim of these practices, as of their worldwide variants, was to ensure (a) the complete *disjunction* of the polar opposite terms of which the universe is composed (earth and sunlight, meat and cooking-fire, wife and husband and so on) in order (b) to make their subsequent *conjunction* all the more emphatic and orderly.

Within this traditional paradigm, storms, thunder, noises of all kinds, blood-flows, rottenness and stench all combine to form a complex of signals performing the function of separators or punctuation marks. All means possible are brought into play to keep the sexes (often coded as earth and sky or sun, game animals and their hunters, raw flesh and cooking-fire) apart. It is as if men and women were disjoined by what stands furthest removed in the universe from fire: the flow of menstrual blood. This blood cannot, of course, be 'heard'. But thunder-claps can be heard, as can their imitation using crashing sticks or clappers, and if the myths say that such things are caused by the spirits (such as monsters, or rainbow snakes) which simultaneously cause the menstrual flow, then conceptually it is *as if* the blood pulse itself could be heard. Thunder, lightning, storms and floods become transformations and amplifications of the simple colour symbolism of the menstrual flow. They are the blood signal translated into a variety of acoustic, meteorological and other codes.

In *The Raw and the Cooked*, Lévi-Strauss points out that in the myths concerning the origin of cooking-fire, this fire is treated as 'negative noise'. People who are cooking – or who are 'stealing' or carrying burning embers from which to make the world's first cooking-fire – must *turn a deaf ear to certain sounds* (in one instance to 'the call of rotten wood'). Lévi-Strauss (1970: 286) asks how we are to interpret 'the curious connection, which is common to all the versions, between the cooking of food and the attitude to noise?' In fact he never gives an explanation, but he discerns a logical pattern built around the following ideas:

1. Noises trigger the *disjunction* of marital partners;
2. Cooking-fire is associated with their *conjunction*;
3. Hence the success of cooking depends on the *avoidance of noise*.

In illustrating this pattern, he enters into a discussion of the institution known as the *charivari*. .

The word 'charivari' refers to the derisive cacophony made at night in traditional European cultures by the community-wide banging of pans, cauldrons, basins and so on, in front of the houses of people suspected of love-making in 'scandalous' incestuous or other circumstances (Lévi-Strauss 1970: 287). Lévi-Strauss links this to the *din* traditionally made by people in many parts of the world at the time of an *eclipse*. A terrific cacophony of banging on various objects gave expression to people's hostility to the 'scandalous' intrusion of night into day, or of a shadow into the full moon when it ought to be clear. Very often, the belief is that a gigantic frog, wolf, dragon or other monster is about to devour the heavenly body. In the case of both 'reprehensible sexual unions' and the 'the excessive intimacy' of a monster in its relations with the moon or sun, the aim seems to be to make sufficient noise to *disjoin* the parties concerned. This is, in any event, the typical native explanation.

But Lévi-Strauss (1970: 295) makes a more subtle point. What is vital is that there should be a regular, predictable, periodic sequence of conjunctions and disjunctions between the polar terms (earth and sky, sun and moon, husbands and wives, cooking-fire and meat) making up the total system of human and cosmic life. The full moon should alternate regularly with the dark moon, just as day should alternate with night, and just as sexual conjunction (marriage) should alternate with disjunction (kinship). Should a celestial 'monster' intervene in this process by plucking the full moon from the sky, there is then the danger of a gap opening up in the sequence, so that unless something is done, dark will alternate . . . with dark. Likewise, if marriage takes place when there ought to be kinship solidarity, the danger is of a similar breaking of the required predictable sequence. It is as if day were to be followed by day.

The *making of loud noises* is designed to prevent such conjunctions of phases which ought to be kept apart. It does this by 'filling in the gap' – putting something in where a void would otherwise open up. The loud noises, in short, do not simply keep apart partners – they are designed to keep apart *periods of time* which should not be conjoined.

This is demonstrated by customs which, to western readers, might seem nearer to home. Even where charivari is no longer practised, writes Lévi-Strauss (1970: 301),

> noise up to a point retains its general function. In twentieth-century Europe, where scientific knowledge is so widespread, it is no longer conceivable that an eclipse should be greeted by noisemaking. Nevertheless the practice still survives in cases where there is a break, or a threatened break, in the cosmological sequence, but only when the interruption in considered as a social, and not a cosmic, event.

In Lithuania, where even up to the present century children were told to beat pans and other metal utensils with sticks in order to drive away evil spirits during eclipses, 'the spring festivities are still marked by a certain rowdyism'. On Good Friday, young Lithuanian men 'create a din by breaking furniture, such as tables, bedsteads. etc.' And in the past, it was customary in the same country *to break the furniture of deceased persons with a great deal of noise.* 'Customs such as these', comments Lévi-Strauss (1970: 301) after his survey,

> are part of a universal system, unmistakable vestiges of which still survive in Western countries – for instance, the smashing of china and exploding of fireworks in Italy on New Year's Eve, and the chorus of automobile horns that ushers in the New Year in Times Square, Piccadilly Circus, and the Champs Elysées. . . .

The old year has to be extinguished in the most emphatic possible way to allow the new year to be born. At all costs, what must be avoided is any merging or confusion between the two.

Silence at Full Moon

While incest, noise and eclipses imply 'anti-cooking', the converse also holds: marital sex, silence and the full moon imply the power and success of the cooking process. And these belong together in the same way. For example, when it is a question, not of charivari, but of endorsing and sustaining a marital union which is approved, the rule of silence may be carried to considerable extremes:

> In various regions of Australia, Oceania, and Africa, young married couples had to remain silent for a period of time varying from two months to a year, according to the locality. A similar custom has been observed in America, the Caucasus, and Sardinia. The ban on speech was usually lifted on the birth of the first child. (Lévi-Strauss 1970: 328)

Discussing the significance of this custom, Frazer (1910; 4: 236–7) concludes that the wife's silence until the birth of her first child 'rests on some superstitious belief touching her first pregnancy which as yet we do not understand'. Lévi-Strauss (1970: 328) comments that the question at issue 'is not pregnancy but birth'. And it is certainly the case that whereas menstrual bleeding implies the inverse of pregnancy and the inverse of birth – playing, between partners who are kin, the role of eclipses or storms 'incestuously' conjoining heaven and earth – the birth of a baby has the opposite effect. It 'plays, between husband and wife, a part similar to that played by cooking fire between sky and earth' (1970: 329).

Sky and earth are linked peacefully as husband and wife in periods when cooking fires are burning and the skies are bright. But they are conjoined 'noisily', 'riotously' and 'incestuously' during 'anti-cooking' periods such as eclipses, storms, moonless nights or floods. Eclipses, and the accompanying din, imply bloodshed. They are a threat to normal human births. By the same token, when the moon is reappearing after its monthly disappearance, its own 'rebirth' requires a cautious attitude to noise:

> The silence that precedes the first birth could correspond to the old Lapp belief that the new moon and the aurora borealis must not be annoyed by any kind of noise. Conversely, in various American communities, eclipses that were marked by noisemaking were also the particular concern of pregnant women and young mothers. (Lévi-Strauss 1970: 329)

During an eclipse, the Micmac of eastern Canada made their women go outside the huts and take care of their children. At Jemez, a pueblo in New Mexico, it was believed that eclipses caused abortions, so pregnant women had to remain indoors or, if they were absolutely obliged to go out, they had to put on a key or an arrowhead in their girdles to prevent the moon from devouring the foetus or to keep the child from being afflicted with a harelip. 'Even today', continues Lévi-Strauss (1970: 329),

> the Maya-speaking Pocomchi have the following rules which must be obeyed during an eclipse: 'First your head is covered. And if you are a (pregnant) girl or even a boy who has just married and has a wife, you should go into the house. . . . It is not good to observe the moon in its struggle.

Pregnant women keep silent because noise is associated with the flowing of
genital blood – with abortions, miscarriages, menstruation and the 'dying' of
the moon. To give birth is analogous to cooking. Normatively it should
occur at full moon. It belongs, with cooking, to the period of the moon's full
and complete 'rebirth', when honeymoon fires are flickering, love-making is
in progress and all is joyful, quiet and calm.

One Myth Only

I have presented a distillation of the logic of *Mythologiques*, emphasising
certain elements and playing down others in order to bring out for the reader
– as briefly and simply as possible – the convergence between Lévi-Strauss'
findings and my own.

It is towards the end of the fourth volume – when Lévi-Strauss (1981:
561–624) is triumphantly demonstrating that his 800 or so stories are all
versions of what he calls 'One Myth Only' – that the fit becomes detailed,
unerring and explicit. The 'bird-nester' turns out to be among other things a
'Naked Man'. He is 'naked' in exactly the same sense that a young girl in her
menstrual seclusion is 'naked'. He is 'raw', and often blood-stained like a
baby. As if returning to the womb – or to the period of infancy before he was
given a name – he has left behind the marks of his normal social identity.
The stories often tell of him leaving his clothes behind as he begins his climb
towards the sky – clothes which are then stolen by a rival. More than a mere
change of apparel is signified here. All Lévi-Strauss' North American bird-
nester stories which centre on an 'exchange of clothes' are in fact depicting
what in other myths is conceptualised as 'skin-change' – the exchange of one
social identity for a different one, this in turn corresponding to a perpetual,
pendulum-like oscillation between a person's marital role and her or his role
as 'blood' or kin.

Lest the reader should feel at this point that matters are getting somewhat
complicated, let me stress once again the remarkable simplicity of the logic
behind all such ideas. It is just that at full moon, one abandons one's identity
(one's role, mask, 'skin', 'clothes' and so on) as 'brother' or 'sister', in order to
assume that of 'spouse' or 'lover'. At dark moon, one throws off one's lover-
identity once more and resumes the role of 'blood' relative or kinsperson. At
each transition point one loses one kind of relative only to gain another,
affines being exchanged for kin and kin for affines in regular succession.
'Rivals' are always involved, because (viewing matters from the standpoint of
a male) when a wife is temporarily abandoned at dark moon, she is 'taken
back' by her brother or other kin, while when a sister is abandoned at full
moon, she is 'taken back' by her lover or husband. The 'quarrel between
antagonists' in all these myths is, then, of the same order as the 'quarrel'
between night and day, wet season and dry, dark moon and full. In such
alternations, first one aspect 'kills' the other, then the 'killed' aspect

resurrects itself and 'kills' its 'opponent' – and so on. Winter reigns; summer
is dead. But then summer regains the ascendancy and kills winter in turn,
before the whole process repeats itself. At a deep level, the seemingly
fraught, often frantic and typically bloody 'conflicts' between 'rivals' in these
myths tell only of such patterns of alternation which are central to the
experience of life in all its forms. Death, murder, incest, cannibalism, rape:
these and similarly drastic deeds and events are memorable code terms whose
function is to help fix in the collective mind the features of a logic of cultural
metamorphosis modelled on the peaceful changes of women and the moon.

The final 'bird-nester' narrative to be presented in full – myth 793a in *The
Naked Man* – 'mainly emphasizes the origin of monthly periods of which
Moon Woman is the instigator' (1981: 574). It is in this Coos Indian story
that the 'quintessential mythic formula' is claimed by Lévi-Strauss to have
been at last extracted (1981: 564). The myth spotlights the bird-nester's
climb in search of the brilliant red feathers of a woodpecker who is busy
pecking at some 'blood-stained faeces' which have been placed at the summit
of a tall tree (p. 564). Meanwhile, the climber's father-in-law, who has
remained down on the ground, assumes the young man's appearance and
takes possession of his wives. In the sky, the climber is threatened by a
cannibalistic Sun Woman who has to be vanquished using an ice-cold penis,
and marries two nocturnal, semi-aquatic women who regulate the synchrony
of all other women's menstrual flows (1981: 564–5). Lévi-Strauss' four-
volume work then culminates (1981: 598–601) in his analysis of an Ojibwa
mythic pattern 'based on a conflict between the two moons' – a set of stories
which combine motifs from the opening Bororo 'bird-nester' myth and
motifs from the Plains Indian 'Wives of the Sun and Moon' narratives central
to Volume 3. The 'two moons' are the heavenly body's dark and light,
waning and waxing aspects whose life and death 'struggle' is depicted – in
myth 810 (the last myth to be given in full) – with the help of an immense
'swing' oscillating to and fro between opposite worlds and also between a
man's wife and his mother.

In the light of all this, one thing at least should be clear. At the core of
American Indian mythology is the depiction of an endless movement – like
that of a pendulum – between darkness and light, 'sky' and 'earth', kinship
and marriage, 'blood' and 'fire'. Central to this in turn is an ancient
sociologically and therefore mythologically necessary equation of cosmic
darkness with the darkness and rawness of both female and animal flesh. Like
Ifi Amadiume's Igbo python, a menstruant should always keep out of the
sun. Such a woman should be not in 'this world' but in the darkness of 'the
world beyond' – inviting cosmic disaster such as the collapse of the sky
should her feet so much as touch the earth upon which ordinary people live
their domestic, marital and other lives. In the 'other world' a menstruant is
symbolically within the domain of all game – in fact, of all living creatures,
to the extent that these are not yet cooked but still have life-blood in their

veins. Here, all intimacies are non-marital. As Lévi-Strauss (1978: 404) puts it:

> a menstruating woman, who has to remain in temporary seclusion, keeps her husband *at a distance*, so that during this period, metaphorically at least, it is as if she had gone back to be near her own people.

'The occurrence of menstruation', Lévi-Strauss continues, 'revives a kind of right of repossession', as if blood kin were temporarily and repeatedly seizing back the woman whom in marriage they had 'given away'. It is not difficult to appreciate how, given the synchronisation of women's periods, the forces exercising these 'rights of marital repossession' might have assumed quite imposing collective proportions and forms. And then, wherever or whenever such synchronisation could be broken down, enabling men to exercise more stable and permananent marital rights in their wives, it is not difficult to appreciate how, in cultures stretching to the outermost corners of the globe, this severing of women's periodic links with 'heaven' or 'the skies' came to be conceptualised as the dismemberment of a 'winged serpent' or woman-seizing 'dragon' by some patriarchal hero who established the present permanence of marriage and order of the world (cf. Fontenrose 1959).

In any event, Woman's blood – its logic identical to that of the great pythons and dragons encountered earlier – in effect 'carries her away'. In this context, according to Lévi-Strauss (1978: 400), a husband unavoidably 'recognises that a wife is never given without some hope of return: each month, during the space of a few days, menstruation deprives the husband of his wife, as if her relatives were reasserting their rights over her'.

During her seclusion a woman is – symbolically – reclaimed if not by a 'dragon' then at least by her *male and female kin*. In this kinship/menstrual role, the woman is 'dead' to her marital life; her husband is therefore 'a widower' (Lévi-Strauss: 1978: 404). Since her kin included her forebears, she is moreover *conjoined with the spirits of the dead*, who – in accordance with the by-now familiar conceptual merging of ancestral blood with the blood of wild animals – may be confused or identified in turn with *'animal husbands'*. All 'kin' – living or dead, animal or human – are now as if swallowed up by the blood which unites them as 'one flesh'. All of this signifies 'incest' in the sense of *a conjuction between those of the same blood*. Yet the logic stipulates that there is nothing wrong with this 'incest' – which is in fact perfectly normal – provided it occurs *at the right time*. Unity between those of the 'same blood' is only indisputably and unambiguously wrong when it occurs *out of phase*.

Christian mythology, as we noted earlier, places Christ, on whose blood the salvation of humanity depends, into the realm of death for three days in every year, and less emphatically once a week on Fridays, when (until recently) Catholics were obliged – as on Good Friday itself – to respect the flesh of their Saviour by abstaining from the consumption of all meat. Traditional ritualism all over the world places menstruating women in the same realm of temporary death – marked in particular by meat avoidances as well as various other forms of abstinence – for three days in every month. The sounds of the 'instruments of darkness' through which Christ's death was once marked are associated inevitably with the realm of decayed and decaying flesh – the 'rotten world'. And the instruments which produce such sounds, like the menstrual flow itself, are conceptualised as emerging from that realm which stands on 'the other side' of life. They come from within ancestral women's wombs, or from within the belly of a monster, or from deep marshes or bogs; and when they are retrieved or first discovered, they are covered in foul-smelling fluids, grease mixed with red ochre or perhaps thick mud. Lévi-Strauss (1973; 414–15) gives an example:

> Let us take the case of the Bororo. They have an instrument of darkness, the parabára, and they also possess the bull-roarer. There is no doubt at all that the latter connotes the rotten world. The bull-roarer, which the Bororo call aigé, mimics the cry of a monster of the same name which is supposed to live in rivers and marshlands. The animal appears in certain rites, in the form of a dancer who is encased in mud from head to foot. The future priest learns of his vocation during a dream in which the aigé embraces him, without his experiencing fear or revulsion either at the monster's smell or at the stench of decayed corpses.

Here, then, as in Northern Australia, a man acquires power through his 'temporary death', when he is embraced by an immense water-monster whose noisy presence is mimicked in the bull-roarer's throbbing sound.

Sounds, Smells – and Blood

Still, however, the reader may be wondering quite why the transition point at dark moon – when a woman abandons her lover to regain her kin – should be marked by the bull-roarer's (or other instrument's) *noise*. Since the aim here is to demonstrate the identity between Lévi-Strauss' findings and my own in connection with dragon legends in general and the Rainbow Snake in particular, let me return at this point briefly to Australia; it is here that our information on the subject of bull-roarers is most complete.

In a review of Buchler's (1978) structuralist analysis of the Rainbow Snake complex, Kolig (1981) criticises the author's view that 'the Snake' is essentially conjured up by female *smells*. Kolig (1981: 316) cites a Western Australian myth about a Rainbow Snake known as *Nginin*:

> two white men noisily ferried down the Fitzroy River in a dinghy, shooting at crocodiles all the while. Enraged by the noise Nginin hooked the boat, hoisted it downriver and drowned the noisy group.

Kolig comments that this story 'rather flatly rebuts Buchler's thesis on the olfactory excellence of the Rainbow Serpent and his antagonism to foul odours'. True, concedes Kolig, the dancing, singing and chanting Wawilak

Sisters were swallowed because of their [menstrual] smells. But, he implies, they might just as well have been swallowed for making such a noise – Buchler's concentration on their smells is one-sided and misleading. If the object is to arouse a Rainbow Snake, smells are not necessary – loud noises work just as well.

Kolig has a point, but it is stretching matters to think of it as 'flatly rebutting' Buchler. It has here been shown that noise, menstrual odours, 'excessive' maternity and many other factors are all possible ways of bringing on the 'anger' of the Rainbow Snake (Chapter 13). Aboriginal myth-makers and narrators have much freedom of choice here. Buchler and other structuralist interpreters are right, however, to see in all this a definite system, in which not everything is allowed, but only some things. The Snake, we have seen, is that force which makes its presence felt, within the model's terms, at the transition point of dark moon, when women as menstruants should be at the height of their sex-strike powers. The Snake extinguishes domestic fire, aborts the cooking process, interrupts marital relations. Wherever it is being aroused, the basic uniformity is that one or several of the linked elements of wetness, flood, storm, thunderous noise, bloodshed, rawness, darkness, menstrual odour, blood-to-blood intimacy and human-with-animal conjuction must be present. The converse of these – dryness, fire, silence, light, cooking, feasting, marital sex and the separation of human from animal forms of life – will be either absent or suppressed. This is an absolute uniformity. There would appear to be no exceptions to these rules.

I have just shown that precisely such a pattern constitutes the essence of the findings of Lévi-Strauss in his *Mythologiques*. If loud noises are made, blood pollution is assumed to be present, and the cooking process is assumed to be threatened or even thrown into reverse. Linked to 'din', as we have seen, is 'stench'. Linked to these in turn we find 'incest' – in particular, the 'excessive' closeness of boys to their mother, or mothers to their own noisy offspring. Linked again with all this we find eclipses or periods of terrifying darkness, including storms. Eclipses are in turn greeted with loud noises – just as in many parts of the world, similar sounds are the appropriate response to unions deemed by the community to be 'incestuous'.

All this seems so totally anomalous within the normal paradigms of social anthropology as to have been successfully ignored until Lévi-Strauss drew such patterns to our attention. Structuralism has uncovered the structures, but it has still left us wondering how and why they came to evolve. There would seem to be no functionalist way of explaining why cooking should be thought incompatible with noise. Neither would it seem that sociobiology can provide an answer. The one dimension which these various contemporary approaches exclude with unanimity is history; it is here that the only possible answers lie. Magico-religious mythology is exceedingly conservative. 'In the life of a society', as the archaeologist Leroi-Gourhan (1968: 48) puts it, 'models of weapons change very often, models of tools less often, and social

institutions seldom, while religious institutions continue unchanged for
millennia'. We have no reason to doubt that at the deepest structural level,
magico-religious myths perpetuate patterns which are as old as human
culture itself. It is not inconceivable, then, that they can tell us something
about how culture came to exist. In this context, the anomalies surveyed in
this chapter are precisely what we would expect. Women once signalled 'no'
in their own blood. Whey they were on sex strike, they were on cooking
strike, too. The blood-triggered 'no' was the basic signal generative of
culture, and it was always switched either 'on' or 'off'. No additional signal
could be allowed to interfere with this one; if the blood signal was
augmented by an auditory accompaniment, it could only be *within* the terms
of the semantic field established already by 'the language of blood'. At the
simplest conceivable level, an auditory signalling system would consist
merely of the *presence or absence of noise of any kind*. So it is clear when the noise
signal would have had to be *present*. If the blood signal was switched 'on', this
had to apply equally to the noise signal. The role of noise was merely to
augment – not conflict with – the primary signal of blood.

   Women declared their sex strike/cooking strike to be 'on' by bleeding as
visibly as possible – and simultaneously by making whatever loud noises
their technology made possible or appropriate for them. Such marriage-
rupturing, tryst-interrupting, tension-inducing noises produced, in effect,
the 'sound' of the blood. Aboriginal Australians know this: they know that
the bull-roarer's sound *is* the sound of their ancestral 'Mother's' blood. Hence
in a variant on the Wawilak Sisters myth, from the Ma:ra tribal group on the
southern banks of the Roper River, the ogress and all-Mother Mumuna is
eventually killed by men who – in the usual way – extract from this
representative of Womankind the secrets of their own ritual power:

> As Mumuna died, she called out *brr*! and that sound went into every tree;
> her blood splashed on to every tree, and it was that blood that contained
> the sound.
>   Afterwards, in memory of Mumuna, the Eaglehawk cut down a big
> tree, and from its'wood he made a bullroarer which is the Mumuna (or
> Mumunga). He tried to get the sound of the dying woman. As he swung
> it, it 'turned into a *mumuna*'; and its sound was the sound contained in the
> wood of the tree, which had in it the Mumuna's blood. (Berndt 1951:
> 151–2)

All over Aboriginal Australia, the sound of the bull-roarer is in effect the
sound of the ancestral Mother's blood. That explains why the instruments are
sounded only on very special occasions – *whenever ancestral blood is flowing*. It
also explains why the instruments and their strings are repeatedly rubbed,
before each ritual use, with 'ancestral' blood and/or red ochre, usually mixed
with an ample supply of grease. The throbbing roar is to replicate and forever
to perpetuate the signal through which culture itself was conjured into
being.

As long as the blood spell lasts, so does the sound, or the possibility of sound. Only when the moon is full – to keep to the model's terms – does marital sex occur. Only then are the cooking-fires lit. Only then is the period of noise replaced by that of silence or auditory calm. Full moon, light, marital sex, cooking and quietness thus all fall together within one and the same segment of lunar time. Dark moon, darkness, blood-intimacy, rawness and noise all fall together in the opposite segment for exactly the same set of reasons.

The Harmony of the Spheres

This book began by arguing that a model of human cultural origins should be testable in relation to the symbolic levels of the relevant archaeological and ethnographic evidence. In Chapter 2, Lévi-Strauss' work on mythology was discussed, and I observed that it would be a point in its favour if a modern origins narrative could explain some of the more unexpected and seemingly bizarre findings made in this vast cross-cultural work. By such a standard, the model presented here seems a strong one.

To anyone who has studied Lévi-Strauss' *Mythologiques* with the thoroughness it deserves, it is clear beyond doubt that the myths of the Americas are all of one piece – facets of a single crystalline object as solid as rock ('of the nature of a thing among things': Lévi-Strauss 1970: 10). In this book I have suggested that the same almost certainly applies to Aboriginal Australian mythology, although – despite the achievements of Kenneth Maddock (1974; 1978a, 1978b: 1985) and a few others in this respect – at present the work of extending Lévi-Strauss' project to this continent has scarcely begun. Even on the basis of the results already achieved, however, it is clear that the Australian myths, no less than the Amerindian ones, are yielding fragments of what is revealing itself to be an unchanging, solid and worldwide 'thing'. But this 'thing' emerges not simply or directly as a reflection of the neurological connections in the human brain. It pertains not only to the mind – but to the body, too. And it is not only, or even primarily, male. It is at least equally female. If the myths and practices we have examined turn out to display one and the same inner logic, it is not because they are constrained by certain mysterious genetically fixed properties of the human intellect. It is because they are transformations worked upon what is invariably one and the same initial paradigm of menstrual solidarity and power.

Lévi-Strauss probably would not endorse the central argument of this book. Nonetheless, his strange cosmological and other findings can be accounted for by the model, whilst they are not explained at all by the patriarchal origins theory which he first put forward in *The Elementary Structures of Kinship* (1969a). Indeed, as one pores over the initially baffling details of *Mythologiques*, the diligent reader becomes increasingly impressed with the extent to which Lévi-Strauss' strange methodology by some unknown mechanism came to facilitate the partial, halting reconstruction of an archaic native paradigm which contradicts Lévi-Strauss' own sexual-political assumptions at almost every point.

It becomes almost exasperating, sometimes, to see how close Lévi-Strauss came to the simple logic he was searching for. Again and again, the materials he marshals and even his own insights point to a set of links between lunar periodicity, menstruation, blood, cooking and marriage rules such as this book has outlined. Almost all of the jigsaw pieces assembled and arranged in this book are items isolated by Lévi-Strauss, and published – from the 1960s onwards – for the academic world to make some kind of sense out of them. Yet the pieces were scrambled so effectively that the four volumes of *Mythologiques*, when they were finally completed, seemed to most readers indecipherable. The dark moon, the full moon; women as menstruants, women as wives; noise, silence; raw meat, cooked – all these logical pairs, along with many others, were painstakingly isolated by Lévi-Strauss, and shown to be the basic conceptual building-blocks of what was revealing itself as the remnants of an awe-inspiring archaic pan-American scientific para-digm. But the paradigm as reconstituted in *Mythologiques* unfortunately does not make sense. No society could ever actually work on the basis of the rules and regulations that Lévi-Strauss suggests. The bizarre composite image he eventually gives us equally relates to nothing very meaningful in our own culture – and perhaps partly for that very reason connotes little which has excited students of history or ethnography either. The *substantive findings* of *Mythologiques* – the transcontinental incompatibility of 'noise' and 'cooking-fire', for example – have not been taken up even by many mythographers or social anthropologists, let alone by evolutionary biologists or palaeoanthro-pologists. It would only have taken a few fairly simple changes to have made the model seem interesting and workable. But these would have involved turning Lévi-Strauss' own deepest personal myth – his 'exchange of women' model – on its head. Despite the immense force of the native logic which often pushed him far in this direction, in the end the founder of structur-alism succeeded in holding the line. Comprehension was finally renounced.

The scale of Lévi-Strauss' achievement cannot be overestimated. In his own way, he (1978: 221–2) confirms that the many hundreds of myths analysed in his vast compilation are all, in the final analysis, variations on the 'Rule of Women' theme. As he puts it: 'the veil lifts to reveal a vast mytho-logical system common to both South and North America, and in which the subjection of women is the basis of the social order. We can now understand the reason for this.'

And what is this reason why women must be 'subjected'? Once again, Lévi-Strauss refers us to menstruation. So powerful are women's flows, and so demanding of cosmic synchrony, that unless carefully controlled they could throw the whole universe into chaos. As Lévi-Strauss (1978: 506) puts it, having touched on the dangers of cycles which are 'too slow' or 'too fast':

The reason why women are most in need of education is that they are periodic creatures. Because of this, they are perpetually threatened – and the whole world with and through them – by the two possibilities that have just been mentioned: their periodic rhythm could slow down and halt the flow of events, or it could accelerate and plunge the world into chaos. It is equally conceivable that women might cease to menstruate and bear children, or that they might bleed continuously and give birth haphazardly. But in either case, the sun and the moon, the heavenly bodies governing the alternation of day and night and of the seasons, would no longer be able to fulfil their function.

Earliest Womankind, the myths allege, simply could not be trusted to menstruate or give birth on time. 'In her pristine innocence, she did not have monthly periods and gave birth suddenly and without warning.' This – according to Lévi-Strauss – was a denial of culture:

The transition from nature to culture demands that the feminine organism should become periodic, since the social as well as the cosmic order would be endangered by a state of anarchy in which regular alternation of day and night, the phases of the moon, feminine menstruation, the fixed period for pregnancy and the course of the seasons did not mutually support one another.

Lévi-Strauss (1978: 222) continues:

So it is as periodic creatures that women are in danger of disrupting the orderly working of the universe. Their social insubordination, often referred to in the myths, is an anticipation in the form of the 'reign of women' of the infinitely more serious danger of their physiological insubordination. Therefore, women have to be subjected to *règles*. And the rules instilled into them by their upbringing, like those imposed on them, even at the cost of their subjection, by a social order willed and evolved by men, are the pledge and symbol of other 'rules', the physiological nature of which bears witness to the correspondence between social and cosmic rhythms.

But it is in this last passage that Lévi-Strauss' sexual-political interpretation departs most starkly from my own. Lévi-Strauss takes chaos as the initial situation which prevailed before male power succeeded in establishing culture. He suggests – or at least allows his Amerindian myth-makers to suggest – that harmony and order were created only when men succeeded in prioritising marriage bonds as the basic building-blocks of the cultural domain, a theory discussed in some detail in Chapter 2. In this book, on the contrary, I have argued that male 'order' embodies no special creativity. Men invented none of the basic principles of kinship, ritual action or cosmological belief which have here been examined. At best, masculinist ritual activity and its associated mythology represents only a politically distorted imprint made from a pre-existent template. It becomes established only through the replacement of its female counterpart, its condition being the collapse of synchrony and harmony between women's menstrual rhythms and the cyclicity of the moon. In place of periodic 'honeymoon' (Lévi-Strauss 1973: 157, 283), male sexual-political hegemony turns marriage into a fixed and permanent bond, devoid of periodicity or scope for renewal. 'The Dragon's' or 'Snake's' periodic hold over Womankind is finally broken, the 'Powers of Darkness' are vanquished – and the world is made safe for patriarchal marriage and family life.

Far from producing culture, as Lévi-Strauss' mythological narrative would have it, male power enters tardily on to the scene, transforming and politically colonising a cultural landscape long since formed by others. Far from enhancing menstrual periodicity in women, it acts as the agency of its suppression as a creative cultural force. Yet tradition holds that without women's bloody periodic rupturing of all marital ties, all order, harmony, balance and renewal in the universe would be in danger of becoming lost. The world, fixed in permanent marriage, might then become fixed, correspondingly, in only one cyclical cosmic phase – in permanent dry season, permanent senility, or permanent day. To avoid this – to bring on night's healing darkness, to invite storms, thunder and the annual rains, to welcome death from which new life must flow – ritual therefore seeks to make amends, preserving the forms of menstrual synchrony and alternation even as the menstrual potency of real women is devalued and denied.

At the root of all ritual in traditional cultures is the notion of harmony. 'Harmony' and 'synchrony' in this context are interchangeable terms. The Karadjeri in western Australia let flow their own blood in the confident belief that this fertilises the local parrot-fish – all hunting and gathering success depending as it does upon the 'harmonizing of natural and social rhythms' (Maddock 1974: 134). Likewise, the Amazonian Barasana who practise *He House* – their version of male menstrual rain-making – do so whenever they fear human society to be 'in danger of becoming separated from, and out of phase with, its generative source' (Hugh-Jones, S. 1979: 249).

It is fitting that the myths accompanying such rituals should so insistently depict their yearned-for synchrony as emanating in some way from ancestral women's wombs (Chapters 12 and 13). This book has shown that such beliefs are in essence good science. As they harmonised their rhythms with those of the world around them, earliest cultural women must have felt the power in their own bodies to be intimately connected with all wider processes of cyclical renewal. It was almost as if their blood – source of all life – made the rains fall, the seasons change, the game animals reproduce and multiply. It would have been logical to feel this – if it really were women's sexual-political combined action which kept the social world so successfully turning in sympathy with wider ecological rhythms. When synchrony with the moon and tides was properly established, social life was successful, adaptation to nature's demands was appropriate, and therefore it seemed that the wind, the rain, the earth, the sky and all of nature was supportive of human life. In this context, we can perhaps imagine the sense of cosmic strength conveyed as women identified their own inner forces with the turning of the moon, with the success of men's hunting efforts, with their own gathering and child-bearing productivities, with the tides, seasons and other manifestions of cyclical change — and in tropical regions with the awesome force of lightning, thunder and the onset of monsoonal rains.

Chapter 15
Becoming Human

All social life is essentially *practical*. All the mysteries which lead theory towards mysticism find their rational solution in human practice and in the comprehension of this practice.

Karl Marx and Friedrich Engels, *Theses on Feuerbach* (1845)

Marx argued that social science could be true to itself only when based on the interests of the working class. This work has been conceived and written in an explicitly Marxist mould, and this could lead to the suggestion that I, too, have produced a model which is politically biased.

My model suggests, however, that culture itself emerged from a comparable bias, having been based on the interests of the most reproductively burdened, materially productive sex.

I would not accept that this makes either Marx's or my own model politically suspect. The only 'bias', as far as I am concerned, is a bias against bias itself. The interests of mothers and their offspring may well have conflicted, prior to the emergence of culture, with male interests. But male dominance had to be overthrown because the unending prioritising of male short-term sexual interests could lead only to the permanence and institutionalisation of behavioural conflict between the sexes, between the generations and also between rival males. If the symbolic, cultural domain was to emerge, what was needed was a political collectivity – an alliance – capable of transcending such conflicts. The overcoming of sexist bias – the establishment between the genders of rational, shared, universally communicable understandings such as those central to human language – presupposed the breaking of male power prerogatives and the establishment of behavioural norms rooted within the domain of general rather than particularistic interests. Only the consistent defence and self-defence of mothers with their offspring could produce a collectivity embodying interests of a sufficiently broad, universalistic kind.

My model suggests that the defence of maternal interests was to the origins of human cultural awareness what the defence of working-class interests was within the project of Marx and Engels, as they fought to establish a science of society which was genuinely free from bias. An implication would be that the first paradigms encoding human cultural knowledge were indeed 'scientific' in that Marxist political sense. They involved the translation of empowering information into universally communicable – rather than merely privatised or sectional – symbolic forms. I have argued in this book that the underlying structures of traditional magico-religious mythology indeed refer us back to those earliest dialectical, revolutionary, world-creating forms of science.

My view of science is not an uninhibitedly social or constructionist one. Although in the Introduction I invited the reader to join with me in exploring my own personal origins myth, I am not one of those who would deny that any meaningful distinction can be drawn between mythology and science. A construct can start out as science, only to become gradually mythologised. Alternatively, one which begins life as a myth can – through collective evaluation, correction and corroboration – turn out to be genuine science.

I am aware that there are Marxist-influenced scholars who *would* construe all human knowledge – including scientific knowledge – as conventional: as 'constructed' rather than 'discovered' (Latour and Woolgar 1979). But an extreme interpretation along these lines, as Donna Haraway (1989: 12) points out, would reduce the sciences to a cynical relativism with no standards beyond arbitrary power. It would imply that there is no world for which we are struggling to give an account, no referent in the system of signs of which each scientific discipline is composed, no hope for such a thing as progress in building better accounts of reality as the generations pass. There would be just political power and its associated myths. When a new paradigm came to prevail (Kuhn 1970), it would not be because it was 'better', or closer to 'the truth'. It would just mean that some new myth-weaving group had succeeded in establishing its dominance for a while.

My understanding of Marxism is more orthodox than this. It holds that although all knowledge *is* socially constructed, science and myth are nonetheless distinct *kinds* of construct. According to Marx, 'the *development of science* . . . is only one aspect, one form in which the *development of the productive forces*, i.e. of wealth, appears' (1973 [1859]: 540–1). This formulation links science with technology, industry and labour. Science becomes just one aspect of the relationship which exists between us, the human species, and the material universe (including our own products) in which we live. This relationship is a practical one. The process by which we acquire knowledge is also a process in which we acquire power – power to channel and to harness natural forces, and power to control those social forces which we as a species have unconsciously created ourselves. 'Science', as an authoritative Marxist nicely put it, 'is knowledge which endows us with power' (Trotsky 1964 [1940]: 344).

According to this reading, scientific revolutions (Kuhn 1970) move knowledge in one direction rather than in the opposite one – in the long run always towards accounts which are objectively 'better' – because humanity's power in relation to its own products and environment is itself an objective phenomenon. When one paradigm replaces another, the conflict between the respective 'scientific communities' reflects a deeper conflict between social and political forces in the wider world. If science eventually wins out over myth – if each new paradigm is objectively closer to 'the truth' than the old – this is because social revolutions themselves are ultimately empowering processes, the classes or forces championing them unerringly choosing information forms which are widely empowering over those which empower only minority groups.

Such a reading would hold that *all* collective mental constructs express relationships of power. The constructs of the natural sciences arise out of humanity's growing power to harness the forces of the world around us. Astronomy made possible the earliest calendars, predictions of eclipses, accurate marine navigation and so on. The development of medical science permitted a measure of freedom from and conquest of disease. The modern advances of physics, chemistry, information technology and the natural sciences generally have today given us collectively an immense power to harness natural forces of all kinds and have utterly transformed the world in which we live.

In this perspective, anything that enhances *our* power – the survival capabilities of the human species as a whole at this stage of our evolution on this planet – can be termed 'science'; any human construct that denies us power, or restricts power only to some sectional interest or ruling élite, is 'ideology' or 'myth'. Of course, most constructs – much of the detailed narrative content of the present book no doubt included – are a bit of both, and as I have just suggested, today's science can very easily become tomorrow's myth. This is a slow, inexorable process of gradual inversion which seems to have given rise to all the more baffling forms of mythology that now exist in the world – from twentieth-century Stalinist and other pseudo-Marxist demonology on the one hand, to so-called 'primitive' mythology on the other. In this context, it certainly does become difficult to disentangle science from mythology, for as Donna Haraway (1989) has shown, even genuine natural science itself, although intrinsically international and of value to the species as a whole, has necessarily been stamped with the birthmark of its development within a politically structured, divided world. Primatology and palaeoanthropology in particular have been so charged with political significance as to have been quite unable to avoid being torn between claims as divergent as the long-term requirements of the human species as such on the one hand, and the felt needs of particular social, racial, gender or otherwise *sectional* interests on the other.

But regardless of the precise proportions of 'myth' to 'science' in any one narrative, it is the extent of the *internationalism* of any construct – the global, species-wide range of the human power it can convey – which gives it whatever scientific status it can ultimately lay claim to. Deference to local religious or other susceptibilities immediately erects barriers to such 'free trade'. 'Must philosophy', as the young Marx (1957: [1842]: 21) once asked,

> adopt different principles for every country, according to the saying 'different countries, different customs,' in order not to contradict the basic truths of dogma? Must it believe in one country that 3 × 1 = 1, in another that women have no soul and in yet another that beer is drunk in heaven? Is there not a *universal human* nature just as there is a universal nature of plants and heavenly bodies?

In stressing that philosophy's truths 'do not know the boundaries of political geography' (1957 [1842]: 26), Marx was simply saying that to the extent that science deserves to be called such, it conveys *distributable, internationally sharable* power. Most of physics, chemistry, astronomy and natural science generally *does* (at least potentially) impart this kind of power, recognising no political frontiers whatsoever – and it is *this* which underlies the ability of paradigm-sharing scientists across the planet to agree with one another in developing their sign systems. It is this scope of agreement in turn which distinguishes science at even the most superficial level from mere local, national or narrowly based (religious, political and so on) forms of consciousness, whose conflict-ridden sign systems are endlessly self-contradictory and incommensurable one with another.

The Conditions of Scientific Objectivity

Marx's general formulation on the relationship between power and knowledge is well known:

> The ideas of the ruling class are in every epoch the ruling ideas: i.e. the class, which is the ruling material force of society, is at the same time its ruling intellectual force. . . . The ruling ideas are nothing more than the ideal expression of the dominant material relationships, the dominant material relationships grasped as ideas, hence of the relationships which make one class the ruling one, therefore the ideas of its dominance. (Marx and Engels 1947 [1846]: 39)

Although I would emphatically extend Marx's argument to include 'gender' every bit as much as 'class', such a formulation has in my view never been bettered. It is not possible to change the prevailing ideas of society – or to produce a universally agreed upon basis for a science of society – without breaking the *material* power of those forces which distort science. The convolutions and contradictions of patriarchal, sexist ideology – to take an example of obvious centrality to this book – cannot be sorted out exclusively through thought. Overcoming such mythology presupposes resisting the *physical* dominance of those masculinist institutions upon which the myth system relies, and without which it would collapse overnight. This is a task which requires the oppressed sex to resort to political – including possibly physical – action. Only when the two sexes can communicate in the absence of one-sided violence or power privileges which exempt men from having to *think at all* in relation to vast areas of sexual, personal and family life – only then will sanity and objectivity in cross-gender communication systems have some chance of arising. Although Marx was thinking in terms more of class than of gender, the same logic of course applies.

It was because Marx saw social contradictions as the source of mythological and ideological contradictions that he was able to insist that *only the removal of the social contradictions themselves could remove their expressions in ideology and science*. This is what Marx meant when he wrote:

> The resolution of *theoretical* contradictions is possible only through *practical* means, only through the practical energy of man. Their resolution is by no means, therefore, the task only of understanding, but is a *real* task of life, a task which *philosophy* was unable to accomplish precisely because it saw there a *purely* theoretical problem. (1963a [1844]: 87)

But Marx at no time advocated tailoring knowledge to suit the felt needs of any sectional interest. The working class was not exempt from this. As Marx himself wrote:

> It is not a matter of knowing what this or that proletarian, or even the proletariat as a whole, *conceives* as its aims at any particular moment. It is a question of knowing *what* the proletariat *is*, and what it must historically accomplish in accordance with its *nature*. (Marx and Engels 1963 [1845]: 237–8)

For Marx, to know 'what the proletariat *is*' constituted a *scientific* question, which could only be given a *scientific* answer in complete independence of any immediate political pressures or concerns. Far from arguing for the subordination of science to politics, Marx insisted on the subordination of politics to science.

Engels (1957 [1888]: 266) wrote: 'the more ruthlessly and disinterestedly science proceeds the more it finds itself in harmony with the interests of the workers'. There can be no doubt but that this accurately expressed Marx's own view. 'Who', the young Marx asked, 'should decide on the bounds of scientific research if not scientific research itself?' (1957 [1842]: 21). Science, as humanity's only universal, international, species-unifying form of knowledge, had to come first. No concessions to political pressure could be allowed. If the maintenance of scientific integrity nonetheless drew strength, according to Marx and Engels, from reliance on *the international working class*, this was only in the sense that both thinkers recognised (a) that all knowledge must be rooted within some social constituency in order to exist at all whilst (b) the wider, the more universalistic and the less subject to prejudice this constituency, the better. The wider and more open the constituency, the greater would be science's freedom to follow its autonomous goals regardless of the consequences.

Marx and Engels felt confident on this score because although workers and their struggles were to them real enough, *the international working class*, in their eyes, was not something which existed preformed and organised already, 'out there', independently of the existence of knowledge of it. It was not telling anyone what to think. It could not conceivably act as a constraint upon scientific thought – any more than 'International Womankind' could so act today. On the contrary, it was itself a scientific construct. It was only in internalising this construct – only in becoming *aware*, through science, of its own planet-changing potential – that *the international working class* could begin existing as an embodied, organised political force for the first time.

Marx and Engels believed that it was possible for there to come into existence a new, revolutionary anthropological science (which of course came to be known as 'Marxism') thanks to the emergence for the first time, and as a direct result of scientific development itself, of a kind of 'anti-class'. There had emerged

> a class in civil society which is not a class of civil society, a class which is the dissolution of all classes, a sphere of society which has a universal character because its sufferings are universal, and which does not claim a *particular redress* because the wrong which is done to it is not a *particular wrong* but *wrong in general*. (Marx 1963b [1843–4]: 58)

Here was a social sphere 'which claimed no *traditional* status but only a *human* status', a sphere which was 'not opposed to particular consequences but is totally opposed to the assumptions of the . . . political system', a sphere, finally, which could not emancipate itself 'without emancipating itself from all these other spheres' since it was 'a *total loss* of humanity' which could only redeem itself 'by a *total redemption of humanity*' (Marx 1963b [1843–4]:58). 'Here', Engels (1957 [1888]: 266) was later to write – referring to the working class – 'there is no concern for careers, for profit-making, or for gracious patronage from above'. Only *here* could science be true to itself, for only here could research be conducted within social surroundings of a truly emancipating, universalising, kind – affording the potential to work for the unity of the species as a whole. Within this scheme of things there was no possibility of science being subordinated to a pre-existing political force. The political force was science's own and could not exist without it. The previously prevailing relationships between science and politics were reversed.

In short, from the standpoint of Marx and Engels it was *in order* to remain true to the interests of science — *in order* to begin solving its internal theoretical contradictions — that they felt obliged, as scientists to identify with that *material* social force which promised to counteract the 'extraneous interests' distorting the objectivity of science, and to take up the leadership of this material force themselves. Their idea was not that science is inadequate, and that politics must replace it or be added to it. It was that science — when fearlessly true to itself — is intrinsically revolutionary, and that it must recognise no other politics than its own.

Marxism and the Dragon

The ancient paradigms of culture-bearing humanity have come down to us in many forms. All of these are in origin woman-empowering, no matter how much they may have undergone patriarchal ideological reworkings and political inversions in the millennia since culture first came into being. The gender-empowering essence of the earliest forms of science can therefore be compared, in the light of my argument in this book, with the class-empowering essence of Marxism. Although in the short term seemingly 'one-sided', this essence has in fact nothing to do with political bias. Rather, it is only through the empowerment of the oppressed that the biases of ruling genders and classes can be overcome. It is only through such empowerment that wider, universalistic interests can be established in place of sectional ones, and that people's collective consciousness of their own strength can be made more and more freely communicable, broadly representative and therefore non-partisan or 'scientific'.

Among the many constructs through which the earliest science has come down to us is one with which the reader will by now be familiar — that of an immense, all-seeing, many-headed, winged, snake-like being or 'dragon', making its presence felt in a multitude of cross-cultural images of composite beings, 'fabulous beasts', 'All-Mothers' and other monsters.

Behind all these images is the awareness that early cultures possessed of their own power. The reason for the paradoxical, dialectical nature of the imagery is the all-embracing, cyclical, conflict-transcending nature of the power itself. As we have seen, the power was collective — and therefore many-headed. It was an immense alliance — and therefore stretched, snake-like, across the landscape. It was dependent on the periodic flowing of blood — and therefore seemed bloodthirsty in its appetites. It involved the harmonisation of menstruation with the periodicity of the moon — and so was experienced as cosmic, umbilical, birth-giving, astrological. Its potency was inseparable from the awesome symbolic potency of menstrual blood — which became encoded as the death-dealing snake venom or poisonous dragon breath emanating from its being. Its rhythm was that of perpetual cyclical alternation between opposite light and dark, marital and kinship, cooked and raw, fire and blood phases or states — and therefore became codified as a rainbow-like, betwixt-and-between entity in which all conceivable opposites were combined.

The science at the root of such images is that which Lévi-Strauss was the first to describe with relative accuracy in his *Mythologiques*. It is not always immediately apparent that it is 'science'. For example, of what conceivable *scientific* value could be the belief, central to all four volumes of *Mythologiques*, that good cooking is ruined by the making of *noise*? Is there anything in functionalism which might explain this? Or in sociobiology?

This notion seems incomprehensible – until it is realised that noise goes with eclipses, with the *dark* moon, and therefore with that time of month when menstrual blood should be flowing and cooking should not be happening at all. *Why* does noise-making accompany eclipses or connote the darkness of the moon? This is merely one of the emergent properties – a logical outcome – of the model. In the initial situation, the blood signal is either 'on' or 'off', and any accompanying signals – such as auditory ones – must be 'on' or 'off' in sympathy, so as to harmonise rather than interfere with the basic rhythmic blood signal (see above, pp. 506–08). When women declared themselves on sex strike, they must have used sound-making instruments to mark this fact, augmenting through loud noises the visual impact of their blood. It is this which ultimately explains why bull-roarers – always said to have been obtained from ancestral menstruating women – are heard throbbing throughout Aboriginal Australia at moments when ancestral blood is flowing.

Humans first became scientific – first learned to share their experiential and other findings so as to compare notes and subject them to collective scrutiny and evaluation – thanks to their discovery of what solidarity can mean. Their science, like ours, was essentially their *consciousness of their own collective strength*. This consciousness could become encoded in shared symbols – 'the Dragon' pre-eminent among them – because understandings themselves could be widely shared. Basic power inequalities and political conflicts – had these existed – would have obstructed such sharing and therefore distorted the objectivity of science. Thanks to the manner in which the human revolution had been achieved, such inequalities and conflicts were not basic to the alliances within which culture evolved. The very earliest cultures therefore had no need for religious myths. Although there was plenty of room for *magic* – for an awareness of the world-changing potency of such activities as dance, poetry and song – religion was not needed because there was no one to mystify, no one to exploit, no one whose conceptual world needed standing on its head.

Mysticism and convoluted theologism emerged only when masculinist institutions began reasserting themselves as the first step in an immensely drawn-out process which was eventually to result in class society and so-called 'civilisation'. Constructs of 'the feminine' became deified only in proportion as real women, in the flesh and blood, were deprived of their power. Goddesses, gods and other miraculous powers could enrich themselves only in proportion as ordinary humans were impoverished – robbed of the magic in their own lives. Only in the course of this process was genuine science – or 'the ancient wisdom', if you prefer to call it that – progressively subjected to the distorting lenses of sectional interest, partisan special pleading and political ideology masquerading as science.

Only when social life had become irretrievably conflict-ridden was the community-wide *sharing* of understandings no longer possible. At this point, humanity's basic capital of accumulated knowledge became increasingly fragmented, pulled in opposite directions, fought over and – in part – monopolised by ruling élites. To the extent that shared symbols could be preserved at all, they now meant one thing to one section of society, quite another to the rest. This is the symbolic essence of all secret or esoteric cults.

We have seen how, in the case of the Australian Aboriginal Rainbow Snake motif, male power succeeded in turning what was once the woman-empowering consciousness-of-strength of society as a whole into the gender-specific exclusive power-knowledge of initiated men. The very same 'All-Mother', 'Snake-Woman' or 'Dragon' which, as a collective construct, had crystallised women's consciousness of their reproductive/menstrual solidarity, now became progressively inverted, to the point at which this blood-empowered monster could be presented as periodically 'angered' by the smell of menstruating women. It was now stated that the Rainbow Snake – born (according to the myths) in women's menstrual solidarity – demanded and insisted upon the marginalisation and isolation of menstruating women. Women now gave birth to male offspring who grew up not only to keep secrets from their own mothers, but through initiation to perpetuate and impose an extraordinary symbolic system in which menstruation and birth were rendered disempowering to women, empowering – in elaborate, male-surrogate symbolic forms – to men.

Within the Marxist political paradigm which I am using here, this may be said to parallel the ultimate paradox at the root of Marx's *Capital*, when Marx finds that Capital and Labour are ultimately one and the same. The one is the other – when turned against itself. The wealth, power and knowledge of the capitalist class is nothing other than the conscious labour of the working class in alienated, politically inverted form – workers now experiencing their atomisation and oppression at the mercy of what in the final analysis is their own co-operative intelligence, productivity and power.

The Structure of Scientific Revolutions

On 21 June 1633, Galileo was interrogated by the Pope and by a tribunal of high officials of the Catholic Church who threatened to torture him unless he withdrew his allegation that the earth circled the sun. As is well known, the conflict between the Ptolemaic and Copernican systems of astronomy was then very much a political one. Anyone supporting Copernicus risked persecution, imprisonment – or even being burnt at the stake.

Darwin more recently was regarded as instigating a theologically danger-ous, politically subversive theory in questioning Genesis by arguing that the human anatomy had evolved by natural selection from that of an ancestral ape. In many parts of Christendom to this day, religious fundamentalism has succeeded in keeping the flames of this particular debate very much alive.

Karl Marx, writing in the same age as Darwin, was viewed as presenting a political rather than scientific theory in arguing that human knowledge itself always expresses the material interests of definite social groups, the funda-mental variable in this context being economic interest.

In the case of both Galileo and Darwin, it was only the political and ideological defeat of the Church on the issues concerned – defeats which formed part of a wider process of social and political change – which eventually lifted the two thinkers' scientific contributions (at least in most parts of the West) from the realm of political controversy. Such cases illustrate that it is only once its initial political coloration has faded away that science becomes generally recognised for what it is. We might say that science *has to conquer politically before it can shed its political cloak.*

Achievements such as those of Copernicus, Darwin or Einstein are termed 'paradigms' by that most frequently cited of all contemporary science historians, T. S. Kuhn. Paradigms are 'universally recognised scientific achievements that for a time provide model problems and solutions to a community of practitioners' (1970: viii).

Once a natural science paradigm has triumphed in its field, the usual course is for it to validate itself again and again, in ever greater detail, by in effect forbidding scientists to investigate problems other than those for which the paradigm offers a solution. Only problems whose solutions, like those of a crossword puzzle, are already 'built in' by their method of formulation are allowed. 'Other problems', as Kuhn (1970: 37) writes, 'including many that had previously been standard, are rejected as meta-physical, as the concern of another discipline, or sometimes as just too problematic to be worth the time'.

However, it is not for us simply to condemn the rigid, conservative paradigms which major scientific advances eventually produce. Kuhn pres-ents instead a subtle, dialectical argument, showing that it is precisely through such conservatism that new, revolutionary scientific breakthroughs are gradually prepared. Only a rigid, conservative but extremely detailed and precise theoretical structure can be disturbed by some small finding which seems 'wrong'. It is only a community of scientists who confidently expect to find everthing 'normal' who will genuinely know what an 'abnormality' or 'novelty' is – and who will be thrown into a state of crisis by it. A more easy going, open-minded community which never expected precise regularities in the first place would not let themselves be bothered by such things.

Scientific revolutions are classically precipitated by anomalies. A planet is in the wrong part of the sky. A photographic plate is clouded when it should not be. A fundamental law of nature is apparently defied. A piece of laboratory equipment designed and constructed merely to add precision to a familiar finding of normal science behaves in a wholly unexpected way. To normal science, such abnormalities are merely an irritation or a nuisance. In attempts to defend the old paradigm, efforts are made to suppress, obliterate or ignore the bothersome findings or events. New observations are made, new experiments are set up – with the sole intention of eliminating the anomaly concerned. But it is precisely these attempts to defend the old paradigm which now begin to shake it to its foundations. Had the old, rigid, paradigm not had its ardent defenders, the anomaly concerned would probably not even have been noticed. Now, however, an entire community of scientists begins to feel challenged by it, and more and more attention is focused upon it. Attempts are made to explain it away. But the more such attempts are made, the more inconsistent and inadequate the old paradigm appears, the more strange the anomaly seems, and the more dissatisfied a section of the scientific community becomes.

It is the *internal inconsistencies* now apparently permeating the old theoretical structure which convince some scientists – at first only a small number – that something is fundamentally wrong. Copernicus, for example, complained that in his day the astronomers who opposed him were so inconsistent 'that they cannot even explain or observe the constant length of the seasonal year'. In all periods immediately preceding what Kuhn terms a *scientific revolution*, similar complaints are made. There is no neat, logical proof that the old paradigm is wrong. Rather, there arises a general sense of dissatisfaction, a feeling – on the part of some – that *absolutely everything is wrong*, and a gradual splintering of the scientific community into schools and factions between whom communication is difficult or even impossible. Few things – not even the most elementary principles – seem to be agreed upon any more. 'The proliferation of competing articulations', writes Kuhn, 'the willingness to try anything, the expression of explicit discontent, the recourse to philosophy and to debate over fundamentals, all these are symptoms of a transition from normal to extraordinary research' (1970: 91). All these are signs that the old theoretical edifice is crumbling and that a new one is about to take its place.

The transition to a new paradigm is achieved, finally, through revolution. A *scientific revolution*, according to Kuhn, is not simply an addition to pre-existing knowledge. It is, within any given field, 'a reconstruction of the field from new fundamentals' – a complete demolition of an old theoretical and conceptual structure and its replacement by a new one based on entirely different interests, aims and premises (1970: 85). During the course of such a revolution, nothing is agreed, everything seems to be ideological and political, and issues are decided by 'unconstitutional' means. The old paradigm is not defeated on the basis of its own rules but is attacked from outside. It cannot be defeated on the basis of its own rules for, as we have seen, and as was discussed in this book in particular in Chapter 1, these rules are not only inadequate to solve the new problems which have begun to arise – *they actually preclude any discussion of these problems at all.*

All of the successful 'scientific revolutions' that Kuhn discusses were accomplished within the natural, not the social, sciences. The reasons for this are not far to seek. In the humanities, social pressures have been far more decisive and enduring than in physics, chemistry or related fields. In the humanities, the power expressed within the competing paradigms has been *directly political.* The paradigm change pressed for by Marx in attempting to introduce objectivity into the historical and social sciences was, for this reason, never consummated.

We have no way of knowing what might have happened had Marxism conquered politically in Europe or even the United States in the period 1905–26 when it apparently stood most chance of doing so. But a possibility consistent with Marx's own vision would be that the late twentieth-century international community would long since have ceased to regard his school of thought as 'politics' rather than 'science'. In fact, of course, capitalism survived, the Russian Revolution which Marx indirectly inspired was contained, Stalinist counter-revolution triumphed within the sealed borders of the Soviet Union, the banner of 'scientific socialism' became mythologised, dogmatised and hopelessly compromised – and for nearly seventy years the world became frozen, paralysed within a mould of mutually antagonistic yet reciprocally dependent 'capitalist' and so-called 'communist' power-blocs. In place of Marx's hoped-for age of scientific enlightenment and human self-emancipation there ensued nearly seventy years of at best postponement and at worst crushing defeat: arms race, balance of terror and – at the deepest level – the kind of intellectual paralysis which only fear can induce. Only since Europe's year of revolutions – that 200th anniversary of the fall of the Bastille when the monstrous edifice of Stalinism finally began crumbling to dust – has this situation begun fundamentally to change, creating vast new economic and other problems but at least freeing conscious humanity to experience these as inescapably *global* challenges and, for the first time in almost a century, to *think.*

In the case of anthropology – despite the political obstacles – there has been perhaps more forward movement throughout the twentieth century than elsewhere in the social sciences. This has been partly, no doubt, because 'other cultures' can be viewed with at least some sense of detachment from one's own. In addition, anthropology owes its existence to the vast amount of often-challenging fieldwork whose accumulating findings have repeatedly prompted movel efforts at interpretation. In effect, anthropological thinkers have been rescued from mental and political oblivion in being subjected to the mental influences of those non-capitalist ordinary people as well as shamanic and other thinkers – many of them scientific geniuses – among whom they have stayed. But without repeating the historical discussion of Chapters 1 and 2, let it be noted simply that in recent decades, with the demise of structuralism and other widely accepted paradigms and the absence of any agreement on alternatives, a sense of impasse, frustration, and widespread dissatisfaction within the discipline has prevailed among social anthropologists for some time.

There has long been no theoretical framework which brings together anthropology's various sub-disciplines – the study of primate behaviour, of human evolution, of archaeology, of pre-capitalist economics, kinship, ritual, mythology and other domains. Nowadays, it is not even believed that there could ever be such a framework. Such paradigms as exist are those of the discipline's fragments; dividing up the field, they validate the permanence of its incommensurable terminologies, its boundaries and its inconsistencies. Each sub-discipline's 'anomalous' findings are for the most part safely ignored – usually by being projected across the nearest disciplinary boundary as someone else's problem.

In fact the 'anomalies' of the science of culture have accumulated since the founding of social anthropology more than a century ago, occasionally finding their way into the centre of a new paradigm (as happened with the marriage rules central to the kinship analyses of Lévi-Strauss) but more often remaining outside the focus of any theoretical framework. When Nadel (1957: 177) wrote that the advance of any science 'is punctuated as much by the disappearance of old problems as by the emergence of new ones', he was particularly thinking of social anthropology. 'The old problems are abandoned', he wrote, not because they are solved but

> because all that can be said has been said; and if certain questions still remain unanswered they are yet shelved in spite of it, or perhaps because of it – because one realises that they are unanswerable and should be replaced by other, more profitable, ones.

The problems abandoned have been precisely those which almost all late nineteenth-century thinkers considered most urgent and significant:

> Think of the controversies, now silent, about the origin of totemism, the distinction of magic and science, the 'meaning' (or 'nature' or 'function') of taboo or sacrifice, and many other, similar topics. These were brave attempts, aiming at final explanations, even though they contained much that was speculative, much that was over-simplified, and a great deal of purely verbal argumentation. Today, we have grown much more modest. . . . And many of the questions which inspired the earlier scholars

are simply no longer asked. Perhaps we shall return to them one day. (Nadel 1957: 189)

Nearly a generation later, Robert Murphy (1972: 37) was to comment: 'We do not just fail to return to the basic questions – we have forgotten what they are.'

This book has set out from the observation that despite decades of attempted explanation, almost everything about traditional human cultures is 'anomalous'. Firstly, the findings of social anthropology are anomalous in a general way in relation to the biological paradigms – Darwinian, neo-Darwininian, sociobiological – which set the parameters for most discussions on human evolution and cultural origins. Secondly, they are anomalous in more specific contexts in relation to what is left of the prevailing paradigms of social anthropology as a discipline.

The dogma of the cultural centrality of 'the family' has been the main generator of such anomalies, burdening western social anthropology from the 1920s onwards. Malinowski (1956: 72, 28) reiterated tirelessly and indeed tiresomely that 'the tradition of individual marriage and the family has its roots in the deepest needs of human nature and of social order', seeing it as his professional task to 'prove to the best of my ability that marriage and the family have been, are, and will remain the foundations of human society'. Whereas, Malinowski noted, W. H. R. Rivers 'would lead us to believe that what I like to call the *initial situation* of kinship is not individual but communal' (1930: 99), his own view was the opposite. The family and marriage, he insisted, 'from the beginning were individual' (1956: 76). Culture's 'initial situation' was dominated by

> the group consisting of father and mother and their children, forming a joint household, co-operating economically, legally united by a contract and surrounded by religious sanctions which make the family into a moral unit. (1956: 80)

Lest anyone imagine that this was a dispassionate 'scientific' rather than thoroughly *politically motivated* judgement, let me quote Malinowski one more time. Here are the words in which he denounced what he termed the 'group motherhood' theory which until recently had been part of the dominant anthropological paradigm:

> I believe that the most disruptive element in the modern revolutionary tendencies is the idea that parenthood can be made collective. If once we came to the point of doing away with the individual family as the pivotal element of our society, we should be faced with a social catastrophe compared with which the political upheavals of the French revolution and the economic changes of Bolshevism are insignificant. The question,

therefore, as to whether group motherhood is an institution which ever existed, whether it is an arrangement which is compatible with human nature and social order, is of considerable practical interest. (Malinowski 1956: 76)

It was in the light of these considerations that Malinowski (1930: 97) came to declare that 'classificatory terminologies do not exist and never could have existed', whilst what he termed the ideas of 'a whole school of anthropologists from Bachofen on' were branded not only wrong but 'positively dangerous' (1956: 76). The family and its kinship terminologies had always been 'individual'. The nuclear, monogamous, family was initially the cellular unit of culture. It has been this politically motivated conception of an 'initial situation' – the reverse of that suggested in this book – which has kept social anthropological kinship theory in a state of crisis for most of the twentieth century.

'I believe', wrote Sir Edmund Leach (1961a: 26) thirty years ago, 'that we social anthropologists are like the mediaeval Ptolemaic astronomers; we spend our time trying to fit the facts of the objective world into the framework of a set of concepts which have been developed *a priori* instead of from observation'. Leach was one of the few to have realised that by far the most damaging of these arbitrarily imposed concepts was the notion of 'the elementary family' as 'a universal institution'. Anthropologists since Malinowski on, he wrote, have insisted that 'the family' in the English-language sense of this word is the logical, necessary and inevitable focal point around which all human kinship systems revolve and from the standpoint of which they must be viewed. Leach observed that the characteristic kinship systems of traditional cultures for the most part become unintelligible when viewed from this standpoint. As a result, he concluded, the mental constructs of modern kinship theory are beginning to look as bewildering and futile as the cycles and epicycles of those Ptolemaic astronomers who could conceptualise the universe only by assuming the centrality of our own Earth.

Some years later, in an evaluation of the contemporary state of kinship theory, Needham (1974: 39) expressed a similar verdict. 'The current theoretical position', he observed, 'is obscure and confused, and there is little clear indication of what future developments we can expect or should encourage.' He concluded, in tones indicating a mood close to despair:

In view of the constant professional attention extending over roughly a century, and a general improvement in ethnographic accounts, this is a remarkably unsatisfactory situation in what is supposed to be a basic discipline. Obviously, after so long a time, and so much field research, it is not just facts that we need. Something more fundamental seems to have gone wrong. What we have to look for, perhaps, is some radical flaw in analysis, some initial defect in the way we approach the phenomena.

Matters have scarcely improved in the years since Leach and Needham wrote.

The Revolution

In this book I have set about *inverting* rather than simply modifying most previous assumptions relating 'norm' to 'anomaly' in human kinship and culture. Whereas most previously prevailing paradigms have regarded 'pair-bonding' or the 'nuclear family' as normative in some basic sense for human culture as a whole, I have set out with a model in which 'the family' is split down the middle. Culture starts with solidarity. This takes the specific form of *gender solidarity* — in effect, women's periodic construction of a sexual 'picket line'. Not only culture but scientific self-awareness is born on this picket line. It is here that 'the Dragon' first flexes her limbs.

Where primary commitments and loyalties are concerned, culture in the first instance places marital partners in opposite camps. Clan organisation, unilineal descent, exogamy, in-law avoidances, rules preventing couples from dancing together, sharing in sacred ceremonial or sharing public meals — these and related features of traditional cultures (see Chapter 9) are expressions of such a norm. From this point of view, menstrual avoidances appear 'normal'. It is the norm for husband and wife to be set apart. Menstrual avoidances periodically help re-establish this norm. Where the contrary obtains — where nuclear family bonding is so strong that husband and wife remain together even during menstruation — this is a deviation from the norm.

In this way, instead of setting out from numerous ideas, I have in this book taken as my point of departure only one — namely, that in order to transcend primate dominance and induce hunters to provide consistent help, evolving human females had to rely on the weapon of the collective strike. Their periodic sexual withdrawal brought women together and had the effect of splitting the nuclear family. I have shown how rules of incest and exogamy, unilineal descent, the existence of moieties and clans, menstrual avoidances and the recurrent formal structures of traditional ritual and myth can be understood as logical consequences and expressions of that starting point alone.

Yet it is necessary to emphasise that the theory presented here — with its stress on 'group parenthood', on matrilineal priority and on the concept of revolution — is not intended as a new paradigm for the anthropological or social sciences. Although some of its logical consequences may seem novel, my model is in fact an orthodox one with respect to the Marxist tradition within anthropology. Let me conclude this book by recalling what this tradition was.

Engels (1972 [1884]: 49) held that in the evolution of the primates, collective bands – ('hordes') on the one hand, 'harem'-type polygamous 'families' on the other – were not complementary 'but antagonistic to each other'. There was a fundamental contradiction between these two *levels* of social and sexual organisation. Systems of primate dominance, according to Engels, have 'a certain value in drawing conclusions regarding human societies – but only in a negative sense'. There are no obvious evolutionary continuities. Where groups of primate females are bound closely to males, in each case 'only one adult male, one husband is permissible'. This individualism is in direct contrast with the incipient primate 'horde', whose full development becomes possible only once the fragmenting influence of male dominance and jealousy is overcome with the transition to humanity.

The system of individualistic male sexual dominance, according to Engels, led to continual sexual conflicts:

> Mutual toleration among the adult males, freedom from jealousy, was, however, the first condition for the building of those large and enduring groups in the midst of which alone the transition from animal to man could be achieved. And indeed, what do we find as the oldest, most primitive form of the family, of which undeniable evidence can be found in history, and which even today can be studied here and there? Group marriage, the form in which whole groups of men and whole groups of women belong to one another, and which leaves but little scope for jealousy. (Engels 1972 [1884]: 49–50)

Contrary to what is sometimes supposed, Engels did not have a gradualistic conception of human origins in which continuities between ape and human social forms were stressed. Had he had such a conception, he would not have been able to insist that 'the animal family and primitive human society are incompatible things . . . ' (1972 [1884]: 49). Extraordinarily in view of the limitations of his sources, and setting him head and shoulders above his contemporaries, Engels' position has survived the test of time. His paradigm has not had to be overturned or transcended in the writing of the present work, although naturally it has been necessary to correct many details and elaborate and document his model on the basis of what we know about primates and human cultures today.

But the relevance of the writings of Marx and Engels is greater than this. In the passages cited, Engels was assuming an important parallel – pregnant with implications on many levels – between the two great revolutions experienced by the human species on what he saw as its journey towards communism. In each case – in the birth of the human species as in its socialist rebirth – the revolution is an emancipation of the 'living instruments of production'. These 'instruments' – women as child-bearers on the one hand, workers as wealth-producers on the other – are human beings who, *because* of their instrumental status, are to that exent denied their full humanity. The materially productive *sex*, according to Engels, achieved its emancipation through the overthrow of male dominance and will do so again; the materially productive *class* will simultaneously achieve its emancipation through the overthrow of Capital. In each case, individualistic and competitive ownership of the instruments of production is or will be replaced by social self-ownership, which transforms the meaning of 'ownership' itself. Within the same paradigm, the socialist revolution, no less than the first human revolution, is a process in which 'for the first time man, in a certain sense, is finally marked off from the rest of the animal kingdom, and emerges from mere animal conditions of existence into really human ones' (Engels 1962 [1887]: 153). The first revolution established communism in its 'primitive' or simple form. The communism of the future will constitute, in the words of Morgan (1877: 552) adopted by Engels (1972 [1884] 166), 'a revival, in a higher form, of the liberty, equality and fraternity of the ancient gentes', in other words, a revival of the kinship solidarity of the matrilineal clan. The future revolution itself is, within this paradigm, a dialectical repetition of the birth process of the human race.

The parallels involved here can be extended indefinitely, and in fact – provided 'the revolution' in its contemporary sense proves more than a mythic construct – would amount to living proof of the theory of origins proposed here. In order to understand the origins of culture, no paradigm shift is required. Although much information-gathering and *learning* is certainly required, it is not necessary to add anything to the *conceptual* model already provided by Marx. The revolutions at both ends of history are in abstract, structural terms the same. It therefore suffices to know how to switch or modulate Marx's conceptual model accurately between the two levels – between the plane of nature and that of culture, the plane of *reproduction* and that of *production proper*, the plane of sex and that of class.

It was crucial to Marx's position that labour *is* procreation – but raised to a different level, and being definable on either level as 'species-life' or 'life producing life' (Marx 1971a [1844]: 139). The labour process is to culture what procreation is to nature. It was crucial to his position that class *is* sex on a higher plane, class oppression actually *beginning* as sexual oppression pure and simple:

> the unequal distribution (both quantitative and qualitative), of labour and its products, hence property: the nucleus, the first form, of which lies in the family, where wife and children are the slaves of the husband. (Marx and Engels 1947 [1846]: 21)

The appearance of exploited classes has taken place in a process whereby oppressed but materially productive males have been treated as 'women' by dominant males, incorporated *within* the category of the 'family' or the 'harem' (see Marx's ethnological notebooks: Krader 1972: 333, 340) in order to be exploited in structurally the same way that patriarchal family heads can exploit their one or several wives. That this process was ultimately connected with the transition from hunting to agriculture was obvious to Marx:

> The modern family contains in embryo not only slavery (*servitus*) but serfdom also, since from the very beginning it is connected with agricultural services. It contains within itself in *miniature* all the antagonisms which later develop on a wide scale within society and its state. (Quoted by Engels (1972 [1884]: 68)

The new system 'makes species-life into a means of individual life' (Marx 1963c [1844]: 127). A married woman, now, must engage in sexual activity – 'species-life' in its natural form – in order to be allowed the things necessary for her physical existence, just as a hired hand must express the human essence through labour, but *only because otherwise there will be no wage-packet*. In this context, '*life activity, productive life*, now appears to man only as *means* for the satisfaction of a need, the need to maintain physical existence' (Marx 1963c [1844]: 127). The manner of exploitation is therefore a form of prostitution, and it is *this* which makes it possible for Marx to insist that 'Prostitution is only a *specific* form of the *universal* prostitution of the worker . . .' (Marx 1963c [1844]: 156n).

The topic of prostitution was discussed in this book at some length in Chapter 5. A system compelling meat-hungry evolving human females to compete in emitting sexual 'yes' signals was there contrasted with a structure allowing them to gain meat by taking the opposite tack and signalling a collective 'no'. The first system tied each performance of the sexual act directly with the struggle for status, privileges or food; the second allowed sex to be postponed and to occur only in its own space, once the hunt had proved successful and anxieties about food had been dispelled. Some loose threads remaining from that discussion can now be tied up.

Prostitution was treated in almost wholly negative terms in our discussion in Chapter 5. Yet among primates it is perfectly natural for sex to be used as a bargaining counter in the search for status, meat or other food. This is a type of sexual activity whose evolutionary *value* is that it involves, as Zuckerman (1932: 232) was among the first to point out, 'the liberation of sexual responses from the function of reproduction'. When sex is used not just reproductively but politically – as a way of negotiating one's way through a conflict-ridden political landscape, or as a way of acquiring privileges or food – then this results in selection pressures placing sex increasingly under cortical rather than hormonal control. Sahlins (1960: 80) comments:

> The evolution of the physiology of sex itself provided a basis for the cultural reorganization of social life. . . . [A] progressive emancipation of

sexuality from hormonal control runs through the primate order. This trend culminates in mankind, among whom sex is controlled more by the intellect – the cerebral cortex – than by glands. Thus it becomes possible to regulate sex by moral rules; to subordinate it to higher, collective ends.

The paradox would be sharp – that the basis for human morality was prepared by prostitution. Yet it would be no more of a paradox than that appreciated by Marx in describing capitalism itself as nothing but the prostitution of labour, a prostitution which divorced labour from its simple, original function – the production of use-values for the reproduction of the community of labourers themselves – whilst subjecting it to quite other forces and purposes operating on an international scale.

It is only when we fail to see it in its dialectical, evolutionary, context that 'prostitution' appears simply as 'prostitution'. In its historical context, as Marx (1971b [1859]: 71) writes, 'universal prostitution appears as a necessary phase in the development of the social character of personal talents, abilities, capacities and activities'. By being prostituted in the service of Capital, labour becomes enormously developed, socialised and – more and more – subjected to global forms of control. This divorce of labour from its attachment to purely local, limited needs and controls is a precondition which has to be met if, eventually, the productive life of humanity is to be brought under our own conscious control in our own interests and those of our planet.

Capitalism, as the most developed system of universal labour prostitution there has ever been, is within this paradigm only a dialectical 'return', on a higher plane, to the competitive sexual systems and forms of dominance of pre-cultural humans and of the higher primates. It is this which *makes* the future revolution the same as the human one: in both epochs, in modern times as in the palaeolithic, the struggle for humanity is directed against *the same kind of thing*.

The most basic teaching of dialectical materialism is that evolutionary time is not linear but curved, like Einstein's space, and that its curves form spiral-like patterns, each return to the point of origin being in fact not a simple return but a 'return on a higher plane'. The period of immense global instability we are going through today – a planet-wide revolution whose immediate precipitating factor was the collapse of Eastern European Stalinism – is not entirely new to us, although it may at first sight appear to be so. The ends of time are being joined together. We have been here – at this point on the spiral – before. The revolution's outcome is not simply in 'the future' conceived as something abstracted from the past. As we fight to become free, it is as if we were becoming *human* for the first time in our lives. But in this sense, because it concerns *becoming human*, the birth process we have got to win – our survival as a species depends on it – has in the deepest sense been won already. None of us would be here had it not been. To understand this may be to understand, and thereby to make ourselves the instruments of, the real strength of our cause and the inevitability of our emancipation as women, as workers and as a species. The working class is the first materially productive class in the history of class society to have acquired the power of the strike. It is the first such class to have acquired the power to say 'no'. When it understands the identity between this 'no' and the 'no' which women have been trying to say for the past several thousand years – a fusion of forces will take place to generate a power which no force on earth will be able to stop.

Bibliography

Aberle, D. F. 1962. Navaho. In D. M. Schneider and K. Gough (eds) *Matrilineal Kinship*. Berkeley & Los Angeles: University of California Press, pp. 96–201.

Abramova, Z. A. 1967. Palaeolithic art in the U.S.S.R. *Arctic Anthropology* 4: 1–179.

Adair, J. 1775. *The History of the American Indians*. London: Dilly.

Adams, D. B., A. R. Gold, and A. D. Burt 1978. Rise in female-initiated sexual activity at ovulation and its suppression by oral contraceptives. *New England Journal of Medicine* 299: 1145–50.

Alexander, R. D. 1989. Evolution of the human psyche. In P. Mellars and C. Stringer (eds) *The Human Revolution. Behavioural and biological perspectives on the origins of modern humans*. Edinburgh: Edinburgh University Press, pp. 455–513.

Alexander, R. D. and K. M. Noonan 1979. Concealment of ovulation, parental care, and human social evolution. In N. Chagnon and W. Irons (eds) *Evolutionary Biology and Human Social Behavior*. North Scituate, MA: Duxbury Press, pp. 436–53.

Allen, M. R. 1967. *Male Cults and Secret Initiations in Melanesia*. Melbourne: Melbourne University Press; London & New York: Cambridge University Press.

Allsworth-Jones, P. 1986. *The Szeletian and the Transition from Middle to Upper Palaeolithic in Central Europe*. Oxford: Oxford University Press.

Altmann, J., S. A. Altmann and G. Haufsater 1978. Primate infant's effects on mother's future reproduction. *Science* 201: 1028–30.

Amadiume, I. 1987. *Male Daughters, Female Husbands. Gender and sex in an African society*. London & New Jersey: Zed Books.

Appell, L. 1988. Menstruation among the Rungus of Borneo: an unmarked category. In Buckley and Gottlieb (eds) *Blood Magic. The anthropology of menstruation*. Berkeley: University of California Press, pp. 94–112.

Arbousset, T. 1846. *Narrative of an Exploratory Tour of the North-east of the Cape of Good Hope*. Cape Town: Robertson & Solomon.

Arcand, B. 1978. Making love is like eating honey or sweet fruit, it causes cavities: an essay on Cuiva symbolism. In E. Schwimmer (ed.) *The Yearbook of Symbolic Anthropology*. London: Hurst. Vol. 1, pp. 1–10.

Archer, M., I. M. Crawford and D. Merrilees 1980. Incisions, breakages and charring, probably man-made, in fossil bones from Mammoth Cave, Western Australia. *Alcheringa* 4(1–2): 115–31.

Ardrey, R. 1969. *The Territorial Imperative*. London: Collins.

Arensburg, B., A. M. B. Vandermeersch, H. Duday, L. A. Schepartz and Y. Rak 1989. A Middle Palaeolithic human hyoid bone. *Nature* 338: 758–60.

Arey, L. B. 1954. *Developmental Anatomy*, 6th edn. Philadelphia: Saunders.

Aristophanes 1973. *The Acharnians; The Clouds; Lysistrata* trans. A. H. Sommerstein. Harmondsworth: Penguin.

Arrhenius, S. 1898. The effect of constant influences upon physiological relationships. *Skandinavisches Archiv für Physiologie* 8: 367–71.

Audouin, F. and H. Plisson 1982. Les ocres et leurs témoins au Paléolithique en France: enquête et expériences sur leur validité archéologique. *Cahiers du Centre de Recherches Préhistoriques* 8: 33–80.

Bachofen, J. J. 1973. *Myth, Religion and Mother-right.* (Selected writings). Princeton, NJ: Princeton University Press.

Bagshawe, F. J. 1925. The peoples of the Happy Valley. Part III, The Sandawe. *Journal of African Society* 24: 328–47.

Bahn, P. 1982. Inter-site and inter-regional links during the Upper Palaeolithic: the Pyrenean evidence. *The Oxford Journal of Archaeology* 1: 247–68.

Bahn, P. 1990. Cave blood dating detects Ice Age art. *Sunday Correspondent*, 8 April.

Bahn, P. and J. Vertut 1988. *Images of the Ice Age.* London: Windward.

Bailey, G. N. 1978. Shell middens as indicators of postglacial economies: a territorial perspective. In P. Mellars (ed.) *The Early Postglacial Settlement of Northern Europe*. London: Duckworth, pp. 37–63.

Bailey, J. and J. Marshall 1970. The relationship of the post-ovulatory phase of the menstrual cycle to total cycle length. *Journal of Biosocial Science* 2: 123–32.

Baldus, H. 1952. Supernatural relations with animals among Indians of Eastern and Southern Brazil. *Proceedings of the Thirtieth International Congress of Americanists*, pp. 195–8.

Bamberger, J. 1974. The myth of matriarchy. In M. Z. Rosaldo and L. Lamphere (eds) *Woman, Culture and Society*. Stanford: Stanford University Press, pp. 263–80.

Bancroft, H. H. 1875. *The Native Races of the Pacific States of North America*. 5 vols. New York: Appleton.

Bar-Yosef, O. 1989. Geochronology of the Levantine Middle Palaeolithic. In P. Mellars and C. Stringer (eds) *The Human Revolution. Behavioural and biological perspectives on the origins of modern humans*. Edinburgh: Edinburgh University Press, pp. 589–610.

Bar-Yosef, O. and A. Belfer-Cohen 1988. The Early Upper Paleolithic in Levantine caves. In J. F. Hoffecker and C. A. Wolf (eds) *The Early Upper Paleolithic. Evidence from Europe and the Near East*. Oxford: BAR International Series, pp. 23–41. 437.

Barbetti, M. 1986. Traces of fire in the archaeological record before one million years ago? *Journal of Human Evolution* 15: 771–81.

Barbetti, M., J. D. Clark, F. M. Williams, and M. A. J. Williams 1980. Paleomagnetism and the search for very ancient fireplaces in Africa. *Anthropologie* 18: 299–304.

Barbot, J. 1746. *A Description of the Coasts of North and South Guinea; and of Ethiopia Inferior, Vulgarly Angola. A new and accurate account of the western maritime countries of Africa*. London: Henry Lintot & Jean Osborn.

Barley, N. 1986. *A Plague of Caterpillars. A return to the African bush*. Harmondsworth: Penguin.

Barnard, A. 1977. Sex roles among the Nharo Bushmen of Botswana, unpublished seminar paper given at London School of Economics Seminar on 'Sex Roles Among Hunter Gatherers', February.

Barnard, A. 1988. Structure and fluidity in Khoisan religious ideas. *Journal of Religion in Africa* 18(3): 216–36.

Bateman, A. J. 1948. Intra-sexual selection in *Drosophila*. *Heredity* 2: 349–68.

Bednarik, R. G. 1989. On the Pleistocene settlement of South America. *Antiquity* 63: 101–11.

Bell, D. 1983. *Daughters of the Dreaming*. Melbourne: McPhee Gribble/Allen & Unwin.

Bennett, J. 1976. *Linguistic Behaviour*. Cambridge: Cambridge University Press.

Benshoof, L. and R. Thornhill, 1979. The evolution of monogamy and concealed ovulation in humans. *Journal of Social and Biological Structures* 2: 95–106.

Bern, J. 1979. Ideology and domination: toward a reconstruction of Australian Aboriginal social formation. *Oceania* 50(2): 118–32.

Berndt, C. H. 1970. Monsoon and honey wind. In J. Pouillon and P. Maranda (eds) *Echanges et Communications*. The Hague: Mouton, pp. 1306–26.

Berndt, C. H. and R. M. Berndt 1945. A preliminary report of field work in the Ooldea region, western south Australia. Sydney: University of Sydney (reprinted from *Oceania* 12–15).

Berndt, C. H. and R. M. Berndt 1951. *Sexual Behaviour in Western Arnhem Land*. Viking Fund Publications in Anthropology 16. New York: Wenner-Gren.

Berndt, C. H. and R. M. Berndt 1964. *The World of the First Australians*. London: Angus & Robertson.

Berndt, C. H. and R. M. Berndt 1970. *Man, Land and Myth in North Australia*. Sydney: Ure Smith.

Berndt, R. M. 1947. Wuradjeri magic and 'clever' men. Parts 1 & 2. *Oceania* 17: 327–65; 18: 60–94.

Berndt, R. M. 1951. *Kunapipi*. Melbourne: Cheshire.

Berndt, R. M. 1952. *Djanggawul*. London: Routledge.

Berndt, R. M. 1976. *Love Songs of Arnhem Land*. Chicago: University of Chicago Press.

Bettelheim, B. 1955. *Symbolic Wounds*. London: Thames & Hudson.

Betzig, L., M. Borgerhoff Mulder and P. Turke (eds) 1988. *Human Reproductive Behaviour. A Darwinian perspective*. Cambridge: Cambridge University Press.

Binford, L. R. 1968. A structural comparison of disposal of the dead in the Mousterian and Upper Paleolithic. *Southwestern Journal of Anthropology* 24: 139–54.

Binford, L. R. 1980. Willow smoke and dogs' tails: hunter-gatherer settlement systems and archaeological site formation. *American Antiquity* 45: 4–20.

Binford, L. R. 1981. *Bones: Ancient Men and Modern Myths*. New York: Academic Press.

Binford, L. R. 1983. *In Pursuit of the Past. Decoding the archaeological record*. London: Thames & Hudson.

Binford, L. R. 1984. *Faunal Remains at Klasies River Mouth*. Orlando: Academic Press.

Binford, L. R. 1987. Were there elephant hunters at Torralba? In M. H. Nitecki and D. V. Nitecki (eds) *The Evolution of Human Hunting*. New York: Plenum Press, pp. 47–105.

Binford, L. R. 1989. Isolating the transition to cultural adaptations: an organizational approach. In E. Trinkaus (ed.) *The Emergence of Modern Humans. Biocultural adaptations in the later Pleistocene*. Cambridge: Cambridge University Press, pp. 18–41.

Binford, L. R. and Chuan Kun Ho 1985. Taphonomy at a distance: Zhoukoudian, 'The cave home of Beijing man?', *Current Anthropology* 26: 413–42.

Binford, L. R. and N. M. Stone 1986. Zhoukoudian: a closer look. *Current Anthropology* 27: 453–75.

Binford, L. R., M. G. L. Mills and N. M. Stone 1988. Hyena scavenging behavior and its implications for the interpretation of faunal assemblages from FLK 22 (the Zinj Floor) at Olduvai Gorge. *Journal of Anthropological Archaeology* 7: 99–135.

Birdsell, J. B. 1953. Some environmental and cultural factors influencing the structuring of Australian Aboriginal populations. *American Naturalist* 87: 171–207.

Blacker, C. 1978. The snake woman in Japanese myth and legend. In J. R. Porter and W. M. S. Russell (eds) *Animals in Folklore*. Totowa, NJ: Rowman Brewer, & Cambridge: Littlefield, for the Folklore Society, pp. 113–25.

Bleek, D. F. 1935. Beliefs and customs of the |Xam Bushmen. Part VII: Sorcerers. *Bantu Studies* 9: 1–47.

Bleek, W. H. I. and L. C. Lloyd, 1911. Specimens of Bushman Folklore. London: Allen.

Blixen, K. 1954. *Out of Africa*. Harmondsworth: Penguin.

Blows, M. 1975. Eaglehawk and crow: birds, myths and moieties in South East Australia. In L. R. Hiatt (ed.) *Australian Aboriginal Mythology*. Canberra: Australian Institute of Aboriginal Studies, pp. 24–45.

Blumenschine, R. J. 1987. Characteristics of an early hominid scavenging niche. *Current Anthropology* 28: 383–407.

Blumenschine, R. J. and M. M. Selvaggio 1988. Percussion marks on bone surfaces as a new diagnostic of hominid behaviour. *Nature* 333: 763–5.

Blurton-Jones, N. G. 1984. A selfish origin for human food sharing: tolerated theft. *Ethology and Sociobiology* 5: 1–3.

Boas, F. 1932. The aims of anthropological research. *Science* 76: 605–13.

Boas, F. 1938. [1911] *The Mind of Primitive Man*. New York: Macmillan.

Boesch, C. 1990. First hunters of the forest. *New Scientist*, 125(1717).

Boesch, C. and H. Boesch 1983. Optimisation of nut-cracking with natural hammers by wild chimpanzees. *Behavior* 83: 265–88.

Boesch, C. and H. Boesch 1989. Hunting behavior of wild chimpanzees in the Taï National Park. *American Journal of Physical Anthropology* 78: 547–73.

Bolton, R. 1976. Comment on Mundkur: The cult of the Serpent in the Americas. *Current Anthropology* 17: 441.

Bolton, R. 1980. Comment on Wreschner: red ochre and human evolution. *Current Anthropology* 21:633–5.

Bonnefille, R. 1984. *The Evolution of East Asian Environment*, ed. R. D. White. Centre of Asian Studies, University of Hong Kong.

Borden, C. E. 1976. Reply to Balaji Mundkur, 'The cult of the serpent in the Americas: Its Asian background'. *Current Anthropology* 17: 441–2.

Boscana, G. 1846. Chinigchinich. In Alfred Robinson, *Life in California*. New York: Wiley & Putnam, pp. 227–341.

Bowdler, S. 1977. The coastal colonisation of Australia. In J. Allen, J. Golson and R. Jones (eds) *Sunda and Sahul: Prehistoric studies in South-East Asia, Melanesia and Australia*. London: Academic Press, pp. 205–46.

Bowdler, S. 1990. Peopling Australasia: the 'coastal colonization' hypothesis re-examined. In P. Mellars (ed.) *The Emergence of Modern Humans*. Edinburgh: Edinburgh University Press, pp. 517–39.

Boyd, R. and P. J. Richerson 1985. *Culture and the Evolutionary Process*. Chicago: University of Chicago Press.

Braidwood, R. J. 1957. *Prehistoric Men*. Chicago Natural History Museum Popular Series, Anthropology, 37. Chicago.

Brain, C. K. 1981. *The Hunters or the Hunted?* Chicago: University of Chicago Press.

Brain, C. K. and A. Sillen 1988. Evidence from the Swartkrans cave for the earliest use of fire. *Nature* 336: 464–66.

Brandenstein, C. G. von 1972. The phoenix 'totemism'. *Anthropos* 67: 586–94.

Brandenstein, C. G. von 1982. *Names and Substance of the Australian Subsection System*. Chicago: University of Chicago Press.

Bräuer, G. 1989. The evolution of modern humans: a comparison of the African and non-African evidence. In P. Mellars and C. Stringer (eds) *The Human Revolution. Behavioural and biological perspectives on the origins of modern humans*. Edinburgh: Edinburgh University Press, pp. 123–54.

Breuil, H. and R. Lantier 1959. *The Men of the Old Stone Age*. New York: St Martin's Press.

Brewer, S. 1978. *The Chimps of Mt. Asserik*. New York: Knopf.

Bridges, E. L. 1948. *Uttermost Part of the Earth*. New York: Duffon.

Briffault, R. 1927. *The Mothers*, 3 vols. London: Allen & Unwin.

Brincker, P. H. 1886. *Wörterbuch und kurzgefasste Grammatik des Otii-Herero*. Leipzig: Weigel.

Bromage, T. D. and M. C. Dean 1985. Re-evaluation of the age at death of immature fossil hominids. *Nature* 317: 525–7.

Buchler, I. R. 1978. The fecal crone. In I. R. Buchler and K. Maddock (eds) *The Rainbow Serpent. A chromatic piece*. The Hague: Mouton, pp. 119–212.

Buckley, T. 1982. Menstruation and the power of Yurok women: methods of cultural reconstruction. *American Ethnologist* 9: 47–60.

Buckley, T. 1988. Menstruation and the power of Yurok women. In T. Buckley and A. Gottlieb (eds) *Blood Magic. The anthropology of menstruation*. Berkeley, Los Angeles and London: University of California Press, pp. 187–209.

Buckley, T. and A. Gottlieb 1988. A critical appraisal of theories of menstrual symbolism. In T. Buckley and A. Gottlieb (eds) *Blood Magic. The anthropology of menstruation*. Berkeley, Los Angeles and London: University of California Press, pp. 3–50.

Bunn, H. T. 1981. Archaeological evidence for meat-eating by Plio-Pleistocene hominids from Koobi Fora and Olduvai Gorge. *Nature* 291: 574–7.

Bunn, H. T. 1983. Evidence on the diet and subsistence patterns of Plio-Pleistocene hominids at Koobi Fora, Kenya, and at Olduvai Gorge, Tanzania. In J. Clutton-Brock and C. Grigson (eds) *Animals and Archaeology: 1. Hunters and their prey*. Oxford: BAR International Series 163, pp. 21–30.

Bunn, H. T. and E. M. Kroll 1986. Systematic butchery by Plio-Pleistocene hominids at Olduvai Gorge, Tanzania. *Current Anthropology* 27: 431–52.

Bunney, S. 1990. First Australians 'were earliest seafarers'. *New Scientist*, 125(1717).

Bünning, E. 1964. *The Physiological Clock*. Berlin: Springer-Verlag.

Burkert, W., R. Girard and J. Z. Smith 1987. *Violent Origins. Ritual killing and cultural formation.* Stanford, CA: Stanford University Press.

Burley, N. 1979. The evolution of concealed ovulation. *The American Naturalist* 114: 835–58.

Butzer, K. W. 1980. Comment on Wreschner: red ochre and human evolution. *Current Anthropology* 21: 635.

Bygott, J. D. 1972. Cannibalism among wild chimpanzees. *Nature* 238: 410–11.

Byrne, R. and A. Whiten 1988. *Machiavellian Intelligence. Social expertise and the evolution of intellect in monkeys, apes, and humans.* Oxford: Clarendon Press.

Cameron, A. 1984. *Daughters of Copper Woman.* London: The Women's Press.

Campbell, A. H. 1967. Aboriginal traditions and the prehistory of Australia. *Mankind* 6: 10.

Campbell, J. 1969. *The Masks of God: Primitive Mythology.* Harmondsworth: Penguin.

Cann, R. L., M. Stoneking and A. C. Wilson 1987. Mitochondrial DNA and human evolution. *Nature* 325: 31–6.

Caro, T. M. 1987. Human breasts: unsupported hypotheses reviewed. *Human Evolution* 2: 271–82.

Carrithers, M. 1990. Why humans have cultures. *Man* (N. S.) 25: 189–206.

Carstens, P. 1975. Some implications of change in Khoikhoi supernatural beliefs. In M. G. Whisson and M. West (eds) *Religion and Social Change in Southern Africa. Anthropological essays in honour of Monica Wilson.* Cape Town: David Philip, pp. 78–95.

Cavalli-Sforza, L. L., and M. W. Feldman 1981. *Cultural Transmission and Evolution.* Princeton, NJ: Princeton University Press.

Cavalli-Sforza, L. L., A. Piazza, P. Menozzi and J. Mountain 1988. Reconstruction of human evolution: Bringing together genetic, archaeological, and linguistic data. *Proceedings of the National Academy of Sciences (USA)* 85: 6002–6.

Cavallo, J. A. and R. J. Blumenschine 1989. Tree-stored leopard kills: expanding the hominid scavenging niche. *Journal of Human Evolution* 18: 393–9.

Chaloupka, G. 1984. *From Paleo Art to Casual Paintings.* Darwin: Northern Territory Museum of Arts and Sciences. Monograph Series 1.

Chamberlain, G. V. P. and M. F. Azam 1988. A time to be born. *British Medical Journal* 297: 1637.

Champion, T., C. Gamble, C. Shennan and A. Whittle 1984. *Prehistoric Europe.* London: Academic Press.

Chance, M. R. A. 1962. The nature and special features of the instinctive social bond of primates. In S. L. Washburn (ed.) *Social Life of Early Man.* Viking Fund Publication in Anthropology 31. New York: Wenner-Gren Foundation for Anthropological Research and Chicago: Aldine, pp. 17–33.

Chance, M. R. A. and A. P. Mead 1953. Social behavior and primate evolution. *Symposia of the Society for Experimental Biology, Evolution* 7: 395–439.

Chase, P. G. and H. A. Dibble 1987. Middle Palaeolithic symbolism: a review of current evidence and interpretations. *Journal of Anthropological Archaeology* 6: 263–96.

Chaseling, W. S. 1957. *Yulengor, Nomads of Arnhem Land.* London: Epworth.

Cheney, D. L. and R. M. Seyfarth 1985. Social and non-social knowledge in vervet monkeys. In L. Weiskrantz (ed.) *Animal Intelligence.* Oxford: Clarendon Press, pp. 187–202.

Chivers, D. J. and J. J. Raemakers 1980. Long-term changes in behavior. In D. J. Chivers (ed.) *Malayan Forest Primates.* New York: Plenum Press, pp. 209–60.

Clark, A. H. 1914. Nocturnal animals. *Journal of the Washington Academy of Sciences* 4: 139–42.

Clark, J. D. 1981. 'New men, strange faces, other minds': an archaeologist's perspective on recent discoveries relating to the origins and spread of Modern Man. *Proceedings of the British Academy* 67: 163–92.

Clark, J. D. 1989. The origins and spread of modern humans: a broad perspective on the African evidence. In P. Mellars and C. Stringer (eds) *The Human Revolution. Behavioural and biological perspectives on the origins of modern humans.* Edinburgh: Edinburgh University Press, pp. 565–88.

Clark, J. H. and M. X. Zarrow 1971. Influence of copulation on time of ovulation in women. *American Journal of Obstetrics and Gynecology* 109: 1083–5.

Clastres, P. 1972. The Guayaki. In M. G. Bicchieri (ed.) *Hunters and Gatherers Today*. New York: Holt, Rinehart & Winston, pp. 138–74.

Clastres, P. 1977. *Society Against the State*, trans. R. Hurley in collaboration with A. Stein. Oxford: Blackwell.

Cloudsley-Thompson, J. L. 1980. *Biological Clocks. Their functions in nature*. London: Weidenfeld & Nicolson.

Cohen, R. 1971. *Dominance and Defiance. A study of marital instability in an Islamic society*. Washington, DC: American Anthropological Association. Anthropological Studies 6.

Cohen S. 1969. Theories of myth. *Man* (N.S.) 4: 337–53.

Colbacchini, A. 1919. *A tribu dos Bororos*. Rio de Janeiro: Papelaria Americana.

Collier, J. F. and M. Z. Rosaldo 1981. Politics and gender in simple societies. In S. B. Ortner and H. Whitehead (eds) *Sexual Meanings. The cultural construction of gender and sexuality*. Cambridge: Cambridge University Press, pp. 275–329.

Collins, D. 1976. *The Human Revolution*. Oxford: Phaidon.

Collins, D. 1986. *Palaeolithic Europe*. Tiverton, Devon: Clayhanger Books.

Conkey, M. W. 1978. Style and information in cultural evolution: toward a predictive model for the palaeolithic. In C. L. Redman, M. J. Berman, E. V. Curtin, W. T. Laughorne Jr, N. Versaggi and J. C. Wasner (eds) *Social Archaeology: Beyond subsistence and dating*. New York: Academic Press, pp. 61–85.

Cords, M. 1984. Mating patterns and social structure in redtail monkeys (*Cercopithecus ascanius*). *Zeitschrift fuer Tierpsychologie* 64: 313–29.

Cory, H. 1961. Sumbwa birth figurines. *Journal of the Royal Anthropological Institute* 91.

Cowgill, U. M., A. Bishop, R. J. Andrew and G. E. Hutchinson 1962. An apparent lunar periodicity in the sexual cycle of certain prosimians. *Proceedings of the National Academy of Sciences (USA)* 48: 238.

Crawford, M. and D. Marsh 1989. *The Driving Force*. London: Heinemann.

Crawford, O. G. S. 1958. *The Eye Goddess*. New York: Macmillan.

Crawley, E. 1927. *The Mystic Rose*, 2 vols. London: Methuen.

Criss, Th. B. and J. P. Marcum 1981. A lunar effect on fertility. *Social Biology* 28: 75–80.

Crocker, J. C. 1985. *Vital Souls. Bororo cosmology, natural symbolism, and shamanism*. Tucson: University of Arizona Press.

Cronin, C. 1977. Illusion and reality in Sicily. In A. Schlegel (ed.) *Sexual Stratification*. New York: Columbia University Press, pp. 67–93.

Crook, J. H. 1972. Social organisation and the environment: aspects of contemporary social ethology. *Animal Behaviour* 18(1970): 197–209. Reprinted in D. D. Quiatt (ed.) *Primates on Primates*. Minnesota: Burgess Publishing, pp. 75–93.

Culver, R., J. Rotton and I. W. Kelly 1988. Moon mechanisms and myths: a critical appraisal of explanations of purported lunar effects on human behavior. *Psychological Reports* 62: 683–710.

Cutler, W. B. 1980. The psychoneuroendocrinology of the ovulatory cycle of woman: a review. *Psychoneuroendocrinology* 5: 89–111.

Cutler, W. B., C. R. Garcia and A. M. Krieger 1979a. Sexual behavior frequency and menstrual cycle length in mature premenopausal women. *Psychoneuroendocrinology* 4: 297–309.

Cutler, W. B., C. R. Garcia and A. M. Krieger 1979b. Luteal phase defects: a possible relationship between short hyperthermic phase and sporadic sexual behavior in women. *Hormones and Behavior* 13: 214–18.

Cutler, W. B., C. R. Garcia and A. M. Krieger 1980. Sporadic sexual behavior and menstrual cycle length in women. *Hormones and Behavior* 14: 163–72.

Cutler, W. B., G. Preti, A. M. Krieger, G. Huggins, C. R. Garcia and H. J. Lawley 1986. Human axillary secretions influence women's menstrual cycles: the role of donor extract from men. *Hormones and Behavior* 20: 463–73.

Cutler, W. B., W. M., Schleidt, E., Friedmann, G. Preti, and R. Stine 1987. Lunar influences on the reproductive cycle in women. *Human Biology* 59: 959–72.

Dahlberg, F. 1981. Introduction. In F. Dahlberg (ed.) *Woman the Gatherer*. New Haven & London: Yale University Press.

Dalton, K. 1971. *The Menstrual Cycle*. New York: Pantheon.

Dalton, K. 1977. *The Premenstrual Syndrome and Progesterone Therapy*. London: Heinemann.

Dalton, K. 1979. *Once a Month*. Pomona, CA: Hunter House.

Daly, M. and M. Wilson 1983. *Sex, Evolution, and Behavior*, 2nd edn. Boston: PWS Publishers.

Darwin, C. 1859. *On the Origin of Species*. London: Murray.

Darwin, C. 1871. *The Descent of Man, and Selection in Relation to Sex*, 2 vols. London: Murray.

Davis, S. 1974. Incised bones from the Mousterian of Kebara Cave (Mount Carmel) and the Aurignacian of Ha-Yonim Cave (Western Gallillee), Israel. *Paleorient* 2: 181–2.

Dawkins, R. 1976. *The Selfish Gene*. Oxford: Oxford University Press.

Dawkins, R. 1988. *The Blind Watchmaker*. Harmondsworth: Penguin.

Dawson, J. 1881. *Australian Aborigines*. Melbourne: Robertson.

Deacon, H. J. 1989. Late Pleistocene palaeoecology and archaeology in the Southern Cape, South Africa. In P. Mellars and C. Stringer (eds) *The Human Revolution. Behavioural and biological perspectives on the origins of modern humans*. Edinburgh: Edinburgh University Press, pp. 547–64.

Dean, M. C., C. B. Stringer, and T. D. Bromage 1986. Age at death of the Neanderthal child from Devil's Tower, Gibralter, and the implications for studies of general growth and development in Neanderthals. *American Journal of Physical Anthropology* 70: 301–9.

Deetz, J. 1972. Hunters in archaeological perspective. In R. B. Lee and I. DeVore (eds) *Man the Hunter*. Chicago: Aldine, pp. 281–5.

de Heusch, L. 1975. What shall we do with the drunken king? *Africa* 45: 363–72.

de Heusch, L. 1982. *The Drunken King, or, The Origins of the State*. Bloomington: Indiana University Press.

Delaney, J., M. J. Lupton and E. Toth 1977. *The Curse. A cultural history of menstruation*. New York: Dutton.

Delluc, B. and G. Delluc 1978. Les manifestations graphiques aurignaciens sur support rocheux des environs des Eyzies (Dordogne). *Gallia Préhistoire* 21: 213–438.

Delporte, H. 1968. L'abri du Facteur à Tursac. *Gallia Préhistoire* 11: 1–112.

Delporte, H. 1979. *L'image de la femme dans l'art préhistorique*. Paris: Picard.

de Lumley, H. 1969. A palaeolithic camp at Nice. *Scientific American* 220(5): 42–50.

D'Errico, F. 1989. Palaeolithic lunar calendars: a case of wishful thinking? *Current Anthropology* 30: 117–18.

De Saussure, F. 1974 [1915]. *Course in General Linguistics*, trans. W. Baskin. London: Fontana/Collins.

Desmond, A. 1979. *The Ape's Reflection*. London: Quartet Books.

Devereux, G. 1950. The psychology of feminine genital bleeding. An analysis of Mohave Indian puberty and menstrual rites. *International Journal of Psychoanalysis* 31: 237–57.

DeVore, I. 1965. The evolution of social life. In S. Tax (ed.) *Horizons of Anthropology*. London: Allen & Unwin, pp. 25–36.

de Waal, F. 1983. *Chimpanzee Politics. Power and sex among apes*. London: Unwin.

de Waal, F. 1991. *Peacemaking Among Primates*. Harmondsworth: Penguin.

Dewan, E. M. and J. Rock 1969. Phase locking of the human menstrual cycle by periodic light stimulation. *Biophysics Journal* 9: A207.

Dewan, E. M., M. F. Menkin and J. Rock 1978. Effect of photic stimulation of the human menstrual cycle. *Photochemistry and Photobiology* 27: 581–5.

Dibble, H. L. 1983. Variability and change in the Middle Paleolithic of Western Europe and the Near East. In E. Trinkaus (ed.) *The Mousterian Legacy: Human biocultural change in the Upper Pleistocene*. Oxford: BAR International Series 16, pp. 53–71.

Dimbleby, G. 1978. *Plants and Archaeology*. New York: Harper & Row.

Dixson, A. F. 1983. Observations on the evolution and behavioral significance of 'sexual skin' in female primates. In J. S. Rosenblatt, R. A. Hinde, C. Beer and M. -C. Busnel (eds) *Advances in the Study of Behavior* 13: 63–106. New York: Academic Press.

Dobkin de Rios, M. 1976. Female odors and the origin of the sexual division of labor in *Homo sapiens. Human Ecology* 4: 261–2.

Dobkin de Rios, M. and B. Hayden 1985. Odorous. differentiation and variability in the sexual division of labor among hunter/gatherers. *Journal of Human Evolution* 14: 219–28.

Doehring, C. H., H. C. Kraemer, H. K. H. Brodie, and D. A. Hamburg 1975. A cycle of plasma testosterone in the human male. *Journal of Clinical Endocrinology and Metabolism* 40: 492–500.

Donelson, E. and J. E. Gullahorn 1977. *Women. A psychological perspective.* New York: Wiley.

Dorsey, G. A. 1903. *The Arapaho Sun Dance. The ceremony of the offerings lodge.* Field Columbian Museum, Publication 75, Anthropological Series, IV. Chicago.

Doty, R. L. 1981. Olfactory communication in humans – a review. *Chemical Senses and Flavor* 6: 351–76.

Douglas, M. 1963. *The Lele of the Kasai.* Oxford: Oxford University Press.

Douglas, M. 1969. Is matriliny doomed in Africa? In M. Douglas and P. M. Kaberry (eds) *Man in Africa.* London: Tavistock, pp. 121–35.

Douglas, M. 1982. *In the Active Voice.* London: Routledge & Kegan Paul.

Dowling, J. H. 1968. Individual ownership and the sharing of game in hunting societies. *American Anthropologist* 70: 502–7.

Driver, H. E. and W. C. Massey 1957. Comparative studies of North American Indians. *Transactions of the American Philosophical Society* (N. S.) 47: Part 2.

Driver, J. C. 1990. Meat in due season: the timing of communal hunts. In L. B. Davis and B. O. K. Reeves (eds) *Hunters of the Recent Past.* London: Unwin Hyman, pp. 11–33.

Dunbar, R. I. M. 1980a. Determinants and evolutionary consequences of dominance among female gelada baboons. *Behavioural Ecology and Sociobiology* 7: 253–65.

Dunbar, R. I. M. 1980b. Demographic and life history variables of a population of gelada baboons (*Theropithecus gelada*). *Journal of Animal Ecology* 49: 485–506.

Dunbar, R. I. M. 1988. *Primate Social Systems.* London & Sydney: Croom Helm.

Dundes, A. 1976. A psychoanalytic study of the bullroarer. *Man* (N. S.) 11: 220–38.

Dundes, A., ed. 1988. *The Flood Myth.* Berkeley & Los Angeles: University of California Press.

Durkheim, E. 1961. [1925] *Moral Education,* trans. E. K. Wilson and H. Schnurner. New York: Free Press.

Durkheim, E. 1963. [1898] La prohibition de l'inceste et ses origines. *L'Année Sociologique* 1: 1–70. Reprinted as *Incest: the nature and origin of the taboo,* trans. E. Sagarin. New York: Stuart.

Durkheim, E. 1965 [1912] *The Elementary Forms of the Religious Life.* New York: Free Press.

Ebling, J. 1985. The mythological evolution of nudity. *Journal of Human Evolution* 14: 33–41.

Eggan, F. 1950. *Social Organization of the Western Pueblos.* Chicago: University of Chicago Press.

Eggan, F., M. B. Duberman and R. O. Clemmer (eds) 1979. Documents in Hopi Indian sexuality: imperialism, culture and resistance. *Radical History Review* Spring/Summer: 99–130.

Eldredge, N. and S. J. Gould, 1972. Punctuated equilibrium: an alternative to phyletic gradualism. In T. J. M. Schopf (ed.) *Models in Paleobiology.* San Francisco: Freeman, pp. 82–115.

Eliade, M. 1958. *Patterns in Comparative Religion.* London: Sheed & Ward.

Eliade, M. 1973. *Australian Religions. An introduction.* Ithaca, NY: Cornell University Press.

Eliade, M. 1978. *A History of Religious Ideas,* 2 vols. Chicago: University of Chicago Press.

Elkin, A. P. 1933. *Studies in Australian Totemism.* Sydney: Australian National Research Council. The Oceania Monographs 2.

Elkin, A. P. 1938. *The Australian Aborigines.* Sydney & London: Angus & Robertson.

Elkin, A. P. 1968. Notes and glossary. In Bill Harney and A. P. Elkin (eds) *Songs of the Songmen. Aboriginal myths retold.* Adelaide: Rigby, pp. 139–78.

Elliot Smith, G. 1919. *The Evolution of the Dragon*. Manchester: Manchester University Press.

Elmendorf, W. W. 1960. *The Structure of Twana Culture with Comparative Notes on the Structure of Yurok Culture by A. L. Kroeber*. Pullman, WA. Washington State University Research Studies 28(3), Monographic Supplement 2.

Ember, M. 1973. An archaeological indicator of matrilocal versus patrilocal residence. *American Antiquity* 38: 177–82.

Engels, F. n.d. [1865]. Letter to F. A. Lange. In K. Marx and F. Engels, *Selected Correspondence, 1843–1895*. Moscow: Foreign Languages Publishing House.

Engels, F. 1957 [1888]. Ludwig Feuerbach and the end of classical German philosophy. In K. Marx and F. Engels, *On Religion*. (Selected Writings). Moscow: Foreign Languages Publishing House.

Engels, F. 1962 [1887]. Socialism: utopian and scientific. In Marx and Engels, *Selected Works*, 2 vols. Vol. 2, pp. 93–155.

Engels, F. 1964 [1873–86] *The Dialectics of Nature*. Moscow: Progress.

Engels, F. 1972 [1884]. *The Origin of the Family, Private Property and the State*. New York: Pathfinder Press.

Evans-Pritchard, E. E. 1946. Applied anthropology. *Africa* 16: 92–8.

Evans-Pritchard, E. E. 1956. *Nuer Religion*. Oxford: Oxford University Press.

Evans-Pritchard, E. E. 1965. *Theories of Primitive Religion*. Oxford: Oxford University Press.

Evans-Pritchard, E. E. 1974. *Man and Woman among the Azande*. London: Faber & Faber.

Fa, J. E. 1986. *Use of Time and Resources by Provisioned Troops of Monkeys*. Basle: Karger.

Fagan, B. 1987. *The Great Journey. The peopling of ancient America*. London: Thames & Hudson.

Farabee, W. C. 1924. *The Central Caribs*. Philadelphia: University of Pennsylvania Anthropological Publications 10.

Fedigan, L. M. 1986. The changing role of women in models of human evolution. *Annual Review of Anthropology* 15: 25–66.

Feuchtwang, S. 1973. The colonial formation of British social anthropology. In Talal Asad (ed.) *Anthropology and the Colonial Encounter*. London: Ithaca, pp. 71–100.

Ffitch, P. 1987. The evolutionary consequences of the use of hands to motor control. Birchtree Farm, Devon: Unpublished.

Fisher, E. 1979. *Woman's Creation*. New York: McGraw-Hill.

Fison, L. and A. W. Howitt 1880. *Kamilaroi and Kurnai*. Melbourne: George Robertson.

Flood, J. 1983. *Archaeology of the Dreamtime*. Sydney & London: Collins.

Flood, J. 1989. Animals and zoomorphs in rock art of the Koolburra region, north Queensland. In H. Morphy (ed.) *Animals into Art*. London: Unwin Hyman, pp. 287–300.

Fock, N. 1963. *Waiwai. Religion and society of an Amazonian tribe*. Copenhagen: The National Museum.

Foley, R. 1987. *Another Unique Species. Patterns in human evolutionary ecology*. Harlow: Longman.

Foley, R. 1988. Hominids, humans and hunter-gatherers: an evolutionary perspective. In T. Ingold, D. Riches and J. Woodburn (eds) *Hunters and Gatherers. 1: History, evolution and social change*. Oxford: Berg, pp. 207–21.

Foley, R. 1989. The ecological conditions of speciation: a comparative approach to the origins of anatomically-modern humans. In P. Mellars and C. Stringer (eds) *The Human Revolution. Behavioural and biological perspectives on the origins of modern humans*. Edinburgh: Edinburgh University Press, pp. 298–318.

Fontenrose, J. 1959. *Python. A study of Delphic myth and its origins*. Berkeley: University of California Press.

Forge, A. 1966. Art and environment in the Sepik: the Curl lecture. *Proceedings of the Royal Anthropological Institute for 1965*.

Fortes, M. 1959. Primitive kinship. *Scientific American* 200(6): 146–158.

Fortes, M. 1966. Totem and Taboo. *Proceedings of the Royal Anthropological Institute*, Presidential Address, pp. 154–9.

Fortes, M. 1970. *Kinship and the Social Order*. London: Routledge.

Forth, G. L. 1981. *Rindi. An ethnographic study of a traditional domain in Eastern Sumba.* The Hague: Martinus Nijhoff.

Fouts, R. S. 1975. Capacities for language in great apes. In R. H. Tuttle (ed.) *Socioecology and Psychology of Primates.* The Hague: Mouton, pp. 371–90.

Fox, R. 1966. *Totem and Taboo* reconsidered. In E. R. Leach (ed.) *The Structural Study of Myth and Totemism.* London: Tavistock, pp. 161–79. A.S.A. Monographs 5.

Fox, R. 1967a. In the beginning: aspects of hominid behavioural evolution. *Man* (N. S.) 2: 415–33.

Fox, R. 1967b. *Kinship and Marriage. An anthropological perspective.* Harmondsworth: Penguin.

Fox, R. 1975a. *Encounter with Anthropology.* Harmondsworth: Penguin.

Fox, R. 1975b. Primate kin and human kinship. In Fox, R. (ed.) *Biosocial Anthropology.* London: Malaby, pp. 9–35.

Frazer, J. G. 1900. *The Golden Bough,* 2nd edn, 3 vols. London: Macmillan.

Frazer, J. G. 1910. *Totemism and Exogamy,* 4 vols. London: Macmillan.

Frazer, J. G. 1926–36. *The Golden Bough. A study in magic and religion,* 3rd edn, 13 vols. London: Macmillan.

Frazer, J. G. 1936. *Aftermath. A supplement to The Golden Bough.* London: Macmillan.

Freeman, L. G. 1975. Acheulian sites and stratigraphy in Iberia and the Meghreb. In K. W. Butzer and G. Isaac (eds) *After the Australopithecines.* The Hague: Mouton, pp. 661–743.

Freud, S. 1965 [1913]. *Totem and Taboo. Some points of agreement between the mental lives of savages and neurotics.* London: Routledge.

Frisch, R. E. 1975. Demographic implications of the biological determinants of female fecundity. *Social Biology* 22(1): 17–22.

Frolov, B. 1965. Stone Age astronomers. *Moscow News,* 4 September.

Frolov, B. 1977–9. Numbers in Paleolithic graphic art and the initial stages in the development of mathematics. *Soviet Anthropology and Archeology* 16 (1977–8): 142–66; and 17(1978–9): 73–93, 41–74, 61–113.

Frolov, B. 1979. Les bases cognitives de l'art paléolithique. In *Valcamonica Symposium III. The intellectual expressions of prehistoric man: art and religion,* pp. 295–8.

Gamble, C. 1982. Interaction and alliance in palaeolithic society. *Man* (N. S.) 17: 92–107.

Gamble, C. 1986a. *The Palaeolithic Settlement of Europe.* Cambridge: Cambridge University Press.

Gamble, C. 1986b. Continents of hunters and gatherers: world models and a comparison of Europe with Australia. Paper delivered at The World Archaeological Congress, Southampton.

Gargett, R. H. 1989. Grave shortcomings. The evidence for Neandertal burial. *Current Anthropology* 30: 157–90.

Gason, S. 1879. The manners and customs of the Dieyerie tribe of Australian Aborigines. In J. D. Woods (ed.) *The Native Tribes of South Australia.* Adelaide: Wigg, pp. 253–307.

Gell, A. 1975. *Metamorphosis of the Cassowaries. Umeda society, language and ritual.* London: Macmillan.

Gennep, A. Van 1946–58. *Manuel de Folklore francaise contemporain,* 9 vols. Paris: Picard.

Ghiglieri, M. P. 1984. Feeding ecology and sociality of chimpanzees in Kibale Forest, Uganda. In P. S. Rodman and J. G. H. Cant (eds) *Adaptations for Foraging in Nonhuman Primates.* New York: Columbia University Press, pp. 161–94.

Gillespie, R., D. R. Horton, P. Ladd, P. G. Macumber, T. H. Rich, A. Thorne and R. V. S. Wright 1978. Lancefield Swamp and the extinction of the Australian megafauna. *Science* 200: 1044–8.

Gillison, G. 1980. Images of nature in Gimi thought. In C. P. MacCormack and M. Strathern (eds) *Nature, Culture and Gender.* Cambridge: Cambridge University Press. pp. 143–73.

Gimbutas, M. 1982. *The Goddesses and Gods of Old Europe, 6,500–3,500 B. C. Myths and cult images.* London: Thames & Hudson.

Gimbutas, M. 1989. *The Language of the Goddess.* London: Thames & Hudson.

Girard, R. 1977. *Violence and the Sacred.* Baltimore, MD & London: Johns Hopkins University Press.

Godelier, M. 1986. *The Making of Great Men*. Cambridge: Cambridge University Press.

Goldenweiser, A. A. 1910. Totemism, an analytical study. *Journal of American Folklore* 23: 179–293.

Goldizen, A. W. 1987. Tamarins and marmosets: communal care of offspring. In B. B. Smuts, D. L. Cheney, R. M. Seyfarth, R. W. Wrangham and T. T. Struhsaker (eds) *Primate Societies*. Chicago & London: University of Chicago Press, pp. 34–43.

Gomez-Tabanera, J. M. 1978. *Les Statuettes Féminines Paléolithiques dites 'Venus'*. Asturias: Love-Gijon.

Goodale, J. C. 1959. The Tiwi women of Melville Island, Australia. Ph. D. thesis, University of Pennsylvania. Ann Arbor, Michigan: University Microfilms International.

Goodale, J. C. 1971. *Tiwi Wives. A study of the women of Melville Island, North Australia*. Seattle & London: University of Washington Press.

Goodall, J. 1977. Infant-killing and cannibalism in free-living chimpanzees. *Folia Primatologica* 28: 259–82.

Goodall, J. 1983. Population dynamics during a 15 year period in one community of free-living chimpanzees in the Gombe National Park, Tanzania. *Zeitschrift fuer Tierpsychologie* 61: 1–60.

Goodall, J. 1986. *The Chimpanzees of Gombe. Patterns of behavior*. Cambridge, MA & London: Belknap Press of Harvard University Press.

Gottlieb, A. 1988. Menstrual cosmology among the Beng of Ivory Coast. In T. Buckley and A. Gottlieb (eds) *Blood Magic. The anthropology of menstruation*. Berkeley: University of California Press, pp. 55–74.

Goudsblom, J. 1986. The human monopoly on the use of fire: its origins and conditions. *Human Evolution* 1: 517–23.

Gould, R. A. 1969. *Yiwara. Foragers of the Australian desert*. London & Sydney: Collins.

Gould, R. A. 1981. Comparative ecology of food-sharing in Australia and Northwest California. In G. Teleki and R. S. O. Harding (eds) *Omnivorous Primates. Gathering and hunting in human evolution*. New York: Columbia University Press, pp. 422–54.

Gourlay, K. A. 1975. *Sound-producing Instruments in Traditional Society. A study of esoteric instruments and their role in male–female relations*. New

Guinea Research Bulletin 60. Port Moresby & Canberra: Australian National University.

Gowlett, J. A. J. 1984. Mental abilities of early man: a look at some hard evidence. In R. Foley (ed.) *Hominid Evolution and Community Ecology: Prehistoric human adaptation in biological perspective*. New York & London: Academic Press, pp. 167–92.

Gowlett, J. A. J., J. W. K. Harris, D. Walton and B. A. Wood 1981. Early archaeological sites, hominid remains and traces of fire from Chesowanja, Kenya. *Nature* 294: 125–9.

Gowlett, J. A. J., J. W. K. Harris and B. A. Wood 1982. Reply to Isaac. *Nature* 296: 870.

Graham, C. A. and W. C. McGrew 1980. Menstrual synchrony in female undergraduates living on a coeducational campus. *Psychoneuroendocrinology* 5: 245–52.

Graham, C. E. 1981. Menstrual cycle physiology of the great apes. In C. E. Graham (ed.) *Reproductive Biology of the Great Apes. Comparative and biomedical perspectives*. New York: Academic Press, pp. 286–383.

Graziosi, P. 1960. *Palaeolithic Art*. London: Faber & Faber.

Gregor, T. 1977. *Mehinaku*. Chicago: University of Chicago Press.

Gregor, T. 1985. *Anxious Pleasures. The sexual lives of an Amazonian people*. Chicago & London: University of Chicago Press.

Griaule, M. 1965. *Conversations with Ogotommêli*. Oxford: Oxford University Press.

Grice, H. 1969. Utterer's meanings and intentions. *Philosophical Review* 78: 147–77.

Groger-Wurm, H. M. 1973. *Australian Aboriginal Bark Paintings and their Mythological Interpretation. Vol. 1. Eastern Arnhem Land*. Canberra: Australian Institute of Aboriginal Studies.

Groves, C. P. 1989. A regional approach to the problem of the origin of modern humans in Australasia. In P. Mellars and C. Stringer (eds) *The Human Revolution. Behavioural and biological perspectives on the origins of modern humans*. Edinburgh: Edinburgh University Press, pp. 274–85.

Guevara, J. 1908–10. *Historia del Paraguay. Rio de la Plata y Tucumán*. Buenos Aires: Anales de la Biblioteca Nacional, Vol. 5.

Guillon, P., D. Guillon, J. Lansac and J. H. Soutoul 1986. Naissances, fertilité, rhythmes et cycle lunaire. *Journal de Gynecologie, Obstetrique, et Biologie de la Reproduction (Paris)* 15: 265–71.

Gunn, D. L., P. M. Jenkin, and A. L. Gunn 1937. Menstrual periodicity: statistical observations on a large sample of normal cases. *Journal of Obstetrics and Gynecology of the British Empire.* 44: 839.

Gusinde, M. 1961 [1937]. *The Yamana. The life and thought of the water nomads of Cape Horn*, trans. F. Schütze, 5 vols. Human Relations Area File. New Haven: Yale University Press.

Haddon, A. C. 1902. Presidential Address to the Anthropological Section, H, of the British Association for the Advancement of Science. Belfast, pp. 8–11.

Hahn, T. 1881. *Tsuni!-Goam. The supreme being of the Khoi-khoi.* London: Trübner.

Haile, B. and M. C. Wheelwright 1949. *Emergence Myth According to the Hanelthnayhe or Upward-Reaching Rite.* Santa Fe, New Mexico: Museum of Navajo Ceremonial Art. Navajo Religion Series 3.

Hallam, S. J. 1975. *Fire and Hearth. A study of Aboriginal usage and European usurpation in South-Western Australia.* Canberra: Australian Institute of Aboriginal Studies.

Hallowell, A. I. 1926. Bear ceremonialism in the northern hemisphere. *American Anthropologist* (N. S.) 28: 1–163.

Hamilton, A. 1980. Dual social systems: Technology, labour and women's secret rites in the eastern Western Desert of Australia. *Oceania* 51: 4–19.

Hamilton, A. 1981. *Nature and Nurture. Aboriginal child-rearing in north-central Arnhem Land.* Canberra: Australian Institute of Aboriginal Studies.

Hamilton, W. D. 1964. The genetical evolution of social behaviour. I, II. *Journal of Theoretical Biology* 7: 1–52.

Hammond, D. and A. Jablow 1975. *Women. Their familial roles in traditional societies.* Menlo Park, CA: Cummings. Cummings Module in Anthropology 57.

Hanbury-Tenison, R. 1982. *Aborigines of the Amazon Rain Forest: The Yanomami.* Amsterdam: Time-Life Books.

Harako, R. 1981. The cultural ecology of hunting behaviour among Mbuti Pygmies in the Ituri Forest, Zaire. In G. Teleki and R. S. O. Harding (eds) *Omnivorous Primates.* New York: Columbia University Press, pp. 499–555.

Haraway, D. 1989. *Primate Visions. Gender, race and nature in the world of modern science.* New York & London: Routledge.

Harcourt, A. H. 1988. Alliances in contests and social intelligence. In R. Byrne and A. Whiten (eds) *Machiavellian Intelligence.* Oxford: Clarendon Press. pp. 132–52.

Harding, R. S. O. 1975. Meat-eating and hunting in baboons. In R. H. Tuttle (ed.) *Socioecology and Psychology of Primates.* The Hague: Mouton.

Hardy, A. 1960. Was man more aquatic in the past? *New Scientist* 7: 642–5.

Harrell, B. B. 1981. Lactation and menstruation in cultural perspective. *American Anthropologist* 83: 796–823.

Harrington, J. P. 1931. Karuk texts. *International Journal of American Linguistics* 6: 121–61, 194–226.

Harrington, J. P. 1933. Annotations. In G. Boscana. *Chinigchinich*, ed. P. Townsend Hanna. Glendale, CA: Clark.

Harris, D. R. 1980. Tropical savanna environments: definition, distribution, diversity and development. In D. R. Harris (ed.) *Human Ecology in Savanna Environments.* New York & London: Academic Press, pp. 3–30.

Harris, M. 1969. *The Rise of Anthropological Theory.* London: Routledge.

Harrison, J. L. 1954. The moonlight effect on rat-breeding. *Bulletin of the Raffles Museum* 25: 166–70.

Harrold, F. B. 1988. The Chatelperronian and the Early Aurignacian in France. In J. F. Hoffecker and C. A. Wolf (eds) *The Early Upper Paleolithic.* Oxford: BAR International Series 437, 157–91.

Harrold, F. B. 1989. Mousterian, Chatelperronian and early Aurignacian in western Europe: continuity or discontinuity? In P. Mellars and C. B. Stringer (eds) *The Human Revolution. Behavioural and biological perspectives on the origins of modern humans.* Edinburgh: Edinburgh University Press, pp. 677–13.

Hauser, M. D. 1988. Invention and social transmission: new data from wild vervet monkeys. In R. Byrne and A. Whiten (eds) *Machiavellian Intelligence. Social expertise and the evolution of intellect in monkeys, apes, and humans*. Oxford: Clarendon Press, pp. 327–43.

Hayden, B. 1979. *Palaeolithic Reflections*. Canberra: Australian Institute of Aboriginal Studies.

Hayden, B. 1981. Subsistence and ecological adaptations of modern hunter/gatherers. In G. Teleki and R. S. O. Harding (eds) *Omnivorous Primates*. New York: Columbia University Press, pp. 344–421.

Hayden, B., M. Deal, A. Cannon, and J. Casey 1986. Ecological determinants of women's status among hunter/gatherers. *Human Evolution* 1(5): 449–74.

Heckewelder, J. 1876. *History, Manners, and Customs of the Indian Nations Who Once Inhabited Pennsylvania and the Neighbouring States* (revised edn). Philadelphia. Memoirs of the Historical Society of Pennsylvania 12.

Henderson, M. E. 1976. Evidence for a male menstrual temperature cycle and synchrony with female menstrual cycle. *New Zealand Medical Journal* 84: 164.

Henry, J. 1964. *Jungle People. A Kaingang tribe of the highlands of Brazil*. New York: Vintage.

Herbert, J. 1968. Sexual preference in the rhesus monkey (*Macaca mulatta*) in the laboratory. *Animal Behavior* 29: 120–8.

Herman, J. L. 1981. *Father–Daughter Incest*. Cambridge, MA: Harvard University Press.

Hewes, G. W. 1974. Language in early hominids. In R. W. Wescott (ed.) *Language Origins*. Maryland: Linstok Press, pp. 1–33.

Hiatt, L. R. 1975a. Introduction. In L. R. Hiatt (ed.) *Australian Aboriginal Mythology. Essays in honour of W. E. H. Stanner*. Canberra: Australian Institute of Aboriginal Studies.

Hiatt, L. R. 1975b. Swallowing and regurgitation in Australian myth and rite. In L. R. Hiatt (ed.) *Australian Aboriginal Mythology*. Canberra: Australian Institute of Aboriginal Studies, pp. 143–62.

Hilger, I. M. 1952. *Arapaho Child Life and its Cultural Background*. Bulletin of the Bureau of American Ethnology 148. Washington DC: Smithsonian Institution.

Hill, J. H. 1974. Commentary three: hominoid proto-linguistic capacities. In R. W. Wescott (ed.) *Language Origins*. Maryland: Linstok Press, pp. 185–95.

Hill, K. 1982. Hunting and human evolution. *Journal of Human Evolution* 11: 521–44.

Hill, K. and H. Kaplan 1988. Tradeoffs in male and female reproductive strategies among the Ache: Part 1. In L. Betzig, M. Borgerhoff Mulder and P. Turke (eds) *Human Reproductive Behaviour. A Darwinian perspective*. Cambridge: Cambridge University Press, pp. 277–89.

Hladik, C. M. 1975. Ecology, diet, and social patterning in Old and New World primates. In R. H. Tuttle (ed.) *Socioecology and Psychology of Primates*. The Hague: Mouton, pp. 3–35.

Hockett, C. F. 1960. The origin of speech. *Scientific American* 203(3): 89–96.

Hockett, C. F. and R. Ascher 1964. The human revolution. *Current Anthropology* 5: 135–68.

Hodge, F. W. (ed.) 1910. *Handbook of American Indians North of Mexico*. Bulletin of the Bureau of American Ethnology 30. Washington DC: Smithsonian Institution. 2 vols.

Hoffecker, J. F. 1988. Early Upper Paleolithic sites of the European USSR. In J. F. Hoffecker and C. A. Wolf (eds) *The Early Upper Paleolithic. Evidence from Europe and the Near East*. Oxford: BAR International Series 437, pp. 237–72.

Hogbin, I. A. 1970. *The Island of Menstruating Men*. Scranton, London & Toronto: Chandler.

Holloway, R. L. 1969. Culture: a human domain. *Current Anthropology* 10: 395–407.

Holloway, R. L. 1981. Culture, symbols and human brain evolution: a synthesis. *Dialectical Anthropology* 5: 287–303.

Holmberg, A. 1948. The Siriono. In J. H. Steward (ed.) *Handbook of South American Indians*. Washington DC: Smithsonian Institution. *Bulletin of the Bureau of American Ethnology* 143(3): 461–4.

Holmberg, A. 1950. *Nomads of the Long Bow. The Siriono of eastern Bolivia*. Washington DC: Smithsonian Institution. Institute of Social Anthropology Publication 10.

Holy, L. 1985. Fire, meat, and children: the Berti myth, male dominance, and female power. In J. Overing (ed.) *Reason and Morality*. London & New York: Tavistock, pp. 180–9.

Hong, S. K. and H. Rahn 1967. The diving women of Korea and Japan. *Scientific American* 216(5): 34–43.

Honigmann, J. J. 1954. *The Kaska Indians. An ethnographic reconstruction*. New Haven: Yale University. Publications in Anthropology 51.

Horton, D. R. 1976. Lancefield: the problem of proof in bone analysis. *Artefact* 1: 129–43.

Horton, D. R. 1979. The great megafaunal extinction debate – 1879–1979. *Artefact* 4: 11–25.

Horton, D. R. and R. V. S. Wright 1981. Cuts on Lancefield bones. *Archaeology in Oceania* 16(2): 78–9.

How, M. W. 1965. *The Mountain Bushmen of Basutoland*. Pretoria: Van Schaik.

Howell, F. C. 1984. Introduction. In F. H. Smith and F. Spencer (eds) *The Origins of Modern Humans. A world survey of the fossil evidence*. New York: Alan R. Liss, pp. xii–xxii.

Howell, S. 1984. *Society and Cosmos. Chewong of Peninsular Malaysia*. Oxford: Oxford University Press.

Howells, W. W. 1988. The meaning of the Neanderthals in human evolution. In Fondation Singer-Polignac (ed.) *L'Evolution dans sa réalité et ses diverses modalités*. Paris: Masson, pp. 221–39.

Howitt, A. W. 1904. *The Native Tribes of South-East Australia*. London: Macmillan.

Hrdy, S. B. 1977. *The Langurs of Abu*. Cambridge, MA: Harvard University Press.

Hrdy, S. B. 1981. *The Woman that Never Evolved*. Cambridge, MA: Harvard University Press.

Hrdy, S. B. and P. L. Whitten 1987. Patterning of sexual activity. In D. L. Cheney, R. M. Seyfarth, R. W. Wrangham and T. T. Struhsaker (eds) *Primate Societies*. Chicago & London: University of Chicago Press, pp. 370–84.

Hubert, H. and M. Mauss 1964. *Sacrifice: Its Nature and Function*, trans. W. D. Halls. London: Cohen & West.

Hugh-Jones, C. 1979. *From the Milk River. Spatial and temporal processes in northwest Amazonia*. Cambridge: Cambridge University Press.

Hugh-Jones, S. 1979. *The Palm and the Pleiades. Initiation and cosmology in northwest Amazonia*. Cambridge: Cambridge University Press.

Hughes, A. L. 1988. *Evolution and Human Kinship*. New York & Oxford: Oxford University Press.

Humphrey, N. K. 1976. The social function of intellect. In P. P. G. Bateson and R. A. Hinde (eds) *Growing Points in Ethology*. Cambridge: Cambridge University Press, pp. 303–17.

Humphrey, N. K. 1982. Peter Evans talking to Dr. Nick Humphrey. *Science Now*. BBC Radio 4, 21 December.

Hunter, J. D. 1957. *Manners and Customs of Several Indian Tribes Located West of the Mississippi*. Minneapolis, MN: Ross & Haines.

Huxley, E. 1962. *The Flame Trees of Thika*. Harmondsworth: Penguin.

Huxley, F. 1957. *Affable Savages. An anthropologist among the Urubu Indians of Brazil*. New York: Viking Press.

Ingersoll, E. 1928. *Dragons and Dragon Lore*. New York: Payson & Clarke.

Ingold, T. 1980. *Hunters, Pastoralists and Ranchers*. Cambridge: Cambridge University Press.

Ingold, T. 1986. *Evolution and Social Life*. Cambridge: Cambridge University Press.

Isaac, G. Ll. 1968. Traces of Pleistocene hunters: an East African example. In R. B. Lee and I. DeVore (eds) *Man the Hunter*. Chicago: Aldine, pp. 253–61.

Isaac, G. Ll. 1969. Studies of early culture in East Africa. *World Archaeology* 1: 1–28.

Isaac, G. Ll. 1971. The diet of early man: aspects of archaeological evidence from lower and middle Pleistocene sites in Africa. *World Archaeology* 21: 278–99.

Isaac, G. Ll. 1978. The food-sharing behavior of protohuman hominids. *Scientific American*, April.

Isaac, G. Ll. 1982. Early hominids and fire at Chesowanja, Kenya. *Nature* 296: 870.

Isaac, G. Ll. 1983. Aspects of human evolution. In D. S. Bendall (ed.) *Evolution from Molecules to Men*. Cambridge: Cambridge University Press, pp. 509–45.

Isaac, G. Ll. and D. Crader 1981. To what extent were early hominids carnivorous? An archaeological pespective. In G. Teleki and R. S. O. Harding (eds) *Omnivorous Primates. Hunting and gathering in human evolution*. New York: Columbia University Press, pp. 37–103.

Isaac, G. L. and J. W. K. Harris 1978. Archaeology. In M. G. Leakey and R. Leakey (eds) *Koobi Fora Research Project*, Vol. 1. Oxford: Clarendon Press, pp. 64–85.

Isaacs, J. (ed.) 1980. *Australian Dreaming. 40,000 years of Aboriginal history*. Sydney: Landsdowne Press.

James, S. R. 1989. Hominid use of fire in the Lower and Middle Pleistocene. *Current Anthropology* 30: 1–26.

James, W. 1973. The anthropologist as reluctant imperialist. In Talal Asad (ed.) *Anthropology and the Colonial Encounter*. London: Ithaca, pp. 41–69.

Jarett, L, 1984. Psychosocial and biological influences on menstruation: synchrony, cycle length, and regularity. *Psychoneuroendocrinology* 9: 21–8.

Jellicoe, M. 1985. Colour and cosmology among the Nyaturu of Tanzania. *Shadow. The Newsletter of the Traditional Cosmology Society* 2(2): 37–44.

Jia Lanpo 1985. China's earliest Palaeolithic assemblages. In Wu Rukang and J. W. Olsen (eds) *Palaeoanthropology and Palaeolithic Archaeology in the People's Republic of China*. Orlando: Academic Press, pp. 135–45.

Jochelson, W. 1926. The Yukaghir and the Yukaghirized Tungus. The Jesup North Pacific expedition, ed. F. Boas. *Memoirs of the American Museum of Natural History* 9. New York.

Jochim, M. A. 1983. Palaeolithic cave art in ecological perspective. In G. N. Bailey (ed.) *Hunter-Gatherer Economy in Prehistory*. Cambridge: Cambridge University Press, pp. 212–19.

Johanson, D. C. and M. A. Edey 1981. *Lucy. The beginnings of humankind*. St Albans, Herts: Granada.

Johanson, D. C. and T. D. White 1979. A systematic assessment of early African hominids. *Science* 203: 321–30.

Johanson, D. C. and T. D. White, 1980. On the status of *Australopithecus afarensis*. *Science* 207: 1104–5.

Johanson, D. C., M. Taieb and Y. Coppens 1982. Pliocene hominids from the Hadar Formation, Ethiopia (1973–1977): stratigraphic, chronologic, and palaeoenvironmental contexts. *American Journal of Physical Anthropology* 57: 373–402.

Jolly, A. 1967, Breeding synchrony in wild Lemur catta. In S. A. Altmann (ed.) *Social Communication Among Primates*. Chicago: University of Chicago Press, pp. 3–14.

Jolly, A. 1972. *The Evolution of Primate Behavior*. New York: Macmillan.

Jolly, C. J. 1966. Lemur social behaviour and primate intelligence. *Science* 153: 501–6.

Jolly, C. J. and F. Plog 1986. *Physical Anthropology and Archaeology*, 4th edn. New York: Knopf.

Jones, C. B. 1985. Reproductive patterns in mantled howler monkeys: estrus, mate choice and copulation. *Primates* 21: 130–42.

Jones, R. 1989. East of Wallace's Line: issues and problems in the colonization of the Australian continent. In P. Mellars and C. Stringer (eds) *The Human Revolution. Behavioural and biological perspectives on the origins of modern humans*. Edinburgh: Edinburgh University Press, pp. 743–82.

Junod, H. A. 1927. *The Life of a South African Tribe*, 2nd edn. 2 vols. London: Macmillan.

Kaberry, P. 1939. *Aboriginal Woman: Sacred and Profane*. London: Routledge.

Kahn, M. 1931. *Djuka: Bush Negroes of Dutch Guiana*. New York: Viking Press.

Kamenka, E. 1962. *The Ethical Foundations of Marxism*. London: Routledge.

Karsten, R. 1926. *The Civilization of the South American Indians*. London: Kegan Paul, Trench, Trubner.

Karsten, R. 1935. *The Head-hunters of Western Amazonas*. Helsingfors: Societas Scientarium Fennica.

Kelly, R. L. 1986. Hunting and menstrual taboos: a reply to Dobkin de Rios and Hayden. *Human Evolution* 1(5): 475–6.

Kerényi, K. 1959. *The Heroes of the Greeks*. London: Thames & Hudson.

Kiltie, R. A. 1982. On the significance of menstrual synchrony in closely associated women. *The American Naturalist* 119: 414–19.

Kinzey, W. G. 1987. Monogamous primates: a primate model for human mating systems. In W. G. Kinzey (ed.) *The Evolution of Human Behavior: Primate Models*. Albany: State University of New York Press, pp. 105–14.

Kitahara, M. 1982. Menstrual taboos and the importance of hunting. *American Anthropologist* 84: 901–3.

Klein, R. G. 1969. *Man and Culture in the Late Pleistocene*. San Francisco: Chandler.

Klein, R. G. 1973. *Ice Age Hunters of the Ukraine*. Chicago & London: University of Chicago Press.

Klima, B. 1957. Übersicht über die jüngsten paläolithischen Forschungen in Mähren. *Quartär* 9: 85–130.

Klima, B. 1963. *Dolni Vestonice*. Prague: Monumenta Archaeologica.

Klima, B. 1968. Das Pavlovian in den Weinbergöhlen von Mauren. *Quartär* 19: 263–73.

Knight, C. D. 1983. Lévi-Strauss and the dragon: *Mythologiques* reconsidered in the light of an Australian Aboriginal myth. *Man* (N. S.) 18: 21–50.

Knight, C. D. 1984. Correspondence: Snakes and dragons. *Man* 19: 150–7.

Knight, C. D. 1985. Menstruation as medicine. *Social Science & Medicine* 21: 671–83.

Knight. C. D. 1987. Menstruation and the origins of culture. A reconsideration of Lévi-Strauss's work on symbolism and myth. Unpublished Ph. D. thesis, University of London, London.

Knight, C. D. 1988. Menstrual synchrony and the Australian rainbow snake. In T. Buckley and A. Gottlieb (eds), *Blood Magic. The anthropology of menstruation.* Berkeley & Los Angeles: University of California Press, pp. 232–55.

Knowlton, N. 1979. Reproductive synchrony, parental investment and the evolutionary dynamics of sexual selection. *Animal Behavior* 27: 1022–33.

Kolig, E. 1981. The Rainbow Serpent in the Aboriginal pantheon: a review article. *Oceania* 51: 312–16.

Kollerstrom, N. 1990. Note on human response to the lunar synodic cycle. In G. J. M. Tomassen, W. de Graaff, A. A. Knoop and R. Hengeveld (eds) *Geo-cosmic Relations. The earth and its macro-environment.* Proceedings of the First International Congress on Geo-cosmic Relations; Amsterdam. Wageningen: Pudoc, pp. 157–60.

Kornietz, N. L. and O. Soffer 1984. Mammoth bone dwellings on the North Russian Plain. *Scientific American* 251(5): 164–75.

Kosłowski, J. K. 1982a. *Excavation in the Bacho Kiro Cave (Bulgaria): Final Report.* Warsaw: Panstwowe Wydawnictwo Naukowe.

Kosłowski, J. K. 1982b. L'Aurignacien dans les Balkans. In *Aurignacien et Gravettien en Europe,* Vol. 1, ed. J. K. Koslowski and B. Klima, pp. 317–21. Etudes et Recherches Archéologiques de l'Université de Liège 13.

Kosłowski, J. K. 1988. L'apparition du Palèolithique supérieur. In *L'homme de Néandertal,* Vol. 8, *La mutation,* ed. M. Otte, pp. 11–21. Etudes et Recherches Archéologiques de l'Université de Liège 35.

Krader, L. 1972. *The Ethnological Notebooks of Karl Marx.* Assen: Van Gorcum.

Kretzoi, M. and L. Vértes, L. 1965. Upper Biharian pebble industry occupation site in western Hungary. *Current Anthropology* 6: 74–87.

Krickeberg, W. 1939. The Indian Sweat Bath. *Ciba Symposia* 1.

Kroeber, A. L. 1901. Decorative symbolism of the Arapaho. *American Anthropologist* 3: 308–36.

Kroeber, A. L. 1908. Appendix: Notes on the Luiseños, pp. 174–86. In C. G. du Bois (ed.) *The Religion of the Luiseño Indians of California.* University of California Publications in American Archaeology and Ethnology 8(3): 69–186.

Kroeber, A. L. 1917. The superorganic. *American Anthropologist* 19: 163–213.

Kroeber, A. L. 1920. Methods and principles. Review of R. H. Lowie's 'Primitive Society'. *American Anthropologist* 22: 377–81.

Kroeber, A. L. 1925. *Handbook of the Indians of California.* Washington: Smithsonian Institution. Bulletin of the Bureau of American Ethnology 78.

Kroeber, A. L. and E. W. Gifford 1949. World renewal: a cult system of native northwest California. *Anthropological Records* 13: 1–155. Berkeley & Los Angeles: University of Califoruia Press.

Kruuk, H. 1984 [1972]. The urge to kill. In G. Ferry (ed.) *The Understanding of Animals.* London: Blackwell & New Scientist, pp. 206–11.

Kuhn, T. 1970. The structure of scientific revolutions. In *International Encyclopedia of Unified Science,* Vol. 2, 2nd edn. Chicago: University of Chicago Press.

Kummer, H. 1967. Tripartite relations in hamadryas baboons. In S. A. Altmann (ed.) *Social Communication among Primates.* Chicago: University of Chicago Press, pp. 63–72.

Kummer, H. 1968. *Social Organization of Hamadryas Baboons.* Basle: Karger.

Kummer, H. 1971. *Primate Societies. Group techniques of ecological adaptation.* Chicago: Aldine Atherton.

Kummer, H. 1982. Social knowledge in free-ranging primates. In D. R. Griffin (ed.) *Animal Mind–Human Mind.* Berlin: Springer, pp. 113–30.

Kupka, K. 1965. *Dawn of Art*. Sydney: Angus & Robertson.

La Barre, W. 1972. *The Ghost Dance. The origins of religion*. London: Allen & Unwin.

Labbé, P. 1903. *Un Bagne Russe, l'Isle de Sakhaline*. Paris.

Lalanne, J. G., and J. Bouyssonie 1946. Le gisement paléolithique de Laussel. *L'Anthropologie* 50: 1–163.

LaLumiere, L. P. 1982 [1981]. The evolution of human bipedalism. *Philosophical Transactions of the Royal Society* B 292: 103–7. Reprinted (shortened) as Appendix I, in E. Morgan, *The Aquatic Ape*, London: Souvenir, pp. 123–35.

Lamp, F. 1988. Heavenly bodies: menses, moon, and rituals of license among the Temne of Sierra Leone. In T. Buckley and A. Gottlieb (eds) *Blood Magic. The anthropology of menstruation*. Berkeley: University of California Press, pp. 210–31.

Lamphere, L. 1974. Strategies, cooperation and conflict. In M. Z. Rosaldo and L. Lamphere (eds) *Woman, Culture and Society*. Stanford, CA: Stanford University press, pp. 97–112.

Lanata, J. L. 1990. Humans and terrestrial and sea mammals at Peninsula Mitre, Tierra del Fuego. In L. B. Davis and B. O. K. Reeves (eds) *Hunters of the Recent Past*. London: Unwin Hyman, pp. 400–6.

Landau, M. 1991. *Narratives of Human Evolution*. New Haven & London: Yale.

Landes, R. 1937. Ojibwa sociology. *Columbia University Contributions to Anthropology* 39: 1–144. New York.

Landes, R. 1938. *The Ojibwa Woman*. New York: Columbia University Press.

Lang, A. 1887. *Myth, Ritual and Religion*, Vol. 1. London: Longman.

Lanman, C. 1856. *Adventures in the Wilds of the United States and British Provinces*. Philadelphia, PA.

Latour, B. and S. Woolgar 1979. *Laboratory Life. The social construction of scientific facts*. London: Sage.

Law, Sung Ping 1986. The regulation of menstrual cycle and its relationship to the moon. *Acta Obstetricia et Gynecologica Scandinavica* 65: 45–8.

Lawrence, D. L. 1988. Menstrual politics: women and pigs in rural Portugal. In T. Buckley and A. Gottlieb (eds.) *Blood Magic. The anthropology of menstruation*. Berkeley: University of California Press, pp. 117–36.

Leach, E. 1954. *Political Systems of Highland Burma*. London: Bell.

Leach, E. 1957. The epistemological background to Malinowski's empiricism. In R. Firth (ed.) *Man and Culture. An evaluation of the work of Bronislaw Malinowski*. London: Routledge, pp. 119–37.

Leach, E. 1961a. *Rethinking Anthropology*. L.S.E. Monographs in Social Anthropology 22. London: University of London Press.

Leach, E. 1961b. Lévi-Strauss in the Garden of Eden: an examiniation of some recent developments in the analysis of myth. *Transactions of the New York Academy of Sciences* 23(2): 386–96.

Leach, E. 1965. Claude Lévi-Strauss – anthropologist and philosopher. *New Left Review* 34: 12–27.

Leach, E. 1967. Brain-twister. *The New York Review of Books* 9: 6. Reprinted in E. N. Hayes and T. Hayes (eds) *Claude Lévi-Strauss: The Anthropologist as Hero*. Cambridge, MA: MIT Press, pp. 123–32.

Leakey, R. E. F. and R. Lewin 1977. *Origins*. New York: Dutton.

Leakey, R. E. F. and R. Lewin. 1979. *People of the Lake. Man: his origins, nature and future*. London: Collins.

Lee, R. B. 1988. Reflections on primitive communism. In T. Ingold, D. Riches and J. Woodburn (eds) *Hunters and Gatherers. 1: History, Evolution and Social Change*. Chicago: Aldine, pp. 252–68.

Lee, R. and I. DeVore (eds) 1968. *Man the Hunter*. Chicago: Aldine.

Leopold, A. C. and R. Ardrey 1972. Toxic substances in plants and the food habits of early man. *Science* 176: 512–14.

Leroi-Gourhan, A. 1968. *The Art of Prehistoric Man in Western Europe*. London: Thames & Hudson.

Leroyer, C. and Arl. Leroi-Gourhan 1983. Problèmes de chronologie: le castelperronien et l'aurignacien. *Bulletin de la Société Préhistorique Française* 80: 41–4.

Letourneau, C. H. 1891. *The Evolution of Marriage*. London: Walter Scott.

Lever, J. with M. G. Brush 1981. *Pre-Menstrual Tension*. New York: Bantam.

Lévi-Strauss, C. 1966 [1962]. *The Savage Mind*. London: Weidenfeld & Nicolson.

Lévi-Strauss, C. 1968. The concept of primitiveness. In R. B. Lee and I. DeVore (eds) *Man the Hunter*. Chicago: Aldine.

Lévi-Strauss, C. 1969a. *The Elementary Structures of Kinship*. London: Eyre & Spottiswoode.

Lévi-Strauss, C. 1969b [1962]. *Totemism*. Harmondsworth: Penguin.

Lévi-Strauss, C. 1970. *The Raw and the Cooked*. Introduction to a Science of Mythology 1. London: Cape.

Lévi-Strauss, C. 1973. *From Honey to Ashes*. Introduction to a Science of Mythology 2. London: Cape.

Lévi-Strauss, C. 1977. *Structural Anthropology*, 2 vols. Harmondsworth: Penguin.

Lévi-Strauss, C. 1978. *The Origin of Table Manners*. Introduction to a Science of Mythology 3. London: Cape.

Lévi-Strauss, C. 1981. *The Naked Man*. Introduction to a Science of Mythology 4. London: Cape.

Lévi-Strauss, C. 1987 [1950]. *Introduction to the Work of Marcel Mauss*. London: Routledge.

Lewis, D. 1988. *The Rock Paintings of Arnhem Land, Australia. Social, ecological and material culture change in the post-glacial period*. Oxford: BAR International Series 415.

Lewis, G. 1980. *Day of Shining Red. An essay on understanding ritual*. Cambridge: Cambridge University Press.

Lewis, J. and B. Towers 1969. *Naked Ape or Homo Sapiens?* London: Garnstone Press.

Lewis-Williams, J. D. 1981. *Believing and Seeing. Symbolic meanings in Southern San rock art*. London: Academic Press.

Lieberman, P. 1988. On human speech, syntax, and language. *Human Evolution* 3: 3–18.

Lieberman, P. 1989. The origins of some aspects of human language and cognition. In P. Mellars and C. B. Stringer (eds) *The Human Revolution. Behavioural and biological perspectives on the origins of modern humans*. Edinburgh: Edinburgh University Press, pp. 309–414.

Lieberman, P. and E. S. Crelin, 1971. On the speech of Neandertal Man. *Linguistic Inquiry* 2: 203–22.

Lienhardt, G. 1961. *Divinity and Experience*. Oxford: Clarendon Press.

Lindenbaum, S. 1976. A wife is the hand of man. In P. Brown and G. Buchbinder (eds) *Man and Woman in the New Guinea Highlands*. Washington DC: American Anthropological Association, pp. 54–62.

Loewenstein, J. 1961. Rainbow and serpent. *Anthropos* 56: 31–40.

Long, J. 1791. *Voyages and Travels of an Indian Interpreter and Trader*. London.

Lorenz, K. 1966. *On Aggression*. New York: Harcourt Brace & World.

Lovejoy, C. O. 1981. The origin of man. *Science* 211: 341–50.

Lowie, R. H. 1919. Family and sib. *American Anthropologist* 21: 28–40. Reprinted in Cora du Bois (ed.) *Lowie's Selected Papers in Anthropology*. Berkeley & Los Angeles: University of California Press.

Lowie, R. H. 1920. *Primitive Society*. New York: Harper.

Lowie, R. H. 1937. *The History of Ethnological Theory*. New York: Holt, Rinehart & Winston.

Lowie, R. H. 1962. The Origin of the State. New York: Russell & Russell.

Luckert, K. W. 1975. *The Navajo Hunter Tradition*. Tucson, AZ: University of Arizona Press.

Lucotte, G. 1989. Evidence for the paternal ancestry of modern humans: evidence from a Y-chromosome specific sequence polymorphic DNA probe. In P. Mellars and C. Stringer (eds) *The Human Revolution. Behavioural and biological perspectives on the origins of modern humans*. Edinburgh: Edinburgh University Press, pp. 39–46.

Lukesch, A. 1976. *Bearded Indians of the Tropical Forest. The Asurini of the Ipiacaba*. Graz: Akademische Druck -ü Verlagsanstalt.

Lumsden, C., and E. O. Wilson 1981. *Genes, Mind, and Culture*. Cambridge, MA: Harvard University Press.

Lyle, E. 1987. Cyclical time as two types of journey and some implications for axes of polarity, contexts, and levels. *Shadow* 4: 10–19.

Maddock, K. 1974. *The Australian Aborigines. A portrait of their society*. Harmondsworth: Penguin.

Maddock, K. 1978a. Introduction. In I. A. Buchler and K. Maddock (eds) *The Rainbow Serpent*. The Hague: Mouton.

Maddock, K. 1978b. Metaphysics in a mythical view of the world. In I. R. Buchler and K. Maddock (eds) *The Rainbow Serpent*. The Hague: Mouton, pp. 99–118.

Maddock, K. 1985. Sacrifice and other models in Australian Aboriginal ritual. In D. E. Barwick, J. Beckett and Marie Reay (eds) *Metaphors of Interpretation. Essays in honour of W. E. H. Stanner*. Canberra: Australian National University Press, pp. 133–57.

Malaiya, S. 1989. Dance in the rock art of central India. In H. Morphy (ed.) *Animals into Art*. London: Unwin Hyman, pp. 357–68.

Malinowski, B. 1912. The economic aspect of the Intichiuma ceremonies. In *Festskrift tillegrad Edvard Westermarck*. Helsingfors, pp. 81–108.

Malinowski, B. 1922. *Argonauts of the Western Pacific*. London: Routledge.

Malinowski, B. 1926. *Crime and Custom in Savage Society*. London: Routledge. Reprinted by Littlefield Adams, New Jersey, 1962.

Malinowski, B. 1927. Lunar and seasonal calendar in the Trobriands. *Journal of the Royal Anthropological Institute* 62: 203–15.

Malinowski, B. 1930. Kinship. *Man* (N.S.) 30(2): 19–29. Reprinted in N. Graburn (ed.) *Readings in Kinship and Social Structure*. New York: Harper & Row, 1971, pp. 95–105.

Malinowski, B. 1932. *The Sexual Life of Savages in North-Western Melanesia*, 3rd edn. London: Routledge.

Malinowski, B. 1945. *The Dynamics of Culture Change. An inquiry into race relations in Africa*, ed. P. Kaberry. New Haven: Yale University Press.

Malinowski, B. 1956. *Marriage: Past and Present. A debate between Robert Briffault and Bronislaw Malinowski*, ed. M. F. Ashley Montagu. Boston: Porter Sargent.

Malinowski, B. 1963 [1913]. *The Family among the Australian Aborigines*. New York: Schocken Books.

Manson, W. C. 1986. Sexual cyclicity and concealed ovulation. *Journal of Human Evolution* 15: 21–30.

March, K. S. 1980. Deer, bears, and blood: a note on nonhuman animal response to menstrual odor. *American Anthropologist* 82: 125–7.

Marean, C. W. 1986. On the seal remains from Klasies River Mouth: an evaluation of Binford's interpretations. *Current Anthropology* 27: 365–8.

Margai, M. A. S. 1965. *Akafa Kolol ka kaKomsir*, trans. H. Kamara. Bo, Sierra Leone: Provincial Literature Bureau.

Margulis, L. 1982. *Early Life*. Boston: Science Books International.

Maringer, J. 1960. *The Gods of Prehistoric Men*. New York: Knopf.

Marks, A. E. 1983. The Middle to Upper Paleolithic transition in the Levant. In F. Wendorf and A. Close (eds) *Advances in World Archaeology*. New York: Academic Press, 2 vols. Vol. 2, pp. 51–98.

Marks, S. A. 1976. *Large Mammals and Brave People. Subsistence hunters in Zambia*. Seattle & London: University of Washington Press.

Marshack, A. 1964. Lunar notation on Upper Paleolithic remains. *Science* 146: 743–5.

Marshack, A. 1972a. Cognitive aspects of Upper Paleolithic engraving. *Current Anthropology* 13: 445–77.

Marshack, A. 1972b. *The Roots of Civilization. The cognitive beginnings of man's first art, symbol and notation*. London: Weidenfeld & Nicolson.

Marshack, A. 1985. On the dangers of serpents in the mind. *Current Anthropology* 26: 139–45.

Marshack, A. 1989. Evolution of the human capacity: the symbolic evidence. *Yearbook of Physical Anthropology* 32: 1–34.

Marshack, A. 1990. The female image: a 'time-factored' symbol. A study in style and modes of image use in the European Upper Paleolithic. *Proceedings of the Prehistoric Society* 56.

Marshall, L. 1961. Sharing, talking, and giving: relief of social tensions among !Kung Bushmen. *Africa* 39: 231–47.

Marshall, L. 1969. The medicine dance of the !Kung Bushmen. *Africa* 39: 347–81.

Martin, E. 1988. Premenstrual syndrome: discipline, work, and anger in late industrial societies. In T. Buckley and A. Gottlieb (eds) *Blood Magic. The anthropology of menstruation*. Berkeley: University of California Press, pp. 161–81.

Martin, R. D. 1977. Translator's preface. In P. Charles-Dominique, *Ecology of Nocturnal Primates*. London: Duckworth, pp. vii–x.

Martin, R. D. 1979. Phylogenetic aspects of prosimian behaviour. In G. A. Doyle and R. D. Martin (eds) *The Study of Prosimian Behaviour*. New York: Academic Press.

Martin, P. S. and H. E. Wright 1967. *Pleistocene Extinctions*. New Haven: Yale University Press.

Marx, K. n.d. [1862]. Letter to Engels, 18 June. In K. Marx and F. Engels, *Selected Correspondence*. Moscow: Foreign Languages Publishing House, pp. 156–7.

Marx, K. 1951 [1875]. Critique of the Gotha programme. In K. Marx and F. Engels, *Selected Works*, 2 vols. Moscow: Foreign Languages Publishing House: Vol. 2.

Marx, K. 1954 [1873]. Afterword to the second German edition. *Capital*. Book 1. London: Lawrence & Wishart, pp. 22–9.

Marx, K. 1957 [1842]. The leading article of No. 179 of *Kölnische Zeitung*. In K. Marx and F. Engels. *On Religion*. Moscow: Foreign Languages Publishing House, pp. 16–40.

Marx, K. 1963a [1844]. Economic and philosophic manuscrips (extract). In T. B. Bottomore and M. Rubel (eds) *Selected Writings in Sociology and Social Philosophy*. Harmondsworth: Penguin, pp. 87–8.

Marx, K. 1963b [1843–4]. Contribution to the Critique of Hegel's Philosophy of Right. Introduction. In T. B. Bottomore (ed.) *Karl Marx: Early Writings*. London: Watts, pp. 43–59.

Marx, K. 1963c [1844]. Economic and Philosophic Manuscripts. In T. B. Bottomore (ed.) *Karl Marx: Early Writings*. London: Watts.

Marx, K. 1963d [1845]. Theses on Feuerbach. In T. B. Bottomore and M. Rubel (eds) *Karl Marx. Selected Writings in Sociology and Social Philosophy*. Harmondsworth: Penguin, pp. 82–4.

Marx, K. 1971a [1844]. The economic and philosophic manuscripts. In D. McLellan (ed.) *Karl Marx: Early Texts*. Oxford: Blackwell, pp. 130–83.

Marx, K. 1971b [1859]. D. McLellan (ed.) *Marx's Grundrisse* (translated extracts). London: Macmillan.

Marx, K. 1972 [1844]. On James Mill. In D. McLellan (ed.) *Karl Marx: Early Texts*. Oxford: Blackwell, pp. 188–203.

Marx, K. 1973 [1859]. *Grundrisse*. Harmondsworth: Penguin.

Marx, K. and F. Engels 1927. *Historisch-kritische Gesamtausgabe. Werke, Schriften, Briefe*, 12 vols, ed. D. Riazanov. Moscow: Marx-Engels Institut. 1927–35.

Marx, K. and F. Engels 1947 [1846]. *The German Ideology*, Parts I & III. New York: International Publishers.

Marx, K. and F. Engels 1963 [1845]. The Holy Family (extract). In T. B. Bottomore and M. Rubel (eds) *Karl Marx. Selected writings in sociology and social philosophy*. Harmondsworth: Penguin, pp. 236–8.

Marx, K. and F. Engels 1967 [1848]. *The Communist Manifesto*. Harmondsworth, Penguin.

Masset, C. 1980. Comment on Wreschner: red ochre in human evolution. *Current Anthropology* 21: 638–9.

Mathews, R. H. 1904. Ethnological notes on the Aboriginal tribes of New South Wales and Victoria. *Royal Society of New South Wales, Journal and Proceedings* 38: 203–381.

Matriarchy Study Group n.d. *Menstrual Taboos*. London: Matriarchy Study Group.

Mauss, M. 1954. *The Gift. Forms and functions of exchange in archaic societies*, trans. I. Cunnison. London: Cohen & West.

Mauss, M. 1979. [1904–5] *Seasonal Variations of the Eskimo. A study in social morphology*. London: Routledge & Kegan Paul.

Maybury-Lewis, D. 1967. *Akwe-Shavante Society*. Oxford: Clarendon Press.

McBurney, C. B. M. 1967. *The Haua Fteah (Cyrenaica) and the Stone Age of the South-East Mediterranean*. Cambridge: Cambridge University Press.

McCarthy, F. D. 1960. The string figures of Yirrkalla. In C. P. Mountford (ed.) *Records of the American-Australian Scientific Expedition to Arnhem Land*, Vol. 2 (*Anthropology and Nutrition*). Melbourne: Melbourne University Press, pp. 415–513.

McClintock, M. K. 1971. Menstrual synchrony and suppression. *Nature* 229: 244–5.

McClintock, M. K. 1978. Estrous synchrony and its mediation by airborne chemical communication (*Rattus norvegicus*). *Hormones and Behavior* 10: 264–76.

McConnel, U. H. 1936. Totemic hero-cults in Cape York Peninsula, north Queensland. Parts 1 & 2. *Oceania* 7: 69–105.

McGrew, W. C. 1979. Evolutionary implications of sex differences in chimpanzee predation and tool use. In D. A. Hamburg and E. R. McCown (eds) *The Great Apes*. Menlo Park, CA: Benjamin/Cummings, pp. 441–64.

McGrew, W. C. 1981. The female chimpanzee as a human evolutionary prototype. In F. Dahlberg (ed.) *Woman the Gatherer*. New Haven & London: Yale University Press, pp. 35–73.

McGrew, W. C. 1989. Comment on S. R. James, Hominid use of fire in the Lower and Middle Pleistocene. *Current Anthropology* 30: 16–17.

McKay, M. 1988. *The Origins of Hereditary Social Stratification*. Oxford: BAR International Series 413.

McKnight, D. 1975. Men, women and other animals. Taboo and purification among the Wik-mungkan. In R. Willis (ed.) *The Interpretation of Symbolism*. London: Malaby, pp. 77–97.

McLellan, J. F. 1869. The worship of animals and plants. Part 1. *The Fortnightly Review* 6(N.S.): 407–27.

Mead, M. 1933. The Marsalai cult of the Arapesh, with special reference to the rainbow serpent beliefs of the Australian Aboriginals. *Oceania* 4: 37–53.

Mead, M. 1935. *Sex and Temperament in Three Primitive Societies*. London: Routledge.

Mead, M. 1941. *The Mountain Arapesh. Part 2. Supernaturalism*. Anthropological Papers of the American Museum of Natural History 37: 317–451.

Mead, M. 1947. *The Mountain Arapesh. Part 3. Socio-economic life*. Anthropological Papers of the American Museum of Natural History 40.

Meehan, B. 1977. Hunters by the seashore. *Journal of Human Evolution* 6: 363–70.

Meggitt, M. J. 1964. Male–female relationships in the Highlands of Australian New Guinea. *American Anthropologist* 66, no 4, part 2, Special Publication.

Meggitt, M. J. 1965. *Desert People. A study of the Walbiri Aborigines of Central Australia*. Chicago & London: University of Chicago Press.

Mellars, P. 1973. The character of the Middle-Upper Palaeolithic transition in southwest France. In C. Renfrew (ed.) *The Explanation of Culture Change*. London: Duckworth, pp. 255–76.

Mellars, P. 1988. The origins and dispersal of modern humans. *Current Anthropology* 29: 186–8.

Mellars, P. 1989. Major issues in the emergence of modern humans. *Current Anthropology* 30: 349–85.

Mellars, P. and C. Stringer (eds) 1989a. *The Human Revolution. Behavioural and biological perspectives on the origins of modern humans*. Edinburgh: Edinburgh University Press.

Mellars, P. and C. Stringer 1989b. Introduction. In P. Mellars and C. Stringer (eds) *The Human Revolution. Behavioural and biological perspectives on the origins of modern humans*. Edinburgh: Edinburgh University Press.

Memmott, P. 1982. Rainbows, story places, and Malkri sickness in the North Wellesley Islands. *Oceania* 53: 163–82.

Menaker, W. 1967. Lunar periodicity with respect to live births. *The American Journal of Obstetrics & Gynecology* 98: 1002–4.

Menaker, W. and A. Menaker, 1959. Lunar periodicity in human reproduction: a likely unit of biological time. *The American Journal of Obstetrics and Gynecology* 77: 905–14.

Merrilees, D. 1968. Man the destroyer: later Quaternary changes in the Australian marsupial fauna. *Journal of the Royal Society of Western Australia* 51: 1–24.

Métraux, A. 1946. *Myths of the Toba and Pilagá Indians of the Gran Chaco*. Philadelphia: Memoirs of the American Folklore Society 40.

Michael, R. P., R. W. Bonsall and D. Zumpe 1978. Consort bonding and operant behavior by female rhesus monkeys. *Journal of Comparative Physiology and Psychology* 92: 837–45.

Milton, K. 1984. The role of food-processing factors in primate food choice. In P. S. Rodman and J. G. H. Cant (eds) *Adaptations for Foraging in Nonhuman Primates. Contributions to an organismal biology of prosimians, monkeys, and apes*. New York: Columbia University Press, pp. 249–79.

Mithen, S. J. 1988. Looking and learning: Upper Palaeolithic art and information gathering. *World Archaeology* 19: 297–327.

Montagu, M. F. A. 1940. Physiology and the origins of the menstrual prohibitions. *Quarterly Review of Biology* 15(2): 211–20.

Montagu, M. F. A. 1957. *Anthropology and Human Nature*. New York: McGraw-Hill.

Montagu, M. F. A. 1965. *The Human Revolution*. Cleveland & New York: World Publishing.

Montagu, M. F. A. 1974. *Coming into Being Among the Australian Aborigines. The procreative beliefs of the Australian Aborigines*. London & Boston: Routledge & Kegan Paul.

Moore-Ede, M. C. 1981. Light: an information source for circadian clocks. *Photochemistry and Photobiology* 34: 237–8.

Morgan, E. 1972. *The Descent of Woman*. London: Souvenir.

Morgan, E. 1982. *The Aquatic Ape. A theory of human evolution*. London: Souvenir.

Morgan, E. 1984. The aquatic hypothesis. *New Scientist* 102(1405): 11–13.

Morgan, E. 1986. Lucy's child. *New Scientist* 112(1540/1541): 13–15.

Morgan, E. 1990. *The Scars of Evolution*. London: Souvenir.

Morgan, L. H. 1871. *Systems of Consanguinity and Affinity of the Human Family*. Washington: Smithsonian Institution.

Morgan, L. H. 1877. *Ancient Society*. London: Macmillan.

Morgan, L. H. 1881. *Houses and House-Life of the American Aborigines*. Chicago & London: University of Chicago Press.

Morphy, H. 1977. 'Too many meanings'. An analysis of the artistic system of the Yolngu of North-east Arnhem Land. Unpublished Ph.D. thesis. Australian National University, Canberra.

Morphy, H. 1984. *Journey to the Crocodile's Nest. An accompanying monograph to the film Madarrpa Funeral at Gurka'wuy*. Canberra: Australian Institute of Aboriginal Studies.

Morris, D. 1967. *The Naked Ape*. London: Cape.

Morris, D. 1977. *Manwatching*. London: Cape.

Mountford, C. P. 1956. *Records of the American-Australian Expedition to Arnhem Land*. Vol. 1 (*Art, Myth and Symbolism*). Melbourne: Melbourne University Press.

Mountford, C. P. 1965. *Ayers Rock*. Sydney: Angus & Robertson.

Mountford, C. P. 1978. The rainbow-serpent myths of Australia. In I. R. Buchler and K. Maddock (eds) *The Rainbow Serpent*. Mouton: The Hague, pp. 23–97.

Movius, H. L. 1966. The hearths of the Upper Perigordian and Aurignacian horizons at the Abri Pataud, Les Eyzies (Dordogne) and their possible significance. *American Anthropologist* 68: 296–325.

Mundkur, B. 1983. *The Cult of the Serpent. An interdisciplinary survey of its manifestations and origins*. Albany: State University of New York Press.

Munn, N. 1973. The spatial representation of cosmic order in Walbiri iconography. In A. Forge (ed.) *Primitive Art and Society*. London: Oxford University Press.

Murdock, G. P. 1949. *Social Structure*. London & New York: Macmillan.

Murdock, G. P. 1959. *Africa. Its peoples and their culture history*. New York: McGraw-Hill.

Murdock, G. P. 1965. *Culture and Society*. Pittsburgh: University of Pittsburgh Press.

Murphy R. F. 1972. *The Dialectics of Social Life. Alarms and excursions in anthropological theory*. London: Allen & Unwin.

Murphy, R. F. 1973. Social structure and sex antagonism. *Southwestern Journal of Anthropology* 15: 89–98. Reprinted in D. R. Gross (ed.) *Peoples and Cultures of Native South America. An anthropological reader*. New York: Doubleday/Natural History Press, pp. 213–24.

Murphy, R. F. and Y. Murphy 1974. *Women of the Forest*. New York & London: Columbia University Press.

Murray, P. and G. Chaloupka 1983–4. The Dreamtime animals: extinct megafauna in Arnhem Land rock art. *Archaeology in Oceania* 18/19: 105–16.

Myers, F. R. 1986. *Pintupi Country, Pintupi Self. Sentiment, place, and politics among Western Desert Aborigines*. Washington & London: Smithsonian Institution Press. Canberra: Australian Institute of Aboriginal Studies.

Nadel, S. F. 1957. Malinowski on magic and religion. In R. Firth (ed.) *Man and Culture. An evaluation of the work of Bronislaw Malinowski*. London: Routledge, pp. 189–208.

Nag, M. 1962. Factors affecting human fertility in nonindustrial societies: a cross-cultural study. *Yale University Publications in Anthropology* 66: 1–227.

Needham, R. 1972. *Belief, Language and Experience*. Oxford: Blackwell.

Needham, R. 1974. *Remarks and Inventions*. London: Tavistock.

Neihardt, J. G. 1961. *Black Elk Speaks*. Lincoln: University of Nebraska Press.

Newman, R. W. 1970. Why man is such a sweaty and thirsty naked animal: a speculative review. *Human Biology* 42: 12–27. Reprinted in M. F.

A. Montagu (ed.) *The Origin and Evolution of Man. Readings in physical anthropology.* New York: Crowell, pp. 374–85.

Nimuendajú, C. 1946. *The Eastern Timbira.* University of California Publications in American Archaeology & Ethnology 41. Berkeley & Los Angeles: University of California Press.

Nishida, T. 1980. Local differences in responses to water among wild chimpanzees. *Folia Primatologica* 33: 189.

Nunley, M. C. 1981. Response of deer to human blood odor. *American Anthropologist* 83: 630–4.

Oakley, K. 1956. Fire as a palaeolithic tool and weapon. *Proceedings of the Prehistoric Society* 21: 36–48.

Oakley, K. P. 1958. Use of fire by Neanderthal man and his precursors. In G. H. R. von Koenigswald (ed.) *Hundert Jahre Neanderthaler.* Cologne & Graz: Böhlau-Verlag, pp. 267–70.

Oosterwal, G. 1961. *People of the Tor. A cultural anthropological study on the tribes of the Tor Territory (northern Netherlands New Guinea).* Assen: Royal Van Corcum.

Osley, M., D. Summerville and L. H. Borst 1973. Natality and the moon. *American Journal of Obstetrics and Gynecology* 117: 413.

Pager, H. 1975. *Stone Age Myth and Magic, as Documented in the Rock Paintings of South Africa.* Gräz, Austria: Akademische Druck-ü. Verlagsanstalt.

Parker, K. L. 1905. *The Euahlayi Tribe.* London: Constable.

Parker, S. T. 1987. A sexual selection model for hominid evolution. *Human Evolution* 2: 235–53.

Parsons, E. C. 1919. Increase by magic: a Zuni pattern. *American Anthropologist* 21.

Pateman, C. 1988. *The Sexual Contract.* Cambridge: Polity Press.

Patterson, C. B. 1986. In the far Pacific at the birth of nations. *National Geographic* 170: 460–99.

Paulme, D. 1963. Introduction. In D. Paulme (ed.) *Women of Tropical Africa.* Berkeley: University of California Press.

Persky, H., H. I. Lief, C. P. O'Brien, D. Strauss, and W. Miller 1977. Reproductive hormone levels and sexual behaviors of young couples during the menstrual cycle. In R. Gemme and C. C. Wheeler (eds) *Progress in Sexology.* New York: Plenum, pp. 293–310.

Pfeiffer, J. E. 1977. *The Emergence of Society. A prehistory of the establishment.* New York: McGraw-Hill.

Pfeiffer, J. E. 1982. *The Creative Explosion.* New York: Harper & Row.

Pilbeam, D. 1986. The origin of *Homo sapiens*: The fossil evidence. In B. Wood and P. Andrews (eds) *Major Topics in Primate and Human Evolution.* Cambridge: Cambridge University Press, pp. 331–8.

Pliny 1942. *Natural History*, trans. H. Rackham. 10 vols. Vol. 2, books III-VII. London: Heinemann.

Pochobradsky, J. 1974. Independence of human menstruation of lunar phases and days of the week. *American Journal of Obstetrics and Gynecology* 118: 1136–8.

Poirier, F. E. 1973. *Fossil Man.* St Louis: Mosby.

Pond, C. 1987. Fat and figures. *New Scientist* 114(1563): 62–6.

Poole, R. 1969. Introduction to C. Lévi-Strauss, *Totemism.* Harmondsworth: Penguin.

Potts, R. 1984a. Hominid hunters? Problems of identifying the earliest hunter/gatherers. In R. Foley (ed.) *Hominid Evolution and Community Ecology. Prehistoric human adaptation in biological perspective.* London: Academic Press, pp. 129–66.

Potts, R. 1984b. Home bases and early hominids. *American Scientist* 72: 338–47.

Potts, R. 1986. Temporal span of bone accumulations at Olduvai Gorge and implications for early hominid foraging behavior. *Palaeobiology* 12: 25–31.

Potts, R. 1987. Reconstructions of early hominid socioecology: a critique of primate models. In W. G. Kinzey (ed.) *The Evolution of Human Behavior: Primate models.* Albany: SUNY Press, pp. 28–47.

Potts, R. 1988. *Early Hominid Activities at Olduvai.* New York: Aldine de Gruyter.

Potts, R. and P. Shipman, 1981. Cutmarks made by stone tools on bones from Olduvai Gorge, Tanzania. *Nature* 291: 577–80.

Potts, R. and A. Walker, 1981. Production of early hominid archaeological sites. *American Journal of Physical Anthropology* 54: 264.

Powers, M. N. 1980. Menstruation and reproduction: an Oglala case. *Signs. Journal of Women in Culture and Society* 6: 54–65.

Praslov, N. D. 1985. L'art du Paléolithique Supérieur à l'est de l'Europe. *L'Anthropologie* 89: 181–92.

Presser, H. B. 1974. Temporal data relating to the human menstrual cycle. In M. Ferin, F. Halberg, R. M. Richart, and R. L. Vande Wiele (eds) *Biorhythms and Human Reproduction.* New York: Wiley, pp. 145–60.

Preti, G., W. B. Cutler, A. Krieger, G. Huggins, C. R. Garcia and H. J. Lawley 1986. Human axillary secretions influence women's menstrual cycles: the role of donor extract from women. *Hormones and Behavior* 20: 474–82.

Propp, V. 1968. *Morphology of the Folktale,* 2nd edn, ed. L. A. Wagner. Austin & London: University of Texas Press.

Quadagno, D. M., H. E. Shubeita, J. Deck and D. Francoeur 1981. Influence of male social contacts, exercise and all-female living conditions on the menstrual cycle. *Psychoneuroendocrinology* 6: 239–44.

Radcliffe-Brown, A. R. 1924. The mother's brother in South Africa. *South African Journal of Science* 21: 542–55.

Radcliffe-Brown, A. R. 1926. The rainbow-serpent myth of Australia. *Journal of the Royal Anthropological Institute* 56: 19–25.

Radcliffe-Brown, A. R. 1929. The sociological theory of totemism. In A. R. Radcliffe-Brown (ed.) *Structure and Function in Primitive Society.* London: Routledge. pp. 117–32. Reprinted from Proceedings of the Fourth Pacific Science Congress, Java.

Radcliffe-Brown, A. R. 1930. The rainbow-serpent myth in south-east Australia. *Oceania* 1: 342–7.

Radcliffe-Brown, A. R. 1931. *The Social Organization of Australian Tribes.* Oceania Monographs 1. Melbourne: Macmillan.

Radcliffe-Brown, A. R. 1940. *Presidential Address on Applied Anthropology.* Delivered to the Anthropology Section of the Australian and New Zealand Association for the Advancement of Science.

Radcliffe-Brown, A. R. 1950. Introduction. In A. R. Radcliffe-Brown (ed.) *African Systems of Kinship and Marriage.* Oxford: Oxford University Press.

Radcliffe-Brown, A. R. 1952. *Structure and Function in Primitive Society.* London: Routledge.

Radcliffe-Brown, A. R. 1960. *Method in Social Anthropology.* Bombay: Asia Publishing House.

Radin, P. 1920. The Autobiography of a Winnebago Indian. *University of California Publications in American Archaeology and Ethnology* 16: 381–473.

Radin, P. 1923. *The Winnebago Tribe.* Washington DC: Thirty-Seventh Report of the Bureau of American Ethnology.

Rajasingham, D., L. P. Marson, A. E. Mills and M. Dooley 1989. There is a tide in the affairs of women. *British Medical Journal* 298: 524.

Rattray, R. S. 1927. *Religion and Art in Ashanti.* Oxford: Oxford University Press.

Rattray, R. S. 1929. *Ashanti Law and Institution.* Oxford: Oxford University Press.

Reefe, T. Q. 1981. *The Rainbow and the Kings. A history of the Luba Empire to 1891.* Berkeley: University of California Press.

Reichel-Dolmatoff, G. 1968. *Amazonian Cosmos. The sexual and religious symbolism of the Tukano Indians.* Chicago & London: University of Chicago Press.

Reid, H. 1939. Dakin, S. B. (ed.), *A Scotch Paisano; Hugo Reid's Life in California, 1832–1852, derived from his correspondence.* Berkeley: University of California Press.

Renfrew, C. 1976. *Before Civilization. The radiocarbon revolution and prehistoric Europe.* Harmondsworth: Penguin.

Renfrew, C. 1987. *Archaeology and Language. The puzzle of Indo-European origins.* London: Cape.

Resek, C. 1960. *Lewis Henry Morgan. American Scholar.* Chicago: University of Chicago Press.

Reynolds, V. 1966. Open groups in hominid evolution. *Man* 4: 441–52.

Reynolds, V. 1976. *The Biology of Human Action.* San Francisco, CA: Freeman.

Richards, A. I. 1932. *Hunger and Work in a Savage Tribe.* London: Routledge.

Richards, A. I. 1956. *Chisungu. A girl's initiation ceremony among the Bemba of Northern Rhodesia.* London: Faber & Faber.

Richards, A. I. 1969. *Land, Labour and Diet in Northern Rhodesia.* Oxford: Oxford University Press.

Richards, G. 1987. *Human Evolution.* London & New York: Routledge & Kegan Paul.

Ridley, M. 1986. The number of males in a primate troop. *Animal Behaviour* 34: 1848–58.

Rightmire, G. P. 1989. Middle Stone Age humans from eastern and southern Africa. In P. Mellars and C. Stringer (eds) *The Human Revolution. Behavioural and biological perspectives on the origins of modern humans.* Edinburgh: Edinburgh University Press, pp. 109–22.

Rindos, D. 1985. Darwinian selection, symbolic variation, and the evolution of culture. *Current Anthropology* 26: 65–88.

Rindos, D. 1986. The evolution of the capacity for culture: sociobiology, structuralism, and cultural selection. *Current Anthropology* 27: 315–32.

Rivière, P. 1969. *Marriage among the Trio.* Oxford: Clarendon Press.

Roberts, N. 1984. Pleistocene environments in time and space. In R. Foley (ed.) *Hominid Evolution and Community Ecology: Prehistoric human adaptation in biological perspective.* London: Academic Press, pp. 25–54.

Robertson-Smith, W. 1914. *The Religion of the Semites.* London: Black.

Robinson, A. 1846. *Life in California, during a Residence of Several Years in that Territory.* New York: Wiley & Putnam.

Robinson, R. 1966. *Aboriginal Myths and Legends.* Melbourne: Sun Books.

Rodman, P. S. 1984. Foraging and social systems of orangutans and chimpanzees. In P. S. Rodman and J. G. H. Cant (eds) *Adaptations for Foraging in Nonhuman Primates. Contributions to an organismal biology of prosimians, monkeys and apes.* New York: Columbia University Press, pp. 134–60.

Róheim, G. 1925. *Australian Totemism.* London: Allen & Unwin.

Róheim, G. 1974. *Children of the Desert.* New York: Basic Books.

Romans, B. 1775. *A Concise Natural History of East and West Florida*, Vol. 1. New York.

Ronen, A. (ed.) 1984. *Sefunim Prehistoric Sites, Mount Carmel, Israel*, 2 vols. Oxford: BAR International Series S230.

Rosaldo, M. Z. 1974. Woman, culture and society: a theoretical overview. In M. Z. Rosaldo and L. Lamphere (eds) *Woman, Culture and Society.* Stanford, CA: Stanford University Press, pp. 17–42.

Rose, S., R. C. Lewontin and L. J. Kamin 1984. *Not in Our Genes. Biology, ideology and human nature.* Harmondsworth: Penguin.

Roth, W. E. 1915. An inquiry into the animism and folk-lore of the Guiana Indians. Extract from the *Thirtieth Annual Report of the Bureau of American Ethnology.* Washington: Government Printing Office.

Rotton, J. and I. W. Kelly 1985. Much ado about the full moon: a meta-analysis of lunar-lunacy research. *Psychological Bulletin* 97: 286–306.

Rowell, T. E. 1963. Behaviour and female reproductive cycles of macaques. *Journal of Reproduction and Fertility* 6: 193–203.

Rowell, T. E. 1967. A quantitative comparison of the behaviour of a wild and caged baboon troop. *Animal Behaviour* 15: 499–509.

Rowell, T. E. 1972. *Social Behaviour of Monkeys.* Harmondsworth: Penguin.

Rowell, T. E. 1978. How female reproduction cycles affect interaction patterns in groups of patas monkeys. In D. J. Chivers and J. Herbert (eds) *Recent Advances in Primatology.* Vol. 1, *Behaviour.* London: Academic Press, pp. 489–90.

Rowell, T. E. and S. M. Richards 1979. Reproductive strategies of some African monkeys. *Journal of Mammalogy* 60: 58–69.

Rubel, P. G. and A. Rosman, 1978. *Your Own Pigs You May Not Eat. A comparative study of New Guinea societies.* Chicago & London: University of Chicago Press.

Rudran, R. 1973. The reproductive cycle of two subspecies of purple-faced langurs (*Presbytis senex*) with relation to environmental factors. *Folia Primatologica* 19: 41–60.

Russell, M. J., G. M. Switz and K. Thompson 1980. Olfactory influences on the human menstrual cycle. *Pharmacology, Biochemistry and Behavior* 13: 737–8.

Ryan, W. M. 1969. *White Man, Black Man.* Milton, Queensland: Jacaranda Press.

Sahlins, M. D. 1960. The origin of society. *Scientific American* 203(3): 76–87.

Sahlins, M. D. 1972. The social life of monkeys, apes and primitive man. *Human Biology* 31 (1959): 54–73. Reprinted in D. D. Quiatt (ed.) *Primates on Primates.* Minneapolis, MN: Burgess, pp. 3–18.

Sahlins, M. D. 1974. *Stone Age Economics.* London: Tavistock.

Sahlins, M. D. 1976. *Culture and Practical Reason*. Chicago: University of Chicago Press.

Sahlins, M. D. 1977. *The Use and Abuse of Biology. An anthropological critique of sociobiology*. London: Tavistock.

Salisbury. R. F. 1962. *From Stone to Steel. Economic consequences of a technological change in New Guinea*. Melbourne: University of Melbourne Press.

Sauer, C. O. 1966. *The Early Spanish Main*. Berkeley: University of California Press.

Schafer, E. H. 1973. *The Divine Woman: Dragon ladies and rain maidens in T'ang literature*. Berkeley, Los Angeles & London: University of California Press.

Schaller, G. B. and G. R. Lowther, 1969. The relevance of carnivore behavior to the study of early hominids. *Southwestern Journal of Anthropology* 25: 307–41.

Schapera, I. 1930. *The Khoisan Peoples of South Africa. Bushmen and Hottentots*. London: Routledge.

Schlenker, C. F. 1861. *A Collection of Temne Traditions, Fables, and Proverbs*. London: Christian Missionary Society.

Schmidt, S. 1979. The rain bull of the South African Bushmen. *African Studies* 38: 201–24.

Schneider, D. M. and K. Gough (eds) 1961. *Matrilineal Kinship*. Berkeley: University of California Press.

Schultz, H. 1950. Lendas dos indios Krahó. *Revista do Museu Paulista* 4. São Paulo.

Schwab, B. 1975. Delivery of babies and the full moon. *Canadian Medical Association Journal* 113: 489–93.

Sears, C. 1990. The chimpanzee's medicine chest. *New Scientist*, 4 August.

Sevitt, S. 1946. Early ovulation. *The Lancet* 2: 448–50.

Sharp, L. 1933. The social organization of the Yir-Yoront tribe, Cape York Peninsula. Part 1. Kinship and the family. *Oceania* 4: 404–31.

Shaw, E. and J. Darling, 1985. *Strategies of Being Female. Animal patterns, human choices*. Brighton: Harvester.

Shea, J. J. 1989. A functional study of the lithic industries associated with hominid fossils in the Kebara and Qafzeh caves, Israel. In P. Mellars and C. Stringer (eds) *The Human Revolution. Behavioural and biological perspectives on the origins*

of modern humans. Edinburgh: Edinburgh University Press, pp. 611–25.

Shimkin, E. M. 1978. The Upper Paleolithic in North-Central Eurasia: evidence and problems. In L. G. Freeman (ed.) *Views of the Past. Essays in old world prehistory and paleoanthropology*. The Hague: Mouton, pp. 193–315.

Shipman, P. 1983. Early hominid lifestyle: hunting and gathering or foraging and scavenging? In J. Clutton-Brock and G. Grigson (eds) *Animals and Archaeology: 1. Hunters and their prey*. Oxford: BAR International Series 163: 31–49.

Shipman, p. 1984. Scavenger hunt. *Natural History* 4: 20–7.

Shipman, P. 1986. Scavenging or hunting in early hominids: theoretical framework and tests. *American Antropologist* 88: 27–43.

Short, R. V. 1976. The evolution of human reproduction. *Proceedings of the Royal Society of London, B: Biological Sciences* 195: 3–24.

Shostak, M. 1983. *Nisa. The life and words of a !Kung woman*. Harmondsworth: Penguin.

Shuttle, P. and P. Redgrove, 1978. *The Wise Wound. Menstruation and everywoman*. London: Gollancz.

Silberbauer, G. B. 1963. Marriage and the girl's puberty ceremony of the G/wi Bushmen. *Africa* 33: 12–24.

Silberbauer, G. B. 1981. *Hunter and Habitat in the Central Kalahari Desert*. Cambridge: Cambridge University Press.

Simmons, L. W. (ed.) 1942. *Sun Chief. The autobiography of a Hopi Indian*. New Haven: Yale University Press.

Singer, R. and J. Wymer 1982. *The Middle Stone Age at Klasies River Mouth in South Africa*. Chicago: University of Chicago Press.

Siskind, J. 1973a. *To Hunt in the Morning*. New York: Oxford University Press.

Siskind, J. 1973b. Tropical forest hunters and the economy. In D. R. Gross (ed.) *Peoples and Cultures of Native South America. An anthropological reader*. New York: Doubleday, pp. 226–40.

Skandhan, K. P., A. K. Pandya, S. Skandhan, and Y. B. Mehta 1979. Synchronization of menstruation among intimates and kindreds. *Panminerva Medica* 21: 131–4.

Smith, F. H. 1984. Fossil hominids from the Upper Pleistocene of Central Europe and the origin of modern Europeans. In F. H. Smith and F. Spencer (eds) *The Origins of Modern Humans: A world survey of the fossil evidence.* New York: Liss, pp. 137–210.

Smith, M. A. 1987. Pleistocene occupation in arid Central Australia. *Nature* 328: 710–11.

Soffer, O. 1985. *The Upper Paleolithic of the Central Russian Plain.* New York: Academic Press.

Solecki, R. 1975. Shanidar IV, a Neanderthal flower burial in Northern Iraq. *Science* 190: 880–1.

Spencer, B. and F. J. Gillen 1899. *The Native Tribes of Central Australia.* London: Macmillan.

Spencer, B. and F. J. Gillen 1904. *The Northern Tribes of Central Australia.* London: Macmillan.

Spencer, B. and F. J. Gillen 1927. *The Arunta,* 2 vols. London: Macmillan.

Stahl, A. B. 1984. Hominid dietary selection before fire. *Current Anthropology* 25: 151–68.

Stanner, W. E. H. 1956. The Dreaming. In T. A. G. Hungerford (ed.) *Australian Signpost.* Melbourne: Cheshire.

Stanner, W. E. H. 1965. Religion, totemism and symbolism. In R. M. and C. H. Berndt (eds) *Aboriginal Man in Australia.* London: Angus & Robertson, pp. 207–37.

Stanner, W. E. H. 1966. *On Aboriginal Religion.* Sydney: University of Sydney Press. Oceania Monograph 11.

Steinen, K. v. d. 1894. *Unter den Naturvölkern Zentral-Brasiliens.* Berlin.

Steiner, F. 1956. *Taboo.* Harmondsworth: Penguin.

Stephen, A. M. 1893. The Navajo. *American Anthropologist* 6(4): 345–62.

Stephens, W. N. 1961. A cross-cultural study of menstrual taboos. *Genetic Psychology Monographs* 64: 385–416.

Stephens, W. N. 1962. *The Oedipus Complex: Cross-cultural evidence.* New York: Free Press.

Stern, J. T. and R. L. Susman 1983. The locomotor anatomy of *Australopithecus afarensis. American Journal of Physical Anthropology* 60: 279–317.

Stoddart, D. M. 1986. The role of olfaction in the evolution of human sexual biology: an hypothesis. *Man* 21: 514–20.

Stoneking, M, and R. L. Cann 1989. African origin of human mitochondrial DNA. In P.

Mellars and C. Stringer (eds) *The Human Revolution. Behavioural and biological perspectives on the origins of modern humans.* Edinburgh: Edinburgh University Press, pp. 17–30.

Strathern, A. and M. Strathern 1968. Marsupials and magic: a study of spell symbolism among the Mbowamb. In E. R. Leach (ed.) *Dialectic in Practical Religion.* Cambridge: Cambridge University Press, pp. 179–202. Cambridge Papers in Social Anthropology 5.

Strathern, M. 1972. *Women in Between. Female roles in a male world: Mount Hagen, New Guinea.* London: Seminar Press.

Straus, L. G. and C. W. Heller 1988. Explorations of the twilight zone: the Early Upper Paleolithic of Vasco-Cantabrian Spain and Gascony. In J. F. Hoffecker and C. A. Wolf (eds) *The Early Upper Paleolithic. Evidence from Europe and the Near East.* Oxford: BAR International Series 437: 97–134.

Stringer, C. 1988. The dates of Eden. *Nature* 331: 565–6.

Stringer, C., J.-J. Hublin and B. Vandermeersch 1984. The origin of anatomically modern humans in Western Europe. In F. H. Smith and F. Spencer (eds) *The Origins of Modern Humans: A world survey of the fossil evidence.* New York: Liss, pp. 51–136.

Strum, S. C. 1981. Processes and Products of change: baboon predatory behaviour at Gilgil, Kenya. In G. Teleki and R. S. O. Harding (eds) *Omnivorous Primates.* New York: Columbia University Press, pp. 255–302.

Strum, S. C. 1987. *Almost Human. A journey into the world of baboons.* London: Elm Tree Books.

Suárez, M. 1968. *Los Warao.* Caracas: Instituto Venozolano de Investigaciones Cientificas.

Sugiyama, Y. 1972. Social characteristics of wild chimpanzees. In F. E. Poirier (ed.) *Primate Socialization.* New York: Random House, pp. 145–63.

Susman, R. L. 1987. Pygmy chimpanzees and common chimpanzees: models for the behavioral ecology of the earliest hominids. In W. G. Kinzey (ed.) *The Evolution of Human Behavior: Primate Models.* Albany: State University of New York Press, pp. 72–86.

Susman, R. L., J. T. Stern and W. L. Jungers 1984. Arboreality and bipedality in the Hadar Hominids. *Folia Primatologica* 43: 113–56.

Suzuki, A. 1975. The origin of hominid hunting: a primatological perspective. In R. H. Tuttle (ed.) *Sociology and Socioecology of Primates*. The Hague: Mouton, pp. 259–78.

Swanton, J. R. 1946. *The Indians of the Southeastern United States*. Washington DC: Smithsonian Institution Bureau of American Ethnology Bulletin 137.

Tanner, J. 1940. *A Narrative of the Captivity and Adventures of John Tanner*, ed. E. James. New York, 1830. Reprinted as *California State Library Occasional Papers*. Reprint Series 20. Parts 1, 2, ed. P. Radin. San Francisco.

Tanner, N. M. 1981. *On Becoming Human*. Cambridge: Cambridge University Press.

Tanner, N. M. 1987. Gathering by females: the chimpanzee model revisited and the gathering hypothesis. In W. G. Kinzey (ed.) *The Evolution of Human Behavior: Primate Models*. Albany: State University of New York Press, pp. 3–27.

Taplin, G. 1879. *The Folklore, Manners, Customs, and Languages of the South Australian Aborigines. Gathered from inquiries made by authority of South Australian Government*. Adelaide: E. Spiller, Acting Government Printer.

Taylor, J. 1985. Chapters 1–10 in L. van der Post and J. Taylor, *Testament to the Bushmen*. Harmondsworth: Penguin.

Teleki, G. 1973. *The Predatory Behavior of Wild Chimpanzees*. E. Brunswick, NJ: Bucknell University Press.

Teleki, G. 1975. Primate subsistence patterns: collector-predators and gatherer-hunters. *Journal of Human Evolution* 4: 125–84.

Ten Raa, E. 1969. The moon as a symbol of life and fertility in Sandawe thought. *Africa* 39: 24–53.

Testart, A. 1978. *Des classifications dualistes en Australie*. Lille: Maison des Sciences de l'Homme, Université de Lille.

Testart, A. 1985. *Le communisme primitif*. Paris: Editions de la Maison des Sciences de l'Homme.

Testart, A. 1986. *Essai sur les fondements de la division sexuelle du travail chez les chasseurs-cueilleurs*. Paris: Editions de l'Ecole des Hautes Etudes en Sciences Sociales.

Testart, A. 1988. Some major problems in the social anthropology of hunter-gatherers. *Current Anthropology* 29: 1–31.

Thomas, N. M. 1959. *The Harmless People*. London: Secker & Warburg.

Thomas, N. W. 1916. *Anthropological Report on Sierra Leone*, Vol. 1. London: Harrison & Sons.

Thomson, D. 1949. *Economic Structure and the Ceremonial Exchange Cycle in Arnhem Land*. Melbourne: Macmillan.

Thurnwald, R. 1932. *Economics in Primitive Communities*. Oxford: Oxford University Press.

Tiger, L. and R. Fox 1974. *The Imperial Animal*. St Albans, Herts: Paladin.

Tillier, A.-M. 1989. The evolution of modern humans: Evidence from young Mousterian individuals. In P. Mellars and C. Stringer (eds) *The Human Revolution. Behavioural and biological perspectives on the origins of modern humans*. Edinburgh: Edinburgh University Press, pp. 286–97.

Timonen, S. and Carpen, E. 1968. Multiple pregnancies and photoperiodicity. *Annales Chirurgiae Gynaecologiae Fenniae* 57: 135–8.

Tomalin, N. 1967. Article in *The New Statesman*. 15 September.

Torrence, R. 1983. Time-budgeting and hunter-gatherer technology. In G. Bailey (ed.) *Hunter-Gatherer Economy in Prehistory: A European perspective*. Cambridge: Cambridge University Press, pp. 11–22.

Trager, G. L. 1972. *Language and Languages*. San Francisco: Chandler.

Treloar, A. E. 1981. Menstrual cyclicity and the premenopause. *Maturitas* 3: 249–64.

Treloar, A. E., R. E. Boynton, B. G. Behn and B. W. Brown 1967. Variation of the human menstrual cycle through reproductive life. *International Journal of Fertility* 12: 77–126.

Trezise, P. J. 1969. *Quinkan Country. Adventures in search of Aboriginal cave paintings in Cape York*. Sydney: Reed & Reed.

Trinkaus, E. 1984. Neandertal pubic morphology and gestation length. *Current Anthropology* 25: 509–14.

Trinkaus, E. 1986. The Neanderthals and modern human origins. *Annual Review of Anthropology* 15: 193–218.

Trinkaus, E. 1989. The Upper Pleistocene transition. In E. Trinkaus (ed.) *The Emergence of Modern Humans. Biocultural adaptations in the later Pleistocene*. Cambridge: Cambridge University Press, pp. 42–66.

Trivers, R. L. 1971. The evolution of reciprocal altruism. *Quarterly Review of Biology* 46: 35–57.

Trivers, R. L. 1972. Parental investment and sexual selection. In B. Campbell (ed.) *Sexual*

Selection and the Descent of Man 1871–1971. Chicago: Aldine, pp. 136–79.

Trotsky, L. D. 1964 [1940]. Dialectical materialism and science. In I. Deutscher (ed.) *The Age of Permanent Revolution. A Trotsky anthology.* New York: Dell, pp. 342–52.

Tsingalia, H. M. and Rowell, T. E. 1984. The behaviour of adult male blue monkeys. *Zeitschrift fuer Tierpsychologie* 64: 253–68.

Turke, P. W. 1984. Effects of ovulatory concealment and synchrony on protohominid mating systems and parental roles. *Ethology and Sociobiology* 5: 33–44.

Turnbull, C. 1959. Legends of the BaMbuti. *Journal of the Royal Anthropological Institute* 89: 45–60.

Turnbull, C. 1966. *Wayward Servants. The two worlds of the African Pygmies.* London: Eyre & Spottiswoode.

Turnbull, C. 1976. *The Forest People.* London: Pan Books.

Turner, V. W. 1957. *Schism and Continuity in an African Society. A study in Ndembu village life.* Manchester: Manchester University Press.

Turner, V. W. 1967. *The Forest of Symbols. Aspects of Ndembu ritual.* Ithaca & London: Cornell University Press.

Turner, V. W. 1969. *The Ritual Process.* Chicago: Aldine.

Tutin, C. E. G. and P. R. McGinnnis 1981. Chimpanzee reproduction in the wild. In C. E. Graham (ed.) *Reproductive Biology of the Great Apes.* New York: Academic Press, pp. 239–64.

Tutin, C. E. G. and W. C. McGrew 1973. Chimpanzee copulatory behavior. *Folia Primatologica* 19: 237–56.

Tylor, E. B. 1899. Remarks on totemism with especial reference to some modern theories concerning it. *Journal of the Royal Anthropological Institute* 28: 138–48.

Ucko, P. 1962. The interpretation of prehistoric figurines. *Journal of the Royal Anthropological Institute* 92.

Ucko, P. 1968. *Anthropomorphic Figurines of Predynastic Egypt and Neolithic Crete with Comparative Material from the Prehistoric Near East and mainland Greece.* London: Andrew Szmidla. Royal Anthropological Institute Occasional Paper 24.

Udry, J. R. and N. M. Morris 1977. The distribution of events in the menstrual cycle. *Journal of Reproduction and Fertility* 51: 419–25.

Ullrich, H. E. 1977. Caste differences between Brahmin and non-Brahmin women in a South Indian village. In A. Schlegel (ed.) *Sexual Stratification.* New York: Columbia University Press.

Valladas, H., J. L. Reyss, J. L. Joron, G. Valladas, O. Bar-Yosef and B. Vandermeersch 1988. Thermoluminiscence dating of Mousterian 'Proto-Cro-Magnon' remains from Israel and the origin of modern man. *Nature* 331: 614–16.

Vandermeersch, B. 1981. *Les hommes fossiles de Qafzeh (Israël).* Paris: Centre National de la Recherche Scientifique.

Vandermeersch, B. 1989. The evolution of modern humans: Recent evidence from Southwest Asia. In C. Stringer and P. Mellars (eds) *The Human Revolution. Behavioural and biological Perspectives on the origins of modern humans.* Edinburgh: Edinburgh University Press, pp. 155–64.

Verhaegen, M. J. B. 1985. The aquatic ape theory: evidence and a possible scenario. *Medical Hypotheses* 16: 17–32.

Villa, P. 1983. *Terra Amata and the Middle Pleistocene Archaeological Record of Southern France.* Berkeley: University of California Press.

Villa, P. 1990. Torralba and Aridos: elephant exploitation in Middle Pleistocene Spain. *Journal of Human Evolution* 19: 299–309.

Vinnicombe, P. 1976. *People of the Eland. Rock paintings of the Drakensberg Bushmen.* Pietermaritzburg: University of Natal Press.

Vogel, C. 1973. Hanuman as an object for anthropologists – field studies of social behavior among the gray langurs of India. In *German Scholars on India: Contributions to Indian Studies.* Varanasi, India: Chowkhamba/Sanskrit Series Office. Vol. 1.

Voget, F. W. 1975. *A History of Ethnology.* New York: Holt, Rinehart & Winston.

Vollman, R. F. 1968. The length of the premenstrual phase by age of women. Proceedings of the Fifth World Congress on Fertility and Sterility. Stockholm, Amsterdam. *Excerpta Medica International Congress Series* 133: 1171–5.

Vollman, R. F. 1970. Conception rates by days of the menstrual cycles, BBT, and outcome of pregnancy. *Sixth World Congress of Gynecology and Obstetrics of the International Federation of Gynecology and Obstetrics,* New York. Abstracts, 112. Baltimore: Williams & Wilkins.

Vollman, R. F. 1977. *The Menstrual Cycle.* New York: Knopf.

Wagener, J. S. 1987. The evolution of man's sense of time. *Human Evolution* 2: 121–33.

Wagner, R. 1972. *Habu. The innovation of meaning in Daribi religion*. Chicago: University of Chicago Press.

Walker, B. G. 1983. *The Woman's Encyclopaedia of Myths and Secrets*. San Francisco: Harper & Row.

Wallis, J. 1985. Synchrony of estrous swelling in captive group-living chimpanzees (*Pan troglodytes*). *International Journal of Primatology* 6: 335–50.

Warner, W. L. 1957. *A Black Civilization*. New York: Harper.

Washburn, S. L. (ed.) 1962. *The Social Life of Early Man*. London: Methuen.

Washburn, S. L. and D. A. Hamburg 1972. Aggressive behaviour in old world monkeys and apes. In P. Dolhinow (ed.) *Primate Patterns*. New York: Holt, pp. 276–96.

Washburn, S. L. and C. S. Lancaster 1968. The evolution of hunting. In R. B. Lee and I. DeVore (eds) *Man the Hunter*. Chicago: Aldine, pp. 293–303.

Weideger, P. 1976. *Menstruation and Menopause*. New York: Knopf.

Wenke, R. J. 1984. *Patterns in Prehistory. Humankind's first three million years*, 2nd edn. Oxford: Oxford University Press.

Werner, A. 1933. *Myths and Legends of the Bantu*. London: Cass.

Wescott, R. W. 1969. *The Divine Animal*. New York: Funk & Wagnalls.

Whallon, R. 1989. Elements of cultural change in the Later Palaeolithic. In P. Mellars and C. Stringer (eds) *The Human Revolution. Behavioural and biological perspectives on the origins of modern humans*. Edinburgh: Edinburgh University Press, pp. 433–54.

Wheeler, P. E. 1984. The evolution of bipedality and loss of functional body hair in hominids. *Journal of Human Evolution* 13: 91–8.

Wheeler, P. E. 1985. The loss of functional body hair in man: the influence of thermal environment, body form and bipedality. *Journal of Human Evolution* 14: 23–8.

Wheeler, P. E. 1988. Stand tall and stay cool. *New Scientist* 118(1612): 62–5.

White, L. 1949. *The Science of Culture*. New York: Grove Press.

White, R. 1989a. Production complexity and standardization in early Aurignacian bead and pendant manufacture: evolutionary implications. In P. Mellars and C. Stringer (eds) *The Human Revolution. Behavioural and biological perspectives on the origins of modern humans*. Edinburgh: Edinburgh University Press, pp. 366–90.

White, R. 1989b. Toward a contextual understanding of the earliest body ornaments. In E. Trinkaus (ed.) *The Emergence of Modern Humans. Biocultural adaptations in the later Pleistocene*. Cambridge: Cambridge University Press, pp. 211–31.

Williams, C. G. 1966. *Adaptation and Natural Selection. A critique of some current evolutionary thought*. Princeton, NJ: Princeton University Press.

Williams, C. G. 1975. *Sex and Evolution*. Princeton, NJ: Princeton University Press.

Williams, F. E. 1936. *Papuans of the Trans-Fly*. Oxford: Clarendon Press.

Williams, N. M. 1986. *The Yolngu and their Land. A system of land tenure and the fight for its recognition*. Canberra: Australian Institute of Aboriginal Studies.

Willis, R. 1982. Introduction. In L. de Heusch (ed.) *The Drunken King, or, The Origin of the State*. Bloomington: Indiana University Press.

Willmott, P. and M. Young 1957. *Family and Kinship in East London*. Harmondsworth: Penguin.

Wilson, E. O. 1975. *Sociobiology. The new synthesis*. Cambridge, MA: Harvard University Press.

Wilson, H. C. 1987. Female axillary secretions influence women's menstrual cycles: a critique. *Hormones and Behavior* 21: 536–46.

Wintle, A. G. and M. J. Aitken 1977. Thermoluminescence dating of burnt flint: application to a Lower Palaeolithic site, Terra Amata. *Archaeometry* 19: 11–30.

Witherspoon, G. 1975. *Navajo Kinship and Marriage*. Chicago: University of Chicago Press.

Wobst, H. M. 1977. Stylistic behaviour and information exchange. In C. E. Cleland (ed.) *Papers for the Director. Research essays in honour of James B. Griffin*. Anthropological Papers, Museum of Anthropology, University of Michigan 61, pp. 317–42.

Wolf, C. A. 1988. Analysis of faunal remains from Early Upper Paleolithic sites in the Levant. In J. F. Hoffecker and C. A. Wolf (eds)

The Early Upper Paleolithic. Oxford: BAR International Series 437, pp. 73–96.

Wolpoff, M. H. 1989. Multiregional evolution. In P. Mellars and C. Stringer (eds) *The Human Revolution. Behavioural and biological perspectives on the origins of modern humans*. Edinburgh: Edinburgh University Press, pp. 62–108.

Wolpoff, M. H., X. Y. Wu and A. G. Thorne 1984. Modern *Homo sapiens* origins: a general theory of hominid evolution involving the fossil evidence from East Asia. In F. H. Smith and F. Spencer (eds) *The Origins of Modern Humans: A world survey of the fossil evidence*. New York: Liss, pp. 411–83.

Wood, B. A. 1984. The origin of Homo erectus. In P. Andrews and J. L. Franzen (eds) *The Early Evolution of Man with Special Emphasis on Southeast Asia and Africa*. Courier Forschunginstitut Senkenberg 69, pp. 99–111.

Woodburn, J. 1968. An introduction to Hadza ecology. In R. B. Lee and I. DeVore (eds) *Man the Hunter*. Chicago: Aldine, pp. 49–55.

Woodburn, J. 1982. Social dimensions of death in four African hunting and gathering societies. In M. Bloch and J. Parry (eds) *Death and the Regeneration of Life*. Cambridge: Cambridge University Press., pp. 187–210.

Worrell, E. 1966. *Reptiles of Australia*. Sydney: Angus & Robertson.

Worthman, C. 1978. Psychoendocrine study of human behavior: some interactions of steroid hormones with affect and behavior in the !Kung San. Unpublished Ph. D. thesis, Harvard University, Cambridge, MA.

Wrangham, R. W. 1979. Sex differences in chimpanzee dispersion. In D. A. Hamburg and E. R. McCown (eds) *The Great Apes. Perspectives on human evolution*. Menlo Park, CA: Benjamin/Cummings, pp. 481–90.

Wrangham, R. W. 1980. An ecological model of female-bonded primate groups. *Behaviour* 75: 269–99.

Wrangham, R. W. 1987. The significance of African apes for reconstructing human social evolution. In W. G. Kinzey (ed.) *The Evolution of Human Behavior: Primate Models*. Albany: State University of New York Press, pp. 51–71.

Wreschner, E. E. 1980. Red ochre and human evolution: a case for discussion. *Current Anthropology* 21: 631–44.

Wright, B. J. 1968. *Rock Art of the Pilbara Region, North-west Australia*. Canberra: Australian Institute of Aboriginal Studies.

Wymer, J. 1982. *The Palaeolithic Age*. London & Sydney: Croom Helm.

Wynn, T. 1988. Tools and the evolution of human intelligence. In E. Byrne and A. Whiten (eds) *Machiavellian Intelligence*. Oxford: Clarendon Press, pp. 271–84.

Yalcinkaya, I. 1987. *Anatolian Studies. Recent work in progress*. Ankara: Institute of Archaeology.

Yalman, N. 1967. 'The raw: the cooked: nature: culture'. Observations on 'Le Cru et le Cuit'. In E. R. Leach (ed.) *The Structural Study of Myth and Totemism*. London: Tavistock.

Yengoyan, A. A. 1972. Pitjandjara of Australia. *Human Relations Area Files*. New Haven: Yale.

Young, F. W. 1965. *Initiation Ceremonies. A cross-cultural study of status dramatization*. New York: Bobbs-Merrill.

Young, F. W. and A. Bacdayan 1965. Menstrual taboos and social rigidity. *Ethnology* 4: 225–40.

Zerries, O. 1968. Primitive South America and the West Indies. In W. Krickeberg, H. Trimborn, W. Müller and O. Zerries (eds) *Pre-Columbian American Religions*. London: Weidenfeld & Nicolson, pp. 230–310.

Zuckerman, S. 1932. *The Social Life of Monkeys and Apes*. London: Kegan Paul, Trench, Trubner.

Author Index

AUTHOR INDEX

Fison, L. 96.
Flood, J. 401–2, 449–50, 453.
Foley, R. 157, 226, 227, 231, 232, 254.
Fontenrose, J. 81.
Fortes, M. 312.
Fouts, R.S. 17.
Fox, R. 1–2, 55, 130, 133, 311.
Frazer, J.G. 56, 65, 104, 118, 119, 381–4, 390, 396, 499, 502.
Freud, S. 26, 54–5, 130, 153, 154, 301, 384.
Frolov, B. 368.

Gamble, C. 196, 278–9, 305, 306, 364, 370, 372.
Gell, A. 99.
Ghiglieri, M.P. 137.
Gillen, F.J. 45, 57, 98, 441–2.
Gillison, G. 430.
Gimbutas, M. 366.
Godelier, M. 376, 432.
Goldenweiser, A.A. 104, 105, 113–15.
Goodale, J.C. 358.
Goodall, J. 159, 161, 211.
Gottlieb, A. 377, 378, 386, 387, 389.
Goudsblom, J. 263.
Gould, R.A. 97, 121, 341.
Graves, R. 81.
Gregor, T. 413.
Gunn, D.L. 248, 249.

Hahn, T. 344, 486–7, 492.
Haraway, D. 2–3, 6–7, 32, 33–4, 515, 516.
Harding, R.S.O. 160.
Harris, M. 58, 62.
Hauser, M.D. 11, 12.
Hayden, B. 121.
Hiatt, L.R. 468.
Hill, K. 177, 179–83, 186, 194, 216.
Hladik, C.M. 159.
Hogbin, I.A. 36, 429.
Holmberg, A. 91.
Holy, L. 139.
How, M.W. 334–6.
Howells, W.W. 275.
Howitt, A.W. 96, 108.
Hrdy, S.B. 8, 33, 131, 132–4, 135, 137, 176, 177–8, 201, 212, 216.
Hugh-Jones, C. 412, 418–19, 435.
Hugh-Jones, S. 434–5.
Hughes, A.L. 309.
Humphrey, N. 253–4.
Huxley, F. 406, 419.

Isaac, G. 163–6, 194.

James, S.R. 264, 265.
Jarett, L. 213.
Jolly, A. 131, 247, 259.
Jones, R. 276.
Junod, H.A. 391.

Kaberry, P. 142.
Kaplan, H. 177.
Karsten, R. 419–20, 489.
Kiltie, R. 214, 221–2.
Kinzey, W.G. 176.
Kitahara, M. 394.
Klein, R. 437.
Knowlton, N. 245.
Kolig, E. 506.
Kroeber, A.L. 60–1, 62–3, 69, 94.
Kruuk, H. 343.
Kuhn, T.S. 515, 516, 523, 524.
Kummer, H. 136, 160.

Lamp, F. 351–4.
Landes, R. 141.
Law, Sung Ping 249–50.
Lawrence, D.L. 376.
Leach, E. 68, 79, 81, 105, 528.
Lee, R. 141, 155.
Leroi-Gourhan, A. 365, 436, 507–8.
Letourneau, C.H. 54.
Lévi-Strauss, C. 30, 38, 39–40, 46, 55, 58, 68, 71–87, 88, 98, 102, 104–7, 109–15, 117, 118, 120, 121, 123–7, 151, 153, 154, 155, 257, 301, 302, 325, 338, 340, 383, 386, 400, 402, 405, 406, 407–9, 412, 416, 429, 432, 472, 474, 493, 494–9, 500–1, 502, 503–6, 509–12, 521.
Lewin, R. 230–1.
Lewis, D. 480, 482.
Lewis, G. 427.
Lewis-Williams, J.D. 332, 333.
Lieberman, P. 267.
Lienhardt, G. 80.
Long, J. 106, 117–18.
Lorenz, K. 154.
Lovejoy, C.O. 162, 169–74, 176–9, 194, 216.
Lowie, R.H. 61–2, 69, 141–2, 297, 304, 312, 384.
Lowther, G.R. 165.
Lupton, M.J. 385.

McClintock, M.K. 36, 213.
McKay, M. 273.
McKnight, D. 381, 399.
McLellan, J.F. 104.
Maddock, K. 455, 456, 473, 509.
Malinowski, B. 55, 58, 63, 64–5, 66, 67–8, 69, 85, 107–8, 178, 186–7, 304, 347–8, 411, 527–8.
Marks, A.E. 319.
Marshack, A. 43, 269, 282, 339, 358–63, 366, 367–70, 371, 373.
Marshall, L. 121.
Marx, K. 1, 7, 50, 51, 53, 56, 62, 71, 88, 122, 154, 198, 200, 256, 281, 327, 374, 417, 499, 480, 514, 517–19, 522–3, 533.
Mauss, M. 27–8.
Mead, M. 61, 99, 109–10.
Menaker, W. and A. 215, 250.
Métraux, A. 489.
Mithen, S.J. 371.

Subject Index

Lightning Source UK Ltd.
Milton Keynes UK
UKOW02f2024140914

9 780300 063080